Basic Arrhythmias

Eighth Edition

Gail Walrave

Brady is an impri

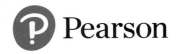

Pearson

330 Hudson Street, NY, NY 10013

Publisher: *Julie Levin Alexander*
Publisher's Assistant: *Sarah Henrich*
Portfolio Manager: *Derril Trakalo*
Portfolio Management Assistant: *Lisa Narine*
Director, Publishing Operations: *Paul DeLuca*
Managing Content Producer: *Melissa Bashe*
Vice President of Sales & Marketing: *David Gesell*
Vice President, Director of Marketing: *Margaret Waples*

Senior Field Marketing Manager: *Brian Hoehl*
Manufacturing Manager: *Vatche Demirdjian*
Manufacturing Buyer: *Mary Ann Gloriande*
Cover Photo: *Lucidio Studio Inc/Photographer's Choice RF/Getty Images*
Composition: *iEnergizer Aptara®, Ltd.*
Printer/Binder: *RR Donnelley Kendallville*
Cover Printer: *Phoenix Color*

Library of Congress Cataloging-in-Publication Data

Names: Walraven, Gail, (Date) author.
Title: Basic arrhythmias/Gail Walraven.
Description: Eighth edition. | Boston: Brady, is an imprint of Pearson, 2016. | Includes index.
Identifiers: LCCN 2016023195 | ISBN 9780134380995 | ISBN 0134380991
Subjects: LCSH: Arrhythmia—Diagnosis—Programmed instruction. | Electrocardiography—Programmed instruction.
Classification: LCC RC685.A65 W33 2016 | DDC 616.1/2807547—dc23 LC record available at https://lccn.loc.gov/2016023195

1   16

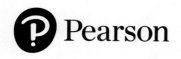

ISBN 13: 978-0-13-438099-5
ISBN 10:   0-13-438099-1

Dedication

To the men in my life: Bruce, Kellen, Dustin, and Case

Contents

Preface

There are many ways to learn electrocardiography and many levels of expertise within this complex field. For ease of reference, the various levels of knowledge/ability can be outlined as follows:

Single-Lead Rhythm Interpretation

Level III: Ability to interpret arrhythmias that include more sophisticated features such as sinus arrest, pacemakers, aberrancy, and blocked beats.

12-Lead EKGs

Level I: Ability to recognize a limited number of familiar patterns, usually the major life-threatening rhythms. No understanding of rules or mechanisms.

Level II: Basic understanding of the rules and mechanisms of common arrhythmias according to pacemaker sites. No familiarity with more sophisticated features that complicate basic arrhythmias.

Level IV: Familiarity with 12-lead EKGs (e.g., bundle branch block, infarction location, axis deviation).

Level V: Ability to distinguish subtle EKG findings (e.g., concealed conduction, reciprocal conduction, trifascicular block, His bundle recordings).

Levels I, II, and III are concerned with interpretation of patterns and use only single-lead EKG tracings. Levels IV and V are multiple leads used to examine both arrhythmias and the greater complexities of the 12-lead EKG.

It is usual for a student to proceed through these levels in a relatively logical progression from simple to complex. Unfortunately, it is also common for a potential student to be prevented from entering this fascinating field for lack of the initial training upon which to build more sophisticated understanding. *Basic Arrhythmias* is designed to provide a sound base of understanding for those interested individuals who have been unable to receive other forms of training. Its primary area of concentration is Level II, the area of basic understanding of the common, uncomplicated rhythms. It is hoped that *Basic Arrhythmias* will provide an enjoyable and interesting way for people to develop the framework that will later support continued learning in the area of electrocardiography.

This self-instructional program is targeted toward several groups of people:

- Those who have previously approached EKGs with "pattern recognition"
- Those who have been unable to participate in more conventional EKG training
- Those who are involved in a formal EKG training program and will use this program concurrently to solidify their learning experience

Because the nature of the book is to provide a foundation for future learning, great care was taken to instill simple, basic concepts without giving the student any misconceptions or erroneous impressions. To this end, some information may have been eliminated or lightly passed over because it was considered to be more sophisticated than necessary, and thus might leave the reader confused and without immediate access to an instructor's help. It is hoped that *Basic Arrhythmias* will open the door for new learners and will provide instructors with more class time for the critical area of reinforcement and refinement.

This text was originally designed to be entirely self-instructional with Chapters 1–8 designed in a programmed format to address basic electrophysiology, waves and measurements, rhythm analysis, and the five major groups of arrhythmias. Over the years, additional sections have been appended to add extra practice strips and to cover cardiac anatomy, clinical manifestations, 12-lead electrocardiography, and cardiac pacemakers. The result is that the first half of the book is self-instructional, while the appendices are generally more traditional narrative text. Together, the two sections provide a good foundation for ongoing learning in the field of electrocardiography.

About the Eighth Edition

Basic Arrhythmias has been well received for many years and has been used successfully by hundreds of thousands of students as they begin to study electrocardiography. It is always a challenge to update and refresh it without detracting from what makes it such a success. With this edition, we've fixed a few bugs, switched out some troublesome EKG strips, added some new illustrations and upgraded some old ones, expanded some sections, and clarified a few ambiguous areas. But for the most part, the body of the text is not changed significantly. Please note that a compiled list of learning objectives is presented later in this front matter section. These objectives outline in depth what you can be expected to learn and do after completing each chapter.

In addition, we have expanded and improved the learning resources for the *Basic Arrhythmias* program. *MyBradyLab*, an online site dedicated to *Basic Arrhythmias*, presents unique study resources and new learning tools to supplement basic text information.

I am very excited about this eighth edition of *Basic Arrhythmias* and hope you find it as enjoyable as I do. With all its upgrades and its fresh new look, it promises to continue the long tradition of helping students embark on their studies of electrocardiography.

What's New in the Eighth Edition

- More 12-leads for practice
- Transition from simplified tracings to more "real-world" 12-leads
- Updated content
- Addition of some new content for clarification
- Standardization of instructor support materials with new edition of text

Acknowledgments

It is impossible to fully acknowledge all the people who have contributed over the years to making *Basic Arrhythmias* what it is today. There have been literally hundreds of people over the years from all across the country who have offered ideas and suggestions, contributed strips, provided clinical reviews, and debated interpretation with me. Without that clinical help, this book would not have achieved the reputation for excellence that it enjoys today. For the eighth edition, I want to again thank Jerrold Glassman, MD, medical director of the Department of Cardiology at Scripps Mercy Hospital, San Diego; he always makes himself available when I come up with a new question. For this edition I am also indebted to Elizabeth Ann Morrell, RN, MSN, NEA-BC, Senior Director, Patient Care, Scripps Mercy Hospitals, Chula Vista and San Diego. And for the tremendous help gathering new EKG strips, I especially want to thank James N. Phan, MBA/HCM, RDCS, RVT, FASE.

Coupled with the clinical excellence, the team at Brady Publishing has set the standard for excellence in the publication of such works. Going all the way back to the original Brady family, countless publishing professionals have added their mark to this book. Most recently, Pearson has moved us to new heights with its print and media

expertise. It is always a joy to work with such professionals. Thank you.

GAIL WALRAVEN
La Jolla, California

Instructor Reviewers

The reviewers of *Basic Arrhythmias* provided excellent suggestions for improving the text. Their reviews were an important aid in the revision and updating of material, and their assistance is greatly appreciated.

Reviewers of the 8th Edition

Ashley Cheryl, BSN, RN, Education Instructor, Saint Francis Hospital, Department of Education and Professional Development, Tulsa, OK

Scott Jones, MBA, EMT-P, EMS Professor, Victor Valley College Regional Public Safety Training Center, Yucaipa, CA

Lawrence Linder, PhD, NREMTP, Program Manager, Hillsborough Community College, Tampa, FL

Reviewers of Previous Editions

Lauri Beechler, RN, MSN, CEN, Director, Paramedic Program, Loyola University Medical Center, Maywood, IL

Jackilyn E. Cypher, RN, MSN, NREMT-P, Paramedic Program Course Director, Lead Instructor, Portland Community College, Cascade Campus, Portland, OR

Deborah Ellis, RN, MSN, NP-C Assistant Professor, Missouri Western State University, Saint Joseph, MO

Mary Fuglaar, PHRN, NREMT-B Training Lieutenant, Fort Bend County EMS Rosenberg, TX

Brian Hess, Star Technical Institute Philadelphia, PA

Bradley K. Jordan, EMT-P EMT-P/Level 1 EMS Instructor, Rockingham Community College, Wentworth, NC

Christine Markut, PhD, RN, BC, CNE, Associate Professor, Stevenson University, Stevenson, MD

Lynette McCullough, NREMT-P, MCH Program Coordinator, Paramedic Technology, Griffin Technical College, Griffin, GA

Jeff McDonald, BS, LP Program Coordinator Tarrant County College, Hurst, TX

Mike McEvoy, EMS Coordinator, Saratoga County, NY

Matthew F. Powers, RN MS CEN MICP EMS Chief, North County Fire Authority Fire/Emergency Nursing, Daly City, CA

Trent Ragsdell, MBA, Life Support Program Manager/ EMS Coordinator, 55th Medical Group Education and Training Department, Offutt AFB, NE

Ken Schoch, Program Director, Yavapai College Prescott, AZ

Douglas P. Skinner, BS, NREMTP, NCEE, Training Officer, Loudoun County Fire Rescue, Leesburg, VA

Michael Smertka, EMT-P, EMS, Assistant Instructor, Cleveland Clinic EMS Academy Cleveland, OH

Kimberly Tew, BSN, RN, University of Iowa College of Nursing, Iowa City, IA

Paul S. Visich, PhD, MPH, Director of the Human Performance Laboratory, Central Michigan University Mt. Pleasant, MI

Carl Voskamp, MBA, LicP, EMS Program Coordinator, The Victoria College Victoria, TX

Michael L. Wallace, MPA, E T-P, CCEMTP, EMS Captain/Educator, Central Jackson County Fire Protection District, Blue Springs, MO

Charlotte A. Wisnewski, PhD, RN, BC, CDE, CNE, Associate Professor, University of Texas Medical Branch School of Nursing, Galveston, TX

Navigating Through the Text

The first eight chapters of this text are structured as a self-instructional unit in a "programmed learning" format. As such, it is an entirely self-contained learning package; the only additional materials you will need are a pencil and a set of EKG calipers, which are available at most medical supply houses and medical bookstores. Everything else is provided here in a format designed to make this learning an enjoyable and worthwhile process. Before you start the program, you should know something about the format of these first eight chapters.

Most of the material has been organized into learning units of approximately similar time frames, so that you can pace yourself as you go along. The first three chapters prepare you with the basic principles of electrocardiography and explain many of the theories and concepts that are the foundation of arrhythmia interpretation. Starting with Chapter 4, you will begin systematically learning arrhythmias according to their site of origin within the heart. Finally, you will be given supplemental practice material to ensure retention of your learning and a self-test to validate your knowledge. The internal structure of each individual chapter is essentially as follows.

Self-Instructional Unit

This programmed narrative will teach you any rules and explanatory materials that you will need to know to interpret arrhythmias. As you read the text, you will be asked to respond to incomplete sentences or direct questions. The answers are given in the right-hand margin directly across from the question. Before reading the text, get into the habit of covering the margin with this book's Heart Rate Calculator bookmark, located on the back cover flap. Then, as you are asked to respond, write your answer in the blank space provided, and slide the bookmark down the page to reveal the desired response. If you have trouble with an answer, go back over the preceding frames to find the solution.

Key Points

Near the end of each chapter, you will find a brief summary of each key point contained in that chapter. This is provided for your review as you complete the chapter and as a reference should you need to look up a point in the future.

Self-Tests

Each chapter closes with a self-test of the important information contained in that chapter. The format of the self-tests is very similar to the format of the text, except that each question is keyed back to the frames in the chapter that specifically provide the answer to the question. Since the self-test is intended to tell you whether or not you learned the material in the chapter, you will want to let a little time pass between completing the chapter and beginning the self-test. If you take the test immediately after finishing the chapter, you might simply be recognizing familiar terms, rather than truly understanding the information. So, once you finish the chapter, take a break from the subject for an hour or two. Then come back to take the test. If you do well on the test, go on to the next chapter. If your results indicate that you did not really learn the material, do not proceed until you remedy that. To do so will merely confuse you and may eventually prevent you from learning future subjects well.

Practice Sheets

Most of the chapters include at least one Practice Sheet of EKG rhythm strips for you to develop skill in analyzing and interpreting arrhythmias. Since practice is probably the single most important element in developing skill at arrhythmia interpretation, it is critical that you take advantage of the practice time provided.

This book is designed to enable you to teach yourself arrhythmia interpretation. However, your learning will be greatly expedited if you have access to an instructor who will guide your learning and stimulate your thinking. If possible, identify a potential instructor before you begin the program, and arrange for tutorial help should you require it. Then your questions can be answered and your horizons expanded as you progress within this self-instructional course.

Flash Cards

Some of the chapters will ask you to take time out from the program to memorize material such as specific rules for each arrhythmia. For your convenience, any material that must be committed to memory has been printed on the flash cards that are provided with this book. This is an effective method of memorizing material in a short period of time. Whenever you are directed to memorize information, stop working on the program and use the flash cards to accomplish this task. Then return to the text. The in-text Flash Card icon, presented in the margin next to corresponding programmed narrative, reminds you to turn to the flash cards.

Learning Objectives

The objectives below outline in depth what you can be expected to learn and do after completing each chapter.

Chapter 1   ELECTROPHYSIOLOGY

1 Describe the electrophysiologic basis of cardiac arrhythmias.
- 1.1 Give the uses and limitations of cardiac arrhythmia monitoring.
  - 1.1.1 Distinguish between the electrical and the mechanical functions of the heart.
  - 1.1.2 Relate cardiac arrhythmia monitoring to pulse/perfusion assessment.
- 1.2 Explain how cardiac impulses are formed.
  - 1.2.1 Briefly describe the sodium pump.
  - 1.2.2 Define polarization and describe the polarized state.
  - 1.2.3 Define depolarization and explain how it occurs.
  - 1.2.4 Define repolarization and explain how it occurs.
- 1.3 Describe the heart's electrical conduction system.
  - 1.3.1 Identify the five major areas of electrical conduction.
  - 1.3.2 Outline the physical layout of the conduction system.
  - 1.3.3 Describe the usual pattern of electrical flow through the conduction system.
  - 1.3.4 Give the inherent rates for the SA node, the AV junction, and the ventricles.
- 1.4 Explain the influence of the nervous system on rate of cardiac impulse formation.
  - 1.4.1 Differentiate between irritability and escape.
  - 1.4.2 Name the nervous system that exerts an influence over rate of cardiac impulse formation.
  - 1.4.3 Identify the two opposing branches of the above-named nervous system, and tell how each would influence the heart if stimulated.
  - 1.4.4 Describe the effect on the heart if one of the branches is blocked.

Chapter 2   WAVES AND MEASUREMENTS

2 Convey cardiac electrical stimuli to a visible graphic medium suitable for arrhythmia interpretation.
- 2.1 Demonstrate the monitoring equipment used to detect cardiac electrical activity.
  - 2.1.1 Prepare equipment/materials for monitoring.
  - 2.1.2 Demonstrate electrode placement for basic arrhythmia monitoring.
  - 2.1.3 Optimize contact between electrode and skin.
  - 2.1.4 Select a lead that gives good wave visibility for arrhythmia interpretation.
- 2.2 Cite specifications of the graph paper used to display cardiac electrical activity.
  - 2.2.1 Given the standardized speed at which EKG graph paper is run through the EKG machine, identify the time intervals associated with each of the following:
    - a. time notches in the margins
    - b. one small box
    - c. one large box
- 2.3 Relate the components of a single cardiac cycle to the electrophysiological events that created them.
  - 2.3.1 Differentiate between the following graphic deflections:
    - a. wave
    - b. segment
    - c. interval
    - d. complex
  - 2.3.2 Given a single cardiac cycle, locate each of the following components and describe the electrical events that created it:
    - a. P wave
    - b. PR segment
    - c. PR interval
    - d. Q wave
    - e. R wave
    - f. S wave
    - g. QRS complex
    - h. ST segment
    - i. T wave
  - 2.3.3 Give the normal time duration for each of the following:
    - a. PR interval
    - b. QRS complex
  - 2.3.4 Identify the two phases of the refractory period.
  - 2.3.5 Identify the vulnerable phase of the cardiac cycle.
  - 2.3.6 Recognize deflections on an EKG tracing that were created by something other than cardiac electrical activity.
- 2.4 Differentiate between a single cardiac cycle and an EKG rhythm strip.

Chapter 3 ANALYZING EKG RHYTHM STRIPS

3 Utilize an organized analysis format to gather necessary data from a rhythm strip to interpret the presenting arrhythmia.

  3.1 Relate the use of a systematic analysis format to the eventual interpretation of an arrhythmia.

  3.2 Outline the five components of an organized approach to rhythm strip analysis.

    3.2.1 Describe the pertinent aspects of a systematic analysis of *regularity*, including R–R intervals, P–P intervals, patterns, and ectopics.

    3.2.2 Describe the pertinent aspects of a systematic analysis of *rate*.

    3.2.3 Describe the pertinent aspects of a systematic analysis of *P waves*, including location, morphology, and patterns.

    3.2.4 Describe the pertinent aspects of a systematic analysis of *PR intervals*, including duration, changes, and patterns.

    3.2.5 Describe the pertinent aspects of a systematic analysis of *ORS complexes*, including duration, morphology, and patterns.

Chapter 4 SINUS RHYTHMS

4 Recognize arrhythmias that originate in the sinus node.

  4.1 Describe the characteristics of a sinus pacemaker.

    4.1.1 Outline the physiologic mechanisms common to the sinus node.

    4.1.2 Describe the expected path of conduction for an impulse originating from a sinus pacemaker.

    4.1.3 Identify EKG features common to all arrhythmias in the sinus category.

  4.2 Outline the identifying features specific to each of the arrhythmias originating in the sinus node.

    4.2.1 Describe *Normal Sinus Rhythm*, including etiology, conduction, and resulting EKG features (regularity, rate, P waves, PR intervals, and QRS complexes).

    4.2.2 Describe *Sinus Bradycardia*, including etiology, conduction, and resulting EKG features (regularity, rate, P waves, PR intervals, and QRS complexes).

    4.2.3 Describe *Sinus Tachycardia*, including etiology, conduction, and resulting EKG features (regularity, rate, P waves, PR intervals, and QRS complexes).

    4.2.4 Describe *Sinus Arrhythmia*, including etiology, conduction, and resulting EKG features (regularity, rate, P waves, PR intervals, and QRS complexes).

Chapter 5 ATRIAL RHYTHMS

5 Recognize arrhythmias that originate within the atria.

  5.1 Describe the characteristics of an atrial pacemaker.

    5.1.1 Outline the physiologic mechanisms common to atrial pacemakers.

    5.1.2 Describe the expected path of conduction for an impulse originating from within the atria.

    5.1.3 Identify EKG features common to all arrhythmias in the atrial category.

  5.2 Outline the identifying features specific to each of the arrhythmias originating within the atria.

    5.2.1 Describe *Wandering Pacemaker*, including etiology, conduction, and resulting EKG features (regularity, rate, P waves, PR intervals, and QRS complexes).

    5.2.2 Describe *Premature Atrial Complexes*, including etiology, conduction, and resulting EKG features (regularity, rate, P waves, PR intervals, and QRS complexes).

    5.2.3 Describe *Atrial Tachycardia*, including etiology, conduction, and resulting EKG features (regularity, rate, P waves, PR intervals, and QRS complexes).

    5.2.4 Describe *Atrial Flutter*, including etiology, conduction, and resulting EKG features (regularity, rate, P waves, PR intervals, and QRS complexes).

    5.2.5 Describe *Atrial Fibrillation*, including etiology, conduction, and resulting EKG features (regularity, rate, P waves, PR intervals, and QRS complexes).

Chapter 6 JUNCTIONAL RHYTHMS

6 Recognize arrhythmias that originate in the AV junction.

  6.1 Describe the characteristics of a junctional pacemaker.

    6.1.1 Outline the physiologic mechanisms common to junctional pacemakers.

    6.1.2 Describe the expected path of conduction for an impulse originating in the AV junction.

    6.1.3 Identify EKG features common to all arrhythmias in the junctional category.

  6.2 Outline the identifying features specific to each of the arrhythmias originating in the AV junction.

    6.2.1 Describe *Premature Junctional Complexes*, including etiology, conduction, and resulting EKG features (regularity, rate, P waves, PR intervals, and QRS complexes).

    6.2.2 Describe *Junctional Escape Rhythm*, including etiology, conduction, and resulting EKG features (regularity, rate, P waves, PR intervals, and QRS complexes).

D.3.2 Describe the appearance of bundle branch block on the EKG.

D.3.3 Differentiate between right and left bundle branch block on the EKG.

D.4 Explain interpreting other abnormalities on the EKG.

D.4.1 Describe the appearance of pericarditis on the EKG.

D.4.2 Describe the appearance of digitalis toxicity on the EKG.

D.4.3 Describe the appearance of hyperkalemia and hypokalemia on the EKG.

D.4.4 Describe the appearance of hypercalcemia and hypocalcemia on the EKG.

D.5 Explain the format for analyzing a 12-lead EKG.

D.5.1 Name the key to easy and effective analysis of the 12-lead EKG.

D.5.2 Name the subjects that the summary analysis of an EKG should address.

Appendix E PACEMAKERS

E.1 Describe pacemakers.

E.1.1 Explain the purpose of artificial pacemakers.

E.1.2 Define capture.

E.1.3 Name the three components of pacemakers.

E.2 Name the chambers of the heart that a pacemaker may pace.

E.3 Describe a "smart" pacemaker.

E.4 Explain the two basic ways in which pacemakers can initiate impulses.

E.4.1 Define triggered pacemaker.

E.4.2 Define inhibited pacemaker.

E.5 Explain the three-letter code system used to classify pacemakers.

E.6 Explain assessment of pacemaker function.

E.6.1 Describe the appearance of pacemakers on the EKG.

E.6.2 Describe the basic sequence of assessing pacemaker function.

E.6.3 Name the information that can be revealed by the relationship between pacemaker spikes and the patient's complexes.

E.7 Name and describe four common types of pacemaker malfunctions.

E.8 Explain how pacemaker malfunction is treated.

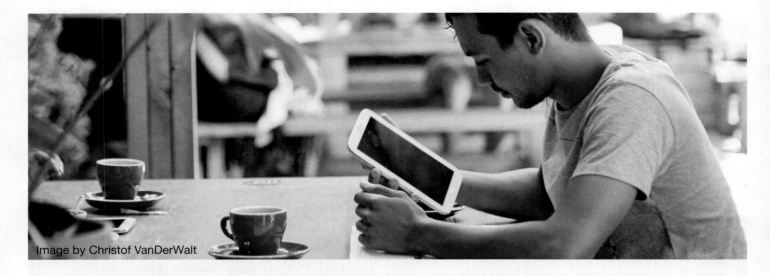

Image by Christof VanDerWalt

MyBRADYLab™

MyBRADYLab gives you the power to reach students on their terms—and to teach however you like. Encourage students to immerse themselves in the Pearson eText on their own time and use your classroom sessions to workshop key concepts. Or enhance your lectures with other engaging content that brings course material to life.

Fostering engagement both within and outside the classroom, MyBRADYLab helps students better prepare for class, quizzes, and exams—resulting in improved performance in the courses.

Features include

- **Gradebook:** A fully functional and customizable gradebook allows instructors to view students results by chapter, outcome, homework and more, to help identify where more classroom time is needed!

- **Multimedia Library:** To help you build assignments, or add an extra engaging element to your lectures, each MyBRADYLab course comes with a Multimedia Library.

- **Pearson eText:** The Pearson eText gives students access to their textbook anytime, anywhere. In addition to note taking, highlighting, and bookmarking, the Pearson eText offers interactive and sharing features.

- **Rhythm Randomizer:** This innovative exercise is for practice, and can be used as a test of your skills. With a database of nearly six hundred randomly generated strips, virtual calipers that you control, and a calculator, you have everything needed to practice reading strips. Test yourself and monitor your progress through the integrated "SCORE" function. There's even a "HINT" button if you need a little help.

- So much more, visit www.bradybooks.com to learn more!

**For more information,
please contact your BRADY sales representative at 1-800-638-0220,
or visit us at www.bradybooks.com**

Chapter 1
Electrophysiology

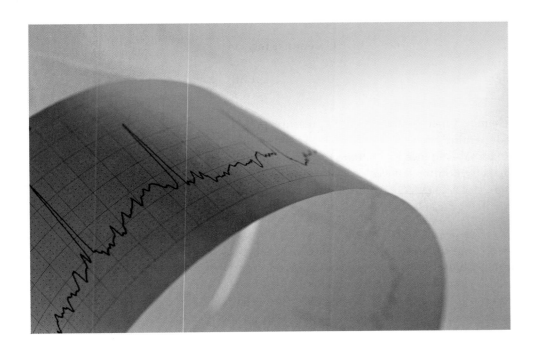

Overview

IN THIS CHAPTER, you'll learn how cardiac arrhythmias reflect what is actually happening electrically in the heart. You will explore the uses and limitations of cardiac arrhythmia monitoring. You will learn how cardiac impulses are formed and how the heart's electrical system conducts electrical impulses throughout the heart. You will also learn how the nervous system can influence the rate at which the heart forms electrical impulses.

Electrical vs. Mechanical Function

1. The human heart is intended to pump blood to the rest of the body. This process has two distinct components:

- The *electrical* impulse that tells the heart to beat
- The *mechanical* beating of the heart in response to the electrical stimulation, resulting in pumping of blood

To perform these two functions, the heart has two distinct types of cells. There are electrical (**conductive**) cells, which initiate electrical activity and conduct it through the heart, and there are mechanical (**contracting**) cells, which respond to the electrical stimulus and contract to pump blood. After the _____ cells initiate   *electrical*

1

the impulse and conduct it through the heart, the _____ _____ cells respond by contracting and pumping blood.

sodium pump

2. The heart will respond with contraction only if it is stimulated by electrical activity. Thus, you cannot have a mechanical response if there is no _____ stimulus.

electrical

3. After the electrical cells have discharged their stimuli, the mechanical cells are expected to respond by _____ .

contracting

4. Without _____ stimulus, the mechanical cells can't be expected to contract.

electrical

5. Since it is not practical to see inside a living patient's heart, we must rely on external evidence to evaluate the status of both electrical and mechanical cardiac function. For a complete assessment of cardiac status, we must evaluate both _____ and _____ functions.

electrical; mechanical

6. As part of our assessment of mechanical function, we use blood pressure, pulses, and other perfusion parameters to determine whether or not the heart is pumping adequately. We must also look for external evidence to evaluate the heart's electrical activity. The best way to do this is to monitor the *electrocardiogram* (EKG). An EKG tracing is used to evaluate the _____ activity of the heart, while the mechanical activity is evaluated by assessing _____ and _____ .

electrical
pulses
blood pressure

7. You might occasionally encounter a situation in which the heart muscle is not able to contract in response to the electrical stimulus. In this case, you could have electrical activity but no _____ response. If you had a functioning electrical system but a failing heart muscle, you could very likely see a viable EKG tracing but the patient might not have palpable _____ or blood pressure.

mechanical

pulses

8. To evaluate a patient's cardiac function, you must assess the mechanical function by examining _____ and _____ and evaluate electrical function by analyzing the _____ tracing.

pulses; blood pressure
EKG

9. An EKG tracing is designed to give a graphic display of the electrical activity in the heart. The pattern displayed on the EKG is called the heart rhythm. Technically, the word **arrhythmia** refers to an abnormal heart rhythm, although the term is often used more generally to refer to all cardiac electrical patterns. The term **dysrhythmia** is synonymous with *arrhythmia*; both are used to refer to patterns of _____ activity within the heart.

electrical

10. An EKG can't tell you about the heart's mechanical activity—you have to assess the patient's pulse and blood pressure to determine that. But an EKG can tell you about the _____ activity, which can be a vital part of your patient assessment. This data is provided in the form of recognizable patterns, called *arrhythmias*. Arrhythmias are graphic representations of the heart's _____ activity.

electrical

electrical

11. To understand and interpret arrhythmias, it is necessary to understand the electrical activity that is occurring within the heart. This is because all arrhythmias are actually graphic displays of electrical activity. The term *electrocardiography* is given to the study of arrhythmias because arrhythmias are manifestations of _____ activity within the heart.

electrical

12. To help you understand and eventually be able to interpret individual arrhythmia patterns, you might want to know a little bit about the electrical processes that take place in the heart to produce the arrhythmia. To do this we'll consider the electrical component independent of the mechanical component. For now, we are discussing only the _____ activity in the heart.

electrical

Impulse Formation

13. The electrical (pacemaking) cells in the heart are distinctive in that they can create their own electrical impulses without an outside stimulus. On the cellular level, they create a change in electrical balance in the cell, causing an electrical current to form. This ability of cardiac cells to initiate electrical impulses on their own is called **automaticity**. Automaticity is the ability of cardiac cells to create their own impulses _____ an outside stimulus. It is not the whole heart that creates the charge, it's the individual pacemaking _____ within the heart's electrical system.

without
cells

14. The creation of an electrical impulse is a function of electrolytes within cardiac cells, or more accurately, the way those electrolytes move across cell walls. The primary electrolytes involved in creating the heart's electrical stimulus are sodium (Na^+) and potassium (K^+). Sodium and _____ are the primary electrolytes that allow the heart to initiate impulses. Both carry a positive electrical charge, but they are not present in equal quantities. The sodium "outweighs" the potassium, making the potassium *relatively* negative to the sodium. It is the *difference* in that potential that allows electrolytes to move through cell membranes. It is movement of these electrolytes through the cell _____ that creates the electrical impulse.

potassium

membrane

Figure 1 The Sodium Pump: Chemical Basis for Impulse Formation

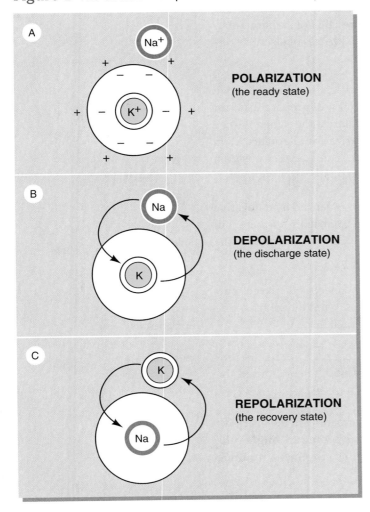

A

Na^+

POLARIZATION
(the ready state)

K^+

B

Na

DEPOLARIZATION
(the discharge state)

K

C

K

REPOLARIZATION
(the recovery state)

Na

15. In a resting cell, the potassium is on the inside and the sodium is on the outside. The outside of the cell is positive, and the inside is *relatively* negative. The charges are _____ , so no electricity flows. (Figure 1A). As the sodium enters the cell, and the potassium leaves, an electrical charge is created. (Figure 1B) The sodium then returns to the outside of the cell and the potassium goes back in. (Figure 1C) This phenomenon is commonly referred to as the **sodium pump**. The cycle is repeated for every heartbeat. The _____ refers to the movement of electrolytes in and out of the cell to create an electrical stimulus. When the positive and negative charges are balanced, no _____ flows. When the positive and negative charges exchange places, an _____ impulse is formed.

balanced

sodium pump

electricity

electrical

16. For an electrical current to form, there must be a difference between the electrical charges. In the resting cell, the charges are balanced; hence no electricity flows. This is called the **polarized** state. The cell charges are _____ and ready for action. Polarization refers to a ready state where the electrical charges are _____ and no _____ current flows. When the cell is in its ready state, it is said to be _____ . When the charges exchange places in the cell, the result is formation of an _____ current. Once the pacemaker cells provide the stimulation, the flow is passed from cell to cell along the conduction pathways until the _____ _____ cells are stimulated to contract.

balanced

balanced

electrical

polarized

electrical

cardiac muscle

Polarization, Depolarization

17. The polarized state is considered a "ready for action" phase. When the two chemical charges (sodium and potassium) trade places, the electricity flows in a wave-like motion throughout the heart. This wave of electrical flow is called **depolarization** and is how the electrical stimulus travels through the heart (Figure 1B). Polarization refers to the "ready" state, and _____ refers to the process of electrical discharge and flow of electrical activity.

depolarization

18. After the cell depolarizes, the positive and negative electrical charges will again return to their original positions around the cell, and the cell will prepare itself for another discharge (Figure 1C). The process that follows depolarization, when the cell charges are returning to their original state, is called **repolarization.** Repolarization refers to the return of the electrical charges to their _____ position. Repolarization occurs _____ depolarization.

original

after

19. If each of the positive charges on the outside of the cell is balanced by a negative charge on the inside of the cell, the electrical charges will be balanced, and there will be no movement of electricity. This state is called _____ and can be considered a "ready" state.

polarization

20. The wave of electrical activity that takes place when the electrical charges surrounding the cell trade places is called _____ , and the return of the electrical charges to their original state is called _____ .

depolarization

repolarization

21. If polarization is considered the *ready* state, and _____ is considered the *discharge* state, then _____ would be considered the *recovery* state.

depolarization

repolarization

22. Now let's relate this cellular activity to what is actually happening in the heart. All of the sequences described in the preceding frames are happening to single cells within the heart, but they do it in a _____ -like movement, resulting in the entire heart responding electrically to the same activity.

wave

Conduction System

23. The electrical cells in the heart are all arranged in a system of pathways called the **conduction system**. The physical layout of the conduction system is shown in Figure 2. This information is an essential part of arrhythmia interpretation and should therefore be memorized now. (*Note:* Flash cards are provided at the back of this book to help you with this and all other memorizing you will need to do as you learn to interpret arrhythmias. The MyKit website also includes activities to make this learning easier.) Normally, the electrical impulse originates in the SA node and travels to the ventricles by way of the AV node. Look at Figure 2 and trace a normal electrical impulse. Where would the impulse go after it left the AV node and the Bundle of His?

MyBRADYLab™

down the left and right bundle branches and then to the Purkinje fibers

24. In the normal heart, the first impulse that starts the flow of electrical current through the heart comes from the SA node. The impulse travels through the atria by way of the intraatrial pathways and to the AV node by means of the internodal pathways. If you look microscopically at the cells along these pathways, you would not see any physical difference between them and the cells in other areas of the atria, so researchers have questioned whether they actually exist. However, current electrophysiologic studies support the concept that these pathways do exist, if only as a preferred route by which impulses travel to the AV node. As it leaves the SA node, where does the current go?

down the internodal and intraatrial pathways

Figure 2 Conduction System

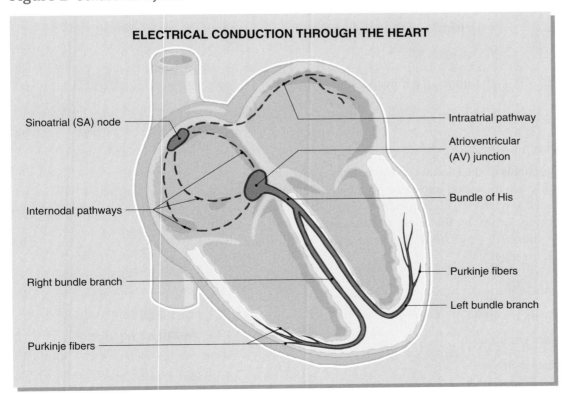

ELECTRICAL CONDUCTION THROUGH THE HEART

Sinoatrial (SA) node
Intraatrial pathway
Atrioventricular (AV) junction
Bundle of His
Internodal pathways
Right bundle branch
Purkinje fibers
Left bundle branch
Purkinje fibers

25. The next area of conductive tissue along the conduction pathway is at the site of the AV node. The AV node is unique in that it does have conductive tissue, but it does not have any pacemaker cells like other areas of the conduction system. The pace-making cells are actually located at the junction between the AV node and the atria, in an area called the **AV Junction.** Thus, the term *AV Node* can be used when talking about conduction, but the term *AV Junction* is more accurate if you are specifically discussing the formation of impulses. Don't let this confuse you. It is simply an explanation of what might otherwise appear to be indiscriminate use of the two phrases. We will use the term *AV Node* if we're talking only about _____ , but if we're specifically discussing pacemaking capabilities, we will call it the AV _____ .

conduction

Junction

26. After leaving the area of the AV node, the impulses go through the _____ to reach the right and left bundle branches. These branches are located within the right and left ventricles, respectively.

Bundle of His

27. At the terminal ends of the bundle branches, smaller fibers distribute the electrical impulses to the muscle cells to stimulate contraction. These terminal fibers are called _____ fibers.

Purkinje

28. Are the muscle cells themselves part of the electrical conduction system?
_____
_____

No, they are made up of mechanical cells, not electrical cells.

29. Rearrange the following parts of the conduction system to place them in the actual order of conduction:

MyBRADYLab™   FLASH CARD

(1) _____   (a) Bundle of His   1. b

(2) _____   (b) SA node   2. f

(3) _____   (c) Purkinje fibers   3. e

(4) _____   (d) left and right bundle branches   4. a

(5) _____   (e) AV node   5. d

(6) _____   (f) intraatrial pathways   6. c

Inherent Rates

30. Each of the three major areas of the conduction system has its own built-in rate, called an **inherent rate,** at which it initiates impulses. An inherent rate means simply that each site has a rate range at which it usually produces impulses. A site can exceed or fall below its inherent rate, indicating that these rates are not concrete rules. But generally speaking, the sites will produce impulses at a rate within their own _____ rate ranges.

inherent

31. The inherent rate ranges of the major sites are as follows:

SA Node   60–100 beats per minute

AV Junction   40–60 beats per minute

Ventricle   20–40 beats per minute

FLASH CARD

MyBRADYLab™

This information would give you a clue that if an EKG rate was between 20 and 40 beats per minute (bpm), the electrical impulse that stimulated the rhythm probably originated in the _____ . If the rate was between 40 and 60 bpm, the impulse probably came from the _____ , and it most likely came from the _____ if the rate was between 60 and 100 bpm.

ventricle

AV junction

SA node

32. These rates are often helpful clues to be used in interpreting arrhythmias, but they can be misleading unless they are understood to be mere guidelines and not concrete _____ .

rules

33. Generally speaking, the fastest inherent rate will become the pacemaker of the heart and override all other stimuli. The inherent rate of the SA node is the fastest and therefore keeps the heart at a rate between _____ and _____ bpm. Thus, the normal EKG is "sinus" in origin. The SA node is the normal pacemaker for the heart because the rate of the SA node is _____ than the other conduction sites.

60

100

faster

Irritability, Escape

34. If, however, a site becomes irritable and begins to discharge impulses at a faster-than-normal rate, it can override the SA node and take over the pacemaking function for the heart. If the SA node is discharging at a rate of 72 and the AV junction begins to fire at a rate of 95, the _____ will become the pacemaker.

AV junction

35. This mechanism of an irritable site speeding up and taking over as pacemaker is called **irritability**. It is usually an undesirable occurrence, since it overrides the normal pacemaker and causes the heart to beat faster than it otherwise would. Irritability occurs when a site below the SA node _____ and takes over the pacemaking role.

speeds up

36. Something very different happens if the normal pacemaker slows down for some reason. If the SA node drops below its inherent rate, or if it fails entirely, the site with the next highest inherent rate will usually take over the pacemaking role. The next highest site is within the _____ , so that site would become the pacemaker if the SA node should fail. This mechanism is called **escape** and is a safety feature that is built into the heart to protect it in case the normal _____ fails.

AV junction

pacemaker

37. Escape mechanism, unlike irritability, is a safety feature to protect the heart. Would you expect an irritable rhythm to be faster or slower than an escape rhythm? _____

faster

38. The inherent rate of different areas of the conduction system refers to the rate at which that site _____ .

initiates impulses

39. The SA node has an inherent rate of _____ to _____ bpm. This means that the normal rate of the heart will usually be within that range.

60;100

40. If the rate of an EKG is between 40 and 60, the impulse for that rhythm is probably coming from the _____ .

AV junction

41. What is the inherent rate of the ventricular conductive tissues? _____

20–40 bpm

42. Because these rates cannot be relied upon as firm rules, they should be viewed only as _____ . If they are used as clues, the rates will be helpful in interpreting arrhythmias, but if they are considered inflexible they will simply confuse the learner.

guidelines

43. A rule regarding the pacemaker function of the heart states that the site that initiates impulses at the _____ rate will usually become the pacemaker.

fastest

44. In the normal heart, the _____ initiates impulses at the fastest rate and therefore becomes the _____ .

SA node

pacemaker

45. If the AV junction or the ventricle became irritable, either could become the pacemaker if it were able to accelerate until it _____ _____ _____ .

became faster than the SA node

46. The process described in the preceding frame is called _____ .

irritability

47. If the SA node failed as pacemaker, or if its rate dropped below the normal range, the _____ would probably take over as pacemaker.

AV junction

48. The safety mechanism described in the preceding frame is called _____ .

escape

Nervous System Influence

49. In addition to the inherent rates, the heart can be influenced by the autonomic nervous system. The two branches of this nervous system oppose each other and thus keep the heart in a relative state of balance. The *sympathetic branch* influences both the atria (i.e., the SA node, the intraatrial and internodal pathways, and the AV junction) and the ventricles. If the sympathetic branch is stimulated, it will cause both the atria and ventricles to react in these ways:

FLASH CARD

MyBRADYLab™

- Increased rate
- Increased conduction through the AV node
- Increased irritability

The *parasympathetic branch* has the opposite effects, but it influences only the atria; it has little or no effect on the ventricles. While stimulation of the parasympathetic branch causes the atria to slow down, as well as decreasing irritability and slowing conduction through the AV node, stimulation of the sympathetic branch would cause what three effects on the atria and ventricles? _____ _____ _____

increased heart rate; increased AV conduction; increased irritability

These nervous influences are outlined in Figure 3.

50. If the vagus nerve (which is part of the parasympathetic branch) is stimulated, you would expect the heart rate to _____ . On the other hand, if both the sympathetic and the parasympathetic branches are balanced, the heart rate would remain normal. What would you expect if you blocked the normal influence of the vagus nerve? _____ _____ _____

decrease

You would get a response similar to stimulation of the sympathetic branch: heart rate would increase as well as irritability and AV conduction.

Figure 3 Innervation of the Heart by the Autonomic Nervous System

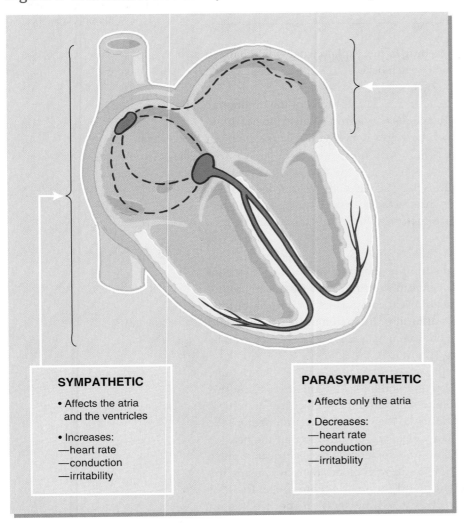

SYMPATHETIC

- Affects the atria and the ventricles

- Increases:
  —heart rate
  —conduction
  —irritability

PARASYMPATHETIC

- Affects only the atria

- Decreases:
  —heart rate
  —conduction
  —irritability

51. If a patient had a heart rate that was too slow, you might try to speed it up by giving a drug that would either stimulate the sympathetic branch or _____ _____ .

block the parasympathetic branch

52. The two branches of the autonomic nervous system that influence heart rate are the _____ branch and the _____ branch.

sympathetic parasympathetic

53. Which of these branches, when stimulated, will produce an increase in heart rate, AV conduction, and irritability? _____

sympathetic

54. One of the branches has control over the atria and the ventricles, while the other influences only the atria. Which one affects both the atria and the ventricles? _____

sympathetic

55. If both branches are exerting equal influence over the heart, what will happen to the rates? _____

They will stay within the ranges of the normal inherent rates.

56. What will happen if one of the branches of the autonomic nervous system is blocked? _____ The heart will respond to the influ-
_____ ence of the opposing branch.

57. Using the reasoning described in the preceding frame, explain what would happen to the heart rate if the parasympathetic branch were blocked. _____ It would increase.

58. The vagus nerve is part of the _____ branch of the autonomic parasympathetic
nervous system. Therefore, stimulation of the vagus nerve would cause the heart rate
to _____ , and blocking of the vagus nerve would cause the heart decrease
rate to _____ . increase

59. All of this discussion is about _____ activity and does not yet electrical
connect with mechanical activity. In order to discuss the heart contracting and producing a pulse, we must connect the electrical activity with _____ mechanical
activity.

60. If the muscle cells receive an electrical stimulus, they will respond to it by contracting. Sometimes, however, the muscle itself can't contract because it is injured or
chemically imbalanced. In these cases the electrical component is all right, but the
_____ component needs attention. In such a patient you would mechanical
expect to find the EKG essentially normal, but the _____ would be pulse
absent or diminished.

61. The opposite situation is more common and is the reason you are reading this
book. This is when the heart muscle is able to respond but the electrical activity is
erratic. Sometimes the electrical stimuli will make the ventricles contract before the
atria do, or maybe there will just be too many electrical stimuli, so that the heart is
not able to respond effectively to any of them. And sometimes the electrical impulse
will discharge before the ventricles have time to fill with blood, thereby causing the
ventricles to contract and eject insufficient blood for an adequate pulse. In all of
these conditions, the erratic electrical activity will be seen on the EKG as an
_____ . arrhythmia

KEY POINTS

- The heart has two types of cells:
  - Electrical cells, which initiate and conduct impulses
  - Mechanical cells, which contract in response to stimulation
- Arrhythmias are graphic representations of electrical activity.
- Electrical activity precedes mechanical activity.
- Electrical activity can occur without mechanical response (pulse).
- If the electrical impulse stimulates the mechanical cells to contract, the heart is expected to contract and pump blood, thus producing a pulse.
- Polarization is when the electrical charges are balanced and ready for discharge.
- Depolarization is the discharge of energy that accompanies the transfer of electrical charges across the cell membrane.
- Repolarization is the return of electrical charges to their original state of readiness.
- Depolarization differs from contraction in that depolarization is an electrical phenomenon, whereas contraction is mechanical and is expected to follow depolarization.
- As shown in Figure 2, electrical flow in the normal heart originates in the SA Node, then travels via the intraatrial and internodal pathways to the AV Node, then through the Bundle of His to the Left and Right Bundle Branches, and finally to the Purkinje Fibers, where the mechanical cells are stimulated.

- The inherent rates of the conduction system are as follows:

SA Node	60–100 bpm
AV Junction	40–60 bpm
Ventricles	20–40 bpm

- The site with the fastest rate will be the pacemaker.
- The SA Node is the normal pacemaker of the heart.
- Irritability is when a site speeds up and takes over as pacemaker.
- Escape is when the normal pacemaker slows down or fails and a lower site assumes pacemaking responsibility.
- The influence of the autonomic nervous system can also affect the heart:
  - *Sympathetic* stimulation causes:

    Increased heart rate
    Increased AV conduction
    Increased irritability
  - *Parasympathetic* stimulation causes:

    Decreased heart rate
    Decreased AV conduction
    Decreased irritability
- The sympathetic branch influences both the atria (i.e., the SA node, the intraatrial and internodal pathways, and the AV junction) and the ventricles; the parasympathetic branch influences only the atria.
- If one branch of the autonomic nervous system is blocked, the effects of the opposing branch will prevail.

SELF-TEST

Directions: Complete this self-evaluation of the information you have learned from this chapter. If your answers are all correct and you feel comfortable with your understanding of the material, proceed to the next chapter. However, if you miss any of the questions, you should review the referenced frames before proceeding. If you feel unsure of any of the underlying principles, invest the time now to go back over the entire chapter. **Do not proceed with the next chapter until you are very comfortable with the material in this chapter.**

Questions

	Referenced Frames	Answers
1. Name the two types of cardiac cells and tell what type of activity each is responsible for.	1, 2, 3, 4	electrical: conduction; mechanical: contraction
2. How do these two types of cells work together to produce cardiac activity?	1, 2, 3, 4	Electrical cells stimulate muscle cells to contract.
3. What physical signs are used to reflect the mechanical function of the heart?	5, 6, 7, 8	pulses, blood pressure, other perfusion parameters

Questions	Referenced Frames	Answers
4. How do you assess electrical activity in the heart?	5, 6, 7, 8, 10	Analyze the EKG.
5. Arrhythmias are manifestations of which type of cardiac activity?	9, 10, 11, 12	electrical
6. What happens when the positive and negative electrical charges exchange places across the cell membrane of a cardiac cell?	13, 14, 15, 16, 17	It initiates the flow of electrical current.
7. Explain the polarized state.	14, 15, 16, 17, 19, 21	when electrical charges are balanced and in a state of readiness for discharge
8. Explain depolarization.	16, 17, 20, 22	the discharge of electrical energy that accompanies the transfer of electrical charges across the cell membrane
9. Is depolarization the same as contraction?	17	No, depolarization is an electrical phenomenon. Contraction is mechanical and is expected to follow depolarization.
10. What is repolarization?	18, 20, 21	the return of the electrical charges to their original state of readiness
11. List the areas of the conduction system in the order in which the impulses travel through the heart.	23, 24, 25, 26, 27, 29	1. SA node 2. intraatrial and internodal pathways 3. AV node 4. Bundle of His 5. Bundle Branches 6. Purkinje Fibers
12. Which site is normally the pacemaker of the heart, and why?	24, 33, 34, 43, 44	The SA node has the fastest inherent rate.
13. Give the inherent rates for each of the following sites: Sinus Node _____ AV Junction _____ Ventricles _____	30, 31, 32, 38, 39, 40, 41, 42	60–100 times per minute 40–60 times per minute 20–40 times per minute
14. What process is responsible for a site speeding up and overriding a higher site, thus taking over as pacemaker?	33, 34, 35, 45, 46	irritability
15. What mechanism is in play if a lower site takes over responsibility for the pacemaking function following failure of a higher site?	33, 36, 37, 47, 48	escape
16. Which nervous system has two branches that control the activities of the heart?	49	autonomic
17. Name the two branches of the nervous system identified in the preceding question.	49, 52	sympathetic; parasympathetic
18. List three things that will happen to the heart if the sympathetic branch is stimulated.	49, 50, 51, 53	increased rate, increased AV conduction, increased irritability
19. List three things that will happen to the heart if the parasympathetic branch is stimulated.	49, 50, 51, 58	decreased rate, decreased AV conduction, decreased irritability

Questions	Referenced Frames	Answers
20. What part of the heart does the sympathetic branch innervate?	49, 54	the atria and ventricles
21. What part of the heart does the parasympathetic branch innervate?	49, 54	only the atria
22. What happens if one branch is blocked?	50, 51, 55, 56, 57, 58	The influence of the opposing branch will control the heart.

Chapter 2
Waves and Measurements

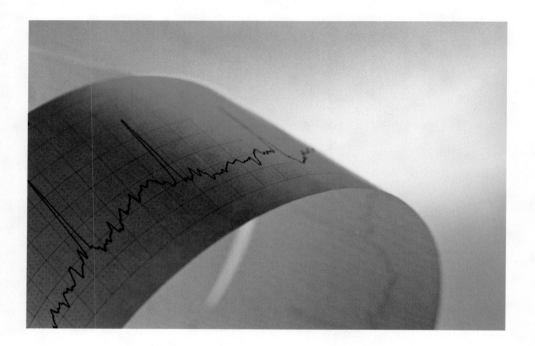

Overview

IN THIS CHAPTER, you will learn how cardiac electrical activity is transferred to graph paper so that it can be seen and analyzed for arrhythmia interpretation. You will learn about the equipment used for monitoring, and you will learn all the specifics of the graph paper upon which EKG images are typically drawn. You will learn the difference between a single cardiac cycle and an EKG rhythm strip. You will find out about the different components that make up a single cardiac cycle on the EKG, and you will learn to identify each component and know what it suggests is happening within the heart.

Introduction

1. In Chapter 1 you learned that arrhythmias are manifestations of the heart's
_____ activity. And you learned that the study of arrhythmias is
called _____ . To study arrhythmias, we have to transform the electrical activity into a format that can be seen.

electrical
electrocardiography

Electrodes

2. The electrical patterns of the heart can be picked up from the surface of the skin by attaching an **electrode** to the skin and connecting it to a machine that will display the electrical activity on graph paper. An electrode is a small item attached to the patient's _____ and then connected by wire to a machine capable of inscribing the patterns on graph _____ .

skin

paper

3. The electrical activity is displayed best if you can ensure good contact between the electrode and the skin. This can be done in several ways:

- By abrading the skin slightly
- By removing any obstacles, such as dirt or hair
- By using a contact medium, such as saline or a commercial gel

All of these measures are intended to improve _____ between the electrode and the skin.

contract

4. An _____ placed on the skin can pick up electrical activity from within the heart and display it on graph paper using an EKG machine. To ensure a good tracing you must provide good contact between the _____ and the _____ .

electrode

skin; electrode

5. Contact between the skin and the electrode can be improved by lightly _____ the skin, by wiping off excess _____ , or possibly by _____ excess hair. An important way to ensure good contact is to use some type of contact medium, such as _____ or a commercial _____ .

abrading; dirt

shaving

saline

gel

6. When an EKG machine is turned on but isn't yet connected to the patient's electrodes, the writing point (stylus) of the machine will simply produce a straight line on the paper. This line is called the **isoelectric line** because all of the electrical forces are equal; no current is flowing. Once the machine is connected to the patient's electrodes, the needle will move up or down on the paper (above or below the isoelectric line) in response to the electrical forces it receives. If no current is flowing, or if the forces balance each other out, the graph paper will show a _____ . If the machine receives a flow of electricity, the needle will move _____ or _____ in response to the current.

straight line

up

down

Rule of Electrical Flow

MyBRADYLab™

7. A very basic rule of electrocardiography refers to the flow of electricity through the heart and out to the electrodes. This rule states that if the electricity flows _toward_ the _positive_ electrode, the patterns produced on the graph paper will be _upright_. The converse of this rule is also true: if the electricity flows _away_ from the _positive_ electrode (or _toward_ the _negative_ electrode), the pattern will be a _downward_ deflection. If the flow of electricity is toward the positive electrode, the machine will produce an _____ deflection on the graph paper (Figure 4).

upright

8. Look at Figure 4. If the electrical flow is toward the negative electrode, would you expect the graph paper to show a positive or a negative deflection? _____

negative

9. If the graph paper shows a positive deflection, you would assume that the electrical activity is flowing primarily toward the _____ electrode.

positive

Figure 4 Rule of Electrical Flow

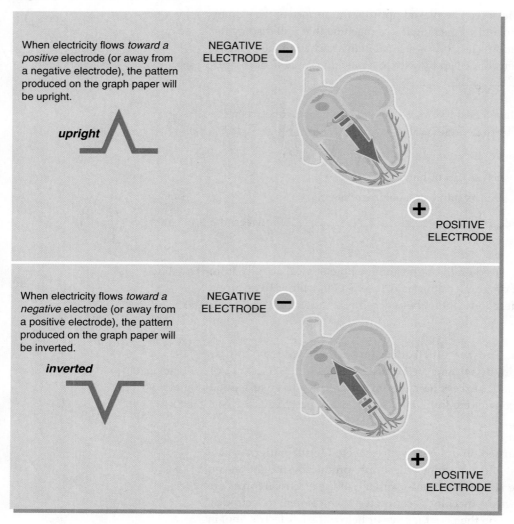

When electricity flows *toward a positive* electrode (or away from a negative electrode), the pattern produced on the graph paper will be upright.

upright

NEGATIVE ELECTRODE **−**

POSITIVE ELECTRODE **+**

When electricity flows *toward a negative* electrode (or away from a positive electrode), the pattern produced on the graph paper will be inverted.

inverted

NEGATIVE ELECTRODE **−**

POSITIVE ELECTRODE **+**

10. If the deflection on the graph paper is negative, you would assume that the electrical flow is toward the _____ electrode and away from the _____ electrode.

negative
positive

11. Thus, we can determine the direction of electrical flow by the type of deflection made on the EKG paper. But to draw any conclusions based on this information, we must be sure that the electrodes are always in the same place on the patient so that the information is not misleading. The placement of the electrodes on patients is always _____ to avoid confusion or misinterpretation of information.

the same (standardized)

Monitoring Leads

12. The positioning of electrodes for monitoring the EKG allows you to see a single view of the heart's electrical pattern. By rearranging electrodes, many such views are possible. (This concept can be compared to a camera that can photograph the heart from many angles, each one giving additional depth to the overall visualization of the heart itself.) Each view of the heart is called a **lead**. Leads can be changed by a knob on the machine that diverts the flow of electricity through different electrodes. For sophisticated EKG interpretation, many leads are inspected to visualize the entire heart. However, for basic arrhythmia interpretation, it is necessary to monitor only a single lead. A monitoring lead shows only one _____ of the heart's electrical activity.

view

Figure 5 Electrode Placement for Monitoring Lead II

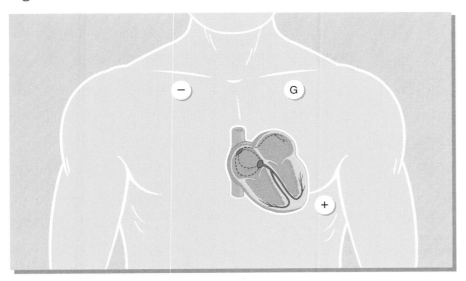

13. When monitoring a patient for patterns of electrical activity such as arrhythmias, a lead is selected to give a clear picture of the basic wave forms. Single leads that give good pictures of the basic waves are called monitoring leads because they are used to _____ patterns such as arrhythmias. The first widely used monitoring lead was Lead II, but now it is common to use other leads as well, especially variations of the chest leads (such as MCL_1). The modified chest leads often give a better view of the heart's atrial activity, which is sometimes needed to differentiate complex arrhythmias. The examples in this book all happen to be Lead II. This does not mean that Lead II is better than MCL_1, nor does it mean that you must always use Lead II for monitoring arrhythmias. The same *patterns* apply whether you view them in Lead II, MCL_1, or any other monitoring lead. Regardless of which lead is used, the _____ remain the same, so it doesn't matter which lead you use to learn basic arrhythmias. Just because the examples in this book are Lead II doesn't mean that it is the only monitoring lead, or even the best. You will encounter other monitoring leads as you learn more about EKGs, but for now you can assume that the information in this book refers to _____ unless otherwise specified.

monitor

patterns

Lead II

14. Figure 5 shows the placement of electrodes to monitor Lead II. Note that the positive electrode is at the apex of the heart, and the negative electrode is below the right clavicle. The third electrode is a ground electrode and does not measure electrical flow in this lead. Since the pacemaker is normally in the _____ and the electrical current flows toward the ventricles, the primary thrust of electrical flow in the heart will be toward the positive electrode in Lead II. Thus, the primary deflections in Lead II will be _____ .

SA node

upright

Graph Paper

15. All EKG interpretation relies on the use of standardized, uniform graph paper. The size of the graph on the paper and the speed at which the paper travels through the EKG machine are both kept constant; all EKG paper is the same, and all EKG machines operate at the same speed. By keeping the paper and the speed standardized, we can look at the patterns created by an individual's heart activity and compare them to what has been established as "normal" activity. If the graph paper was not _____ , we would not be able to compare one person's EKG to any

standardized

Figure 6 Sample EKG Graph Paper

The three vertical lines in the upper margin are measures of time standard to all EKG graph paper. The distance between two "tic" marks is 3 seconds; thus, this strip measures 6 seconds in duration.

other EKG, nor would we be able to compare several EKGs taken on one person at different times. Similarly, if all EKG machines ran at different _____ , we would not have a constant "norm" for comparing individual EKGs.

speeds

16. Since all graph paper has _____ markings, we must learn what these markings mean so that we will be able to interpret the EKG tracings that are superimposed on the graph paper. Look at the sample graph paper shown in Figure 6. You will notice that there are lines going up and down (vertical) and lines going across (horizontal). Also notice that every fifth line is heavier than the other lighter lines. How many light lines are there between two heavy ones? _____

standardized

four

17. The lines on the graph paper can help determine both the direction and the magnitude of deflections. When all electrical forces are equal, there is neither an upright nor a downward deflection; an isoelectric line is created. If the electrical force is toward the positive electrode, the stylus will draw an _____ wave. If the force travels primarily toward the negative electrode, the wave will be _____ . If no current is present, or if positive and negative forces are equal, the graph paper will show a _____ line, called an isoelectric line.

upright

downward (inverted)

straight

Voltage Measurements

18. It is the strength of the current, or its voltage, that will determine the magnitude of the deflection. If it is a very strong positive wave, it will create a high spike above the isoelectric line. If it is a very weak positive charge, the deflection will go only slightly above the isoelectric line in response to the amplitude of the charge. Therefore, the height of the deflection will indicate the _____ of the electrical charge that produced the deflection. The same principle holds for negative deflections: the stronger the charge, the deeper the wave will go below the isoelectric line.

voltage (or amplitude)

19. Since voltage produces either an upright or a downward deflection on the EKG, the magnitude of the current can be measured by comparing the height of the spike against the horizontal lines on the graph paper (Figure 7). Voltage can be measured quantitatively (in millivolts), but you need not concern yourself with these figures for basic arrhythmia interpretation. On the graph paper, the horizontal lines measure _____ .

voltage

Figure 7 Using Graph Paper Markings to Measure Voltage and Time

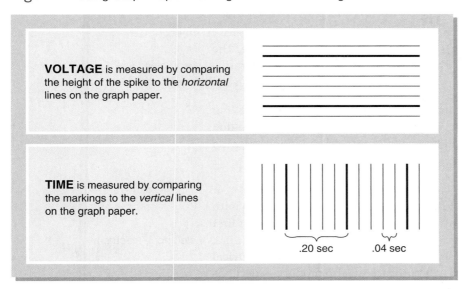

VOLTAGE is measured by comparing the height of the spike to the *horizontal* lines on the graph paper.

TIME is measured by comparing the markings to the *vertical* lines on the graph paper.

.20 sec   .04 sec

Time Measurements

20. The second, and more important, thing that the graph paper can provide is a determination of time. The vertical lines can tell you just how much time it took for the electrical current within the heart to travel from one area to another. The vertical lines are the most important markings for simple arrhythmia identification because they can tell you about the _____ it takes for the current to travel about within the heart.

time

21. The standard rate at which the EKG machine runs paper past the stylus is 25 millimeters per second. At this standard rate we know that it takes 0.20 second to get from one *heavy* vertical line to the next *heavy* vertical line. Therefore, if a deflection began on one heavy line and ended on the next heavy line, we would know that the electrical current within the heart that caused the deflection lasted _____ second. This is an essential figure to remember because it is the basis for many of the rates, rules, and normal values you will learn in later sections. The distance (in time) between two heavy vertical lines on the EKG graph paper is _____ second.

0.20

0.20

22. If the time frame between two heavy vertical lines is 0.20 second and there are five small squares within this same area, it would follow that each of these small squares is equivalent to one-fifth of 0.20 second, or 0.04 second each. The distance (in time) between two light vertical lines, or across one small square, is _____ second.

0.04

23. You now can see that graph paper can be used to measure _____ and _____ .

voltage
time

Cardiac Cycle

24. As you know, the heart has four chambers. The upper two are the atria and the lower two are the ventricles. In most cases the atria function as a team and contract together, and the ventricles also operate as a single unit. So for nearly all of our discussions we will consider the atria as a single unit and the ventricles as a single unit, even

though we realize that they are actually the _____ separate cham-   four
bers that make up the heart.

25. The upper chambers of the heart are called the _____ ,   atria
and they will be considered a single _____ . Likewise, the   unit
_____ are the lower chambers and will be considered a   ventricles
_____ unit.   single

26. In the normal heart, blood enters both atria simultaneously and then is forced into
both ventricles simultaneously as the atria contract. All of this is coordinated so that
the atria fill while the ventricles contract, and when the ventricles are filling, the atria
contract. In considering a cardiac cycle, we would expect the _____   atria
to contract first.

27. Before the atria can contract, they must first receive an electrical stimulus to initiate the muscle cell response. In fact, for any myocardial cell to contract, it must first
receive an _____ stimulus. We know that the _____   electrical; electrical
cells have the ability to initiate an impulse. And we know that the same electrical
impulses that eventually produce contraction of the heart can also produce deflections
on the EKG graph paper. It is by careful scrutiny of these wave patterns that we are
able to determine the _____ activity that is present in the heart, and   electrical
sometimes we can even speculate on the type of _____ activity that   mechanical
could be expected. But to make these determinations, we must first investigate the
_____ patterns produced by the heart's electrical activity.   wave

28. During each phase of the cardiac electrical cycle, a distinct pattern is produced on
the EKG _____ paper. By learning to recognize these wave patterns   graph
and the cardiac activity each represents, we can study the relationships between the
different areas of the heart and begin to understand what is taking place within the
heart at any given time. For each pacemaker impulse, the electrical flow travels down
the _____ pathways, depolarizing the atria and then the ventricles   conduction
as it goes. Following this, the pattern begins again with another impulse from the
pacemaker. Each cardiac cycle includes all of the electrical activity that would normally be expected to produce a single heart beat. The cardiac cycle begins with the
initiating impulse from the pacemaker and encompasses all phases until the ventricles
are repolarized. On the EKG graph paper, the cardiac cycle includes all of the wave
patterns produced by electrical activity, beginning with the _____   pacemaker
impulse and including ventricular _____ .   repolarization

29. On the EKG, each of these phases is displayed by a specific wave pattern. Figure 8
shows a series of cardiac electrical cycles that makes up a typical EKG rhythm strip. In

Figure 8 A Typical EKG Rhythm Strip

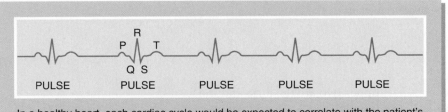

In a healthy heart, each cardiac cycle would be expected to correlate with the patient's
individual pulse beats.

Figure 9 The EKG Complex

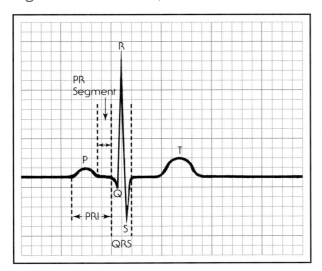

Figure 9, a single cardiac cycle has been enlarged so that we can see each of the individual patterns more closely. A single cardiac cycle is expected to produce one _____ beat. An EKG rhythm strip is composed of more than one _____ cycle.

heart
cardiac

Waves, Intervals, Segments

30. In labeling the activity on the graph paper, the deflections above or below the isoelectric line are called *waves*. In a single cardiac cycle there are five prominent waves, and each is labeled with a letter. Look at Figure 9 and find the P, Q, R, S, and T waves. An **interval** refers to the area between (and possibly including) waves, and a **segment** identifies a straight line or area of electrical inactivity between waves. Find the PR segment and the PR interval (PRI) on Figure 9. Does the PR segment include any waves?_____ Does the PR interval include any waves? _____

No.
Yes. The PRI includes the P wave and the PR segment.

P Wave and PRI

31. The first wave you see on the cardiac cycle is the P wave. Locate it in Figure 9. The P wave starts with the first deflection from the isoelectric line. The _____ wave is indicative of atrial depolarization.

P

32. When you see a P wave on the EKG, does that mean that the atria contracted?

No, not necessarily. It means the atria were depolarized, but it is possible that the muscle cell did not contract in response. It is impossible to tell whether or not the atria contracted simply by looking at the EKG.

33. As the impulse leaves the atria and travels to the AV node, it encounters a slight delay. The tissues of the node do not conduct impulses as fast as other cardiac electrical tissues. This means that the wave of depolarization will take a longer time to get through the AV node than it would in other parts of the heart. On the EKG, this is translated into a short period of electrical inactivity called the **PR segment**. This is the straight line between the P wave and the next wave. Locate the PR segment on Figure 9. The PR segment is indicative of the delay in the

_____ .

AV node

34. The AV node is the area of the heart with the slowest conduction speed. That is, the conductive tissues of the sinus node, the atria, and the ventricles all conduct impulses faster than the AV node does. This is necessary to allow time for atrial contraction and complete filling of the ventricles. On the EKG tracing, this delay at the AV _____ is seen as a short isoelectric segment between the _____ wave and the next wave. This segment is called the _____ segment.

node
P
PR

35. If you wished to refer to all of the electrical activity in the heart before the impulse reached the ventricles, you would look at the PR interval. This includes both the P wave and the PR segment. The P wave displays _____ depolarization, and the PR segment is caused by the _____ in the AV node. Therefore, the PR _____ includes all atrial and nodal activity.

atrial
delay
interval

QRS Complex

36. By definition, the PR interval begins at the first sign of the P wave and ends at the first deflection of the next wave, called the **QRS complex**. The PR interval includes all _____ activity and all _____ activity but does not include ventricular activity.

atrial; nodal

37. The ventricular depolarization is shown on the EKG by a large complex of three waves: the Q, the R, and the S. Collectively, these are called the QRS complex. This complex is significantly larger than the P wave because ventricular depolarization involves a greater muscle mass than atrial depolarization. The QRS complex starts with the Q wave. The Q wave is defined as the first negative deflection following the P wave but before the R wave. Locate the Q wave on Figure 9. The Q wave flows immediately into the R wave, which is the first positive deflection following the P wave. Next comes the S wave, which is defined as the second negative deflection following the P wave, or the first negative deflection after the R wave. Collectively, the QRS complex signifies _____ depolarization.

ventricular

38. The QRS complex is larger and more complicated than the P wave, primarily because it involves a larger part of the heart. Very often, the QRS complex looks different from the complex shown in Figure 9, but it is still called the QRS complex. Several different configurations of the QRS complex are shown in Figure 10. Regardless of appearance, these still indicate depolarization of the _____ .

ventricles

39. After the ventricles depolarize, they begin their repolarization phase, which results in another wave on the EKG. The T wave is indicative of ventricular repolarization. The atria also repolarize, but their repolarization is not significant enough to show up on the EKG, so you do not see an atrial equivalent of the T wave. Ventricular repolarization is much more prominent and is seen on the EKG as the _____ wave.

T

Figure 10 Various QRS Configurations

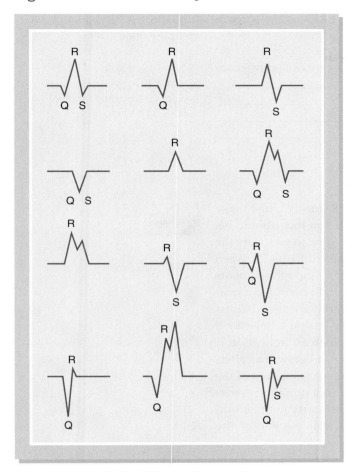

40. Now that you have learned the definitions of all of the waves on the EKG and what each one means, turn to the Practice Strips at the end of this chapter and label each wave on each practice strip in Part I (strips 2.1–2.12). Be sure to recall what each wave means as you mark it on the EKG. When you finish marking the waves, go back and identify the PR interval, the PR segment, and the QRS complex for each strip.

Practice Strips (Part I)

41. To interpret arrhythmias you must be able to measure the duration of the PR interval and the QRS complex. The grid markings on the graph paper are used to determine just how many seconds it took for the impulse to create those intervals. To make these measurements, you will use EKG calipers. Let's measure the PRI first. You can use Figure 9 for practice. Place one point of the calipers on the very first deflection that marks the beginning of the P wave. Then place the other point of the calipers on the final point of the PR interval, which you will recall is actually the very beginning of the _____ complex. Make sure you don't have any part of the QRS complex included in your measurement. Now, count the number of small boxes within your caliper points, and multiply that number by _____ second, which is the amount of time allotted to each small box. What is your measurement? _____ second.

QRS

0.04

0.16

42. For the PR interval to be considered normal, it must be between 0.12 and 0.20 second. If it is less than 0.12 second, it is considered a short PRI, and if it is greater than 0.20 second, it is said to be prolonged. The P wave itself does not contribute to a long

PRI; it is actually the delay in the AV node, or the PR _____ , that varies according to how long the node held the impulse before transmitting it. The normal PRI should be _____ second; a long PRI would suggest a _____ in the _____ .

segment

0.12–0.20

delay; AV node

43. Is the PRI measurement you determined for the complex shown in Figure 9 considered to be normal? _____

Yes. It is 0.16 second, which is within the normal range of 0.12–0.20 second.

ST Segment and T Wave

44. You measure the QRS complex in the same way as the PR interval. Just make sure your caliper points are exactly where the definitions tell you they should be. The Q wave should be measured where the deflection first begins to go below the isoelectric line. This part usually isn't so hard. The S wave is more difficult. Between the S wave and the T wave is a section called the **ST segment**. Although segments are supposed to be straight lines, the ST segment often gets caught up in the transition between the QRS complex and the T wave and is very rarely a cut-and-dried configuration. So you must look for some clue that indicates to you where the S wave stops and the _____ wave begins. If such an indication is present, it will usually be a very small notch or other movement suggesting an alteration of electrical flow. At any rate, this should be the outside measurement of the QRS complex. Include in your measurement the entire S wave, but don't let it overlap into the ST segment or the T wave. The QRS complex measurement should include the beginning of the _____ wave and the end of the _____ wave.

T

Q
S

Measurements

45. For practice, measure the QRS complex shown in Figure 9. What is your measurement? _____ second.

0.08

46. People very rarely agree on what a normal time range is for the QRS measurement. It is usually considered to be between 0.06 and 0.11 second. For simplicity, we'll define the normal QRS complex measurement as anything less than 0.12 second. This means that the ventricles took a normal amount of time to depolarize if they did it in less than _____ second.

0.12

47. Is the QRS measurement shown in Figure 9 considered to be normal?

Yes. It measures 0.08 second, which is less than 0.12 second.

Practice

48. Now that you know how to measure PRIs and QRSs, the rest is up to you. All it takes is practice, practice, and more practice. It is particularly helpful if you can get someone to check your measurements in the beginning so you don't develop bad habits. You can start by measuring PRI and QRS intervals on each of the strips in Part II of the Practice Strips at the end of the chapter (strips 2.13–2.30). The answer key shows you where the calipers were placed to obtain the answers, so if your measurements

Practice Strips (Part II)

differ from those given, look to see where the complex was measured to arrive at the answer shown.

Artifact, Interference

49. The complexes on an EKG tracing are created by electrical activity within the heart. But it is possible for things other than cardiac activity to interfere with the tracing you are trying to analyze. Some common causes of interference, or artifact, are:

- Muscle tremors, shivering
- Patient movement
- Loose electrodes
- The effect of other electrical equipment in the room (called 60-cycle interference)

Each of these situations can cause _____ on the EKG tracing, which   artifact
may interfere with your interpretation of the arrhythmia. When such external factors cause deflections on an EKG strip, those deflections are considered to be artifact and are important to recognize because they can _____ with your inter-   interfere
pretation of the arrhythmia.

50. Figure 11 shows you what each of these types of interference can look like on an EKG tracing. As you can see, _____ can often confuse you and   artifact

Figure 11 Types of Interference

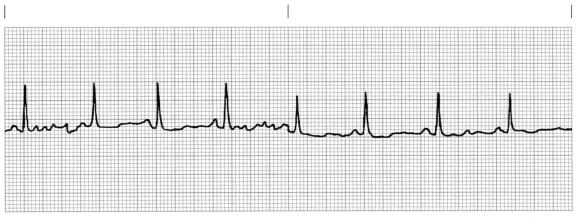

Muscle Tremors

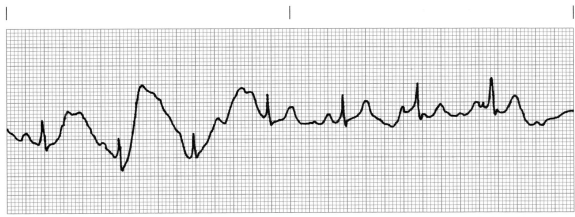

Patient Movement

Figure 11 (*Continued*)

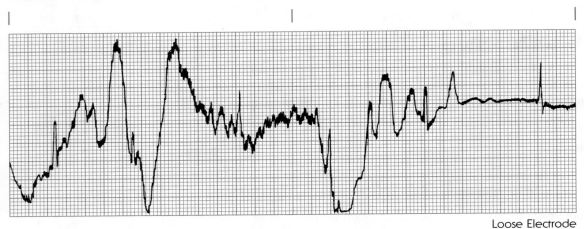

Loose Electrode

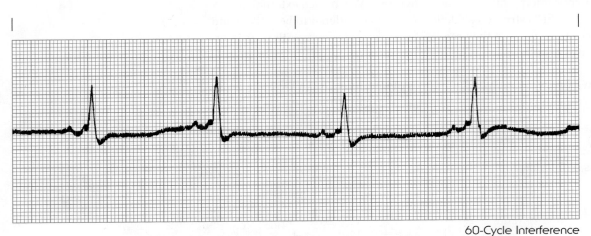

60-Cycle Interference

lead you to believe that the deflection was caused by cardiac activity when it was not. As you practice identifying the P waves and QRS complexes, you will become more and more familiar with the normal configurations of these wave forms and will be more apt to distinguish them from artifact. When trying to determine whether or not a deflection was caused by artifact, you should try to identify the _____ waves and _____ complexes of the P; QRS underlying rhythm and compare these configurations with the questionable deflections.

Refractory Periods

51. Let's go back to electrophysiology to make one final point. Since depolarization takes place when the electrical charges begin their wave of movement by exchanging places across the cell membrane, it would follow that this process cannot take place unless the charges are in their original position. This means that the cell cannot depolarize until the _____ process is complete. For depolarization to repolarization take place, repolarization must be _____ . complete

52. When the charges are depolarized and have not yet returned to their polarized state, the cell is said to be electrically "refractory" because it cannot yet accept another impulse. If a cell is _____ , it cannot accept an impulse because it isn't yet _____ .

refractory
repolarized

53. On the EKG, the refractory period of the ventricles is when they are depolarizing or repolarizing. Thus, the QRS and the T wave on the EKG would be considered the _____ period of the cardiac cycle, since it signifies a period when the heart would be unable to respond to an impulse.

refractory

54. Sometimes an electrical impulse will try to discharge the cell before repolarization is fully complete. In most cases nothing will happen because the cells aren't back to their original position and therefore can't _____ . But once in a while, if the stimulus is strong enough, an impulse might find several of the charges in the right position and thus discharge them before the rest of the cell is ready. This results in abnormal depolarization and hence is an undesirable occurrence. This premature depolarization can occur only if most of the cell charges are back to the _____ position. Thus, there is a small part of the refractory period that is not absolutely refractory. This small section is called the *relative* refractory period because some of the charges are polarized and thus can be _____ if the impulse is strong enough.

depolarize

original

depolarized

55. So there are actually two refractory periods: an *absolute* refractory period, when no impulse can cause depolarization, and a *relative* refractory period, when a strong impulse can cause a premature, abnormal discharge. The _____ refractory period would allow depolarization if the impulse were strong enough, while the _____ refractory period would not allow any response at all.

relative

absolute

56. Figure 12 shows you where these refractory periods are located on the EKG. Notice that while all of the T wave is considered a refractory period, the downslope of the T wave is only relatively refractory. This means that if a strong impulse fell on the downslope of the T wave, it could result in ventricular _____ . This fact will become more important to you when we begin to look at specific arrhythmias.

depolarization

57. You now have all of the information you need to begin analyzing EKG rhythm strips. You can identify all of the different waves that make up a cardiac cycle, and you can measure the PRI and the QRS complex. You are now ready to turn to Chapter 3 and learn how to apply this knowledge as you develop a technique for analyzing EKG rhythm strips.

Figure 12 Refractory Periods

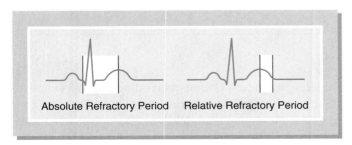

Absolute Refractory Period   Relative Refractory Period

KEY POINTS

- Electrodes are devices that are applied to the skin to detect electrical activity and convey it to a machine for display.
- Electrode contact can be improved by:
  - Abrading the skin
  - Cleaning or drying the skin
  - Using a contact medium
- If electricity flows toward the positive electrode, the patterns produced on the graph paper will be upright; if the electrical flow is toward the negative electrode, the patterns will be inverted.
- Electrode placement is standardized to avoid confusion in EKG interpretation (Figure 5).
- A lead is a single view of the heart, often produced by a combination of information from several electrodes.
- A monitoring lead is one that clearly shows individual waves and their relationship to other waves. All the examples in this book are Lead II (although this is only one of many monitoring leads).
- Graph paper is standardized to allow comparative analysis of EKG wave patterns.
- The isoelectric line is the straight line made on the EKG when no electrical current is flowing.
- Vertical lines on the graph paper measure time; horizontal lines measure voltage (Figure 7).
- A small square on the graph paper (the distance between two light vertical lines) is 0.04 second.
- A large square on the graph paper (the distance between two heavy vertical lines) is 0.20 second.
- The atria normally contract before the ventricles do.
- A single cardiac cycle on the EKG includes everything from depolarization of the atria up to and including repolarization of the ventricles.
- A single cardiac cycle is expected to produce a single heart beat (a pulse).
- The P wave represents atrial depolarization.

- The PR segment represents delay in the AV node.
- The PR interval includes the P wave and the PR segment and represents both atrial depolarization and delay in the AV node.
- The PRI is measured from the beginning of the P wave to the beginning of the QRS complex.
- The PRI is normally between 0.12 and 0.20 second.
- The QRS complex represents ventricular depolarization.
- The QRS interval is measured from the beginning of the Q wave to the end of the S wave.
- The Q wave is the first negative deflection following the P wave but before the R wave.
- The R wave is the first positive wave following the P wave, or the first positive wave of the QRS complex.
- The S wave is the second negative deflection following the P wave, or the first negative deflection following the R wave.
- The QRS interval is normally less than 0.12 second.
- External factors capable of producing artifact on the EKG tracing include muscle tremors, shivering, patient movement, loose electrodes, and 60-cycle electrical current.
- A cell is electrically refractory when it has not yet repolarized and thus cannot accept and respond to another stimulus.
- The absolute refractory period occurs when the cells cannot respond to any stimulus at all.
- The relative refractory period occurs when some of the cells are capable of responding if the stimulus is strong enough.
- If an impulse falls during the relative refractory period, the heart might be depolarized, but in an abnormal way.
- The absolute refractory period encompasses the QRS and the first part of the T wave.
- The relative refractory period is the downslope of the T wave.

SELF-TEST

Directions: Complete this self-evaluation of the information you have learned from this chapter. If your answers are all correct and you feel comfortable with your understanding of the material, proceed to the next chapter. However, if you missed any of the questions, you should review the referenced frames before proceeding. If you feel unsure of any of the underlying principles, invest the time now to go back over the entire chapter. **Do not proceed with the next chapter until you are very comfortable with the material in this chapter.**

Questions	Referenced Frames	Answers
1. What is an electrode used for?	1, 2, 4	to pick up electrical activity from the skin surface
2. List three ways to improve contact between the electrode and the skin.	2, 3, 4, 5	abrade skin; clean skin; use contact medium
3. If the electrical current flows toward the positive electrode, will the deflection on the graph paper be upright or downward?	6, 7, 8, 9, 10, 17	upright
4. Why is it important to standardize electrode placement?	11, 12	to avoid confusion when interpreting EKG patterns
5. What is a lead, and how does it differ from an electrode?	12, 13	A lead is a single view of the heart, often produced by a combination of information from several electrodes.
6. How many leads do you need to know to interpret arrhythmias?	12, 13	one; only a monitoring lead
7. Which lead will be discussed throughout this book?	13	Lead II
8. What are the electrode positions for the lead identified in the preceding question?	14	negative electrode below right clavicle; positive electrode at the apex; ground electrode below the left clavicle.
9. What features are important for a good monitoring lead?	12, 13	clear visualization of the basic waves
10. In Lead II, will the primary deflections be upright or downward on the EKG?	14	Upright, because the current is flowing toward the positive electrode.
11. Why is it important to use standardized EKG graph paper?	15, 16	Standardized markings enable you to measure the EKG and compare it to "normal."
12. What is an isoelectric line?	17	It is the straight line on the EKG made when no electrical current is flowing.
13. What do the vertical lines on the graph paper tell you?	16, 17, 20, 21, 22, 23	time
14. What do the horizontal lines on the graph paper tell you?	16, 17, 18, 19, 23	voltage
15. How much time is involved between two heavy lines on the graph paper?	16, 21, 22	0.20 second
16. How much time is involved in one small square on the graph paper?	16, 21, 22	0.04 second
17. Which chambers contract first in a single cardiac cycle?	24, 25, 26	the atria
18. What must occur for the heart to contract?	27	The muscle cells must receive an electrical stimulus.

Questions	Referenced Frames	Answers
19. What cardiac activity is included in a single cardiac cycle on the EKG?	28	everything from depolarization of the atria up to and including repolarization of the ventricles
20. How many heart beats would you expect a single cardiac cycle to produce?	28, 29	one
21. What are the five waves found in a single cardiac cycle on the EKG?	30, 40	P, Q, R, S, and T
22. Differentiate between waves, segments, and intervals.	30	Waves are deflections, segments are straight lines, and intervals include both waves and segments.
23. What does the P wave represent, and how is it found on the EKG?	31	atrial depolarization; it is measured from the first deflection on the cardiac cycle until the deflection returns to the isoelectric line
24. What does the PR segment represent?	33, 34	delay in the AV node
25. What is the PR interval, how is it measured, and what is its normal duration?	35, 36, 41, 42, 43, 48	The PRI includes the P wave and the PR segment. It is measured from the beginning of the P wave to the very beginning of the QRS complex. It is normally 0.12–0.20 second.
26. What does the QRS represent, how is it measured, and what is its normal duration?	37, 38, 44, 45, 46, 47, 48	ventricular depolarization; measure from the beginning of the Q wave to the end of the S wave; normally less than 0.12 second
27. What does the T wave represent?	39	ventricular repolarization
28. List four external factors capable of producing artifact on the EKG tracing.	49, 50	muscle tremors, shivering; patient movement; loose electrodes; 60-cycle electrical current
29. What is meant by *electrical refractoriness?*	51, 52, 53	The cells are not yet repolarized and thus cannot accept and respond to another stimulus.
30. Differentiate between absolute refractory period and relative refractory period.	54, 55, 56	Absolute refractory period means that the heart cannot accept any stimulus at all. Relative refractory period means that some of the cells are capable of responding to a strong stimulus.
31. What is so important about the relative refractory period?	54, 55, 56	If an impulse hits on the relative refractory period, the heart can be discharged in an abnormal way.
32. What part of the EKG complex signifies the relative refractory period?	56	the downslope of the T wave

PRACTICE STRIPS (answers can be found in the Answer Key on page 541)

PART I: LABELING WAVES

Directions: For each of the following rhythm strips, label the P, Q, R, S, and T waves of a single cardiac cycle. (Some of the tracings may not have all of these waves.) As you finish each strip, check your answers. They start on page 541.

2.1

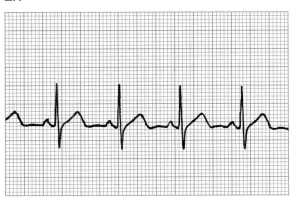

2.2

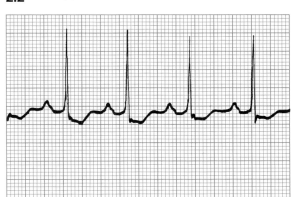

2.3

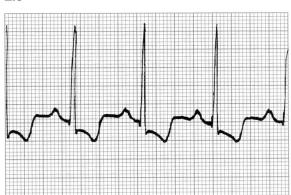

2.4

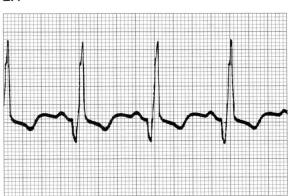

2.5

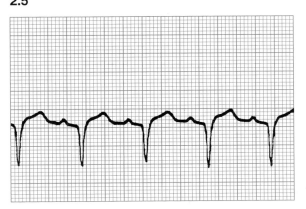

2.6

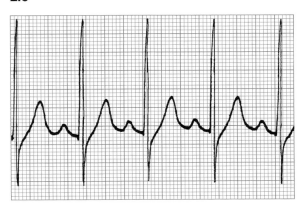

2.7

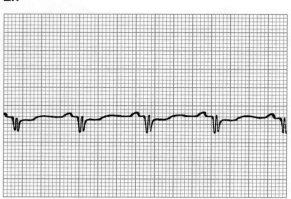

2.8

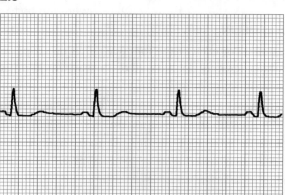

2.9

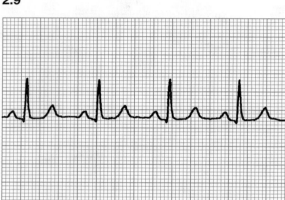

2.10

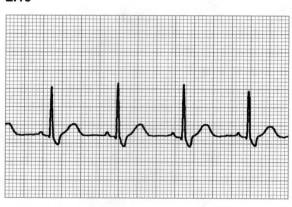

2.11

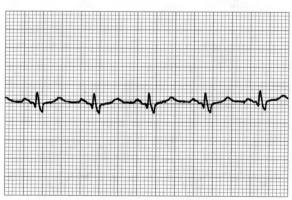

2.12

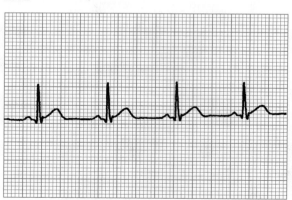

When you have completed this exercise, check your answers. They start on page 543. Then return to Frame 41 in this chapter (page 23).

PART II: MEASURING INTERVALS

Directions: For each of the following rhythm strips, measure the PR interval and the QRS complex. As you do each strip, check your answers. They start on page 543.

2.13

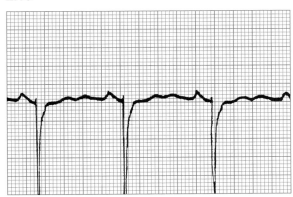

PRI: _____ second

QRS: _____ second

2.14

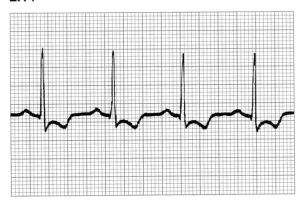

PRI: _____ second

QRS: _____ second

2.15

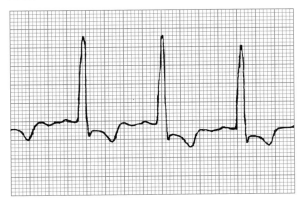

PRI: _____ second

QRS: _____ second

2.16

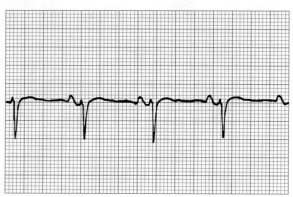

PRI: _____ second

QRS: _____ second

2.17

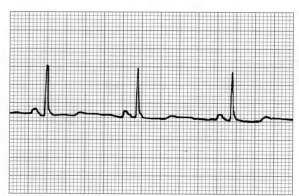

PRI: _____ second

QRS: _____ second

2.18

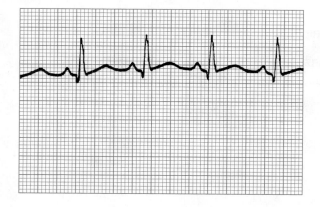

PRI: _____ second

QRS: _____ second

2.19

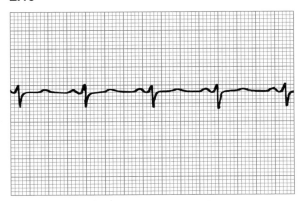

PRI: _____ second

QRS: _____ second

2.20

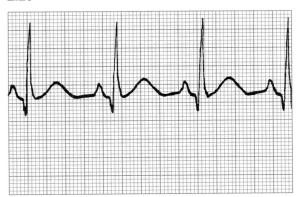

PRI: _____ second

QRS: _____ second

2.21

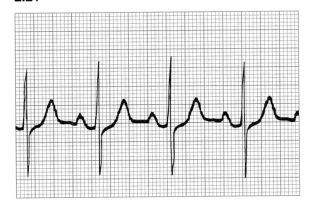

PRI: _____ second

QRS: _____ second

2.22

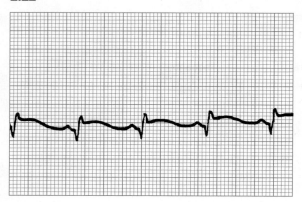

PRI: _____ second

QRS: _____ second

2.23

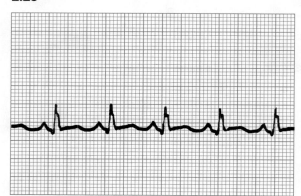

PRI: _____ second

QRS: _____ second

2.24

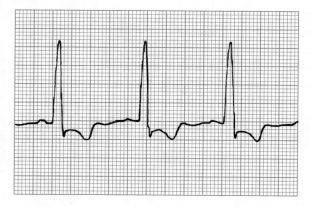

PRI: _____ second

QRS: _____ second

2.25

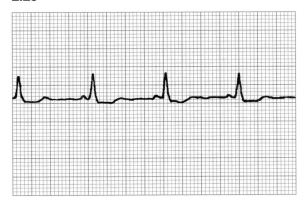

PRI: _____ second

QRS: _____ second

2.26

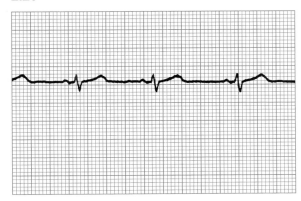

PRI: _____ second

QRS: _____ second

2.27

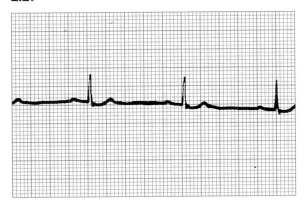

PRI: _____ second

QRS: _____ second

2.28

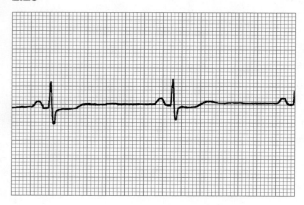

PRI: _____ second

QRS: _____ second

2.29

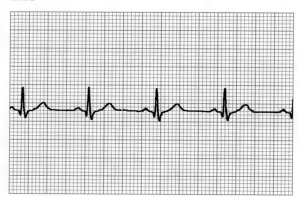

PRI: _____ second

QRS: _____ second

2.30

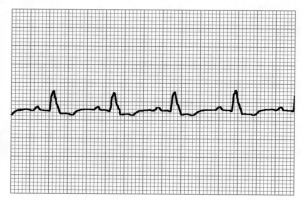

PRI: _____ second

QRS: _____ second

When you complete this exercise, return to Frame 49 in this chapter (page 25).

Chapter 3
Analyzing EKG Rhythm Strips

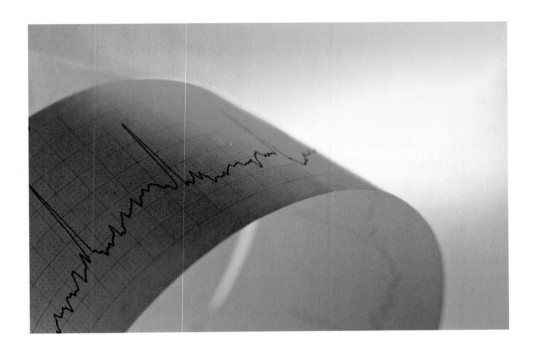

Overview

IN THIS CHAPTER, you will learn to use an organized analysis format to gather data from a rhythm strip. You will learn that a systematic format, consistently applied, will provide the data you need to identify the presenting arrhythmia. You will then learn such a systematic format and begin to use it consistently to gather data from EKG strips.

Analysis Format

1. In Chapter 2 you learned that there are five distinct wave patterns that make up a single _____ on the EKG. You also learned that a beating heart will produce a series of these _____ , which together become an EKG rhythm strip.

cardiac cycle
cardiac cycles

2. EKGs are even more complex than fingerprints. Not only does every person on earth have his or her own individual EKG, distinct from all others, but one person's EKG can look very different from one moment to the next. This is why it is inadequate simply to memorize eight or ten of the most common EKG patterns and hope you can recognize one the next time you see it. This type of EKG analysis is called *pattern recognition* and is a common but haphazard way to approach arrhythmias. A much more reliable way to approach an EKG tracing is to take it apart, wave by wave, and interpret exactly what's happening within the heart. This method of EKG interpretation is more sophisticated than _____ and will be far more valuable to you because it's more reliable.

pattern recognition

3. Arrhythmias can be categorized into groups according to which pacemaker site initiates the rhythm. The most common sites, and thus the major categories of arrhythmias, are:

- Sinus

- Atrial

- Junctional

- Ventricular

Arrhythmias are categorized this way because the _____ impulse for that rhythm came from one of these sites.

pacemaker

4. The most common cardiac rhythm is sinus in origin, because the _____ node is the usual pacemaker of the heart. Therefore, a normal, healthy heart would be in **Normal Sinus Rhythm** (NSR) because the rhythm originated in the _____ node.

sinus (SA)

SA

5. To get an idea of the variety of EKG patterns possible, look at the Practice Strips at the end of this chapter. All of the EKG tracings shown are sinus rhythm. You can see why it is necessary to have an organized format for approaching arrhythmia interpretation. Without a format for deciphering EKGs, you could easily be intimidated even by a group of "normal" tracings. To develop competency and confidence in interpreting EKGs, you must have an organized _____ for approaching arrhythmias.

format

6. Each EKG tracing provides a multitude of clues as to what is happening in that heart. These clues include wave configurations, rates, measurements, and wave relationships. Experts have compiled this data and found that each cardiac arrhythmia has its own set of clues. That is, each specific arrhythmia will repeatedly give off the same set of clues. By looking at the clues available from the strip, you can tell what the rhythm is, but only if you know in advance the kinds of clues that any specific arrhythmia is known to produce. We call these clues the "rules" for a specific arrhythmia. For example, NSR has a set of rules, including a specific relationship between P waves and QRS complexes, and a range for both rate and wave measurements. If you memorize these rules in advance and then come across a rhythm that meets these rules, you have reason to believe that this rhythm is NSR. Therefore, it is necessary to memorize the rules for each rhythm strip and then look for the _____ available from each strip you approach.

clues

7. EKG interpretation is a true "gray" area; there is no black and white to any of the information you will learn here. When it comes right down to naming a rhythm, you'll find that this isn't always possible, particularly in the more complex tracings. However, the clues you get from the strip should collectively eliminate most of the possibilities and point to one or two specific patterns. From there, it is a matter of which possibility has the most clues in its favor. Even though you can't always identify the rhythm exactly, the _____ you get from the strip should fit the rules of one or two arrhythmias, thus suggesting the category of arrhythmia you are trying to identify.

clues

Figure 13 Systematic Approach to Arrhythmia Interpretation

REGULARITY
(also called *Rhythm*)

- Is it regular?
- Is it irregular?
- Are there any patterns to the irregularity?
- Are there any ectopic beats? If so, are they early or late?

RATE

- What is the exact rate?
- Is the atrial rate the same as the ventricular rate?

P WAVES

- Are the P waves regular?
- Is there one P wave for every QRS?
- Is the P wave in front of the QRS or behind it?
- Is the P wave normal and upright in Lead II?
- Are there more P waves than QRS complexes?
- Do all the P waves look alike?
- Are the irregular P waves associated with ectopic beats?

PR INTERVAL

- Are all the PRIs constant?
- Is the PRI measurement within normal range?
- If the PRI varies, is there a pattern to the changing measurements?

QRS COMPLEX

- Are all the QRS complexes of equal duration?
- What is the measurement of the QRS complex?
- Is the QRS measurement within normal limits?
- Do all the QRS complexes look alike?
- Are the unusual QRS complexes associated with ectopic beats?

8. Let's repeat the point we just made in the preceding frame, because it will be important as we go over the analysis process. As you approach an arrhythmia, look at the _____ and compare them to the rules for arrhythmias. If there are two possibilities, or two people who disagree on the interpretation, it will be decided by whoever has the most clues in his or her favor. Therefore, it is critical to pick up the clues from the strip and compare them to the _____ for each arrhythmia. Now you can see why it will be essential to memorize the rules for each arrhythmia and have them comfortably available for recall as you begin arrhythmia interpretation.   clues   rules

9. Although EKG interpretation is acknowledged to be a very negotiable field, and everyone is entitled to a personal opinion of each arrhythmia's true identity, we have been able to agree on a fairly standard format for approaching arrhythmias. This format is outlined in Figure 13 and will be discussed point by point in the next several frames. Look at Figure 13 and determine which item we will look at first when starting to analyze an EKG. _____   regularity

Regularity

10. The regularity, or _____ , of an EKG pattern is determined by looking at the R-to-R interval (R–R, or RRI). This interval is measured by placing one point of the calipers on one R wave (or any other fixed, prominent point on the QRS complex) and placing the other point on the same spot of the next QRS complex. The R wave is indicative of ventricular _____ and thus *should* correspond to the patient's _____ .   rhythm   depolarization   pulse

11. When looking to see if the rhythm is regular or irregular, measure the _____ *across the entire strip.* If the pattern is regular, the RRI should remain constant throughout. A constant RRI would mean that the rhythm is _____.

R–R intervals

regular

12. A key point in determining regularity is to measure *all* the RRIs across the rhythm strip. If you skip around and don't measure _____ the RRIs, you will frequently miss a pattern of irregularity.

all

13. If the pattern is not regular, you must determine whether it is:

- *Regularly irregular*
  (it has a pattern of irregularity)
- *Basically regular*
  (it is a regular rhythm that has a beat or two that interrupts it)
- *Totally irregular*
  (it has no patterns at all)

If the rhythm has a pattern to the irregularity, it is said to be _____ irregular; if it has a beat or two that interrupts the regular pattern, it would be basically _____ ; if it is totally irregular, it would have _____ patterns.

regularly

regular

no

14. If the rhythm is regular across the entire strip, you can consider it a _____ rhythm. Sometimes a rhythm will be very nearly regular but will be "off" by one or even two small squares. This can be especially disconcerting to the student, who is usually still looking for everything to fit exactly. However, as you now know, EKG interpretation isn't always exact, and regularity determination is no exception. It is not uncommon for a rhythm, especially a slow one, to be "off" by a small square and still be considered regular. A general guideline is that faster rates should be more exactly _____ , while slower rates can sometimes have a little more leeway. The key issue is to make sure that there are no other areas of irregularity. If there are other areas of irregularity, or if there are patterns of irregularity, you really can't consider the rhythm to be _____ .

regular

regular

regular

15. If the rhythm is not regular, measure all combinations of RRIs to see if there is a pattern to the irregularity. Possible patterns include:

- A regular rhythm with one or more disrupting (ectopic) beats
- A combination of normal beats and ectopic beats that produces a pattern of "grouped" beats

If these possibilities are eliminated, you should consider the rhythm totally irregular. An irregular EKG strip will be considered totally irregular if it has no _____ of irregularity.

patterns

Rate

16. The next major step in the analysis process (as shown in Figure 13) is rate. There are several common ways to calculate heart rate, and the method you choose depends primarily on the regularity of the rhythm. To select the method of calculating rates, you must first determine whether or not the rhythm is _____ .

regular

17. If the rhythm is regular, the most accurate way to calculate heart rate is to count the number of small squares between two R waves and divide the total into 1,500. A

Figure 14 Calculating Heart Rates

METHOD	DIRECTIONS	FEATURES
A	Count the number of R waves in a 6-second strip and multiply by 10.	• Not very accurate • Used only with very quick estimate
B	Count the number of large squares between two consecutive R waves and divide into 300. **or** *Memorize this scale:* 1 large square = 300 bpm 2 large squares = 150 bpm 3 large squares = 100 bpm 4 large squares = 75 bpm 5 large squares = 60 bpm 6 large squares = 50 bpm	• Very quick • Not very accurate with fast rates • Used only with regular rhythms
C	Count the number of small squares between two consecutive R waves and divide into 1,500.	• Most accurate • Used only with regular rhythms • Time-consuming

faster way is to count the number of large squares between two R waves and divide the total into 300. If you count small squares, you would divide the total into _____ , but if you count large squares, you divide the total into _____ , since there are five small squares in each large square.

1,500
300

18. There is an even simpler (but less accurate) way to calculate the rate of a regular rhythm. There is a small ruler on the inside back cover of your book. It is based on the system of dividing the number of large squares into 300, but it requires that you memorize the simple rate scale shown in Figure 14. This rate scale is well worth memorizing, since it will probably be the method you use most often. It is a quick and fairly accurate way to calculate rate, but to use this method, the rhythm must be _____ .

regular

19. If the rhythm is irregular, it's very easy to estimate the rate. Look at the sample rhythm strip in Figure 15. On each strip you will notice small vertical notches in the upper margin of the paper. Each of these notches is 3 seconds away from the next. So if you count the number of QRS complexes in a 6-second span, you can multiply that by 10 to get the heart rate for 1 minute. This method of estimating rate for irregular rhythms requires that you count the number of QRS complexes in a 6-second span and multiply by _____ to get the heart rate in beats per minute (bpm).

10

20. The method described in the preceding frame is the quickest and easiest way to estimate rate, but it is not very accurate and shouldn't be used unless the rhythm is irregular and can't be calculated any other way. For regular rhythms, you should count the number of small squares between two R waves and divide the total into _____ , or count the number of large squares between two R waves and divide the total into _____ . Again, the most convenient way to estimate rate for a regular rhythm is to memorize the chart shown in Figure 14.

1,500
300

Figure 15 Figuring Rates Based on the Number of QRS Complexes in a 6-Second Strip

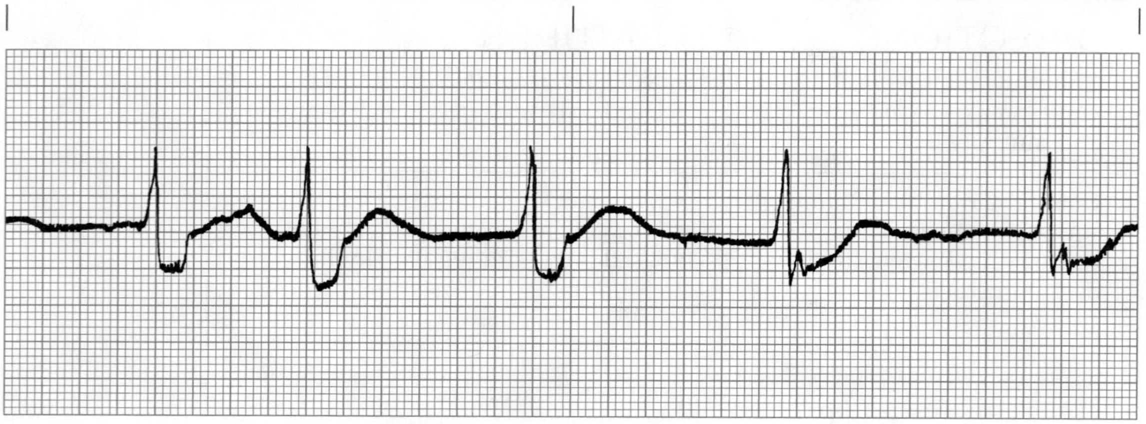

This sample strip has five R waves within the 6-second period defined by the notches in the margin. To figure the heart rate, multiply the R waves by 10 for a rate of 50 beats in 60 seconds.

21. By now, you would have looked at the rhythm strip and decided whether or not it was regular and then would have determined the heart rate. Turn to the Practice Strips at the end of this chapter and make both of those determinations for each strip in Part I (strips 3.1–3.6).

Practice Strips (Part I)

MyBRADYLab™

22. Now that you have determined regularity and rate for the strip you are analyzing, the next step is to begin figuring out the wave patterns. This is a very basic step that you should always follow when approaching arrhythmias. Before you can interpret the arrhythmia, you must first locate and identify each _____ so that you can understand what's happening in the heart.

wave

P Waves

23. To begin marking waves, first identify the P wave. The QRS complex is tempting because it is usually the largest and most conspicuous, but you will soon learn that the P wave can be your best friend because it's more reliable than the other waves. To begin identifying the waves, look first for the _____ waves.

P

24. The P wave has a characteristic shape that will often stick out even among a lot of unidentifiable waves. The morphology (shape) of the P wave is usually rounded and uniform. Sometimes P wave morphology can change if the pacemaker begins moving out of the sinus node. But if the sinus node is the pacemaker, and it isn't diseased or hypertrophied (enlarged), the P wave will have a smooth, rounded, uniform _____ .

morphology (shape)

25. Another characteristic of the _____ P wave is that it is upright and uniform. If you look back at Figure 5 in Chapter 2, you will see that the electrical flow is toward the positive electrode in Lead II, which explains why the P wave will be upright as long as the impulse begins in the sinus node and travels toward the ventricles. As you get more sophisticated in your understanding of arrhythmias, you will learn that a P wave can sometimes be negative. But for now, you need to remember that a normal sinus P wave will always be upright. If the P wave originates in the _____ node, it will be a smooth, rounded, _____ wave.

sinus

SA; upright

26. Now you know that P waves usually come before _____ complexes, so look at Part 1 of the Practice Strips (strips 3.1–3.6) at the end of this chapter and label each P wave. It might help you keep things straight if you mark the P above the wave directly on the strip. (*Note:* This is a helpful way to learn arrhythmias, but be careful not to mark up an EKG if it's the patient's only original.)

QRS
Practice Strips
MyBRADYLab™

27. Were you able to locate each P wave all across each strip? If you ever have trouble finding a P wave, or if you can't decide whether or not a wave is a P wave, there are several tips to remember. First, you know that the normal PRI is _____ second. So set your calipers at 20 seconds and measure that distance in front of the QRS complex. If there is a wave there, it's likely to be a _____ wave. To determine whether or not a P wave precedes the QRS, look for the P wave between _____ and _____ second in front of the QRS complex, since that is the normal PRI measurement.

0.12–0.20

P

0.12; 0.20

28. P waves are the most reliable of the waves, so map out the Ps across the strip. If most of them are regular but a space is missing near the T wave, it is probable that a P is hidden in another wave. Because P waves are reliably _____ , you can often assume that a P wave is present just by noting the patterns of the visible P waves.

regular

29. Let's take a minute to talk about "losing" waves. This is a phenomenon that occurs when two electrical activities take place at the same time. For instance, if the atria depolarize at the same time the ventricles repolarize, the P wave will be in the same spot on the EKG as the _____ . When this happens, the largest wave will usually obscure all or most of the smaller wave. In this situation, the P wave would be said to be "lost" or "hidden" in the T wave. If the P wave is _____ in the T wave, you may be able to tell it's there by mapping out the other P waves or by looking for a suspicious notch on the T wave where you expect the P wave to be.

T wave

lost (hidden)

30. Once all the P waves are marked, it is usually not as difficult to identify the other waves. Go to the Practice Strips for Chapter 3 and mark the Q, R, S, and T waves for the strips in Part I (strips 3.1–3.6). As you're doing this, make a mental note of the relationships between the waves. That is, does a P wave precede every QRS complex? Is there only one P wave for every QRS, or are there more P waves than QRS complexes?

Practice Strips

PR Intervals and QRS Complexes

31. Now that all the waves are identified, go back through the rhythm strips Part I (strips 3.1–3.6) and measure the PRIs and QRS complexes to determine whether or not they are within the normal ranges. If you've forgotten the normal measurements, review the Key Points for Chapter 2 (page 00).

Practice Strips
MyBRADYLab™

32. You now have all the data you need from these arrhythmias in order to identify them. The reason you can't name them now is that you have not yet learned the necessary rules and thus do not know into which category each tracing falls. To identify an arrhythmia, you must first collect the data from the strip and then compare that data to the _____ for each arrhythmia.

rules

33. In the next chapter you will begin learning the rules for each of the arrhythmias. Before you go on to that, there are one or two more points that must be covered for you to be able to interpret arrhythmias, rather than just recognize them. For example, the measurements you have just learned are actually measurements of time. As we go on to the next chapters, it will become increasingly important for you to think of measurements such as PRI and QRS as actual activity within the heart and not just normal or abnormal figures. That is, a PRI is considered abnormal if an impulse took too long to get from the sinus node through the _____ and the _____ ; similarly, a QRS is considered abnormal if the impulse took too long to travel through the _____ . The actual figure is not as critical as being able to understand what occurred within the heart to produce that figure.

atria

AV node

ventricles

34. Let's carry this point a bit further. We know from information gathered during research that it takes 0.12–0.20 second for an impulse to get from the sinus node through the atria and AV node of a normal heart. On the EKG, this time frame is depicted as the _____ interval. If this time is extended and the PRI is elongated, we can deduce that there was some delay somewhere in the atria or the node.

PR

35. The _____ includes the P wave and the PR segment. The P wave itself indicates the amount of time it took the impulse to travel through the _____ and depolarize them. The isoelectric component of the PRI, or the PR segment, shows the delay in the AV node. Together, these two parts of the cardiac cycle show us what happened to the impulse *before* it reached the _____ . Therefore, the PRI represents the cardiac activity that takes place above the ventricles in the atria and AV node; this category of activity is referred to as **supraventricular** activity. Supraventricular refers to the part of the heart _____ the ventricles.

PRI

atria

ventricles

above

Role of the AV Node

36. In Chapter 2 you learned that the _____ is the area of the heart with the slowest conduction speed. That is, the conductive tissues of the sinus node, the atria, and the ventricles all conduct impulses _____ than the AV node. There is one more thing you should know about the AV node. Because it is the doorway between the atria and ventricles, the node has the responsibility of "holding" impulses until the ventricles are able to receive them. This is why there is a slight delay at the node before each impulse passes through to the ventricles. In the normal heart, this is not a particularly critical feature, but occasionally the atria will become irritable and begin firing impulses very rapidly. The ventricles cannot respond effectively to all these impulses, so the AV node "screens" some of them, allowing only a few to get through. This vital function of the node is called the heart's "fail-safe" mechanism, and you will learn much more about it later as you learn about the more complex arrhythmias. The AV node is a vital structure within the heart because it protects the _____ from having to respond to too many impulses.

AV node

faster

ventricles

Ventricular vs. Supraventricular

37. When a rhythm originates in the sinus node, the atria, or the AV junction, it is considered to be in the general category of supraventricular arrhythmias because it originated above the ventricles. _____ rhythms include all those that originate above the ventricles; in fact, the only rhythms *not* included in the supraventricular category are those that originate in the ventricles. This basic categorization separates rhythms that originate in the ventricles from those that originate _____ the ventricles.

Supraventricular

above

38. The major EKG finding that can help you distinguish between supraventricular and ventricular rhythms is the width of the QRS complex. This is because research data show us that the only way an impulse can get all the way through the ventricles in less than 0.12 second is if it follows normal conduction pathways; all other means of depolarizing the ventricles will take a longer time. Therefore, if a rhythm has a normal QRS measurement of less than 0.12 second, it must have been conducted normally and thus would have to be _____ in origin. This tells us that a rhythm is known to be supraventricular, meaning it originated above the ventricles, if it has a QRS measurement of less than _____ second.

supraventricular

0.12

39. Unfortunately, this rule does not apply in the reverse. That is, just because the QRS is wide does not mean that the rhythm is ventricular. A wide QRS complex can be caused by:

- A supraventricular impulse that reaches an obstruction in the bundle branches
- A supraventricular impulse that cannot be conducted normally through the ventricles because they are still refractory from the preceding beat
- An irritable focus in the ventricles that assumes pacemaking responsibility

Of these possibilities, the third is by far the most common, telling us that a _____ very frequently is caused by a ventricular impulse. However, it can get you into trouble if you assume that all wide QRSs are ventricular in origin. So a normal QRS complex *must* be supraventricular, whereas a wide QRS complex can be ventricular, but it can also be supraventricular with a conduction defect. A wide QRS can be either ventricular or supraventricular, but a QRS of less than 0.12 second must be _____ in origin.

wide QRS

supraventricular

40. By definition, supraventricular arrhythmias must have a normal QRS measurement of less than _____ second. However, as was shown in the preceding frame, they can frequently have prolonged ventricular _____ . When this happens, you must note it along with your interpretation of the rhythm. For example, a Normal Sinus Rhythm should have a QRS of _____ than 0.12 second, but if it had a _____ disturbance in the ventricles, it would fit all the rules of NSR except that the QRS would be too _____ . It should then be called Sinus Rhythm *with a wide QRS complex*. It is not necessary for you to be more specific in identifying which type of disturbance is present; if you choose to learn more about EKGs at a later time, you will most likely also learn to distinguish between these conduction irregularities. For now, you will simply call attention to an abnormal QRS complex by calling it a _____ . Regardless of whether or not ventricular conduction is normal, you must give primary attention to identifying the basic arrhythmia.

0.12
conduction

less
conduction

wide

wide QRS complex

41. You now have the necessary knowledge to begin learning specific arrhythmias. The secret to arrhythmia interpretation is practice. So if you have time now, turn to the Practice Strips at the end of this chapter and practice gathering data from the tracings in Part II (strips 3.7–3.15).

Practice Strips (Part II)

MyBRADYLab™

KEY POINTS

- The beating heart produces a series of cardiac cycles, which together become an EKG rhythm strip.

- Arrhythmias are categorized according to which pacemaker site initiates the rhythm.

- The normal heart rhythm originates in the sinus node and thus is called Normal Sinus Rhythm.

- It is necessary to memorize the rules for each arrhythmia in order to interpret it.

- EKG interpretation is based on how closely the clues gathered from the rhythm strip comply with the rules for a given arrhythmia.

- Because EKG interpretation can be so complex, it is essential to develop a routine format for analyzing rhythm strips and then use it consistently when identifying arrhythmias. An example of such a format is as follows:

  - Rhythm (also called regularity)
  - Rate
  - P Wave
  - PR Interval (PRI)
  - QRS Complex (QRS)

- Rhythm, or regularity, is determined by measuring the R–R intervals, or possibly the P–P intervals, across the entire strip. If the pattern is not regular, note whether it is regularly irregular, basically regular, or totally irregular. Look for patterns to the irregularity that could indicate ectopics or grouped beating.

- *Rate* can refer to either the ventricular rate (most common) or the atrial rate, if they differ. Rate can be calculated in one of three ways:

  1. Count the number of small squares between two R waves and divide the total into 1,500.

  2. Count the number of large squares between two R waves and divide the total into 300. Standard tables giving this information are available and can be memorized for quick reference.

  3. Count the number of R waves in a 6-second strip and multiply by 10. This last method should be used only on irregular arrhythmias because it is the least accurate.

- The P wave should be found preceding the QRS complex. It should be upright and uniform. The P waves should be regular across the entire strip, and there should be only one P wave for each QRS complex. It is possible for the P wave to be hidden in the T wave of the preceding complex.

- The PR interval is an indication of the electrical activity taking place within the atria and the AV node. It encompasses all electrical activity above the ventricles. The PRI consists of the P wave and the PR segment. The PR segment is caused by the delay of the impulse at the AV node. The PRI should be constant across the strip and should measure between 0.12 and 0.20 second.

- The QRS complex can help you determine whether the rhythm originated from a supraventricular focus or from the ventricles. A supraventricular focus normally produces a QRS complex measuring less than 0.12 second. However, it is possible for a supraventricular rhythm to have a wider QRS complex if there was a conduction disturbance within the ventricles. If the rhythm originated in the ventricles, the QRS complex will be 0.12 second or greater. A narrow QRS complex indicates that the impulse is supraventricular, while a wide QRS complex can be either supraventricular with a conduction disturbance, or it can be ventricular.

SELF-TEST

Directions: Complete this self-evaluation of the information you have learned in this chapter. If your answers are all correct and you feel comfortable with your understanding of the material, proceed to the next chapter. However, if you miss any of the questions, you should review the referenced frames before proceeding. If you feel unsure of any of the underlying principles, invest the time now to go back over the entire chapter. **Do not proceed with the next chapter until you are very comfortable with the material in this chapter.**

Questions	Referenced Frames	Answers
1. What is a cardiac cycle on the EKG?	1	the electrical impulses associated with a single heart beat: the P, Q, R, S, and T waves
2. What is the name of the normal cardiac rhythm associated with a healthy heart?	4	Normal Sinus Rhythm
3. Why is it necessary to have an organized format for approaching arrhythmia interpretation?	2, 5, 9	There are so many possible configurations of EKGs that you would never be able to memorize all of them. You must be able to systematically gather all of the available information and then compare it to the rules for the rhythms. With-out a routine format, you could overlook important clues.
4. Why do you have to memorize the rules for each of the arrhythmias?	2, 6, 7, 8, 9	so that you can compare them to the findings on an EKG strip and thus determine the identity of the arrhythmia
5. What are the five parts of the analysis format that you learned in this chapter?	9	Regularity (rhythm), Rate, P Wave, PR Interval, QRS complex
6. How can you tell whether or not an arrhythmia is regular?	10, 11, 12, 14	Measure the R–R interval or the P–P interval.
7. What does the phrase "regularly irregular" mean?	13, 15	There is a pattern to the irregularity.
8. What does the phrase "basically regular" mean?	13, 15	The underlying rhythm is regular, but it is interrupted by ectopics.
9. What does it mean when you call an arrhythmia "totally irregular"?	13, 15	There is no pattern to the irregularity.
10. If you wanted to calculate accurately the rate of a regular rhythm, you could count the number of *small* squares between two R waves and divide it into what number?	16, 17, 18, 20	1,500
11. If you counted the number of *large* squares between two R waves, what number would you divide that total into to determine the heart rate?	16, 17, 18, 20	300
12. When an arrhythmia is irregular, you should determine the heart rate by counting the number of R waves in 6 seconds and multiplying that total by what number?	19, 20	10
13. What is the first wave you should try to locate and map out when analyzing a rhythm strip?	22, 23	the P wave
14. What does a normal sinus P wave look like?	23, 24, 25	It has a smooth, rounded shape; it is upright and uniform.
15. Where can you normally find the P wave?	26	It is usually located immediately in front of the QRS complex.

Questions	Referenced Frames	Answers
16. Are P–P intervals usually regular or irregular?	23, 28	They are usually very regular.
17. What is meant when a P wave is said to be "lost" in the T wave?	29	It means that the P wave occurred on or near the T wave and is thus obscured beyond clear identification.
18. In your analysis of a rhythm strip, what waves should you look for after you have located the P waves?	30, 31	the QRS and the T waves
19. Why is it important for you to know all these waves and measurements?	32, 33	because they reflect cardiac activity
20. What is a "supraventricular" arrhythmia?	33, 34, 35, 36, 37, 38, 39, 40	an arrhythmia that originates above the ventricles
21. If a QRS complex measures less than 0.12 second, where can you assume that it originated?	38, 39, 40	from a supraventricular focus
22. If a QRS complex measures 0.12 second or greater, it could possibly be a supraventricular rhythm with a ventricular conduction disturbance. What is the other possible explanation for a wide QRS complex?	38, 39, 40	A rhythm that originates in the ventricles will have a QRS measurement of 0.12 second or more.

PRACTICE STRIPS (answers can be found in the Answer Key on page 552)

PART I: ANALYZING EKG STRIPS

3.1

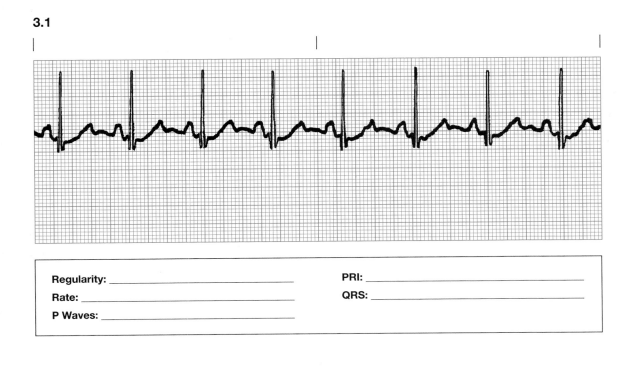

Regularity: _____	**PRI:** _____
Rate: _____	**QRS:** _____
P Waves: _____	

3.2

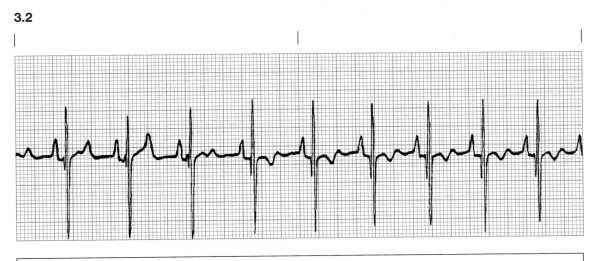

Regularity: _____	**PRI:** _____
Rate: _____	**QRS:** _____
P Waves: _____	

3.3

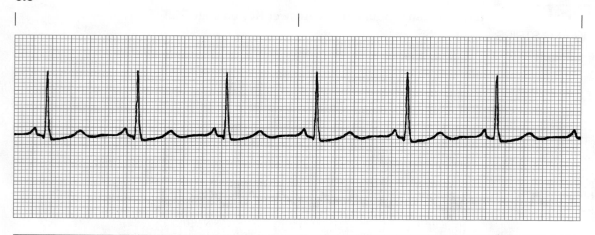

Regularity: _____	PRI: _____
Rate: _____	QRS: _____
P Waves: _____	

3.4

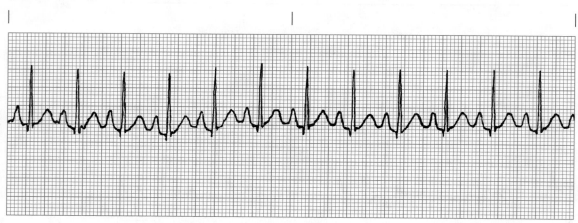

Regularity: _____	PRI: _____
Rate: _____	QRS: _____
P Waves: _____	

3.5

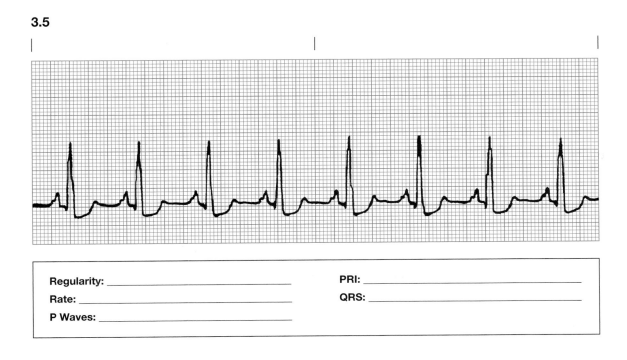

Regularity: _____   PRI: _____

Rate: _____   QRS: _____

P Waves: _____

3.6

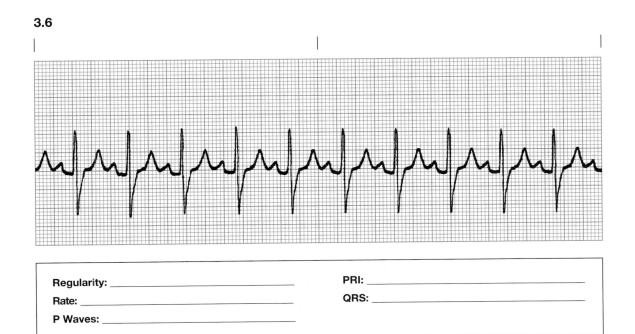

Regularity: _____   PRI: _____

Rate: _____   QRS: _____

P Waves: _____

3.7

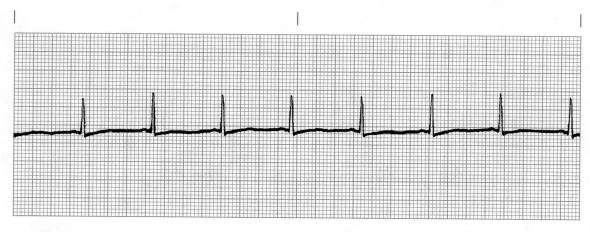

Regularity: _____   PRI: _____

Rate: _____   QRS: _____

P Waves: _____

PART II: GATHERING INFORMATION FROM STRIPS

3.8

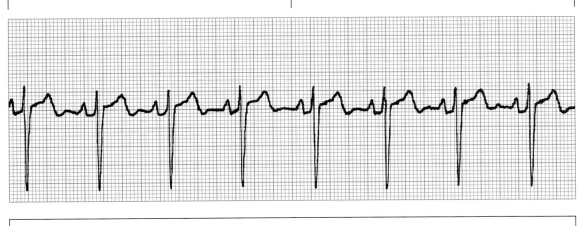

Regularity: _____   PRI: _____

Rate: _____   QRS: _____

P Waves: _____

3.9

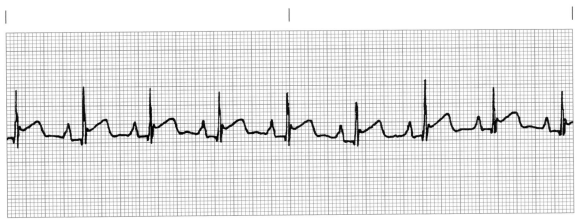

Regularity: _____   PRI: _____

Rate: _____   QRS: _____

P Waves: _____

3.10

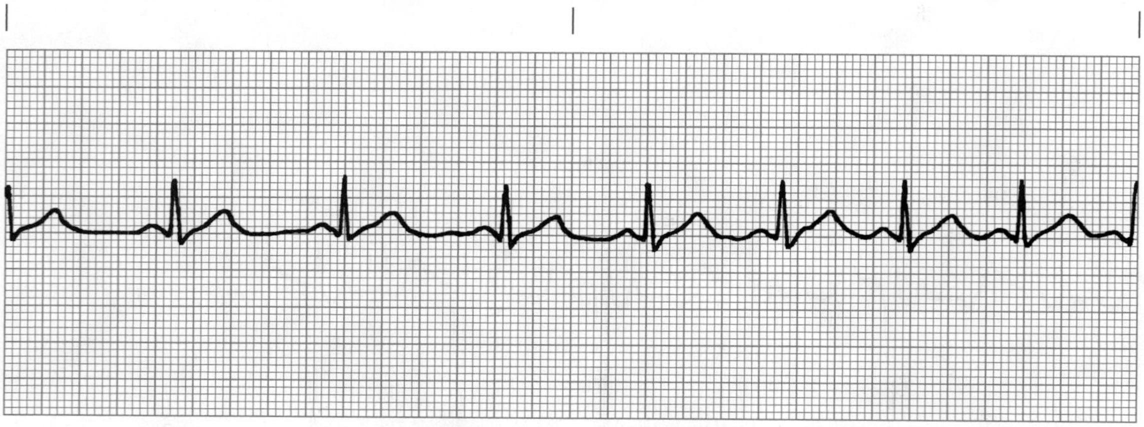

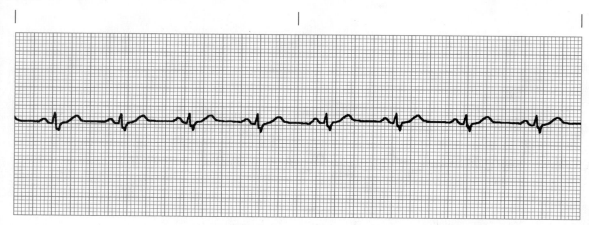

Regularity: _____ PRI: _____

Rate: _____ QRS: _____

P Waves: _____

3.11

Regularity: _____ PRI: _____

Rate: _____ QRS: _____

P Waves: _____

3.12

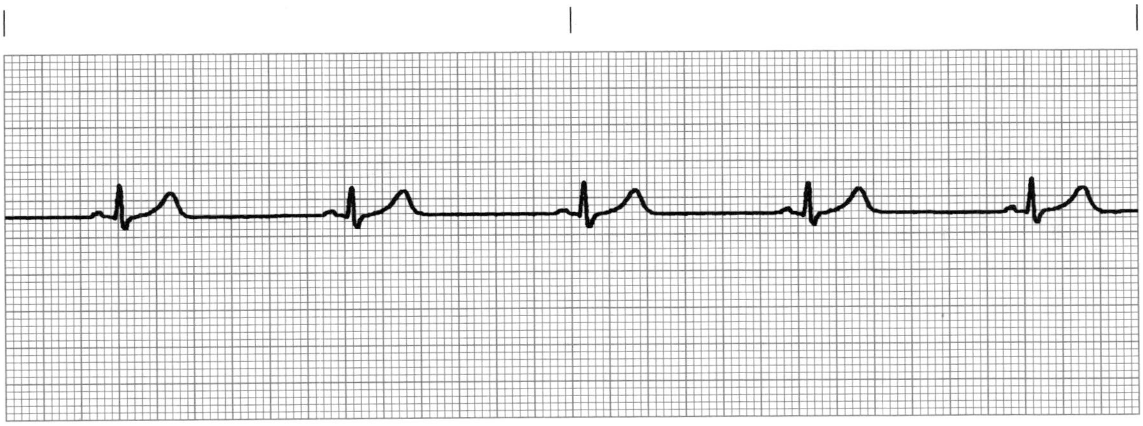

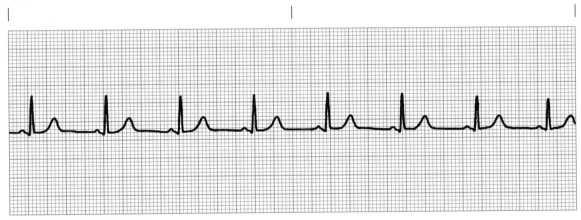

Regularity: _____   PRI: _____

Rate: _____   QRS: _____

P Waves: _____

3.13

Regularity: _____   PRI: _____

Rate: _____   QRS: _____

P Waves: _____

3.14

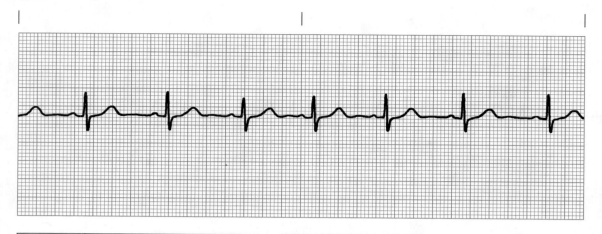

Regularity: _____		**PRI:** _____
Rate: _____		**QRS:** _____
P Waves: _____		

3.15

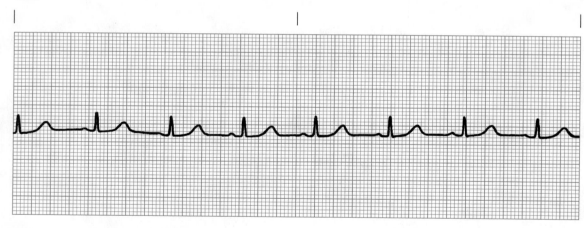

Regularity: _____		**PRI:** _____
Rate: _____		**QRS:** _____
P Waves: _____		

Chapter 4
Sinus Rhythms

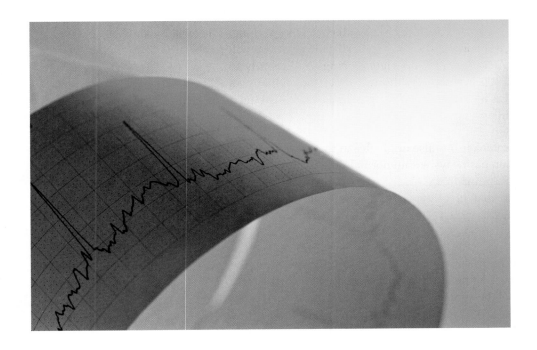

Overview

IN THIS CHAPTER, you will learn the characteristics of rhythms produced by a sinus pace-maker and features that are shared by all rhythms originating in the sinus node. You will then learn the names and features of four different arrhythmias that originate in the sinus node. For each of these arrhythmias, you will learn about the etiology, conduction, and resulting EKG features (regularity, rate, P waves, PR intervals, and QRS complexes).

Introduction

1. The first category of arrhythmias you will learn is the category of rhythms that originate in the sinus node. This group includes:

- Normal Sinus Rhythm (NSR)
- Sinus Bradycardia
- Sinus Tachycardia
- Sinus Arrhythmia

Each of these arrhythmias will be discussed individually. You will need to memorize the information provided because it will give the rules necessary for you to be able to identify that arrhythmia again. You will eventually need to memorize the _____ for all of the arrhythmias, but we will begin just with those originating in the _____ node.

rules

sinus

Normal Sinus Rhythm

2. First, we will discuss Normal Sinus Rhythm (Figure 16). We will look at what a normal rhythm is and what defines it as normal, and then we will begin looking at arrhythmias and how they differ from _____ . Technically speaking, NSR is not an arrhythmia because it is a normal, rhythmic pattern. However, you will often hear phrases like *arrhythmia, dysrhythmia,* and *rhythm* being used loosely to describe both normal and abnormal EKG patterns. Although NSR is not actually an _____ because it has a normal, rhythmic pattern, we will include it in general discussions of all arrhythmias.

normal

arrhythmia

3. In Normal Sinus Rhythm, the pacemaker impulse originates in the sinus node and travels through the normal conduction pathways within normal time frames. Because the pacemaker originates in the _____ node, the P waves will be uniform, and since conduction is normal, one P wave will be in front of every QRS complex. In NSR, there will be _____ P waves, one in front of every _____ complex.

sinus

uniform
QRS

4. In NSR, the atria are stimulated by the sinus impulse and depolarize before the ventricles do. Because the major thrust of the electrical current is traveling *toward* the positive electrode in Lead II, there will be an upright _____ wave.

P

5. Since the SA node inherently fires at a rate of 60–100 times per minute, a Normal Sinus Rhythm must, by definition, fall within this rate range. If an EKG rhythm is slower than _____ beats per minute (bpm) or faster than _____ bpm, it is not _____ .

60
100; Normal Sinus Rhythm

6. NSR is defined as being a regular rhythm. That is, the _____ interval must be regular across the entire strip. Even if a normal sinus rhythm is interrupted by an ectopic beat, the underlying pattern must have a regular R–R measurement to be called _____ .

R–R

Normal Sinus Rhythm

Figure 16 Mechanism of Normal Sinus Rhythm

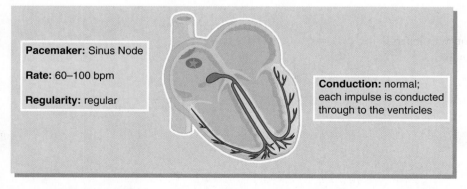

Pacemaker: Sinus Node

Rate: 60–100 bpm

Regularity: regular

Conduction: normal; each impulse is conducted through to the ventricles

The sinus node is the pacemaker, firing at a regular rate of 60–100 times per minute. Each impulse is conducted normally through to the ventricles.

7. You now know that a Normal Sinus Rhythm must be a regular pattern, at a rate between _____ and _____, with an upright P wave in front of every QRS complex. When you measure the PR interval, it must fall between 0.12 and 0.20 second, and it must be of the same duration across the entire strip. That is, if it is less than _____ second or greater than _____ second, it is outside the normal range and not defined as _____ . Further, if the PRI is, for instance, 0.16 second, then each PRI on the strip must be 0.16 second. If the PRI changes from one complex to the next, even if it stays within the normal range, it would not be considered a Normal Sinus Rhythm. In NSR, the PRI must be between _____ and _____ second and must be constant across the _____ strip.

60; 100

0.12

0.20

NSR

0.12

0.20

entire

8. Finally, the QRS measurement for a true NSR must be within the normal range; that is, _____ than 0.12 second. This can be a little tricky, because a sinus rhythm might fit all the other rules but still have a wide QRS complex. When this happens, the rhythm must be qualified by calling it a "Sinus Rhythm with a wide _____ ." Notice that the pattern is no longer called "Normal" Sinus Rhythm, but simply "Sinus Rhythm." If you go on to study EKGs to greater depth, you will learn the reasons behind this phenomenon of the wide QRS complex and will learn the proper terminology for identifying it, but for now, just remember that unless the QRS is less than _____ second, the rhythm is not a _____ Sinus Rhythm.

less

QRS complex

0.12

Normal

9. To summarize the rules for the EKG findings in NSR (Figure 17):

Regularity: regular

Rate: 60–100 bpm

P Wave: uniform shape; one P wave in front of every QRS complex

PRI: 0.12–0.20 second and constant

QRS: less than 0.12 second

FLASH CARD

MyBRADYLab™

Figure 17 Rules for NSR

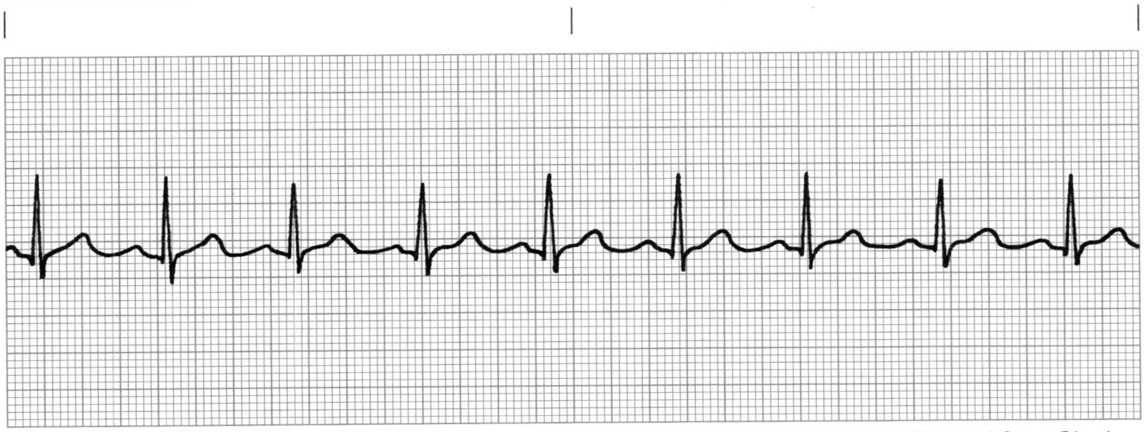

Normal Sinus Rhythm

Regularity: The R–R intervals are constant; the rhythm is regular.

Rate: The atrial and ventricular rates are equal; heart rate is between 60 and 100 bpm.

P Wave: The P waves are uniform. There is one P wave in front of every QRS complex.

PRI: The PR interval measures between 0.12 and 0.20 second; the PRI measurement is constant across the strip.

QRS: The QRS complex measures less than 0.12 second.

Figure 18 Mechanism of Sinus Bradycardia

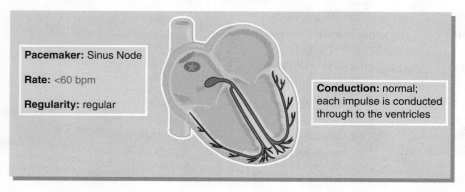

Pacemaker: Sinus Node

Rate: <60 bpm

Regularity: regular

Conduction: normal; each impulse is conducted through to the ventricles

The sinus node is the pacemaker, firing regularly at a rate of less than 60 times per minute. Each impulse is conducted normally through to the ventricles.

For a rhythm to be called NSR, it must have _____ P waves, one in front of every QRS complex; the rate must be _____ to _____ bpm, with a _____ R–R interval across the entire strip. It must have a PRI that measures between _____ and _____ second, and the PRI must be _____ across the entire strip. Finally, the QRS measurement must be less than _____ second, or if it is not, the interpretation must be qualified by calling it a Sinus Rhythm with a wide QRS complex.

uniform

60

100; regular

0.12

0.20; constant

0.12

10. Now go back to the Practice Strips for Chapter 3. Look at all the data available from each strip. Each of these strips has been identified as Sinus Rhythm. Compare your findings with the rules for NSR to see which patterns comply with the rules for NSR.

Practice Strips; (Chapter 3, Parts I and II)
All are NSR except 3.4, 3.6, 3.10, 3.12, 3.14

Sinus Bradycardia

11. If a rhythm originates in the sinus node, but doesn't follow one or more of the rules for NSR, it might fall into one of the other categories of sinus rhythms. If the rate is lower than 60 bpm, it is called a bradycardia, meaning *slow heart*. When a rhythm originating in the sinus node has a normal, upright P wave in front of every QRS complex, a normal PRI and QRS, and it is regular, it is called Sinus Bradycardia since the only reason it doesn't fit into NSR is because the rate is too slow (Figure 18). A rhythm can be identified as Sinus Bradycardia when it fits all of the rules for NSR except that the rate is less than _____ bpm.

60

12. Here are the rules for the EKG findings in Sinus Bradycardia (Figure 19):

Regularity: regular

Rate: less than 60 bpm

P Wave: uniform shape; one P wave in front of every QRS complex

PRI: 0.12–0.20 second and constant

QRS: less than 0.12 second

MyBRADYLab™

Sinus Tachycardia

13. The same thing is true for a rhythm that fits all of the rules for NSR except that the rate is too fast. When the heart beats too fast, it is called tachycardia, meaning *fast*

Figure 19 Rules for Sinus Bradycardia

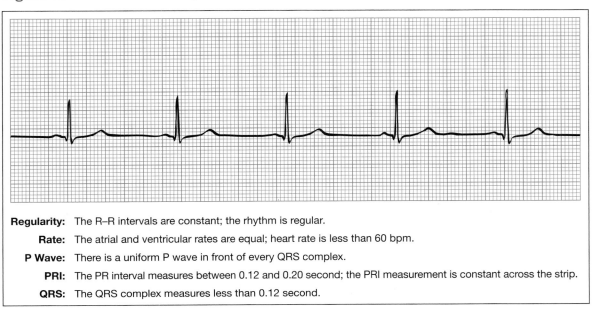

Regularity:	The R–R intervals are constant; the rhythm is regular.
Rate:	The atrial and ventricular rates are equal; heart rate is less than 60 bpm.
P Wave:	There is a uniform P wave in front of every QRS complex.
PRI:	The PR interval measures between 0.12 and 0.20 second; the PRI measurement is constant across the strip.
QRS:	The QRS complex measures less than 0.12 second.

heart. So a rhythm that originates in the sinus node and fits all rules for NSR except that the rate is too _____ would be called a **Sinus Tachycardia** (Figure 20). When a rhythm is regular, has a uniform P wave in front of every QRS complex, has a normal and constant PRI and QRS, but the rate is greater than 100 bpm, it is called _____ .

fast

Sinus Tachycardia

14. The rules for Sinus Tachycardia (Figure 21) are:

Regularity:	regular
Rate:	greater than 100 bpm (usually does not exceed 160 bpm)
P Wave:	uniform shape; one P wave in front of every QRS complex
PRI:	0.12–0.20 second and constant
QRS:	less than 0.12 second

FLASH CARD

MyBRADYLab™

Figure 20 Mechanism of Sinus Tachycardia

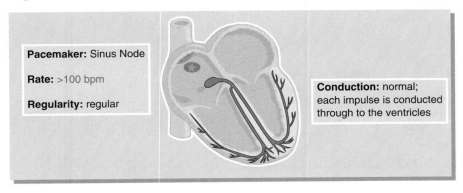

Pacemaker: Sinus Node

Rate: >100 bpm

Regularity: regular

Conduction: normal; each impulse is conducted through to the ventricles

The sinus node is the pacemaker, firing regularly at a rate of greater than 100 bpm. Each impulse is conducted normally through to the ventricles.

Figure 21 Rules for Sinus Tachycardia

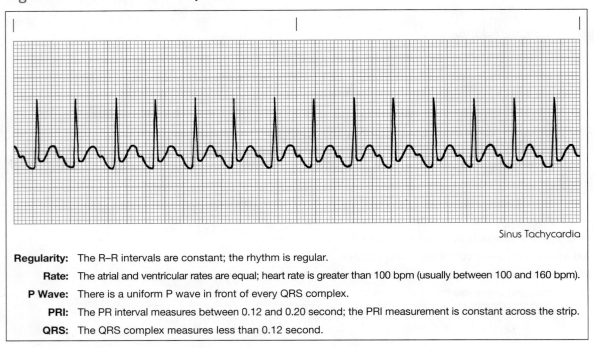

Sinus Tachycardia

Regularity: The R–R intervals are constant; the rhythm is regular.

Rate: The atrial and ventricular rates are equal; heart rate is greater than 100 bpm (usually between 100 and 160 bpm).

P Wave: There is a uniform P wave in front of every QRS complex.

PRI: The PR interval measures between 0.12 and 0.20 second; the PRI measurement is constant across the strip.

QRS: The QRS complex measures less than 0.12 second.

Sinus Arrhythmia

15. The last of the sinus rhythms we will learn is Sinus Arrhythmia (Figure 22). This rhythm is characterized by a pattern that would normally be considered NSR, except that the rate changes with the patient's respirations. When the patient breathes in, the rate increases, and when he or she breathes out, the rate slows. This causes the _____ to be irregular across the strip. The result is a pattern with an   R–R interval
upright P wave in front of every QRS complex, a normal and constant PRI, a normal
QRS complex, but an _____ R–R interval. The difference between   irregular
NSR and Sinus Arrhythmia is that NSR is regular and Sinus Arrhythmia is
_____ . A true Sinus Arrhythmia will have an obvious pattern of   irregular
irregularity across the entire strip. If the rhythm is only very slightly irregular (off by
only 1 or 2 small squares), that can be noted, but the rhythm would be considered only
slightly _____ , and thus not a Sinus Arrhythmia.   irregular

Figure 22 Mechanism of Sinus Arrhythmia

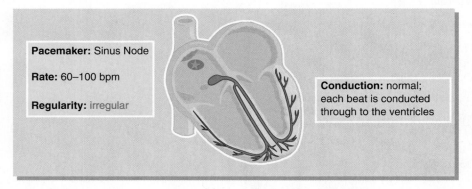

Pacemaker: Sinus Node

Rate: 60–100 bpm

Regularity: irregular

Conduction: normal; each beat is conducted through to the ventricles

The sinus node is the pacemaker, but impulses are initiated in an irregular pattern. The rate increases as the patient breathes in and decreases as the patient breathes out. Each impulse is conducted normally through to the ventricles.

Figure 23 Rules for Sinus Arrhythmia

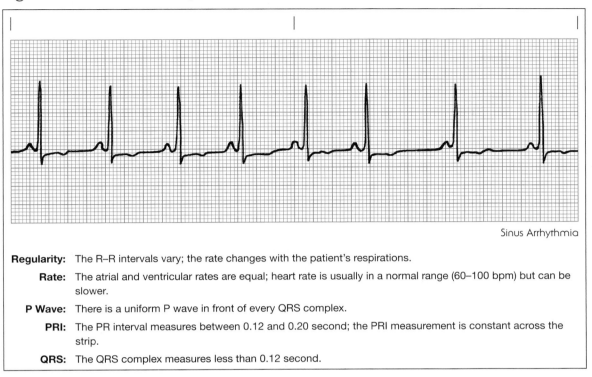

Sinus Arrhythmia

Regularity: The R–R intervals vary; the rate changes with the patient's respirations.

Rate: The atrial and ventricular rates are equal; heart rate is usually in a normal range (60–100 bpm) but can be slower.

P Wave: There is a uniform P wave in front of every QRS complex.

PRI: The PR interval measures between 0.12 and 0.20 second; the PRI measurement is constant across the strip.

QRS: The QRS complex measures less than 0.12 second.

16. Here are the rules for the EKG findings in Sinus Arrhythmia (Figure 23):

Regularity:	irregular
Rate:	60–100 bpm (usually)
P Wave:	uniform shape; one P wave in front of every QRS complex
PRI:	0.12–0.20 second and constant
QRS:	less than 0.12 second

FLASH CARD

MyBRADYLab™

Review

17. You now know the rules for the first four arrhythmias. Normal Sinus Rhythm originates in the _____ node and has normal conduction within normal time frames. This means that the _____ wave will be uniform in front of every QRS complex, the PRI and QRS measurements will be within _____ limits, and the _____ will be constant. For NSR, the rate must fall between _____ and _____ bpm. If the rate drops below 60 bpm but all the other rules to NSR apply, the rhythm is called _____ ; if the rate is faster than 100 bpm, the rhythm is called _____ . If the rhythm fits all the rules of NSR except that it is irregular, the rhythm is called _____ .

sinus

P

normal; PRI
60; 100

Sinus Bradycardia
Sinus Tachycardia
Sinus Arrhythmia

18. If a rhythm originates in the sinus node, it will have uniform, upright _____ waves because the electrical impulses are traveling from the atria downward through the ventricles, and thus are heading toward the _____ electrode in Lead II.

P

positive

19. With NSR, Sinus Tachycardia, Sinus Bradycardia, and Sinus Arrhythmia, the PRI will always be between _____ and _____ second and constant.

0.12; 0.20

20. Of the four sinus rhythms you have learned, the only one that does not have a regular R–R interval is _____ .

Sinus Arrhythmia

21. With all rhythms that originate in the sinus node, the QRS measurement should be _____ . If it is greater than 0.12 second, it cannot be considered _____ , and this should be noted along with your interpretation of the underlying pattern. For the time being, you can qualify your interpretation by naming the rhythm and including "_____ ." If you continue to study EKGs, you will learn the proper terminology for this phenomenon.

less than 0.12 second

normal with a wide QRS

22. Now you must memorize all of the rules for each of the sinus arrhythmias. Then you can begin gathering data from the strips shown in the Practice Strips at the end of this chapter and compare them to the rules for each pattern. You should be able to identify each of the strips. If you have any trouble, or are unsure about the process, you should seek help before going on to the next section. If you would like more practice after you finish, go back to the Practice Strips at the end of Chapter 3. With the information you now know, you should be able to identify each of those rhythm strips. Check your results with the answer key (on page 84). If you missed any of these arrhythmias, spend the time *now* to review this section. Do not go on until you are very comfortable with the information in this chapter.

Practice Strips

MyBRADYLab™

KEY POINTS

- Rhythms that originate in the sinus node include:
  - Normal Sinus Rhythm
  - Sinus Bradycardia
  - Sinus Tachycardia
  - Sinus Arrhythmia

- All rhythms that originate in the sinus node will have upright P waves. This is because the electrical current flows from the atria toward the ventricles, which is toward the positive electrode in Lead II.

- Here are the rules for *NSR*:

Regularity:	regular
Rate:	60–100 bpm
P Wave:	normal and upright; one P wave in front of every QRS complex
PRI:	0.12–0.20 second and constant
QRS:	less than 0.12 second

- Here are the rules for *Sinus Bradycardia*:

Regularity:	regular
Rate:	less than 60 bpm
P Wave:	normal and upright; one P wave in front of every QRS complex

PRI:	0.12–0.20 second and constant
QRS:	less than 0.12 second

- Here are the rules for *Sinus Tachycardia*:

Regularity:	regular
Rate:	greater than 100 bpm (usually 100–160 bpm)
P Wave:	normal and upright; one P wave in front of every QRS complex
PRI:	0.12–0.20 second and constant
QRS:	less than 0.12 second

- Here are the rules for *Sinus Arrhythmia*:

Regularity:	irregular
Rate:	60–100 bpm (usually)
P Wave:	normal and upright; one P wave in front of every QRS complex
PRI:	0.12–0.20 second and constant
QRS:	less than 0.12 second

- When a rhythm is determined to have originated in the sinus node but has a QRS measurement greater than 0.12 second, this should be noted in the interpretation by calling it a Sinus Rhythm with a wide QRS complex.

SELF-TEST

Directions: Complete this self-evaluation of the information you have learned from this chapter. If your answers are all correct and you feel comfortable with your understanding of the material, proceed to the next chapter. However, if you miss any of the questions, you should review the referenced frames before proceeding. If you feel unsure of any of the underlying principles, invest the time now to go back over the entire chapter. **Do not proceed with the next chapter until you are very comfortable with the material in this chapter.**

Questions	Referenced Frames	Answers
1. Why do sinus rhythms have upright P waves?	3, 4, 7, 17, 18	Because an impulse that originates in the sinus node will travel downward through the atria to the ventricles. In Lead II, the positive electrode is placed below the apex, thus the major electrical flow is toward the positive electrode in Lead II, creating an upright wave form.
2. In a Normal Sinus Rhythm, what will the rate range be?	5, 7, 9, 17	60–100 bpm
3. What is the defined PRI for an NSR?	3, 7, 9, 17, 19	0.12–0.20 second and constant
4. Is NSR defined as being regular or irregular?	6, 7, 9, 17, 20	regular

Questions	Referenced Frames	Answers
5. What should the QRS measurement be to be called a Normal Sinus Rhythm?	8, 9, 17, 21	less than 0.12 second
6. What would you call a rhythm that originated in the sinus node and fits all the rules for NSR except that the QRS was too wide?	8, 9, 21	Sinus Rhythm with a wide QRS
7. What will the P wave be like for Sinus Bradycardia?	3, 11, 17, 18	normal and upright; one P wave in front of every QRS complex
8. In Sinus Bradycardia, what is the rate range?	11, 12	less than 60 bpm
9. Is Sinus Bradycardia regular or irregular?	11, 12, 20	regular
10. What will the PRI measurement be in Sinus Bradycardia?	11, 12, 19	0.12–0.20 second and constant
11. What is the normal QRS measurement in Sinus Bradycardia?	11, 12, 21	less than 0.12 second
12. How does Sinus Bradycardia differ from Normal Sinus Rhythm?	11, 12	The rate in Sinus Bradycardia is slower than NSR.
13. Is Sinus Tachycardia regular or irregular?	13, 14, 20	regular
14. What is the rate range for Sinus Tachycardia?	13, 14	greater than 100 bpm (usually does not exceed 160 bpm)
15. What is the PRI for Sinus Tachycardia?	13, 14, 19	0.12–0.20 second and constant
16. What is the normal QRS measurement for Sinus Tachycardia?	13, 14, 21	less than 0.12 second
17. What do the P waves look like in Sinus Tachycardia?	13, 14, 18	normal and upright; one P wave in front of every QRS complex
18. How does Sinus Tachycardia differ from NSR?	13, 14	The rate in Sinus Tachycardia is faster than NSR.
19. Describe the rhythm (regularity) of Sinus Arrhythmia.	15, 16, 20	It is irregular. The rate increases with each respiratory inspiration and decreases with each expiration.
20. What is the rate range for Sinus Arrhythmia?	15, 16	usually 60–100 bpm
21. What is the PRI measurement in Sinus Arrhythmia?	15, 16, 19	0.12–0.20 second and constant
22. What is the normal QRS measurement in Sinus Arrhythmia?	15, 16, 21	less than 0.12 second
23. How does Sinus Arrhythmia differ from NSR?	15, 16, 20	Sinus Arrhythmia is irregular, whereas NSR is regular.

PRACTICE STRIPS (answers can be found in the Answer Key on page 552)

4.1

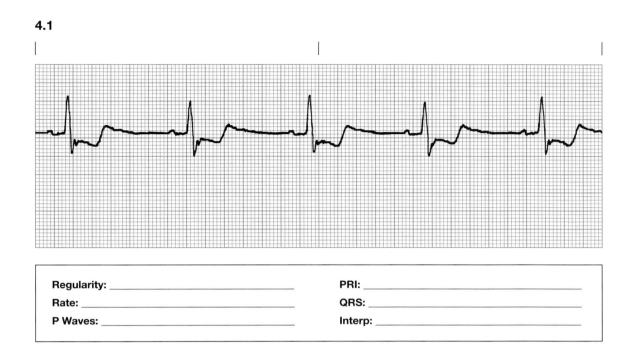

Regularity: _____	**PRI:** _____
Rate: _____	**QRS:** _____
P Waves: _____	**Interp:** _____

4.2

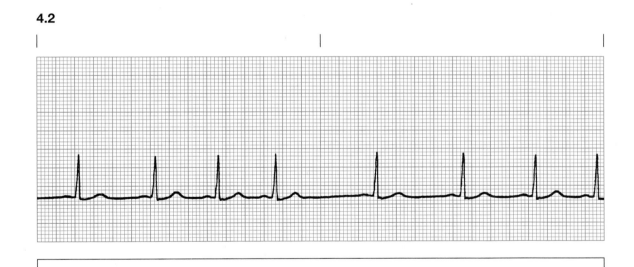

Regularity: _____	**PRI:** _____
Rate: _____	**QRS:** _____
P Waves: _____	**Interp:** _____

4.3

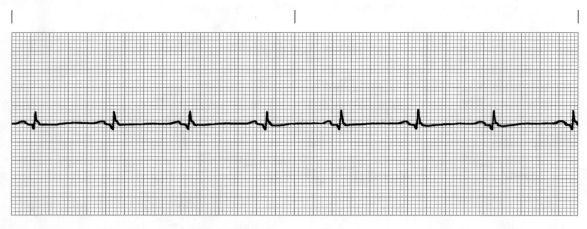

Regularity: _____	PRI: _____
Rate: _____	QRS: _____
P Waves: _____	Interp: _____

4.4

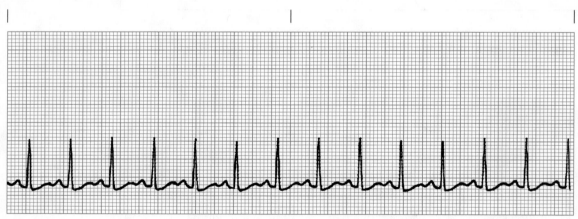

Regularity: _____	PRI: _____
Rate: _____	QRS: _____
P Waves: _____	Interp: _____

4.5

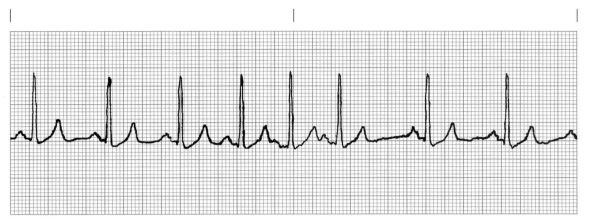

Regularity: _____	PRI: _____
Rate: _____	QRS: _____
P Waves: _____	Interp: _____

4.6

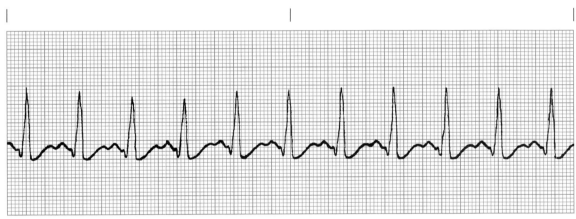

Regularity: _____	PRI: _____
Rate: _____	QRS: _____
P Waves: _____	Interp: _____

4.7

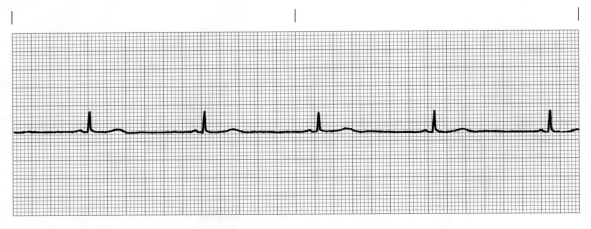

Regularity: _____	PRI: _____
Rate: _____	QRS: _____
P Waves: _____	Interp: _____

4.8

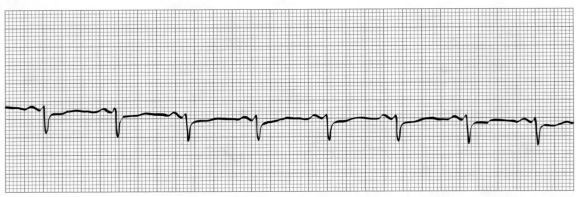

Regularity: _____	PRI: _____
Rate: _____	QRS: _____
P Waves: _____	Interp: _____

4.9

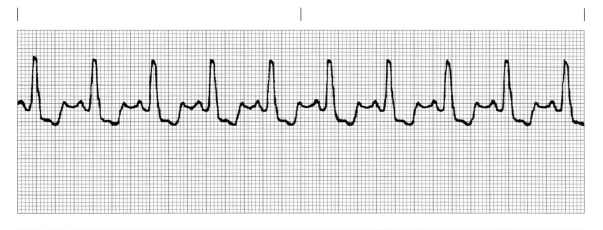

Regularity: _____	**PRI:** _____
Rate: _____	**QRS:** _____
P Waves: _____	**Interp:** _____

4.10

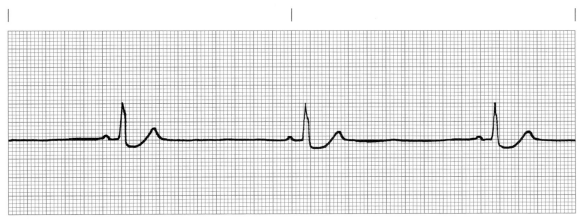

Regularity: _____	**PRI:** _____
Rate: _____	**QRS:** _____
P Waves: _____	**Interp:** _____

4.11

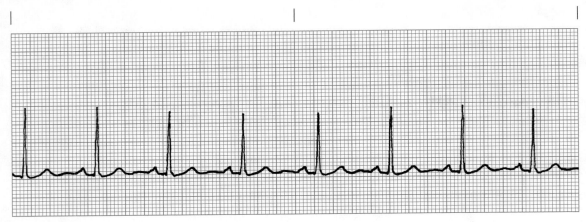

Regularity: _____	**PRI:** _____
Rate: _____	**QRS:** _____
P Waves: _____	**Interp:** _____

4.12

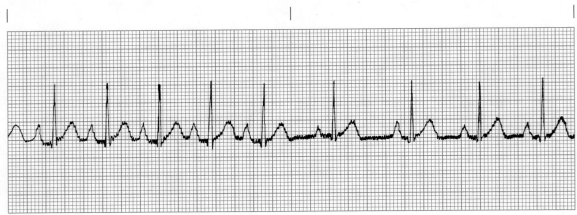

Regularity: _____	**PRI:** _____
Rate: _____	**QRS:** _____
P Waves: _____	**Interp:** _____

4.13

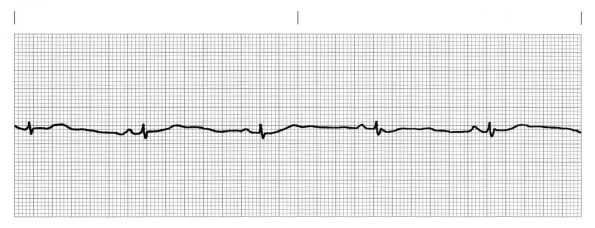

Regularity: _____	PRI: _____
Rate: _____	QRS: _____
P Waves: _____	Interp: _____

4.14

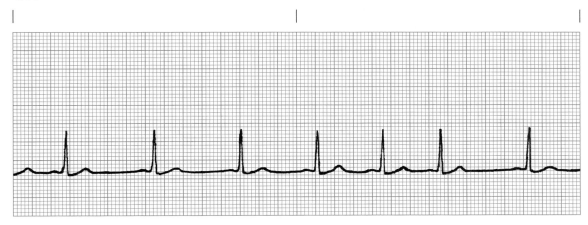

Regularity: _____	PRI: _____
Rate: _____	QRS: _____
P Waves: _____	Interp: _____

4.15

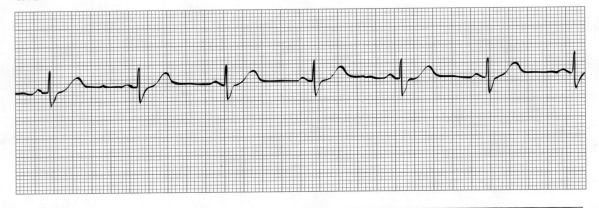

Regularity: _____	PRI: _____
Rate: _____	QRS: _____
P Waves: _____	Interp: _____

4.16

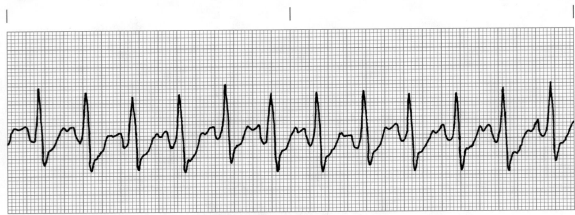

Regularity: _____	PRI: _____
Rate: _____	QRS: _____
P Waves: _____	Interp: _____

4.17

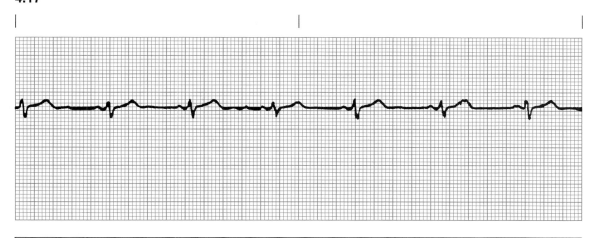

Regularity: _____	**PRI:** _____
Rate: _____	**QRS:** _____
P Waves: _____	**Interp:** _____

4.18

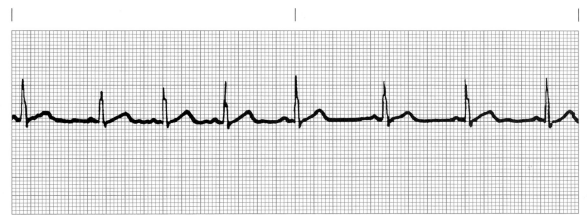

Regularity: _____	**PRI:** _____
Rate: _____	**QRS:** _____
P Waves: _____	**Interp:** _____

4.19

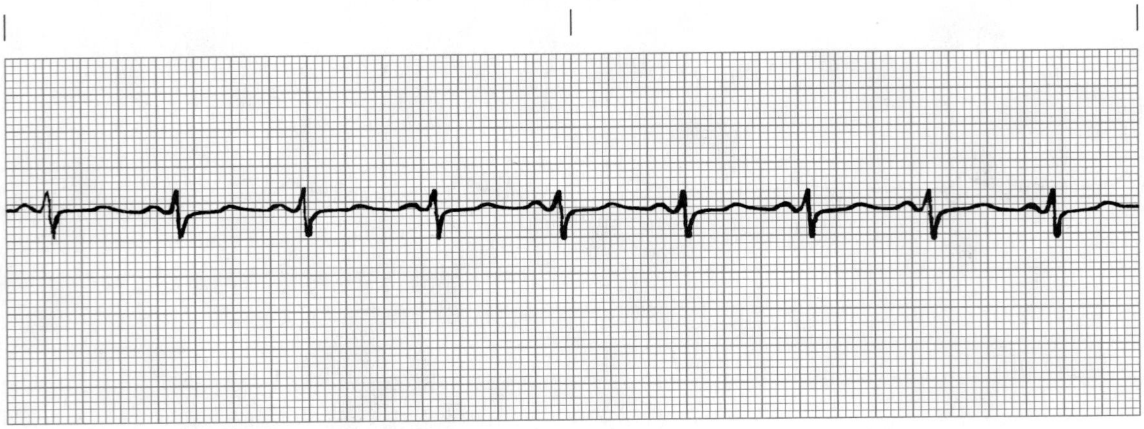

Regularity: _____	PRI: _____
Rate: _____	QRS: _____
P Waves: _____	Interp: _____

4.20

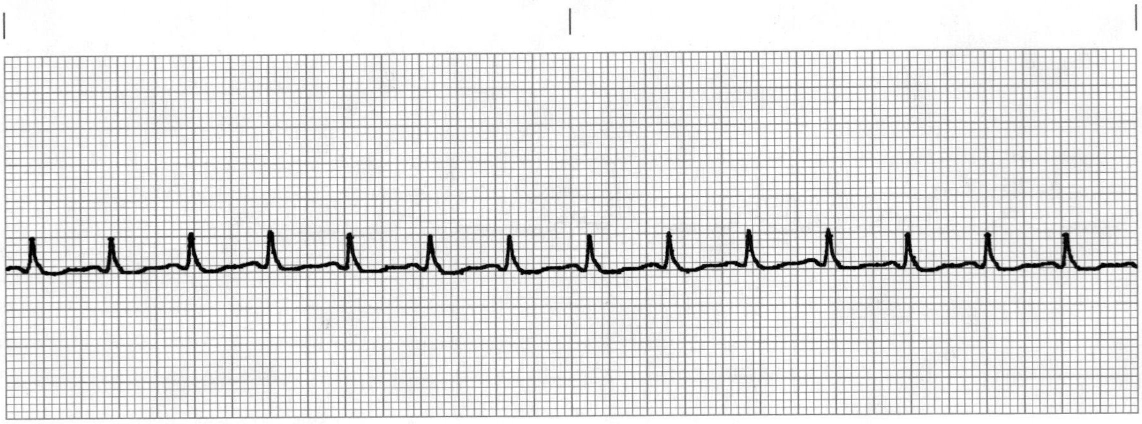

Regularity: _____	PRI: _____
Rate: _____	QRS: _____
P Waves: _____	Interp: _____

4.21

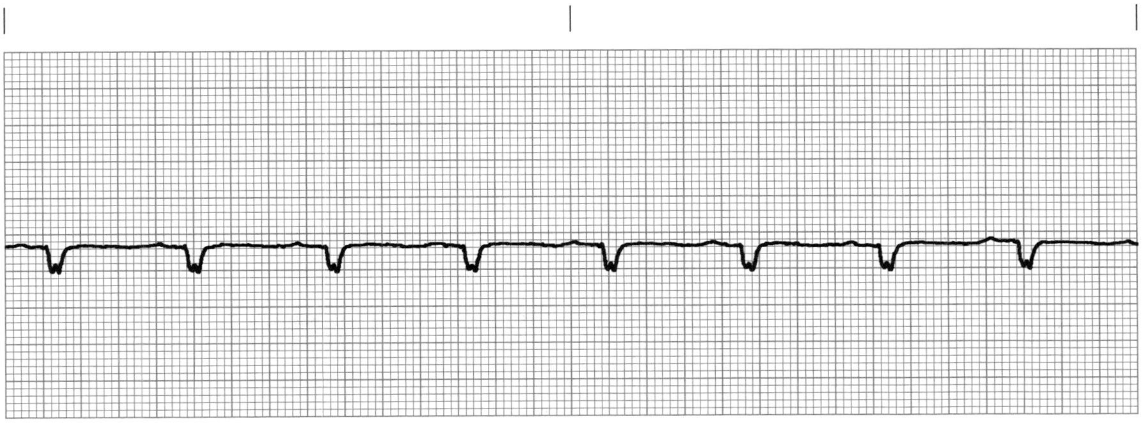

Regularity: _____	PRI: _____
Rate: _____	QRS: _____
P Waves: _____	Interp: _____

4.22

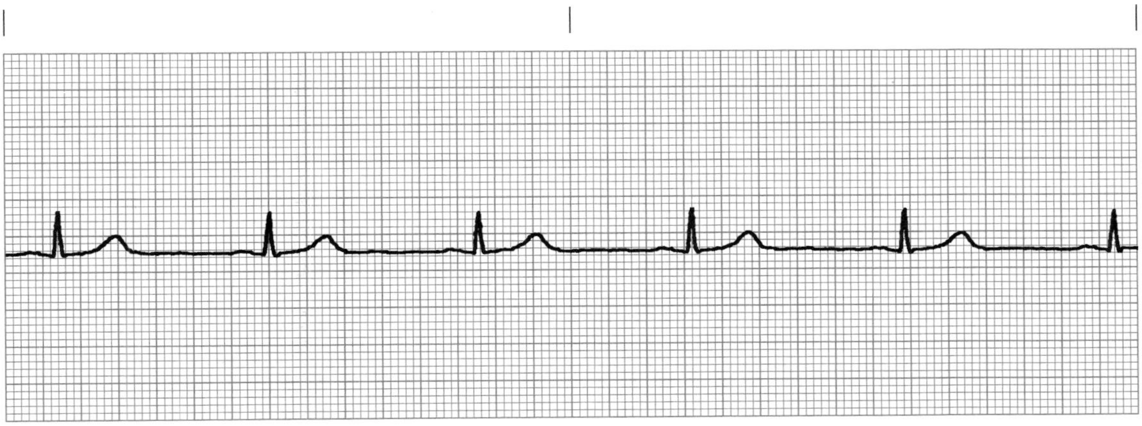

Regularity: _____	PRI: _____
Rate: _____	QRS: _____
P Waves: _____	Interp: _____

4.23

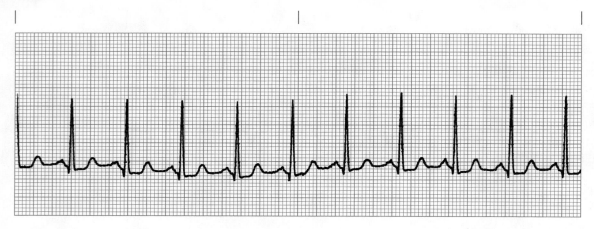

Regularity: _____	PRI: _____
Rate: _____	QRS: _____
P Waves: _____	Interp: _____

4.24

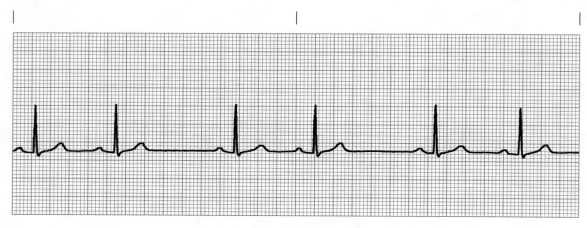

Regularity: _____	PRI: _____
Rate: _____	QRS: _____
P Waves: _____	Interp: _____

4.25

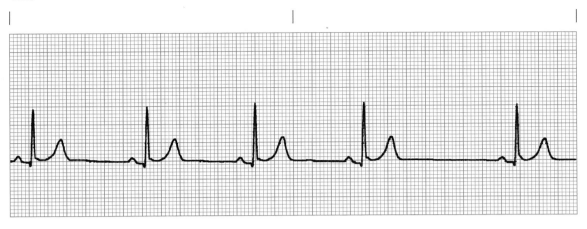

Regularity: _____ PRI: _____

Rate: _____ QRS: _____

P Waves: _____ Interp: _____

4.26

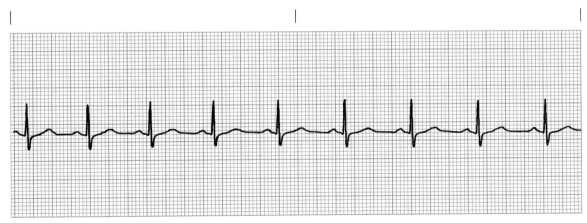

Regularity: _____ PRI: _____

Rate: _____ QRS: _____

P Waves: _____ Interp: _____

4.27

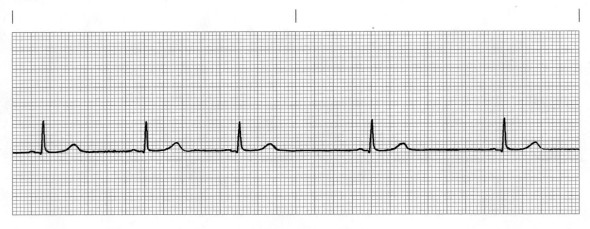

Regularity: _____	PRI: _____
Rate: _____	QRS: _____
P Waves: _____	Interp: _____

4.28

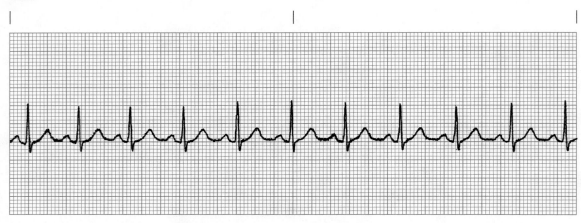

Regularity: _____	PRI: _____
Rate: _____	QRS: _____
P Waves: _____	Interp: _____

4.29

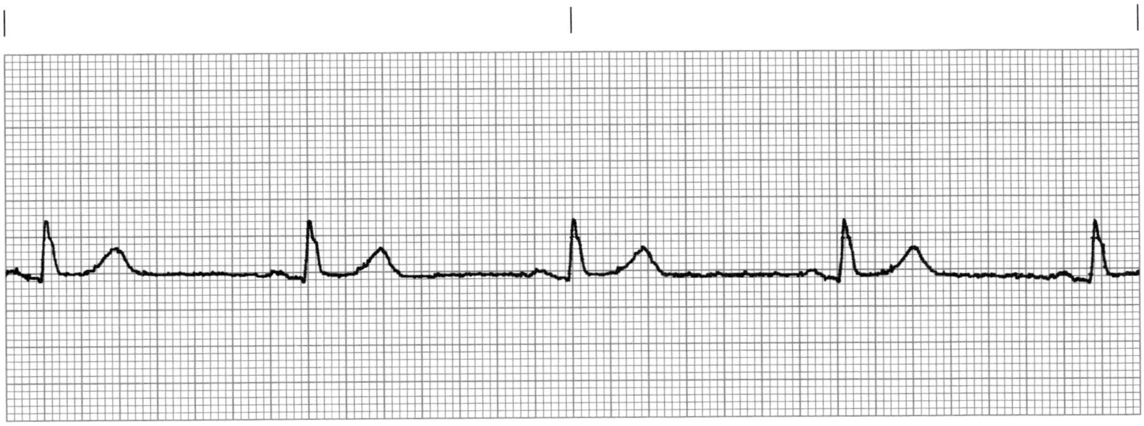

Regularity: _____   PRI: _____

Rate: _____   QRS: _____

P Waves: _____   Interp: _____

4.30

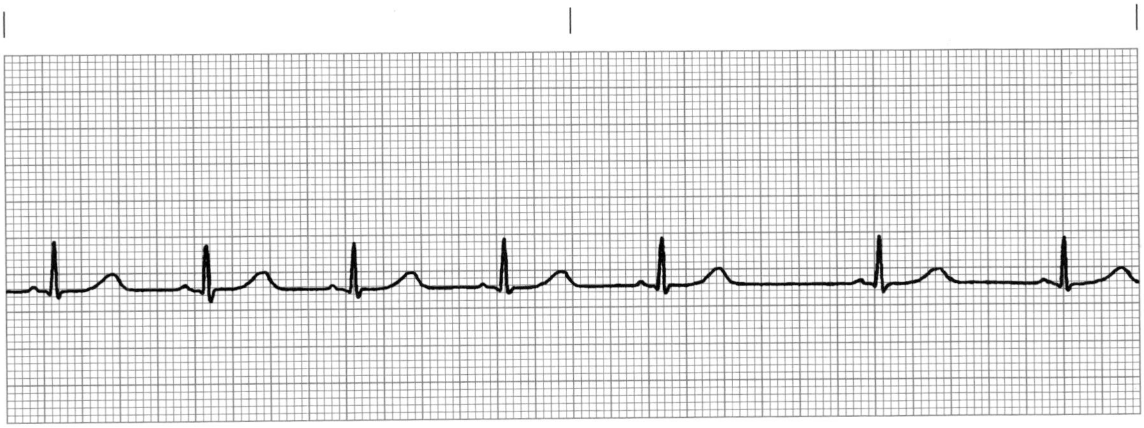

Regularity: _____   PRI: _____

Rate: _____   QRS: _____

P Waves: _____   Interp: _____

Interpretation of Chapter 3 Rhythm Strips

3.1	Normal Sinus Rythm
3.2	Normal Sinus Rhythm (only very slightly irregular)
3.3	Normal Sinus Rhythm
3.4	Sinus Tachycardia
3.5	Normal Sinus Rhythm
3.6	Sinus Tachycardia
3.7	Normal Sinus Rhythm
3.8	Normal Sinus Rhythm
3.9	Normal Sinus Rhythm
3.10	Sinus Arrhythmia
3.11	Normal Sinus Rhythm
3.12	Sinus Bradycardia
3.13	Normal Sinus Rhythm
3.14	Sinus Arrhythmia
3.15	Normal Sinus Rhythm

Chapter 5
Atrial Rhythms

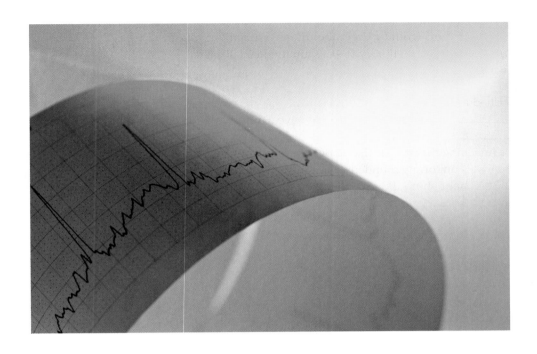

Overview

IN THIS CHAPTER, you will learn the characteristics of an atrial pacemaker and features that are shared by all rhythms originating in the atria. You will then learn the names and features of five different arrhythmias that originate within the atria. For each of these arrhythmias, you will learn about the etiology, conduction, and resulting EKG features (regularity, rate, P waves, PR intervals, and QRS complexes).

Atrial Rhythms

1. In Chapter 4 you learned that NSR, Sinus Bradycardia, Sinus Tachycardia, and Sinus Arrhythmia all originate in the _____ node. These are all rhythms that originate in the normal pacemaker of the heart. Sometimes, for one reason or another, the _____ node loses its pacemaking role, and this function is taken over by another site along the conduction system. The site with the fastest inherent rate usually controls the _____ function. Since the atria have the next highest rate after the SA node, it is common for the atria to take over from the SA node. Rhythms that originate in the atria are called **atrial arrhythmias.**

sinus

sinus

pacemaking

2. Atrial _____ are caused when the atrial rate becomes faster than the sinus rate, either by irritability or by escape, and an impulse from somewhere along the atrial _____ pathways is able to override the SA node and stimulate _____ . When an atrial impulse is able to take over the pacemaking function from the SA node and initiate depolarization, the resulting pattern is termed an _____ arrhythmia.

arrhythmias

conduction

depolarization

atrial

3. As with a sinus rhythm, an impulse that originates in the atria will travel through the atria to the AV junction and then through the _____ conduction pathways to the Purkinje fibers. The only difference is in the atria, where the conduction will be a little slower and rougher than it is with sinus rhythms. Since atrial depolarization is seen on the EKG as a P wave, you would expect the unusual atrial depolarization seen with _____ arrhythmias to show up in unusual or atypical _____ waves.

ventricular

atrial
P

4. The normal sinus P wave is described as having a nice, rounded, uniform wave shape that precedes the _____ . An atrial P wave will have a different morphology than the _____ P wave. It can be flattened, notched, peaked, sawtoothed, or even _diphasic_ (meaning that it goes first above the isoelectric line and then dips below it). A P wave that is uniformly rounded would most likely be coming from the _____ node, but a P wave that is notched, flattened, or diphasic would be called an _____ P wave.

QRS complex
sinus

sinus
atrial

5. Atrial arrhythmias have several features in common. They originate above the ventricles and would therefore have a _____ QRS complex. The impulse has a little trouble getting through the atria, since it originated outside the SA node, and would thus produce an atrial P wave rather than a typical _____ P wave. We will be discussing five atrial arrhythmias, each of which will have a _____ QRS complex and a _____ wave that has a different shape than the _____ P wave.

narrow

sinus

normal (narrow); P
sinus

Wandering Pacemaker

6. The first atrial arrhythmia we'll learn is called **Wandering Pacemaker** (Figure 24). Wandering Pacemaker is caused when the pacemaker role switches from beat to beat from the SA node to the atria and back again. The result is a rhythm made up of interspersed sinus and atrial beats. The sinus beats are preceded by nice, rounded P waves,

Figure 24 Mechanism of Wandering Pacemaker

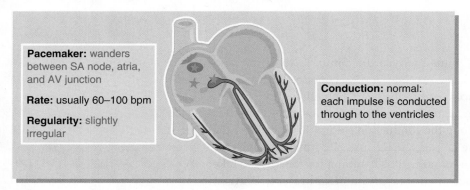

Pacemaker: wanders between SA node, atria, and AV junction

Rate: usually 60–100 bpm

Regularity: slightly irregular

Conduction: normal: each impulse is conducted through to the ventricles

The pacemaker site wanders between the sinus node, the atria, and the AV junction. Although each impulse originates from a different focus, the rate usually remains within a normal range, but it can be slower or faster. Conduction through to the ventricles is normal.

Figure 25   Rules for Wandering Pacemaker

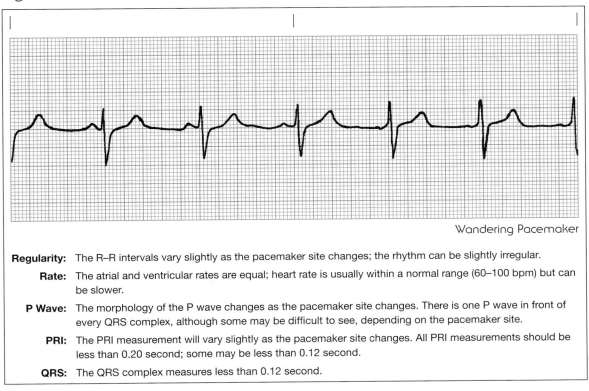

Wandering Pacemaker

Regularity: The R–R intervals vary slightly as the pacemaker site changes; the rhythm can be slightly irregular.

Rate: The atrial and ventricular rates are equal; heart rate is usually within a normal range (60–100 bpm) but can be slower.

P Wave: The morphology of the P wave changes as the pacemaker site changes. There is one P wave in front of every QRS complex, although some may be difficult to see, depending on the pacemaker site.

PRI: The PRI measurement will vary slightly as the pacemaker site changes. All PRI measurements should be less than 0.20 second; some may be less than 0.12 second.

QRS: The QRS complex measures less than 0.12 second.

but the P wave changes as the pacemaker drops to the atria. The P waves of the atrial beats are not consistent and can be any variety of atrial configuration (e.g., flattened, notched, diphasic). Sometimes the pacemaker site will drop even lower, into the AV junction, resulting in inverted or even absent P waves. This concept is dealt with in greater detail in Chapter 6. Wandering Pacemaker is categorized as an atrial arrhythmia characterized by _____ in the _____ waves from one beat to the next.

changes; P

7. Because the pacemaker site is changing between beats, each of the impulses will vary in the time it takes to reach the ventricles. Therefore, the PRI may be slightly different from one beat to the next. This can also cause a slightly irregular R–R interval. In Wandering Pacemaker, the rhythm is usually slightly _____ , and the _____ can vary somewhat from one beat to the next, but it will always be less than 0.20 second. Both the R–R interval and the PR interval are usually slightly _____ .

irregular

PRI

irregular

8. The rules for Wandering Pacemaker (Figure 25) are:

Regularity: slightly irregular

Rate: usually normal, 60–100 bpm

P Wave: morphology changes from one complex to the next

PRI: less than 0.20 second; may vary

QRS: less than 0.12 second

MyBRADYLab™

Ectopics

9. The next atrial arrhythmia is not really a rhythm at all, but is actually a single beat. When a single beat arises from an ectopic focus (a site outside of the SA node) within

the conduction system, that beat is called an **ectopic** beat. An _____ ectopic
beat is a single beat that arises from a focus outside of the _____ . SA node

10. When an ectopic beat originates in the atria, it is called an atrial ectopic. An ectopic beat arises when a site somewhere along the _____ system conduction
becomes irritable and overrides the SA node for a single beat. By definition, an ectopic
can also be caused when an ectopic focus initiates an impulse as an escape mechanism, but the most common use of the term suggests that the site became irritable
_____ and overrode the _____ node. sinus

11. When you see a single ectopic beat interrupting a rhythm, you can easily tell
whether it is caused by irritability or escape. An irritable beat will come earlier than
expected, while an escape beat will be delayed because it fires only after the expected
beat is skipped. An early, or premature, beat would be an indication of
_____ , while an _____ beat would be preceded irritability; escape
by a prolonged R–R cycle.

Premature Atrial Complex

12. An atrial ectopic that is caused by irritability is called a **Premature Atrial Complex**
(PAC) (Figure 26). A PAC is an ectopic beat that comes _____ in the early
cardiac cycle and originates in the _____ . atria

13. When you look for a PAC on an EKG tracing, keep in mind that it is a single beat,
not an entire rhythm. So you really have two jobs: to identify the underlying rhythm
and to locate any ectopics. When interpreting an arrhythmia that has ectopics in it,
you must identify both the _____ and the _____ . underlying rhythm; ectopics

14. The first thing you will notice about a PAC is that it comes prematurely; that is, it
comes _____ you would expect the next beat. This causes a normally before
regular rhythm to be _____ , since the ectopic(s) will interrupt the reg- irregular
ular underlying rhythm. A rhythm with PACs will be _____ because irregular
the ectopics come prematurely and interrupt the _____ rhythm. underlying

15. However, in identifying the _____ rhythm, you should deter- underlying
mine whether or not it is regular in places where there are no ectopics to interrupt it. It

---

Figure 26 Mechanism of Premature Atrial Complex

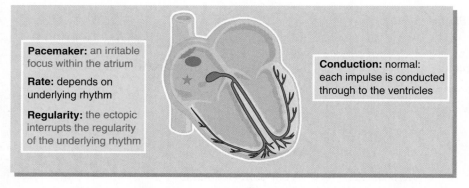

Pacemaker: an irritable focus within the atrium

Rate: depends on underlying rhythm

Regularity: the ectopic interrupts the regularity of the underlying rhythm

Conduction: normal: each impulse is conducted through to the ventricles

The pacemaker is an irritable focus within the atrium that fires prematurely and produces a single ectopic beat. Conduction through to the ventricles is normal. *This is a single beat, not an entire rhythm; the underlying rhythm also must be identified.*

would be inaccurate to label a normally regular rhythm as irregular simply because it is interrupted by PACs. To determine whether or not the underlying rhythm is regular, you should measure the R–R intervals on a section of the strip where there are no _____ .

ectopics (PACs)

16. Because PACs originate in the atria, they will have a characteristic atrial P wave that differs in morphology from the _____ P waves. An atrial P wave will usually be _____ .

sinus

flattened, notched, peaked, or diphasic

17. As with Wandering Pacemaker, conduction through the AV node and the ventricles is usually _____ with a PAC; therefore, the PRI will usually be _____ – _____ second, and the QRS will be less than _____ second. It is possible, though, for the PRI to be prolonged if the AV node is refractory.

normal

0.12; 0.20

0.12

18. Since a PAC comes _____ in the cardiac cycle, it will usually fall very close to the end of the preceding QRS complex. This often means the atrial P wave that initiated the PAC will fall very near the T wave and may be "lost" in it entirely. If visible, the PAC will have a typical atrial P wave, but it might not be visible, since it can be _____ in the preceding _____ .

early

lost; T wave

19. As with all other supraventricular rhythms, a PAC should have normal _____ through the AV node and ventricles and therefore have a QRS complex of normal duration. It is possible, though, for any of these arrhythmias to have a conduction problem, thus causing a prolonged QRS complex. For all of our purposes, it is sufficient simply to call attention to this abnormality by calling it a PAC with a wide QRS complex. However, for an ectopic with a wide QRS complex to fit the rule of a PAC, it must have an atrial P wave in front of it. A PAC with a QRS complex greater than 0.12 second in duration should be called a PAC with a _____ .

conduction

wide QRS complex

20. When an atrial focus becomes irritable and fires a pacemaker impulse to override the sinus node, the premature ectopic beat is called a _____ . This beat will be characterized by P waves with a morphology that is different from _____ P waves. However, the PRI and QRS measurements will be _____ . PACs cause an _____ rhythm because they come earlier than expected and interrupt the regularity of the underlying rhythm.

PAC

sinus

normal; irregular

21. The rules for PACs (Figure 27) are:

Regularity:	depends on the underlying rhythm; regularity will be interrupted by the PAC
Rate:	depends on the underlying rhythm
P Wave:	P wave of early beat differs from the sinus P waves; can be flattened or notched; may be lost in the preceding T wave
PRI:	0.12–0.20 second; can exceed 0.20 second
QRS:	less than 0.12 second

FLASH CARD

MyBRADYLab™

Atrial Tachycardia

22. A PAC is caused when an irritable focus in the _____ takes over the pacemaking function for a single beat. It is also possible for a single focus in the atria to become so irritable that it begins to fire very regularly and thus overrides the SA node for the entire rhythm. This arrhythmia is called **Atrial Tachycardia** (AT) (Figure 28). AT

atria

Figure 27   Rules for Premature Atrial Complex

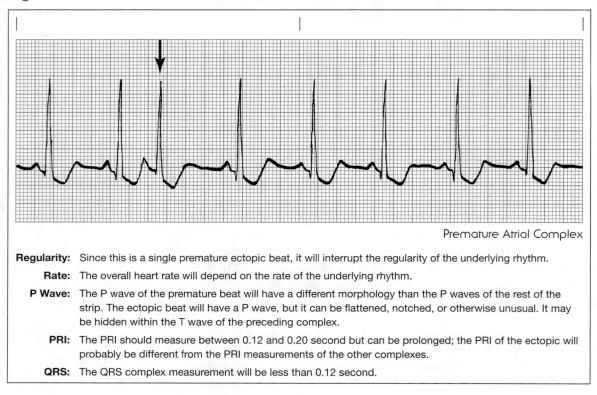

Premature Atrial Complex

Regularity: Since this is a single premature ectopic beat, it will interrupt the regularity of the underlying rhythm.

Rate: The overall heart rate will depend on the rate of the underlying rhythm.

P Wave: The P wave of the premature beat will have a different morphology than the P waves of the rest of the strip. The ectopic beat will have a P wave, but it can be flattened, notched, or otherwise unusual. It may be hidden within the T wave of the preceding complex.

PRI: The PRI should measure between 0.12 and 0.20 second but can be prolonged; the PRI of the ectopic will probably be different from the PRI measurements of the other complexes.

QRS: The QRS complex measurement will be less than 0.12 second.

Figure 28   Mechanism of Atrial Tachycardia

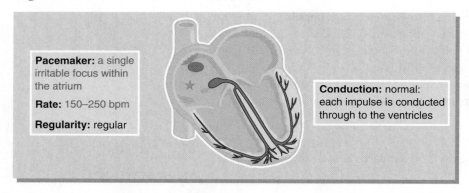

Pacemaker: a single irritable focus within the atrium

Rate: 150–250 bpm

Regularity: regular

Conduction: normal: each impulse is conducted through to the ventricles

The pacemaker is a single irritable site within the atrium that fires repetitively at a very rapid rate. Conduction through to the ventricles is normal.

is caused by a single focus in the _____ that fires rapidly to override   atria
the SA node and thus assumes pacemaking responsibility for the entire rhythm.

23. Atrial Tachycardia will have all of the characteristics of a PAC, except that it is an
entire _____ instead of a single beat. All of the P waves in AT will   rhythm
have an atrial configuration; they will be peaked, flattened, notched, or diphasic. The PRI
is usually normal, and the QRS should be normal. As with PACs, Atrial Tachycardia will
have a normal _____ interval and a normal _____   PR; QRS
duration. The P waves will be typically _____ in configuration and   atrial
hence different from sinus P waves.

Figure 29 Rules for Atrial Tachycardia

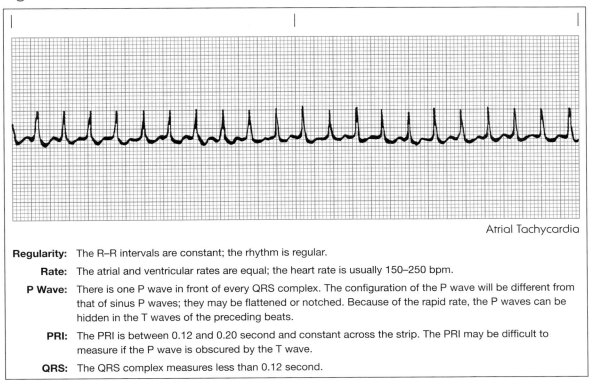

Atrial Tachycardia

Regularity: The R–R intervals are constant; the rhythm is regular.

Rate: The atrial and ventricular rates are equal; the heart rate is usually 150–250 bpm.

P Wave: There is one P wave in front of every QRS complex. The configuration of the P wave will be different from that of sinus P waves; they may be flattened or notched. Because of the rapid rate, the P waves can be hidden in the T waves of the preceding beats.

PRI: The PRI is between 0.12 and 0.20 second and constant across the strip. The PRI may be difficult to measure if the P wave is obscured by the T wave.

QRS: The QRS complex measures less than 0.12 second.

24. Atrial tachycardia is characteristically a very regular arrhythmia. It is usually very rapid, with a rate range between 150 and 250 bpm. At this rate it is very common for the P waves to be hidden on the preceding T waves. The usual rate for AT is _____ bpm, and the rhythm is characteristically very _____ .

150–250

regular

25. When you see a very regular supraventricular rhythm that has atrial P waves and a rate between 150 and 250 bpm, you should suspect that it is _____ .

Atrial Tachycardia

26. The rules for Atrial Tachycardia (Figure 29) are:

Regularity: regular

Rate: 150–250 bpm

P Wave: atrial P wave; differs from sinus P wave; can be lost in T wave

PRI: 0.12–0.20 second

QRS: less than 0.12 second

MyBRADYLab™

Atrial Flutter

27. When the atria become so irritable that they fire faster than 250 bpm, they are said to be **fluttering**. It is theorized that an area in the atrium initiates an impulse that is conducted in a repetitive, cyclic pattern, creating a series of atrial waves with a sawtooth appearance (called *Flutter* or *F waves*). This rhythm is called **Atrial Flutter** (Figure 30). Atrial Flutter is an atrial arrhythmia that occurs when ectopic foci in the atria exceed a rate of _____ bpm; the atrial rate is usually in the range of 250–350 bpm.

250

28. The problem with a heart rate this rapid is that the ventricles don't have enough time to fill with blood between each beat. The result is that the ventricles will continue

Figure 30 Mechanism of Atrial Flutter

Pacemaker: a single irritable focus within the atrium

Rate: atrial rate 250–350 bpm; ventricular rate varies depending on conduction ratio, will be less than atrial rate

Regularity: atria are beating regularly; ventricles can be regular or irregular, depending on conduction ratio

Intermittent Block

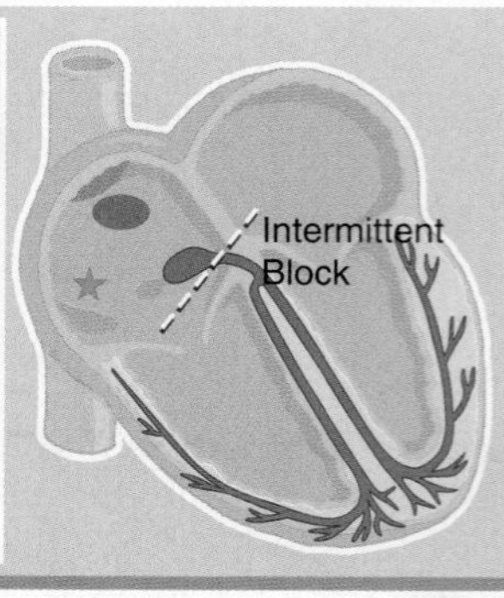

Conduction: AV node blocks some impulses but allows others through to the ventricles; those that do get through are conducted normally.

A single irritable focus within the atria issues an impulse that is conducted in a rapid, repetitive fashion. To protect the ventricles from receiving too many impulses, the AV node blocks some of the impulses from being conducted through to the ventricles. Those that do get through are conducted normally.

to pump but they won't be ejecting adequate _____ volume to meet body needs. The heart has a built-in protective mechanism to prevent this from happening: the AV node. The AV _____ is responsible for preventing excess impulses from reaching the ventricles. So when the heart beats too fast, the _____ will prevent some of the impulses from reaching the _____ . This blocking action allows the ventricles time to fill with blood before they have to contract.

blood

node

AV node

ventricles

29. In Atrial Flutter, the atrial rate is between 250 and 350 bpm. Therefore, the AV node seeks to block some of these impulses and slow the ventricular rate. This will be seen on the EKG as a very rapid series of P waves (Flutter waves) with an atrial rate of 250–350, but not every one is followed by a QRS complex. The ventricular rate will thus be quite a bit slower than the atrial rate. In Atrial Flutter the atrial rate will be between _____ and _____ bpm, but the ventricular rate will be _____ .

250; 350

slower

30. The AV node usually allows only every second, third, or fourth impulse to be conducted through to the ventricles. On the EKG this will look like two, three, or four sawtooth F waves between each QRS complex. If the node is consistent in how it lets the impulses through, the ventricular rhythm will be regular. However, the node can be very erratic about conducting impulses. When this happens, the ratio between F waves and QRS complexes can vary between 2:1, 3:1, and 4:1, thus creating an irregular R–R interval. This is called variable block, and it causes the R–R interval in Atrial Flutter to be _____ .

irregular

31. When the atria are fluttering, it is virtually impossible to determine the PRI accurately. So when you gather data from the strip, the PRI is not measured. In an Atrial Flutter, the _____ is not measured.

PRI

32. The QRS complex is normal in Atrial Flutter. As with other supraventricular arrhythmias, if the rhythm is normal, the QRS complex will be less than 0.12 second. If the QRS is greater than 0.12 second, the arrhythmia should be considered abnormal and should be labeled Atrial Flutter with a _____ .

wide QRS complex

33. When you see an EKG tracing that has more than one P wave for every QRS complex, with an atrial rate of 250–350 bpm, particularly if the P waves have a sawtooth

Figure 31 Rules for Atrial Flutter

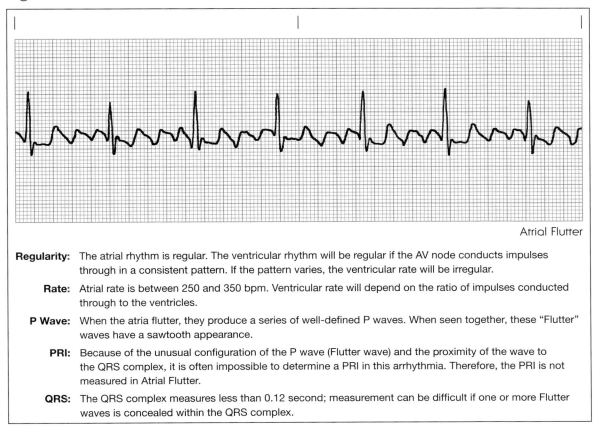

Atrial Flutter

Regularity: The atrial rhythm is regular. The ventricular rhythm will be regular if the AV node conducts impulses through in a consistent pattern. If the pattern varies, the ventricular rate will be irregular.

Rate: Atrial rate is between 250 and 350 bpm. Ventricular rate will depend on the ratio of impulses conducted through to the ventricles.

P Wave: When the atria flutter, they produce a series of well-defined P waves. When seen together, these "Flutter" waves have a sawtooth appearance.

PRI: Because of the unusual configuration of the P wave (Flutter wave) and the proximity of the wave to the QRS complex, it is often impossible to determine a PRI in this arrhythmia. Therefore, the PRI is not measured in Atrial Flutter.

QRS: The QRS complex measures less than 0.12 second; measurement can be difficult if one or more Flutter waves is concealed within the QRS complex.

configuration, you would know that there is a lot of irritability in the atria and that they are fluttering. This rhythm is called _____ .

Atrial Flutter

34. The rules for Atrial Flutter (Figure 31) are:

Regularity: atrial rhythm is regular; ventricular rhythm is usually regular but can be irregular if there is variable block

Rate: atrial rate 250–350 bpm; ventricular rate varies

P Wave: characteristic sawtooth pattern

PRI: unable to determine

QRS: less than 0.12 second

MyBRADYLab™

Atrial Fibrillation

35. The last atrial arrhythmia you will learn about is called **Atrial Fibrillation** (Figure 32). This rhythm results when the atria become so irritable that they are no longer beating but are merely quivering ineffectively. This ineffective quivering is called **fibrillation**. On the EKG tracing it is seen as a series of indiscernible waves along the isoelectric line. In most arrhythmias the P wave is reliably present, and nearly always regular, thus providing a helpful clue for interpreting the rhythm. But in Atrial Fibrillation, there are no discernible P waves, and when you do see one or two here or there, they cannot be mapped out across the strip. Atrial Fibrillation characteristically has no discernible _____ waves. The fibrillatory waves characteristic of Atrial Fibrillation are called *f waves.*

P

Figure 32 Mechanism of Atrial Fibrillation

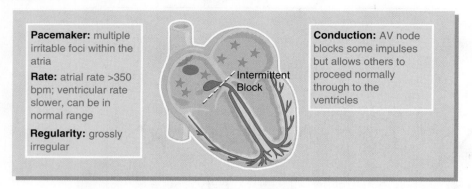

Pacemaker: multiple irritable foci within the atria

Rate: atrial rate >350 bpm; ventricular rate slower, can be in normal range

Regularity: grossly irregular

Intermittent Block

Conduction: AV node blocks some impulses but allows others to proceed normally through to the ventricles

The atria are so irritable that a multitude of foci initiate impulses, causing the atria to depolarize repeatedly in a fibrillatory manner. The AV node blocks most of the impulses, allowing only a limited number through to the ventricles.

36. In Atrial Fibrillation, the atria are quivering at a rate in excess of 350 times per minute. But this is an academic point, since there are no _____ waves with which we can measure the atrial rate. We do know, though, that the atria are fibrillating so rapidly that the AV _____ must block some of the impulses in order to keep the ventricular rate reasonable. Unlike Atrial Flutter, where the sawtooth P waves are conducted through in a semiregular fashion, the fibrillatory waves of Atrial Fibrillation are conducted in an extremely chaotic pattern, producing a grossly irregular _____ interval. The rhythm of Atrial Fibrillation is grossly _____ because the fibrillatory waves are conducted in a very chaotic way.

P

node

R–R
irregular

37. The two most characteristic features of Atrial Fibrillation, and the reasons why this arrhythmia is so easily recognized, are that there are no discernible P waves and the rhythm is grossly irregular. As the ventricular rate becomes faster, the R waves get closer together on the EKG paper, which makes the rhythm appear more regular. But even with rapid rates, Atrial Fibrillation is grossly _____ and has no discernible _____ waves. Whenever you encounter an irregular rhythm with no obvious P waves, you should consider the possibility of Atrial Fibrillation.

irregular
P

38. Because Atrial Fibrillation originates above the ventricles, conduction through to the ventricles will proceed within normal time frames (for those impulses that are conducted), thus resulting in a _____ QRS measurement. The QRS measurement in Atrial Fibrillation will normally be less than 0.12 second.

normal (narrow)

39. One other thing is important to note about Atrial Fibrillation. There is a big difference between an Atrial Fibrillation with a ventricular response within a normal rate range (100 bpm or less) and an Atrial Fibrillation with an excessively rapid ventricular response. This is because the rapid rate will create symptoms in the patient, whereas the slower rate is less likely to cause problems. If the ventricular rate is 100 bpm or less, the rhythm is called Atrial Fibrillation with a controlled ventricular response, or Atrial Fibrillation, controlled. If the rate is greater than 100 bpm, the rhythm is called Atrial Fibrillation with a rapid ventricular response, or Atrial Fibrillation, uncontrolled. A controlled ventricular response indicates that the ventricular rate is 100 bpm _____ , while a rapid ventricular response (uncontrolled) means that the ventricles are beating at _____ than 100 bpm.

or less

more

Figure 33 Rules for Atrial Fibrillation

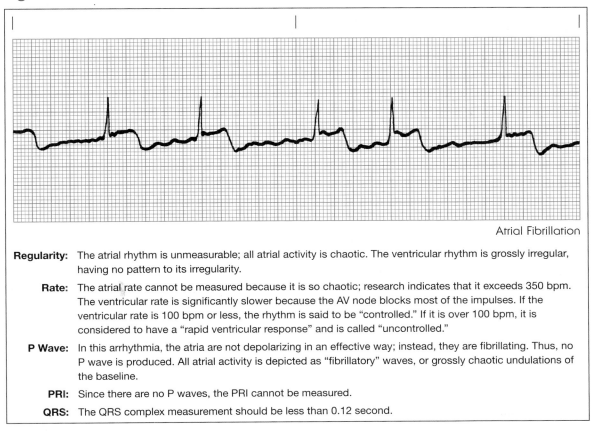

Atrial Fibrillation

Regularity: The atrial rhythm is unmeasurable; all atrial activity is chaotic. The ventricular rhythm is grossly irregular, having no pattern to its irregularity.

Rate: The atrial rate cannot be measured because it is so chaotic; research indicates that it exceeds 350 bpm. The ventricular rate is significantly slower because the AV node blocks most of the impulses. If the ventricular rate is 100 bpm or less, the rhythm is said to be "controlled." If it is over 100 bpm, it is considered to have a "rapid ventricular response" and is called "uncontrolled."

P Wave: In this arrhythmia, the atria are not depolarizing in an effective way; instead, they are fibrillating. Thus, no P wave is produced. All atrial activity is depicted as "fibrillatory" waves, or grossly chaotic undulations of the baseline.

PRI: Since there are no P waves, the PRI cannot be measured.

QRS: The QRS complex measurement should be less than 0.12 second.

40. Since you can't identify legitimate P waves in an Atrial Fibrillation, it is impossible to determine a _____ interval. You would note this on your data sheet as "not able to measure," or "unable," or "none." In an Atrial Fibrillation, the PRI is not _____ .

PR

measurable

41. The rules for Atrial Fibrillation (Figure 33) are:

Regularity: grossly irregular

Rate: atrial rate greater than 350 bpm; ventricular rate varies greatly

P Wave: no discernible P waves; atrial activity is referred to as *fibrillatory waves* (f waves)

PRI: unable to measure

QRS: less than 0.12 second

MyBRADYLab™

42. You now know five atrial arrhythmias and four sinus rhythms. You know that rhythms originating in the sinus node have a characteristic, _____ P wave. The P wave associated with atrial arrhythmias can be flattened, peaked, notched, diphasic, or even inverted. But all of these patterns should have a normal QRS measurement since they originate _____ the ventricles.

uniform

above

43. As with the sinus rhythms, you must now memorize all of the rules for each of the atrial arrhythmias. Then you can begin gathering data from the strips shown in the Practice Strips at the end of this chapter and compare them to the rules for each pattern. You should be able to identify each of the strips with relative ease. If you have any trouble, or are unsure about the process, you must seek help before going on to the next chapter.

MyBRADYLab™

Practice Strips

KEY POINTS

- All supraventricular arrhythmias should have a normal QRS measurement; if they don't, the anomaly should be noted by naming the rhythm but saying that it has "a wide QRS complex."

- Atrial arrhythmias occur when an ectopic focus in the atria assumes responsibility for pacing the heart, either by irritability or escape.

- An ectopic focus is one that originates outside of the SA node.

- Because an atrial focus is outside of the SA node, any impulse coming from it would cause an unusual depolarization wave, thus causing the P wave to have an unusual configuration; this atrial P wave can be either flattened, notched, peaked, or diphasic.

- In Wandering Pacemaker the pacemaker shifts between the SA node and the atria, causing each P wave to differ slightly from those around it.

- Here are the rules for *Wandering Pacemaker:*

Rhythm:	slightly irregular
Rate:	usually normal, 60–100 bpm
P Wave:	morphology changes from beat to beat
PRI:	less than 0.20 second; may vary
QRS:	less than 0.12 second

- Premature Atrial Complexes (PACs) are single beats that originate in the atria and come early in the cardiac cycle.

- Ectopic beats that come early in the cardiac cycle are caused by irritability; ectopic beats that come later than expected in the cardiac cycle are caused by escape mechanism.

- When confronted with ectopics, you must identify both the ectopic and the underlying rhythm.

- A rhythm with ectopics in it will be irregular, even if the underlying rhythm is characteristically regular; this is because the ectopic(s) interrupt the regularity of the underlying pattern.

- Here are the rules for *Premature Atrial Complexes:*

Rhythm:	depends on the underlying rhythm; will usually be regular except for the PAC
Rate:	usually normal; depends on underlying rhythm
P Wave:	P wave of early beat differs from sinus P waves; can be flattened or notched; may be lost in preceding T wave
PRI:	0.12–0.20 second; can be greater than 0.20 second
QRS:	less than 0.12 second

- Atrial Tachycardia is caused when a single focus in the atria fires very rapidly and overrides the SA node.

- Here are the rules for *Atrial Tachycardia:*

Rhythm:	regular
Rate:	150–250 bpm
P Wave:	atrial P wave; differs from sinus P wave; can be lost in preceding T wave
PRI:	0.12–0.20 second
QRS:	less than 0.12 second

- In Atrial Flutter and Atrial Fibrillation the atria are beating too rapidly for the ventricles to respond, so the AV node blocks some of the impulses.

- Here are the rules for *Atrial Flutter:*

Rhythm:	atrial rhythm is regular; ventricular rhythm is usually regular but can be irregular if there is variable block
Rate:	atrial rate 250–350 bpm; ventricular rate varies
P Wave:	characteristic sawtooth pattern (F waves)
PRI:	unable to determine
QRS:	less than 0.12 second

- Here are the rules for *Atrial Fibrillation:*

Rhythm:	grossly irregular
Rate:	atrial rate greater than 350 bpm; ventricular rate varies greatly; 100 bpm or less is considered "controlled," while more than 100 bpm is called "uncontrolled"
P Wave:	no discernible P waves; atrial activity is referred to as fibrillatory waves (f waves)
PRI:	unable to measure
QRS:	less than 0.12 second

SELF-TEST

Directions: Complete this self-evaluation of the information you have learned from this chapter. If your answers are all correct and you feel comfortable with your understanding of the material, proceed to the next chapter. However, if you miss any of the questions, you should review the referenced frames before proceeding. If you feel unsure of any of the underlying principles, invest the time now to go back over the entire chapter. **Do not proceed with the next chapter until you are very comfortable with the material in this chapter.**

Questions	Referenced Frames	Answers
1. How does an atrial P wave differ from a sinus P wave?	3, 4, 5, 42	Sinus P waves are upright and uniform. Atrial P waves can be flattened, notched, irregular, or even inverted.
2. What two basic mechanisms can cause an atrial focus to take over pacemaking responsibilities?	1, 2, 11	irritability or escape
3. What is an ectopic focus?	9, 10	It is a site of electrical activity *other than* the SA node.
4. Which atrial arrhythmia is characterized by a pacemaker that shifts between the SA node and various foci in the atria, sometimes even dropping down to the AV junction?	6, 7, 8	Wandering Pacemaker
5. What is a PAC (Premature Atrial Complex)?	9, 10, 11, 12, 13, 14, 20, 21, 22	It is a single beat that originates in the atrium and comes early in the cardiac cycle.
6. Is a PAC an ectopic?	9, 10, 11, 12, 13, 22	Yes, because it originates outside of the SA node.
7. If an ectopic is caused by irritability, will it come earlier than expected or later than expected?	11, 14, 18, 22	Earlier; if the ectopic comes later than expected, it was caused by escape mechanism.
8. Is Wandering Pacemaker a single ectopic beat?	6, 9	No, it is an entire arrhythmia.
9. What is the most characteristic feature of Wandering Pacemaker?	6	It is the changing shapes of the P waves as the pacemaker site shifts locations.
10. What should the QRS measurement be for a PAC?	5, 17, 19, 21, 42	less than 0.12 second
11. What will the P wave look like on a PAC?	5, 16, 19, 20, 21, 42	It would have the characteristic look of atrial P waves. It could be flattened, notched, diphasic, or peaked.
12. If the P wave of a PAC was not clearly visible, where might you consider looking for it?	18	in the T wave of the preceding complex
13. Is Atrial Tachycardia caused by one irritable focus or by many?	22	Only one, which is why it is usually so regular.
14. What is the usual rate range for Atrial Tachycardia?	24, 25, 26	150–250 bpm
15. Does Atrial Tachycardia have a P wave in front of every QRS complex?	26	Yes, although you may have some trouble seeing them if they are superimposed on the T waves of the preceding complexes.
16. What does the P wave look like in an Atrial Tachycardia?	5, 23, 26, 43	It looks just like the P wave of a PAC. In fact, AT looks very much like a lot of PACs connected together.
17. What happens if the atria begin beating too rapidly for the ventricles to respond to them?	28, 29, 30	The AV node may block some of the impulses so that they aren't conducted to the ventricles. This results in more P waves than QRS complexes.

Questions	Referenced Frames	Answers
18. Which two atrial arrhythmias do you know that involve the phenomenon described in the preceding question?	29, 36	Atrial Flutter and Atrial Fibrillation
19. What's the atrial rate in Atrial Flutter?	27, 29, 33, 34	250–350 bpm
20. Is the ventricular rhythm regular or irregular in Atrial Flutter?	30, 34	This depends on how the AV node is blocking impulses. If atrial impulses are being conducted in a regular pattern (e.g., 2:1 or 4:1), the ventricular rhythm would be regular. But if the conduction ratio varied (e.g., 2:1, 3:1, 2:1, etc.), the ventricular rhythm would be irregular.
21. In Atrial Flutter, would the ventricular rate be faster or slower than the atrial rate?	29, 30, 33, 34	The ventricular rate would always be slower, unless the conduction ratio was 1:1. This is because not all of the P waves are able to produce QRS complexes.
22. What does the atrial activity look like in an Atrial Flutter?	29, 30, 33, 34	The Flutter waves usually take on a characteristic sawtooth appearance, although not always.
23. How would you describe the atrial activity in Atrial Fibrillation?	35, 36, 41	The atria are not contracting; instead, they are quivering chaotically. This causes the isoelectric line to undulate in a very irregular fashion. There are no visible P waves, only fibrillatory waves (f waves).
24. What is the atrial rate in Atrial Fibrillation?	36, 41	over 350 bpm (typically not measurable)
25. Is there a relationship between atrial activity and ventricular activity in Atrial Fibrillation?	36, 38, 41	Yes, there is. Some of the impulses are conducted through to the ventricles, but it is not possible to determine a PRI because there is no clear P wave.
26. What is the ventricular rate for Atrial Fibrillation?	36, 39, 41	That depends on how many of the impulses are conducted through to the ventricles. If the ventricular rate is 100 bpm or less, the rhythm is called Atrial Fibrillation with "controlled ventricular response," or "Atrial Fibrillation, controlled." If the rate is over 100 bpm, it is called a "rapid ventricular response," or "Atrial Fibrillation, uncontrolled."
27. What are the two most characteristic features of Atrial Fibrillation?	36, 37, 41	It has no discernible P waves, and the R–R interval is grossly irregular.

PRACTICE STRIPS (answers can be found in the Answer Key on page 554)

5.1

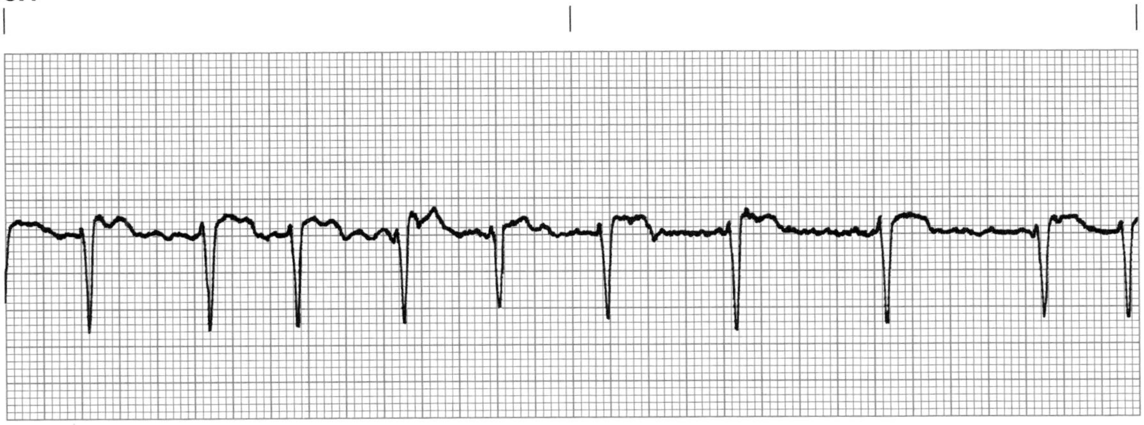

Regularity: _____   PRI: _____

Rate: _____   QRS: _____

P Waves: _____   Interp: _____

5.2

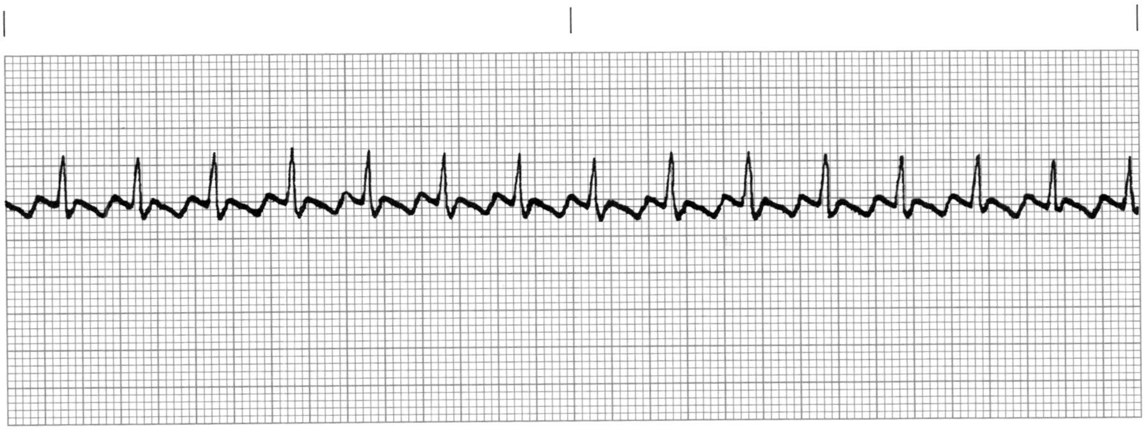

Regularity: _____   PRI: _____

Rate: _____   QRS: _____

P Waves: _____   Interp: _____

5.3

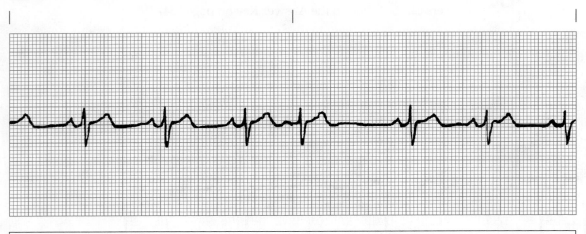

Regularity: _____	PRI: _____	
Rate: _____	QRS: _____	
P Waves: _____	Interp: _____	

5.4

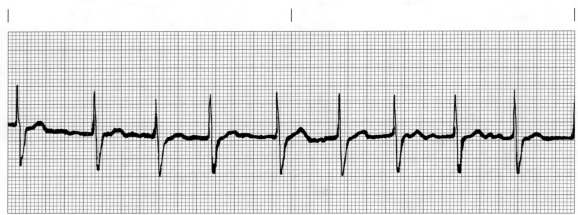

Regularity: _____	PRI: _____	
Rate: _____	QRS: _____	
P Waves: _____	Interp: _____	

5.5

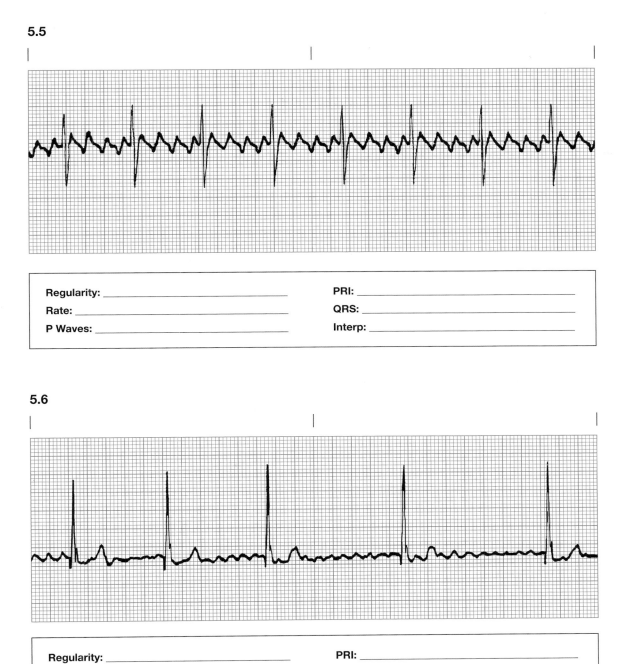

Regularity: _____	PRI: _____
Rate: _____	QRS: _____
P Waves: _____	Interp: _____

5.6

Regularity: _____	PRI: _____
Rate: _____	QRS: _____
P Waves: _____	Interp: _____

5.7

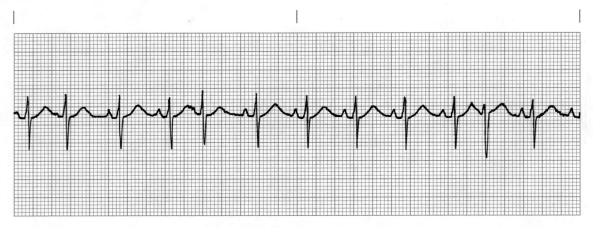

Regularity: _____	PRI: _____
Rate: _____	QRS: _____
P Waves: _____	Interp: _____

5.8

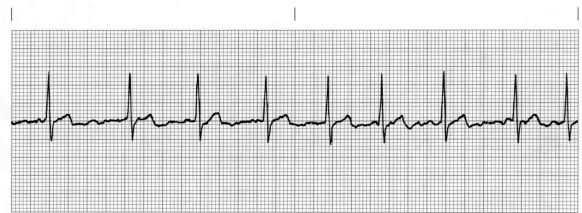
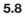

Regularity: _____	PRI: _____
Rate: _____	QRS: _____
P Waves: _____	Interp: _____

5.9

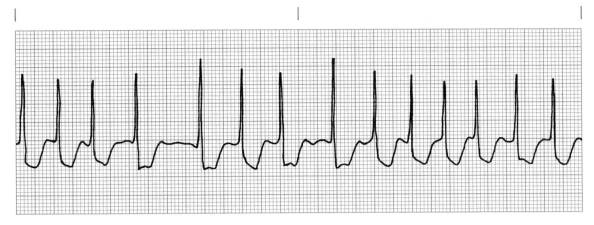

Regularity: _____	PRI: _____
Rate: _____	QRS: _____
P Waves: _____	Interp: _____

5.10

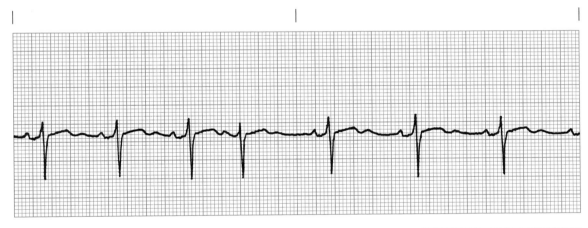

Regularity: _____	PRI: _____
Rate: _____	QRS: _____
P Waves: _____	Interp: _____

5.11

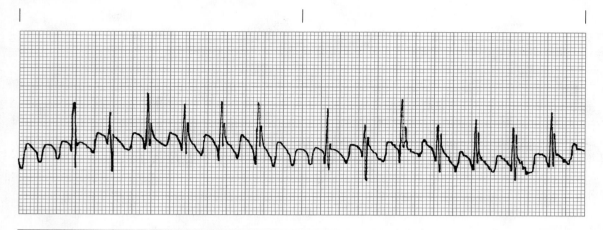

Regularity: _____	PRI: _____
Rate: _____	QRS: _____
P Waves: _____	Interp: _____

5.12

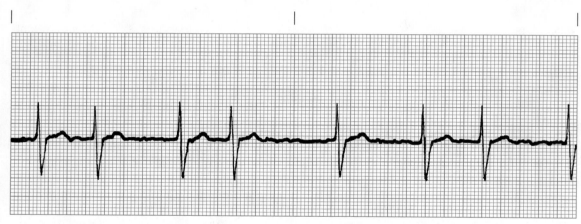

Regularity: _____	PRI: _____
Rate: _____	QRS: _____
P Waves: _____	Interp: _____

5.13

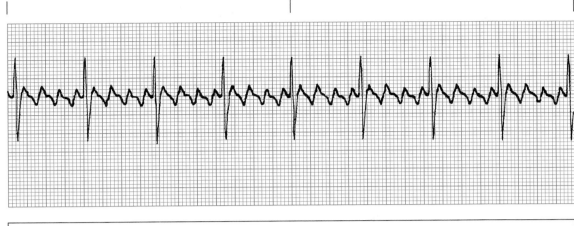

Regularity: _____	PRI: _____
Rate: _____	QRS: _____
P Waves: _____	Interp: _____

5.14

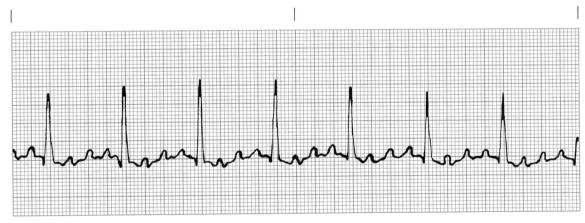

Regularity: _____	PRI: _____
Rate: _____	QRS: _____
P Waves: _____	Interp: _____

5.15

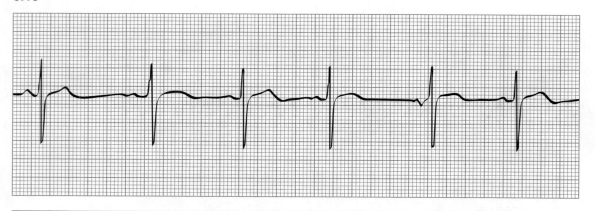

Regularity: _____	PRI: _____
Rate: _____	QRS: _____
P Waves: _____	Interp: _____

5.16

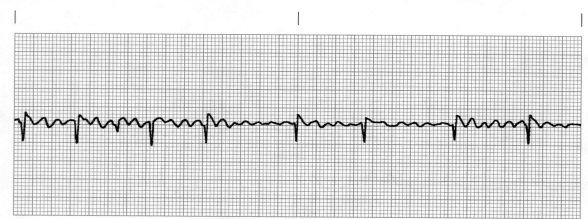

Regularity: _____	PRI: _____
Rate: _____	QRS: _____
P Waves: _____	Interp: _____

5.17

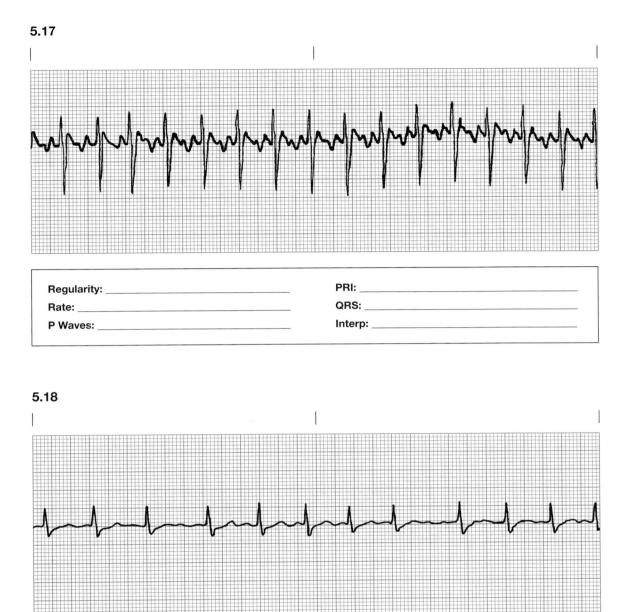

Regularity: _____	PRI: _____
Rate: _____	QRS: _____
P Waves: _____	Interp: _____

5.18

Regularity: _____	PRI: _____
Rate: _____	QRS: _____
P Waves: _____	Interp: _____

5.19

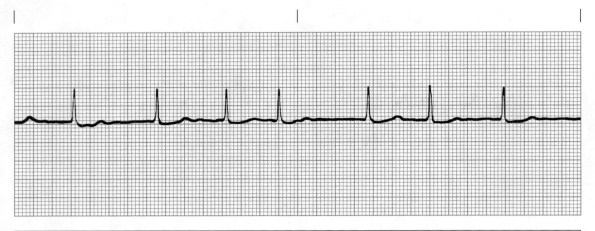

Regularity: _____	PRI: _____
Rate: _____	QRS: _____
P Waves: _____	Interp: _____

5.20

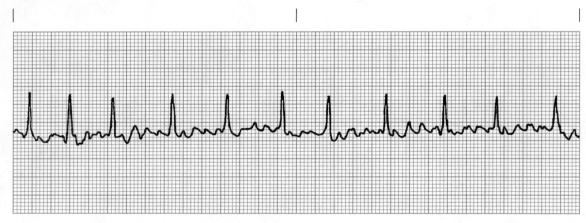

Regularity: _____	PRI: _____
Rate: _____	QRS: _____
P Waves: _____	Interp: _____

5.21

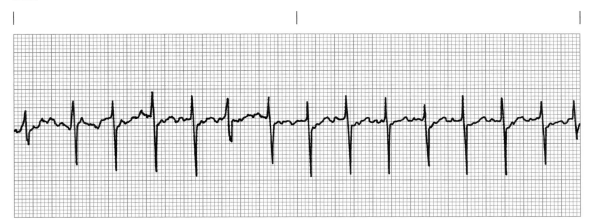

Regularity: _____		PRI: _____	
Rate: _____		QRS: _____	
P Waves: _____		Interp: _____	

5.22

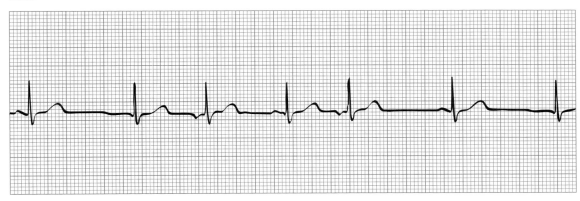

Regularity: _____		PRI: _____	
Rate: _____		QRS: _____	
P Waves: _____		Interp: _____	

5.23

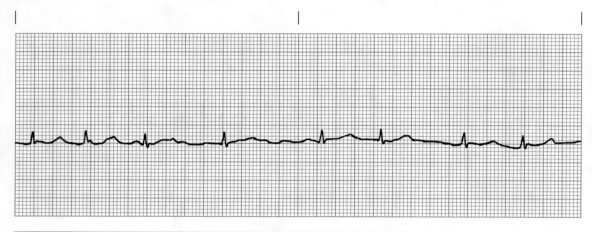

Regularity: _____	PRI: _____
Rate: _____	QRS: _____
P Waves: _____	Interp: _____

5.24

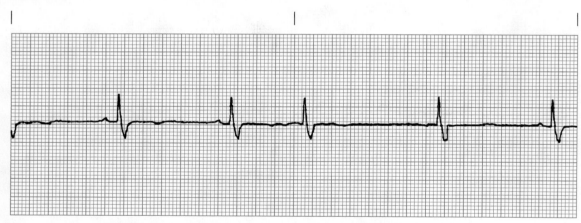

Regularity: _____	PRI: _____
Rate: _____	QRS: _____
P Waves: _____	Interp: _____

5.25

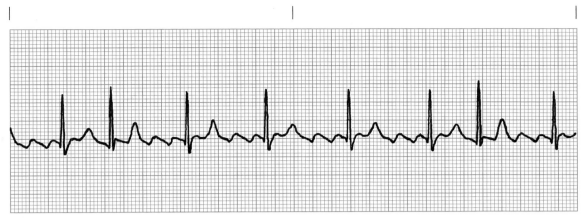

Regularity: _____

Rate: _____

P Waves: _____

PRI: _____

QRS: _____

Interp: _____

5.26

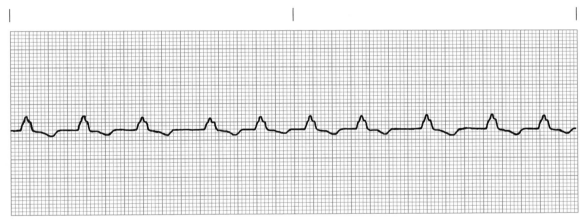

Regularity: _____

Rate: _____

P Waves: _____

PRI: _____

QRS: _____

Interp: _____

5.27

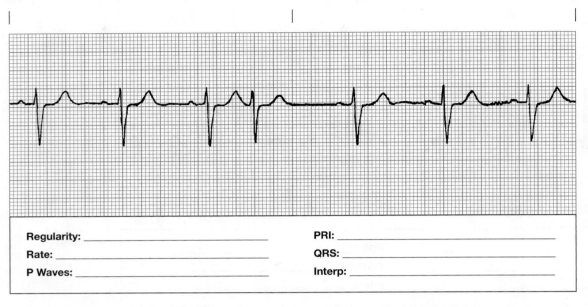

Regularity: _____	PRI: _____
Rate: _____	QRS: _____
P Waves: _____	Interp: _____

5.28

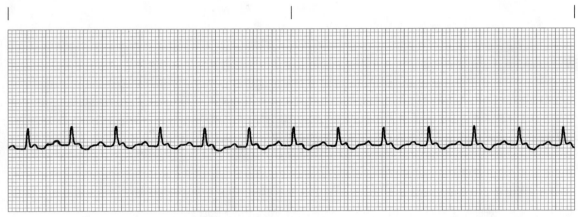

Regularity: _____	PRI: _____
Rate: _____	QRS: _____
P Waves: _____	Interp: _____

5.29

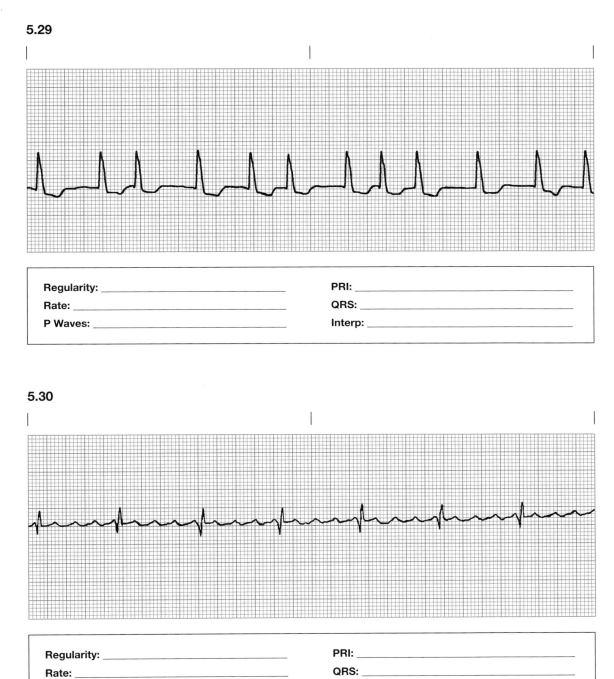

Regularity: _____	PRI: _____
Rate: _____	QRS: _____
P Waves: _____	Interp: _____

5.30

Regularity: _____	PRI: _____
Rate: _____	QRS: _____
P Waves: _____	Interp: _____

5.31

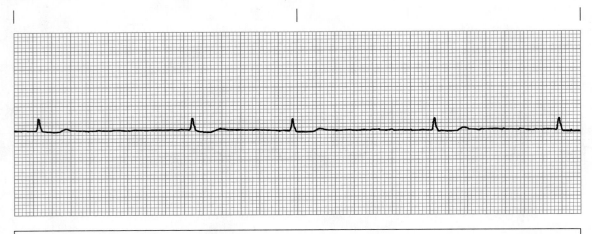

Regularity: _____	**PRI:** _____
Rate: _____	**QRS:** _____
P Waves: _____	**Interp:** _____

5.32

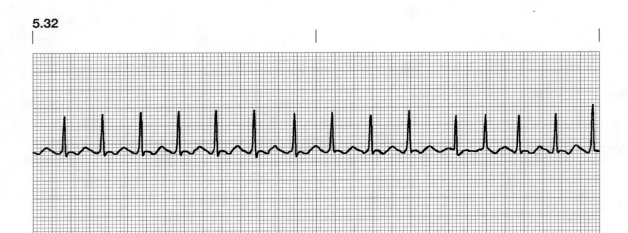

Regularity: _____	**PRI:** _____
Rate: _____	**QRS:** _____
P Waves: _____	**Interp:** _____

5.33

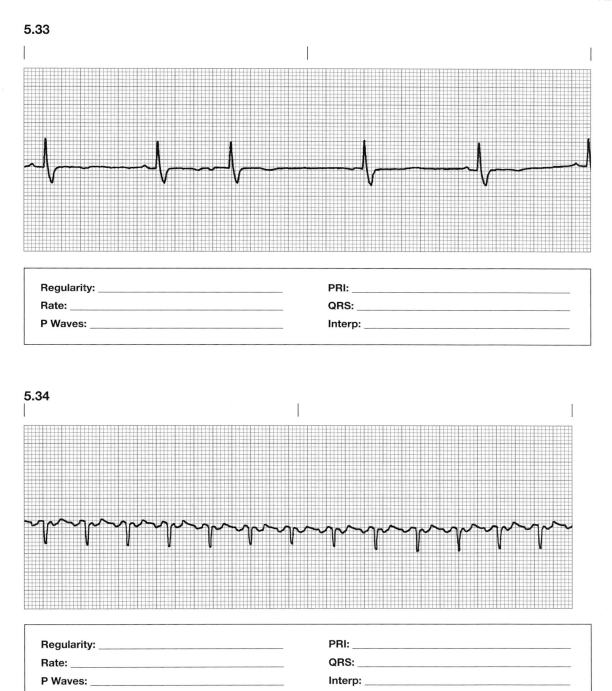

Regularity: _____	PRI: _____
Rate: _____	QRS: _____
P Waves: _____	Interp: _____

5.34

Regularity: _____	PRI: _____
Rate: _____	QRS: _____
P Waves: _____	Interp: _____

5.35

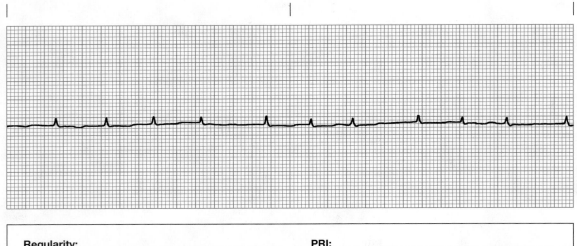

Regularity: _____	PRI: _____
Rate: _____	QRS: _____
P Waves: _____	Interp: _____

5.36

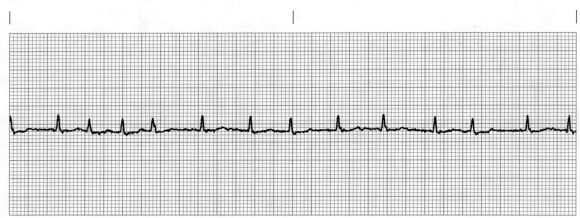

Regularity: _____	PRI: _____
Rate: _____	QRS: _____
P Waves: _____	Interp: _____

5.37

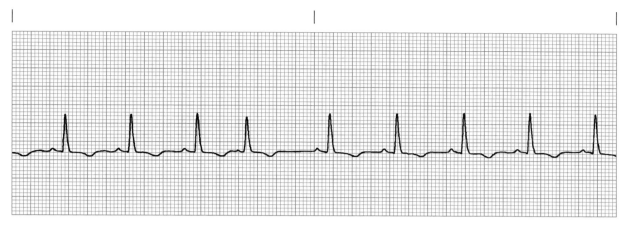

Regularity: _____	**PRI:** _____
Rate: _____	**QRS:** _____
P Waves: _____	**Interp:** _____

5.38

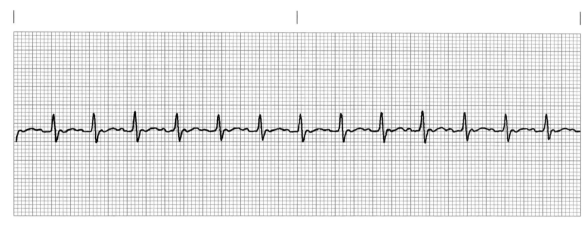

Regularity: _____	**PRI:** _____
Rate: _____	**QRS:** _____
P Waves: _____	**Interp:** _____

5.39

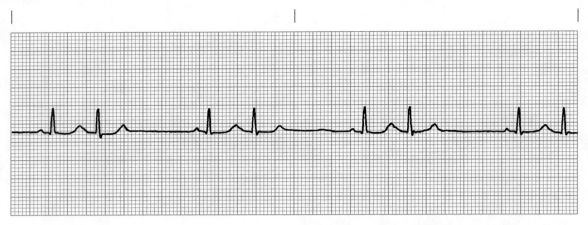

Regularity: _____	PRI: _____
Rate: _____	QRS: _____
P Waves: _____	Interp: _____

5.40

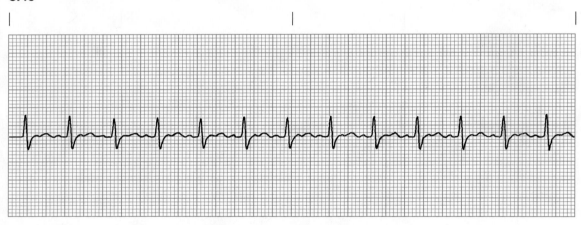

Regularity: _____	PRI: _____
Rate: _____	QRS: _____
P Waves: _____	Interp: _____

5.41

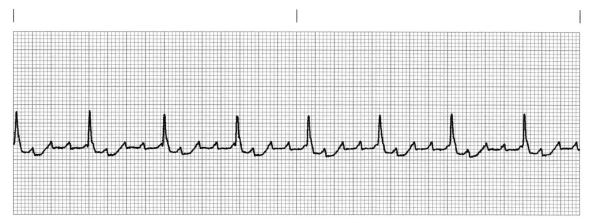

Regularity: _____   PRI: _____

Rate: _____   QRS: _____

P Waves: _____   Interp: _____

5.42

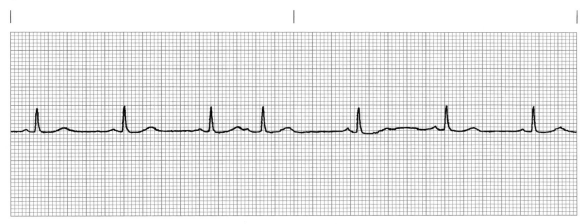

Regularity: _____   PRI: _____

Rate: _____   QRS: _____

P Waves: _____   Interp: _____

5.43

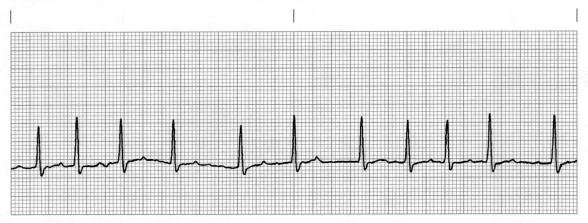

Regularity: _____   PRI: _____

Rate: _____   QRS: _____

P Waves: _____   Interp: _____

5.44

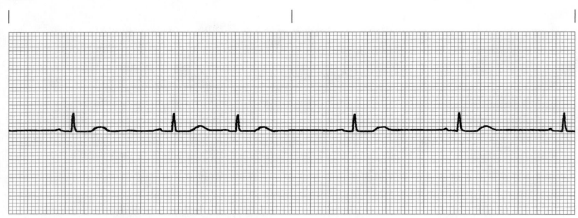

Regularity: _____   PRI: _____

Rate: _____   QRS: _____

P Waves: _____   Interp: _____

5.45

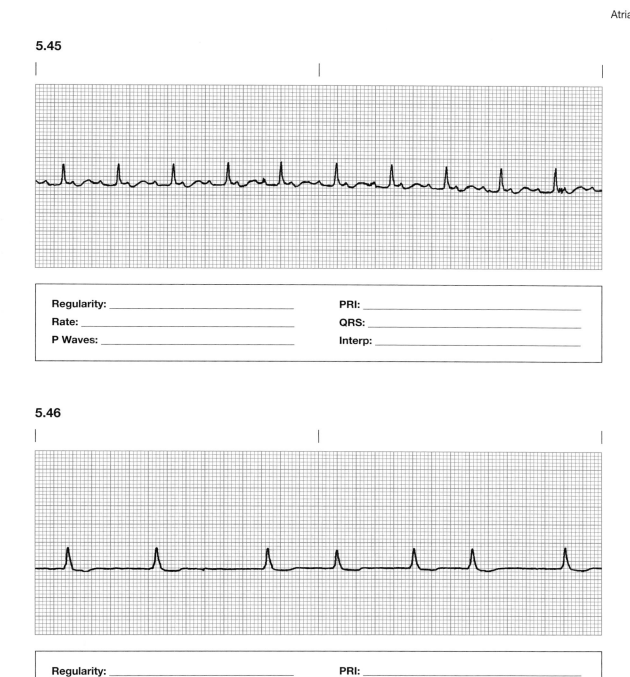

Regularity: _____	**PRI:** _____
Rate: _____	**QRS:** _____
P Waves: _____	**Interp:** _____

5.46

Regularity: _____	**PRI:** _____
Rate: _____	**QRS:** _____
P Waves: _____	**Interp:** _____

5.47

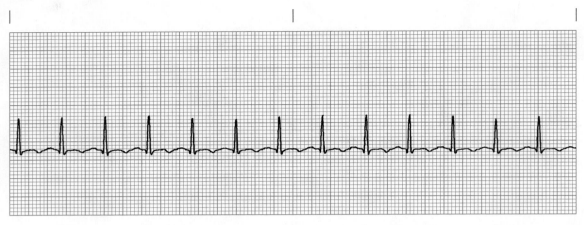

Regularity: _____ PRI: _____

Rate: _____ QRS: _____

P Waves: _____ Interp: _____

5.48

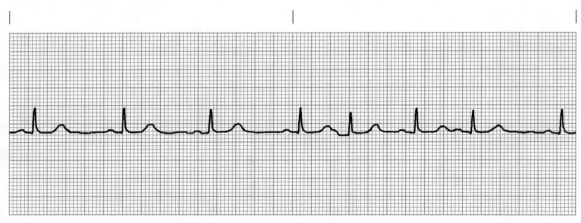

Regularity: _____ PRI: _____

Rate: _____ QRS: _____

P Waves: _____ Interp: _____

5.49

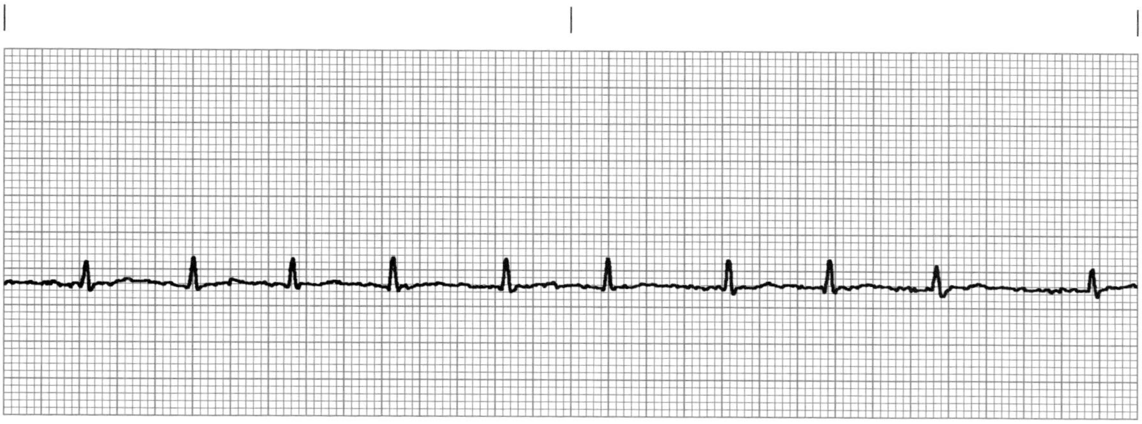

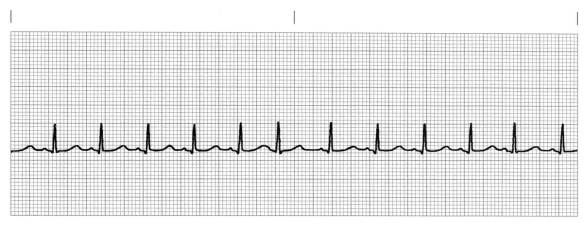

Regularity: _____	PRI: _____
Rate: _____	QRS: _____
P Waves: _____	Interp: _____

5.50

Regularity: _____	PRI: _____
Rate: _____	QRS: _____
P Waves: _____	Interp: _____

5.51

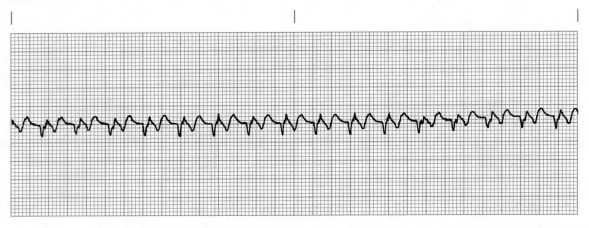

Regularity: _____	PRI: _____
Rate: _____	QRS: _____
P Waves: _____	Interp: _____

5.52

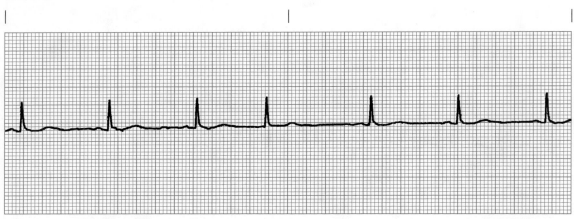

Regularity: _____	PRI: _____
Rate: _____	QRS: _____
P Waves: _____	Interp: _____

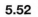

5.53

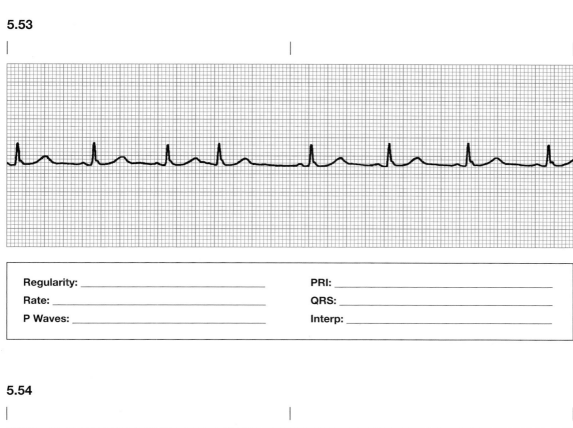

Regularity: _____	**PRI:** _____
Rate: _____	**QRS:** _____
P Waves: _____	**Interp:** _____

5.54

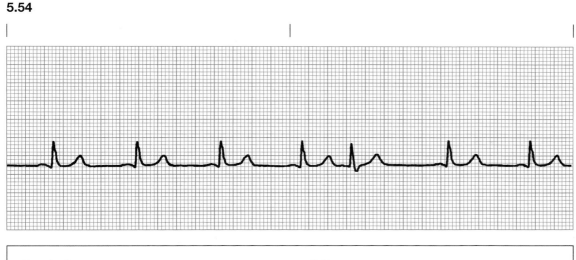

Regularity: _____	**PRI:** _____
Rate: _____	**QRS:** _____
P Waves: _____	**Interp:** _____

5.55

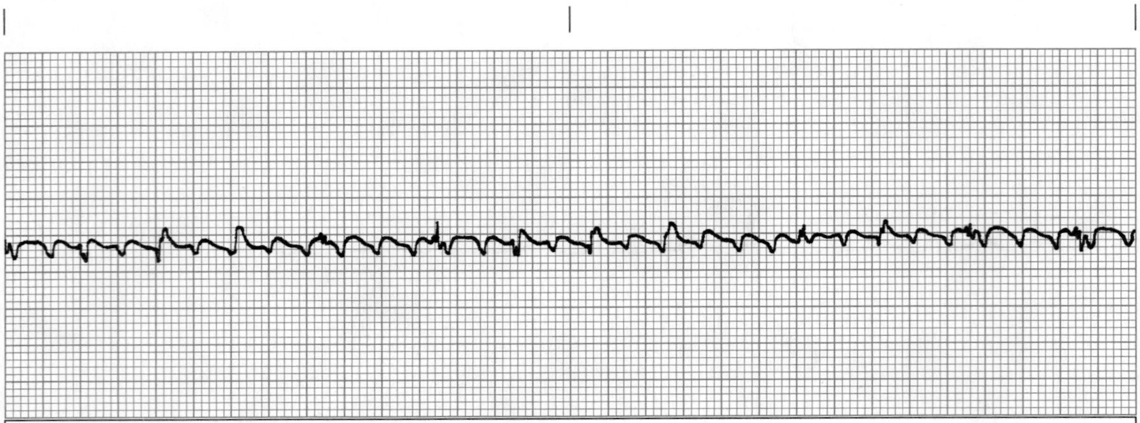

Regularity: _____   PRI: _____

Rate: _____   QRS: _____

P Waves: _____   Interp: _____

5.56

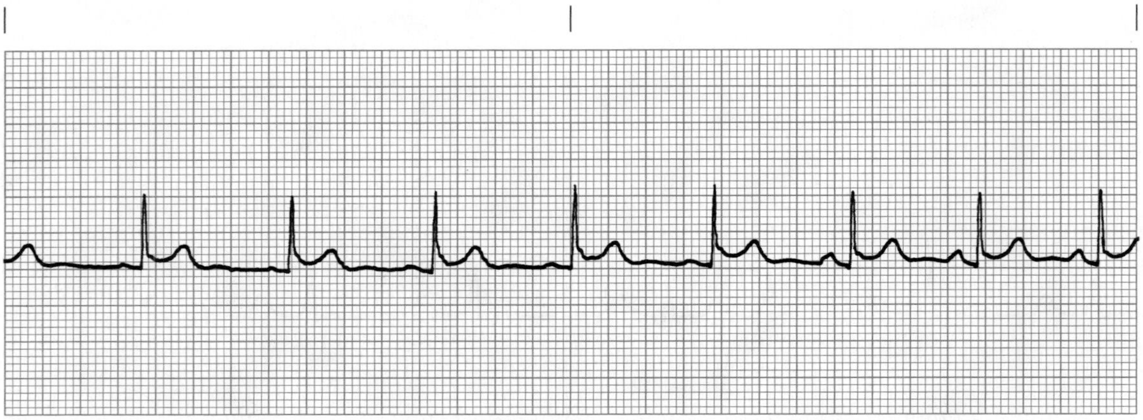

Regularity: _____   PRI: _____

Rate: _____   QRS: _____

P Waves: _____   Interp: _____

5.57

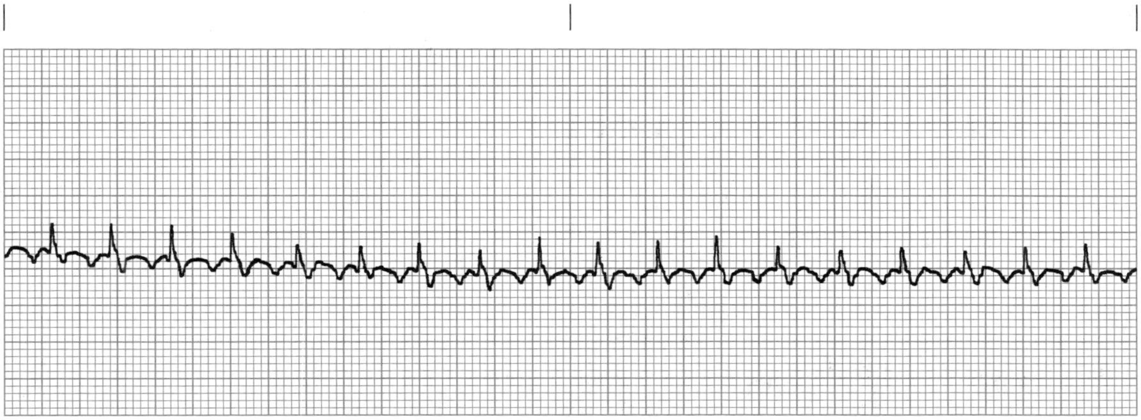

Regularity: _____	**PRI:** _____
Rate: _____	**QRS:** _____
P Waves: _____	**Interp:** _____

Chapter 6
Junctional Rhythms

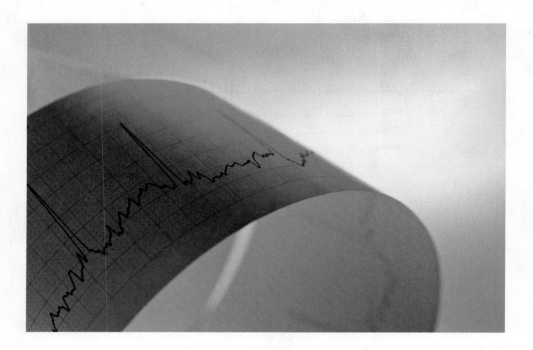

Overview

IN THIS CHAPTER, you will learn the characteristics of an AV junctional pacemaker and the features that are shared by rhythms originating in the AV junction. You will then learn the names and characteristics of five different arrhythmias that originate within the AV junction. For each of these arrhythmias, you will learn about the etiology, conduction, and resulting EKG features (regularity, rate, P waves, PR intervals, and QRS complexes).

Junctional Pacemaker

1. You learned in Chapter 1 that the AV junction consists of the AV node and the Bundle of His. This unique part of the conduction system is responsible for conducting impulses from the _____ down the conduction pathways to the ventricles. The *body* of the AV node is responsible for delaying each impulse just long enough to give the ventricles time to fill before contracting. The lower region of the AV junction—where the node merges with the Bundle of His—houses the pacemaking cells that initiate the group of arrhythmias called *junctional* rhythms. Arrhythmias that originate in the area of the AV node come from the tissues at the junction between the lower node and the Bundle of His; thus, they are called AV _____ rhythms.

SA node

junctional

2. When electrical impulses originate in the AV junction, the heart is depolarized in a somewhat unusual fashion. With the pacemaker located in the middle of the heart, the electrical impulses spread in two directions simultaneously. This is unusual because the heart is normally depolarized by a single force spreading downward toward the _____ . However, when the AV junction assumes _____ responsibility, the atria and the ventricles will be depolarized at very nearly the same time because the impulse spreads in _____ directions at one time. This concept is pictured in Figure 34.

ventricles

pacemaking

two

3. As you recall, electrode positions for Lead II place the _____ electrode above the right atria and the _____ electrode below the ventricle (see Figure 35). In the normal heart, the major thrust of electrical flow is toward the ventricles (and toward the positive electrode in Lead II), thus producing an upright P wave and an upright QRS complex. In a junctional rhythm, the ventricles are depolarized by an impulse traveling down the conduction system toward the positive electrode; thus, the QRS complex usually is _____ . But at the same time, the impulse can spread upward through the atria toward the _____ electrode. When the atria are depolarized in this "backward" fashion, it's called **retrograde** conduction because the electrical impulse travels in the opposite direction it usually takes. The mechanism that enables the AV junction to depolarize the atria with a backward flow of electricity is called _____ conduction.

negative

positive

upright

negative

retrograde

4. In junctional rhythms, the impulse that depolarizes the ventricles is traveling toward the _____ electrode (in Lead II), thus producing a QRS complex that usually is upright. When retrograde conduction occurs in AV junctional rhythms, the electrical impulse that depolarizes the atria is traveling toward the _____ electrode. Thus, we can deduce that the atrial activity will produce a *negative* deflection on the EKG. In other words, the P wave of an AV junctional arrhythmia should be inverted because it was produced by an impulse traveling toward the _____ electrode.

positive

negative

negative

5. In AV junctional arrhythmias, the atria are depolarized via _____ conduction at approximately the same time as the ventricles are depolarized normally. The two simultaneous electrical force flows, one retrograde and the other normal, result in an inverted _____ wave and an upright _____ complex.

retrograde

P

QRS

6. In junctional arrhythmias, a single impulse originates in the AV junction and causes electricity to flow in two directions. One electrical force flows upward (retrograde) to depolarize the _____ , while the other flows downward to

atria

Figure 34 Electrical Flow in Junctional Arrhythmias

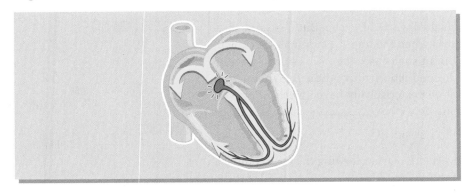

Figure 35 Normal Electrical Flow in Lead II

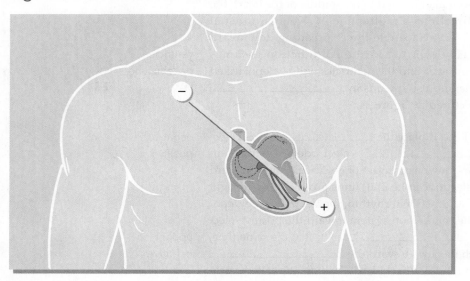

depolarize the _____ . Even though both electrical forces originate from a single impulse in the junction, the force that depolarizes the atria is not the same force that depolarizes the ventricles. For this reason, you will not always see a consistent relationship between the inverted P wave and the QRS complex. The _____ wave will not have a consistent relationship to the _____ complex because the force that depolarizes the atria is not the same force that depolarizes the _____ .

ventricles

P
QRS
ventricles

Junctional P Wave

7. In junctional arrhythmias, the P wave does not always have to precede the QRS complex because it is possible for the ventricles to be depolarized before the atria, if the force reaches them first. The position of the P wave in relation to the QRS complex will depend on whether the atria or the ventricles were _____ first. If the ventricles are depolarized before the atria, the QRS will come before the P wave. If the atria depolarize first, the P wave will precede the QRS complex. If they both depolarize simultaneously, the _____ wave will be hidden within the QRS complex. In junctional arrhythmias, the P wave isn't always visible, but when it is, it will be _____ because the atria are depolarized via retrograde conduction. The P wave in junctional rhythms can come before, during, or after the _____ complex, depending on which depolarize first, the atria or the ventricles (see Figure 36).

depolarized

P

inverted

QRS

8. The biggest clue to a junctional rhythm is the inverted P wave. But this same phenomenon occurs with some atrial arrhythmias when the impulse originates so low in the atria that it is very near the AV junction. In such cases the impulse will have to depolarize parts of the atria with retrograde conduction, thus producing an inverted P wave. Therefore, while junctional rhythms characteristically have inverted P waves, a rhythm with an inverted P wave can be either _____ or _____ in origin.

atrial
junctional

9. When you see an arrhythmia with an inverted P wave following the QRS complex, you know that the rhythm originated in the AV _____ . But if the

junction

Figure 36 P Wave Placement in Junctional Rhythms

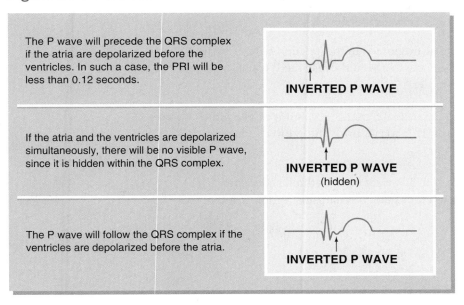

The P wave will precede the QRS complex if the atria are depolarized before the ventricles. In such a case, the PRI will be less than 0.12 seconds.

INVERTED P WAVE

If the atria and the ventricles are depolarized simultaneously, there will be no visible P wave, since it is hidden within the QRS complex.

INVERTED P WAVE
(hidden)

The P wave will follow the QRS complex if the ventricles are depolarized before the atria.

INVERTED P WAVE

inverted P wave precedes the QRS complex, you need to determine whether it originated in the AV junction or in the _____ . The important clue will   atria
come from the PR interval. If the impulse originated in the atria, the impulse would
take the normal length of time getting through the node and into the ventricles. Thus,
the PRI would be normal, or _____ second. But if the impulse origi-   0.12–0.20
nated in the AV junction, it would take less time to get to the ventricles and thus would
have a PRI of less than 0.12 second. If the rhythm has an inverted P wave and a normal
PRI measurement, you would know that it originated in the _____ ;   atria
whereas if the PRI is less than 0.12 second, it must have originated in the

_____ .   AV junction

10. You now know quite a bit about junctional rhythms in general. You know that the
QRS measurement is _____ and that the P wave will be   normal
_____ . The P wave can be seen before, during, or after the QRS   inverted
complex but may not be visible at all if it is hidden within the QRS complex. Finally,
you know that the PRI must be less than 0.12 second; if it is greater than 0.12 second,
the arrhythmia would be _____ in origin. All of these rules pertain   atrial
to every junctional rhythm, regardless of whether it is a tachycardia, bradycardia, or a
single ectopic beat. For each of the four AV junctional arrhythmias you will now learn,
you already know that all of the preceding rules apply.

11. All junctional arrhythmias will have an inverted P wave because the atria are
depolarized via _____ conduction.   retrograde

12. Atrial arrhythmias can also have _____ P waves since they can   inverted
be produced by retrograde conduction.

13. Junctional arrhythmias will have a PRI of less than _____ sec-   0.12
ond; atrial arrhythmias will have a PRI of _____ second.   0.12–0.20

14. An inverted P wave that precedes the QRS complex and has a PRI of less than 0.12
second indicates that the pacemaker impulse originated in the _____ ,   AV junction
and the atria depolarized _____ the ventricles.   before

15. If the junctional impulse reached the ventricles first and depolarized the ventricles before the atria, it would produce an inverted P wave _____ the QRS complex.

following

16. You would not see a P wave if the impulse originated in the junction but reached the atria and the ventricles simultaneously, since this would cause the P wave to be _____ within the QRS complex.

hidden

17. If visible, a junctional P wave will be _____ , but it can be hidden within the QRS complex if both the atria and the ventricles are _____ simultaneously.

inverted

depolarized

18. The junctional pacemaker site can produce a variety of arrhythmias, depending on the mechanism employed. We will discuss four basic mechanisms common to the AV junction:

- Premature Junctional Complex
- Junctional Escape Rhythm
- Accelerated Junctional Rhythm
- Junctional Tachycardia

Although these are four different mechanisms, each of these arrhythmias originates in the AV _____ .

junction

Premature Junctional Complex

19. The first junctional arrhythmia we will learn about is called a **Premature Junctional Complex**, or PJC (Figure 37). A PJC is not an entire rhythm; it is a single ectopic beat. A PJC is similar in many ways to a PAC. In the case of the PJC, the irritable focus comes from the AV junction to stimulate an early cardiac cycle, which interrupts the underlying rhythm for a single _____ .

beat

When such a premature ectopic originates in the atria, it is called a Premature Atrial Complex, or PAC. But when the irritable focus is in the AV junction, it is called a PJC, or _____ . A PJC is a single ectopic beat that comes _____ in the cardiac cycle to interrupt the underlying rhythm.

Premature Junctional Complex

early

Figure 37 Mechanism of Premature Junctional Complex

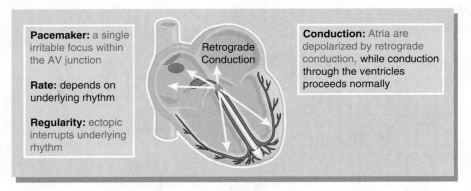

The pacemaker is an irritable focus within the AV junction that fires prematurely and produces a single ectopic beat. The atria are depolarized via retrograde conduction. Conduction through the ventricles is normal. *This is a single beat, not an entire rhythm; the underlying rhythm also must be identified.*

20. Since a PJC is a single beat, it will interrupt the rhythm of the underlying pattern. The R–R interval will be regular or irregular, depending on the regularity of the underlying rhythm, but the PJC will come earlier than expected and thus will cause the overall rhythm to be irregular. Because a PJC is a single early beat, it will cause the overall rhythm to be _____ .

irregular

21. As with regularity, the rate will depend on the rate of the underlying arrhythmia. Being a single beat, a PJC does not have a rate of its own. To determine heart rate, you would have to look at the overall rate of the _____ rhythm.

underlying

22. The P wave of a PJC will be consistent with the P waves of all other junctional arrhythmias. Because atrial depolarization is retrograde, the P wave will be _____ and can fall before, during, or after the _____ complex.

inverted; QRS

23. If the P wave of the PJC precedes the QRS complex, the PRI will be less than _____ second.

0.12

24. Conduction through the ventricles should be normal with a PJC. Therefore, the QRS complex should have a normal duration of _____ .

less than 0.12 second

25. The rules of PJCs (Figure 38) are:

Regularity: depends on regularity of underlying arrhythmia

Rate: depends on rate of underlying arrhythmia

P Wave: will be inverted; can fall before, during, or after the QRS complex

PRI: can be measured only if the P wave precedes the QRS complex; if measurable, will be less than 0.12 second

QRS: less than 0.12 second

Figure 38 Rules for Premature Junctional Complex

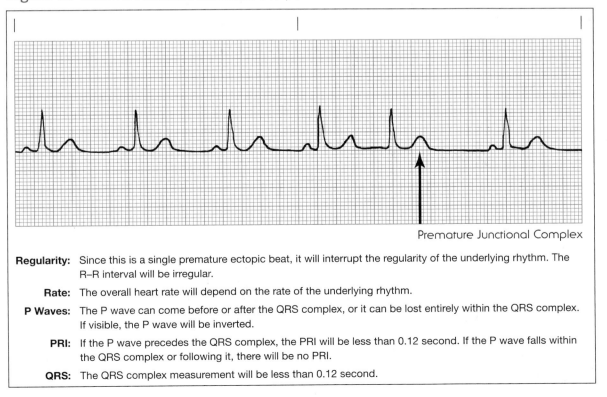

Premature Junctional Complex

Regularity: Since this is a single premature ectopic beat, it will interrupt the regularity of the underlying rhythm. The R–R interval will be irregular.

Rate: The overall heart rate will depend on the rate of the underlying rhythm.

P Waves: The P wave can come before or after the QRS complex, or it can be lost entirely within the QRS complex. If visible, the P wave will be inverted.

PRI: If the P wave precedes the QRS complex, the PRI will be less than 0.12 second. If the P wave falls within the QRS complex or following it, there will be no PRI.

QRS: The QRS complex measurement will be less than 0.12 second.

26. The normal, inherent rate for the AV junction is 40–60 bpm. A PJC occurs when the junction becomes irritable and overrides higher sites. But the junction can also take over pacemaking responsibility if higher sites fail. The junction would then "escape" and assume pacemaking functions at its own inherent rate of _____ bpm.

40–60

27. As you recall, a premature beat is a sign of irritability, whereas an _____ beat comes later than you would expect it and is a fail-safe mechanism to protect the heart. When the AV junction is allowed to assume that pacemaking functions at its inherent rate of 40–60 bpm, this is an example of _____ mechanism rather than irritability.

escape

escape

Junctional Escape Rhythm

28. When you see **Junctional Escape Rhythm** (Figure 39), you would expect it to have a rate of _____ bpm, since this is the inherent rate of the AV junction. Junctional Escape Rhythm is sometimes referred to as "Passive" Junctional Rhythm.

40–60

29. The AV junction is normally a very regular pacemaker. In a Junctional Escape Rhythm, you would find a regular R–R interval. AV Junctional Escape Rhythm is a _____ rhythm with a rate of 40–60 bpm.

regular

30. As with other junctional arrhythmias, Junctional Escape Rhythm has inverted P waves, which can fall before or after the QRS complex. It is also possible that there would be no P wave, since the P wave can be hidden within the QRS complex. Junctional Escape Rhythm always has inverted P waves, either before or after the QRS complex, or the P wave might be hidden within the _____ complex.

QRS

31. If the P wave precedes the QRS complex, the PRI will be less than _____ second. If the PRI is greater than 0.12 second, you would suspect that the rhythm originated in the _____ .

0.12
atria

32. As with other junctional arrhythmias, you would expect ventricular conduction to be _____ , and thus the QRS measurement should be less than _____ second in a Junctional Escape Rhythm.

normal
0.12

Figure 39 Mechanism of Junctional Escape Rhythm

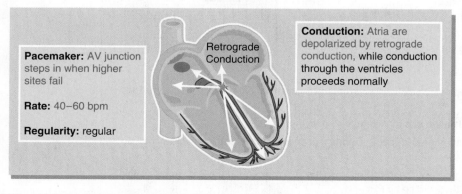

Pacemaker: AV junction steps in when higher sites fail

Rate: 40–60 bpm

Regularity: regular

Retrograde Conduction

Conduction: Atria are depolarized by retrograde conduction, while conduction through the ventricles proceeds normally

When higher pacemaker sites fail, the AV junction is left with pacemaking responsibility. The atria are depolarized via retrograde conduction. Conduction through the ventricles is normal.

Figure 40 Rules for Junctional Escape Rhythm

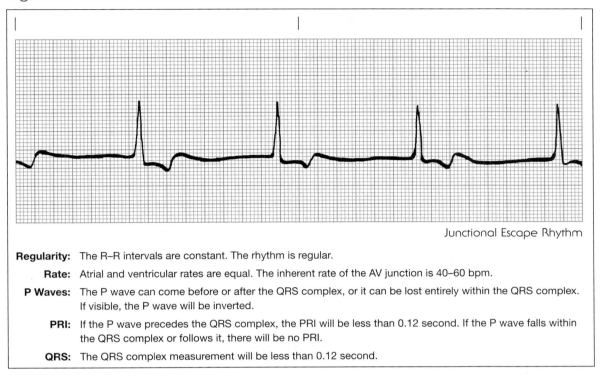

Junctional Escape Rhythm

Regularity: The R–R intervals are constant. The rhythm is regular.

Rate: Atrial and ventricular rates are equal. The inherent rate of the AV junction is 40–60 bpm.

P Waves: The P wave can come before or after the QRS complex, or it can be lost entirely within the QRS complex. If visible, the P wave will be inverted.

PRI: If the P wave precedes the QRS complex, the PRI will be less than 0.12 second. If the P wave falls within the QRS complex or follows it, there will be no PRI.

QRS: The QRS complex measurement will be less than 0.12 second.

33. The rules of Junctional Escape Rhythm (Figure 40) are:

Regularity: regular

Rate: 40–60 bpm

P Wave: will be inverted: can fall before or after the QRS complex or can be hidden within the QRS complex

PRI: can be measured only if the P wave precedes the QRS complex; if measurable, will be less than 0.12 second

QRS: less than 0.12 second

Junctional Tachycardia

34. Junctional Escape Rhythm is a fail-safe mechanism rather than an irritable arrhythmia. However, the AV junction is capable of irritability and is known to produce an irritable arrhythmia called **Junctional Tachycardia**. This rhythm occurs when the junction initiates impulses at a rate _____ than its inherent rate of 40–60 bpm, thus overriding the SA node or other higher pacemaker sites for control of the heart rate. Junctional Escape Rhythm is an escape mechanism, whereas Junctional Tachycardia is an _____ rhythm.

faster

irritable

35. Junctional Tachycardia is usually divided into two categories, depending on how fast the irritable site is firing. If the junction is firing between 60 and 100 bpm, the arrhythmia is termed an **Accelerated Junctional Rhythm** (Figure 41) because a rate below 100 can't really be considered a tachycardia. When the junctional rate exceeds 100 bpm, the rhythm is considered a Junctional Tachycardia (Figure 42). Junctional Tachycardia can be as fast as 180 bpm, but at this rapid rate, it is extremely difficult to identify positively since P waves are superimposed on preceding T waves. When an AV junctional focus fires at a rate of 60–100 bpm, it is termed an _____

Accelerated

Figure 41 Mechanism of Accelerated Junctional Rhythm

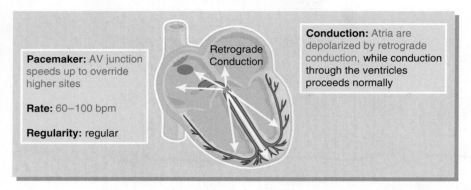

An irritable focus in the AV junction speeds up to override the SA node for control of the heart. The atria are depolarized via retrograde conduction. Conduction through the ventricles is normal.

Figure 42 Mechanism of Junctional Tachycardia

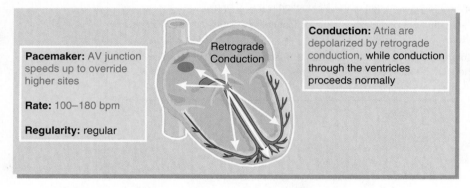

A very rapid irritable focus in the AV junction overrides the SA node for control of the heart. The atria are depolarized via retrograde conduction. Conduction through the ventricles is normal.

Junctional Rhythm. If the rate exceeds 100 bpm, up to a rate of 180 bpm, the rhythm is called a Junctional _____ .

Tachycardia

Accelerated Junctional Rhythm

36. Let's take Accelerated Junctional Rhythm separately first. This is an irritable arrhythmia that originates in the AV junction and fires at a rate of _____ bpm. It will have the inverted P wave typical of junctional arrhythmias, or it may have no P wave if the atria and ventricles depolarize _____ . If the P wave precedes the QRS complex, the PRI should be less than _____ second. Conduction through the ventricles is normal, so the QRS complex should have a _____ measurement of less than 0.12 second.

60–100

simultaneously

0.12

normal

37. Here are the rules for Accelerated Junctional Rhythm (Figure 43):

Regularity: regular

Rate: 60–100 bpm

P Wave: will be inverted; can fall before or after the QRS complex or can be hidden within the QRS complex

PRI: can be measured only if the P wave precedes the QRS complex; if measurable, will be less than 0.12 second

QRS: less than 0.12 second

Figure 43 Rules for Accelerated Junctional Rhythm

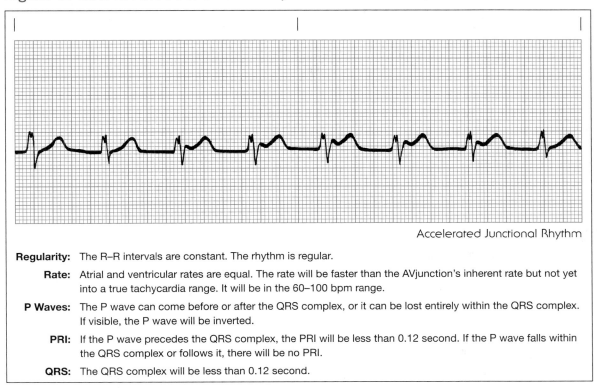

Accelerated Junctional Rhythm

Regularity: The R–R intervals are constant. The rhythm is regular.

Rate: Atrial and ventricular rates are equal. The rate will be faster than the AVjunction's inherent rate but not yet into a true tachycardia range. It will be in the 60–100 bpm range.

P Waves: The P wave can come before or after the QRS complex, or it can be lost entirely within the QRS complex. If visible, the P wave will be inverted.

PRI: If the P wave precedes the QRS complex, the PRI will be less than 0.12 second. If the P wave falls within the QRS complex or follows it, there will be no PRI.

QRS: The QRS complex will be less than 0.12 second.

38. When the AV junction fires in the tachycardia range (100–180 bpm) the rhythm will remain regular. The P waves will be inverted and can fall before or after the QRS complex, or they might be absent if they are _____ within the QRS complex. When the P wave precedes the QRS complex, the PRI will be _____ than 0.12 second. Since conduction through the ventricles is normal, the QRS complex will be less than _____ second.

hidden

less

0.12

39. The rules for **Junctional Tachycardia** (Figure 44) are:

Regularity: regular

Rate: 100–180 bpm

P Wave: will be inverted; can fall before or after the QRS complex or can be hidden within the QRS complex

PRI: can be measured only if the P wave precedes the QRS complex; if measurable, will be less than 0.12 second

QRS: less than 0.12 second

40. The only difference you will see on the EKG among Junctional Escape Rhythm, Accelerated Junctional Rhythm, and Junctional Tachycardia is the rate. The rates are:

Junctional Escape Rhythm   40–60 bpm

Accelerated Junctional Rhythm   60–100 bpm

Junctional Tachycardia   100–180 bpm

Each of these rhythms originates in the _____ , and will thus produce an inverted P wave because of retrograde conduction. Depending on whether the atria or ventricles depolarize first, the P wave can come before, during, or after the

AV junction

Figure 44 Rules for Junctional Tachycardia

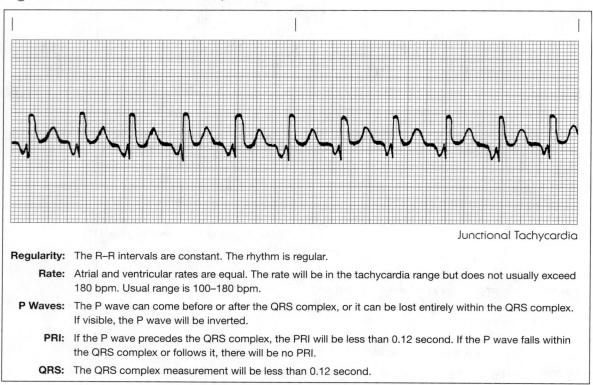

Junctional Tachycardia

Regularity: The R–R intervals are constant. The rhythm is regular.

Rate: Atrial and ventricular rates are equal. The rate will be in the tachycardia range but does not usually exceed 180 bpm. Usual range is 100–180 bpm.

P Waves: The P wave can come before or after the QRS complex, or it can be lost entirely within the QRS complex. If visible, the P wave will be inverted.

PRI: If the P wave precedes the QRS complex, the PRI will be less than 0.12 second. If the P wave falls within the QRS complex or follows it, there will be no PRI.

QRS: The QRS complex measurement will be less than 0.12 second.

QRS complex. If the P wave precedes the QRS complex, the PRI will be less than 0.12 second. The QRS measurement will be normal. If the rate is 40–60 bpm, the rhythm is called _____ Rhythm. If the rate is between 60 and 100 bpm, the rhythm is termed _____ Junctional Rhythm, and the rhythm is called Junctional Tachycardia if the rate is _____ bpm.

Junctional Escape
Accelerated
100–180

41. A junctional impulse that reaches the atria before the ventricles will produce an inverted P wave that falls _____ the QRS complex. Such a beat would have a PRI of less than _____ second. If the PRI were greater than 0.12 second, you would suspect that the impulse originated in the _____ .

before
0.12

atria

42. A regular rhythm with a QRS complex of less than 0.12 second and a rate of 50 bpm, which did not have any visible P waves, would fit the rules for a _____ Rhythm.

Junctional Escape

43. A single premature ectopic beat originating from an irritable focus in the AV junction would be called a PJC, or _____ . Such a beat would have an inverted P wave _____ , _____ , or _____ the QRS complex.

Premature Junctional Complex
before; during
after

44. All junctional arrhythmias have the same general characteristics; that is, they all have _____ P waves that can occur before, during, or after a QRS complex; the PRI will be _____ ; and the QRS will be _____ . However, not all junctional arrhythmias have the same mechanism. PJCs, Junctional Tachycardia, and Accelerated Junctional Rhythm are all caused by irritability, whereas a junctional rhythm within its inherent rate of 40–60 bpm would be an indication of an _____ mechanism.

inverted
shortened
normal

escape

Supraventricular Tachycardia

45. You have now learned several arrhythmias that are regular and beat at such a rapid rate that the P wave might not be discernible from the T wave. If you include Junctional Tachycardia, which might not have a visible P wave, you have a group of tachycardias that are regular and don't have visible P waves. The ventricular rates for these arrhythmias are:

Sinus Tachycardia	100–160 bpm
Atrial Tachycardia	150–250 bpm
Atrial Flutter	150–250 bpm
Junctional Tachycardia	100–180 bpm

From these rate ranges you can see that as the rate exceeds 150 or 160 bpm, a rate at which the P wave could very well be encroaching on the preceding _____ wave, you would have no way to distinguish between these   T arrhythmias. Since you can't accurately identify the rhythm, you would instead give it a descriptive identification. The term that's used to describe this category of indistinguishable arrhythmias is **Supraventricular Tachycardias** (Figure 45).

46. A Supraventricular Tachycardia (SVT) is not the name of a specific _____ . It is a term that's used to _____ a category   arrhythmia; describe of several regular tachyarrhythmias that can't be identified more accurately because they have indistinguishable _____ waves and fall within a common   P _____ range.   rate

47. The rates at which you most commonly need to use the term _Supraventricular Tachycardia_ is the 150–250 range, although sometimes a slower rate will still have obscured P waves. An SVT is usually a toss-up between Atrial Tachycardia and Junctional Tachycardia, although Sinus Tachycardia and, less commonly, Atrial Flutter can also be in the running. These arrhythmias can only be called SVT if they cannot be identified more accurately. It is not a catch-all phrase. To be called SVT, an arrhythmia must be _____ , have no visible   regular _____ waves, and have a _____ range common   P; rate to other arrhythmias, thereby making further and more accurate identification _____ .   impossible

Figure 45 Overlapping Rates in Supraventricular Tachycardia

	RATE (bpm)															
	100	110	120	130	140	150	160	170	180	190	200	210	220	230	240	250
Sinus Tachycardia																
Atrial Tachycardia																
Atrial Flutter																
Junctional Tachycardia																

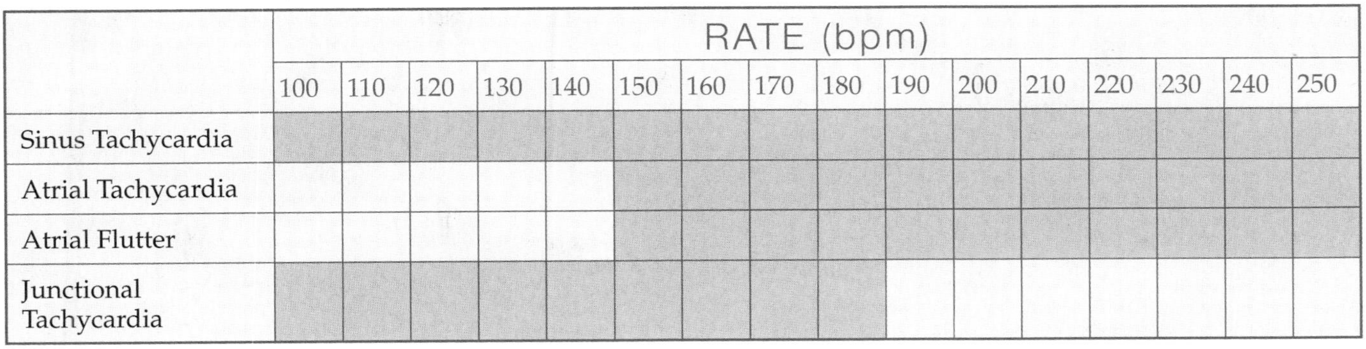

48. You now know about four more arrhythmias—those that originate in the AV junction. You have learned the characteristics that these arrhythmias share and how they differ from rhythms that originate in other pacemaker sites. You also learned that several of the tachycardias cannot always be differentiated, because they might have similar rate ranges and obscured P waves. When this situation exists, you can only describe the rhythm as a Supraventricular Tachycardia, rather than giving it a specific name. Now you must practice applying this knowledge to actual interpretation of rhythm strips. Turn to the Practice Strips at the end of this chapter and practice applying your new knowledge until you feel very comfortable in this area.

Practice Strips

KEY POINTS

- Rhythms that originate in the AV junction include:
  - Premature Junctional Complex
  - Junctional Escape Rhythm
  - Accelerated Junctional Rhythm
  - Junctional Tachycardia

- Junctional arrhythmias will create an inverted P wave because the atria are depolarized via retrograde conduction.

- A junctional impulse will depolarize the ventricles in a normal manner at about the same time that the atria are being depolarized with retrograde conduction.

- A junctional rhythm can have the inverted P wave occurring before, during, or after the QRS complex.

- All junctional arrhythmias will create an inverted P wave, but some low atrial impulses can also cause inverted P waves.

- All junctional arrhythmias will have a PRI of less than 0.12 second.

- The rules for *Premature Junctional Complex* are:

Regularity:	depends on regularity of underlying arrhythmia
Rate:	depends on rate of underlying arrhythmia
P Waves:	will be inverted; can fall before, during, or after the QRS complex
PRI:	can only be measured if the P wave precedes the QRS complex; if measurable, will be less than 0.12 second
QRS:	less than 0.12 second

- A PJC is an irritable ectopic.

- The normal inherent rate of the AV junction is 40–60 bpm.

- If higher pacemaker sites fail, a junctional escape pacemaker might take over control of the heart. This is called Junctional Escape Rhythm.

- The rules for *Junctional Escape Rhythm:*

Regularity:	regular
Rate:	40–60 bpm
P Waves:	will be inverted; can fall before, during, or after the QRS complex
PRI:	can be measured only if the P wave precedes the QRS complex; if measurable, will be less than 0.12 second
QRS:	less than 0.12 second

- If the AV junction becomes irritable, it can speed up and override higher pacemaker sites. This arrhythmia is called Junctional Tachycardia.

- Junctional Tachycardia is usually divided into two categories, depending on rate:

60–100 bpm	Accelerated Junctional Rhythm
100–180 bpm	Junctional Tachycardia

- The rules for *Accelerated Junctional Rhythm* are:

Regularity:	regular
Rate:	60–100 bpm
P Waves:	will be inverted; can fall before, during, or after the QRS complex
PRI:	can be measured only if the P wave precedes the QRS complex; if measurable, will be less than 0.12 second
QRS:	less than 0.12 second

- The rules for *Junctional Tachycardia* are:

Regularity:	regular
Rate:	100–180 bpm
P Waves:	will be inverted; can fall before, during, or after the QRS complex
PRI:	can be measured only if the P wave precedes the QRS complex; if measurable, will be less than 0.12 second
QRS:	less than 0.12 second

- If a rapid arrhythmia is regular, has no visible P waves, and has a rate range common to other arrhythmias, thereby making more accurate identification impossible, the arrhythmia is termed Supraventricular Tachycardia.

SELF-TEST

Directions: Complete this self-evaluation of the information you have learned from this chapter. If your answers are all correct and you feel comfortable with your understanding of the material, proceed to the next chapter. However, if you miss any of the questions, you should review the referenced frames before proceeding. If you feel unsure of any of the underlying principles, invest the time now to go back over the entire chapter. **Do not proceed with the next chapter until you are very comfortable with the material in this chapter.**

Questions	Referenced Frames	Answers
1. What does the P wave look like in a junctional rhythm?	5, 6, 7, 8, 10, 11, 17, 44	The P is always inverted, even though it is often hidden in the QRS complex.
2. How do you explain the unusual configuration of the P wave in junctional rhythms?	2, 3, 4, 5, 6, 7	The atria are depolarized via retrograde conduction. Since the electrical flow will be traveling away from the positive electrode in Lead II, the wave form will be negative.
3. Will the QRS complex be normal in a junctional rhythm?	3, 5, 10	Yes, even though atrial depolarization is retrograde, ventricular depolarization will be normal. The QRS complex should measure less than 0.12 second.
4. Does an inverted P wave always indicate a junctional rhythm?	8, 9, 12, 13, 14	No, atrial rhythms can also have inverted P waves if the impulse originated low enough in the atria. You can differentiate between the two by looking at the PRI; in a junctional rhythm it will be less than 0.12 second.
5. Where will the P wave be located in a junctional rhythm?	6, 7, 10, 15, 16, 17, 41	It can fall before or after the QRS complex, or it can be hidden within the QRS complex. In the latter, it will appear as if the rhythm has no P wave at all.
6. What is the biggest clue to a junctional rhythm?	8	the inverted P wave
7. What is a PJC?	19, 20, 21, 25, 43	A Premature Junctional Complex is a single beat that originates from an irritable focus in the AV junction.
8. Will a PJC have a P wave?	22, 23, 25	Yes, the P wave will be inverted, either before or after the QRS complex or it can be hidden within the QRS complex.
9. What will the PRI be for a PJC?	23, 25	If the P wave is in front of the QRS complex, the PRI will be less than 0.12 second. Otherwise, there will be no PRI.
10. Does a PJC come earlier or later than expected in the cardiac cycle?	19, 20, 25	earlier
11. What will the QRS measurement be for a PJC?	24, 25	Since conduction through the ventricles is normal, the QRS measurement should be less than 0.12 second.
12. What is the normal, inherent rate for the AV junction?	26, 27, 28, 44	40–60 bpm
13. What is a Junctional Escape Rhythm?	26, 27, 28, 33, 34, 42	It is an escape mechanism that occurs when a higher pacemaking site fails and the AV junction has to take over at its own inherent rate of 40–60 bpm.
14. Is Junctional Escape Rhythm regular or irregular?	29, 33	regular

Questions	Referenced Frames	Answers
15. What will the P waves look like for this arrhythmia?	30, 33	They will be inverted: they can fall before or after the QRS complex or can be hidden within the QRS complex.
16. Will the PRI measurement be normal for a Junctional Escape Rhythm?	31, 33	No, if the P wave precedes the QRS, the PRI will be less than 0.12 second. If it falls within the QRS or after the QRS, there will be no PRI.
17. What is the rate range for an Accelerated Junctional Rhythm?	35, 36, 37, 40	60–100 bpm
18. Is Accelerated Junctional Rhythm regular or irregular?	37, 40	regular
19. What is the P wave like in Accelerated Junctional Rhythm?	36, 37, 40	Just like the P wave in all other junctional rhythms: it is inverted and can fall before, during, or after the QRS complex.
20. Is the QRS measurement normal for Accelerated Junctional Rhythm?	36, 37, 40	Yes, since the conduction through to the ventricles is normal, the QRS should measure less than 0.12 second.
21. What is the rate range for Junctional Tachycardia?	35, 39, 40	100–180 bpm
22. Is a Junctional Tachycardia regular or irregular?	38, 39, 40	regular
23. What does the P wave look like in Junctional Tachycardia?	38, 39, 40	It is probably not visible since the rate is so fast that it might be hidden in the T waves, or it might be occurring within the QRS complex. If it is visible, it will be inverted either before or after the QRS complex.
24. Is the QRS measurement normal for Junctional Tachycardia?	38, 39, 40	Yes, it should be less than 0.12 second.
25. Is the PRI measurement normal for Junctional Tachycardia?	38, 39, 40	No, if the P wave precedes the QRS complex, the PRI will be less than 0.12 second. Otherwise, there will be no PRI.
26. When can you call an arrhythmia a Supraventricular Tachycardia?	45, 46, 47, 48	only when you have a regular rhythm, in a tachycardia range with no visible P waves, and at a rate that is common to more than one arrhythmia, thereby making more accurate identification impossible
27. Which arrhythmias commonly need to be described as Supraventricular Tachycardias?	45, 46, 47, 48	The most common ones are Atrial Tachycardia and Junctional Tachycardia, although the term is also used to describe Sinus Tachycardia and Atrial Flutter.
28. At what rate would you expect to have trouble discerning P waves and might consider calling an arrhythmia Supraventricular Tachycardia?	47	usually 150–250 bpm, although you may lose the P waves at slower rates

PRACTICE STRIPS (answers can be found in the Answer Key on page 556)

6.1

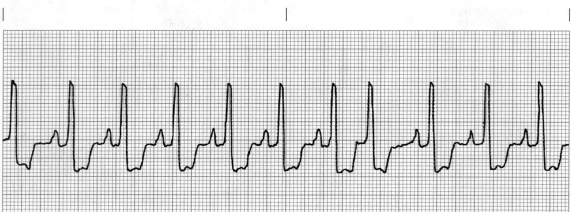

Regularity: _____	**PRI:** _____
Rate: _____	**QRS:** _____
P Waves: _____	**Interp:** _____

6.2

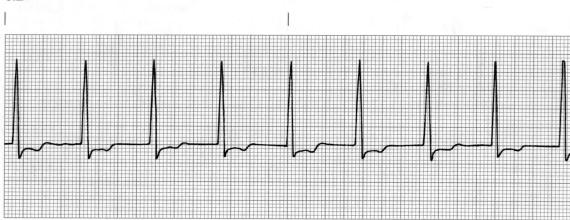

Regularity: _____	**PRI:** _____
Rate: _____	**QRS:** _____
P Waves: _____	**Interp:** _____

6.3

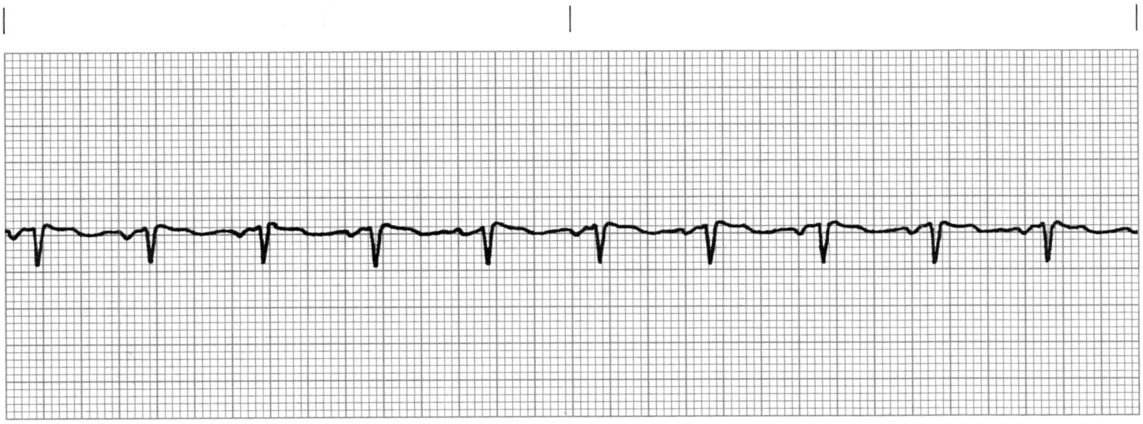

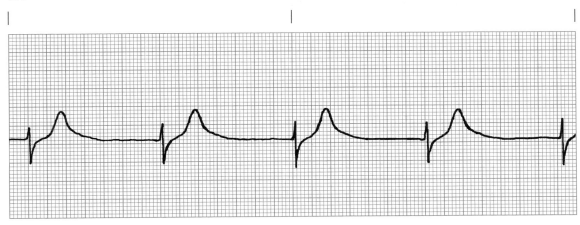

Regularity: _____   PRI: _____

Rate: _____   QRS: _____

P Waves: _____   Interp: _____

6.4

Regularity: _____   PRI: _____

Rate: _____   QRS: _____

P Waves: _____   Interp: _____

6.5

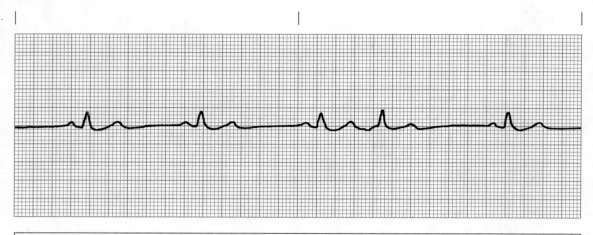

Regularity: _____   PRI: _____

Rate: _____   QRS: _____

P Waves: _____   Interp: _____

6.6

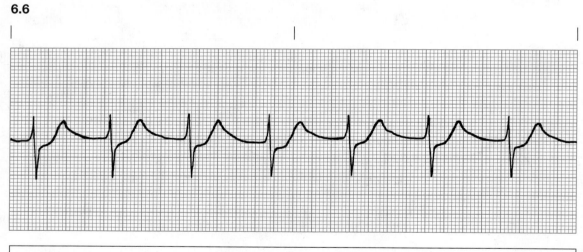

Regularity: _____   PRI: _____

Rate: _____   QRS: _____

P Waves: _____   Interp: _____

6.7

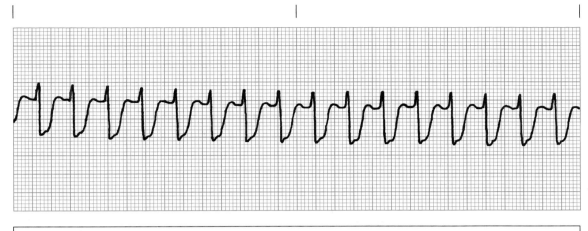

Regularity: _____   PRI: _____

Rate: _____   QRS: _____

P Waves: _____   Interp: _____

6.8

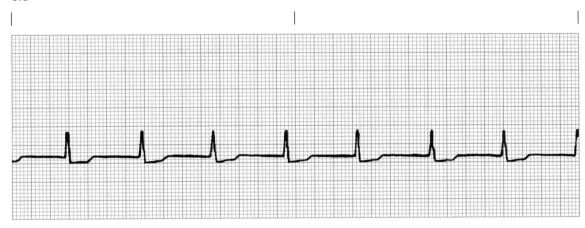

Regularity: _____   PRI: _____

Rate: _____   QRS: _____

P Waves: _____   Interp: _____

6.9

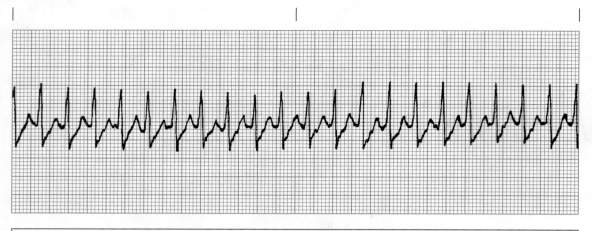

Regularity: _____ PRI: _____

Rate: _____ QRS: _____

P Waves: _____ Interp: _____

6.10

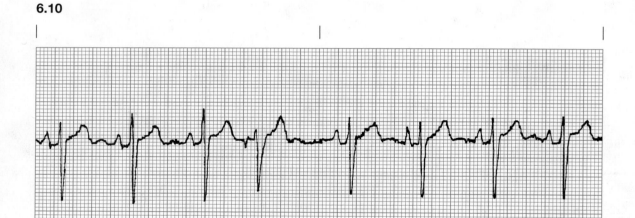

Regularity: _____ PRI: _____

Rate: _____ QRS: _____

P Waves: _____ Interp: _____

6.11

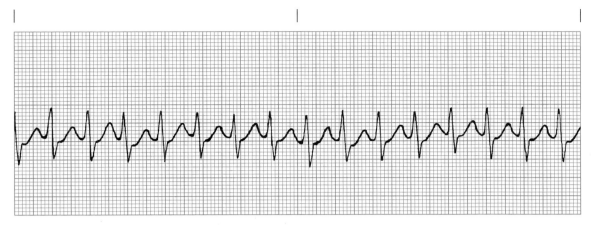

Regularity: _____	PRI: _____
Rate: _____	QRS: _____
P Waves: _____	Interp: _____

6.12

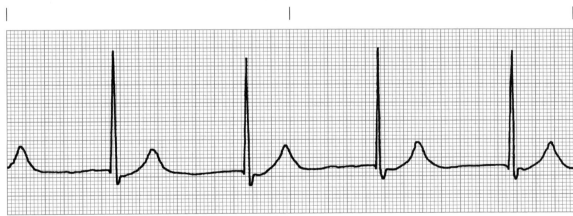

Regularity: _____	PRI: _____
Rate: _____	QRS: _____
P Waves: _____	Interp: _____

6.13

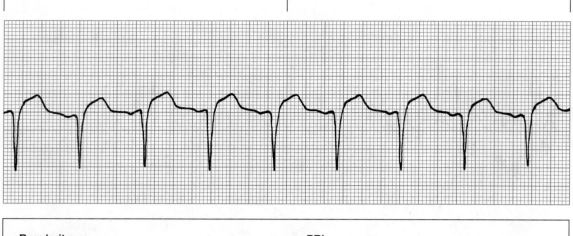

Regularity: _____   PRI: _____

Rate: _____   QRS: _____

P Waves: _____   Interp: _____

6.14

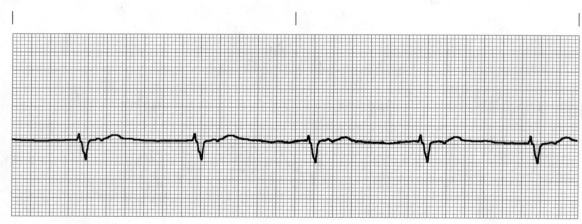

Regularity: _____   PRI: _____

Rate: _____   QRS: _____

P Waves: _____   Interp: _____

6.15

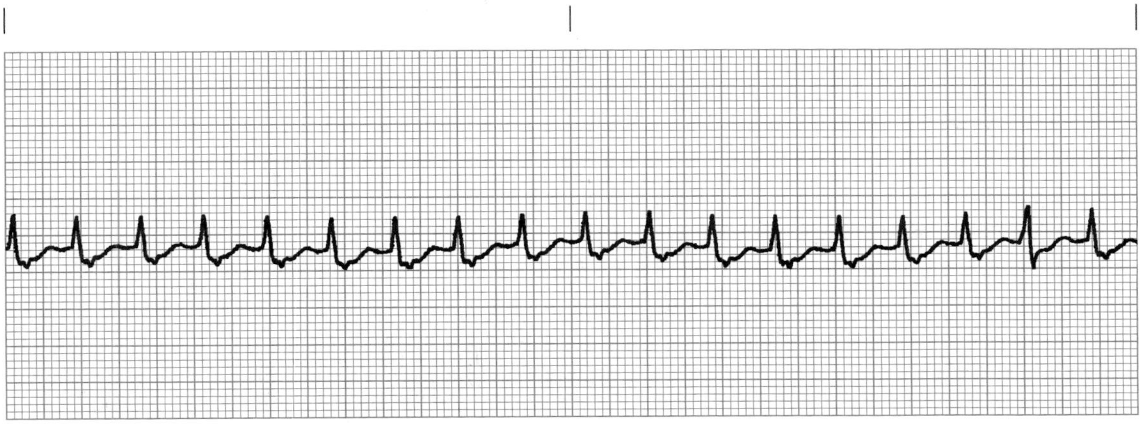

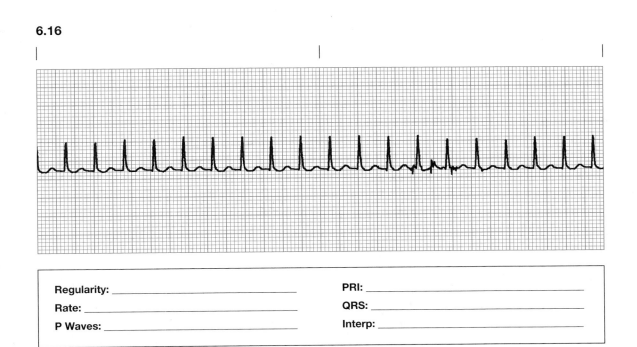

Regularity: _____	PRI: _____
Rate: _____	QRS: _____
P Waves: _____	Interp: _____

6.16

Regularity: _____	PRI: _____
Rate: _____	QRS: _____
P Waves: _____	Interp: _____

6.17

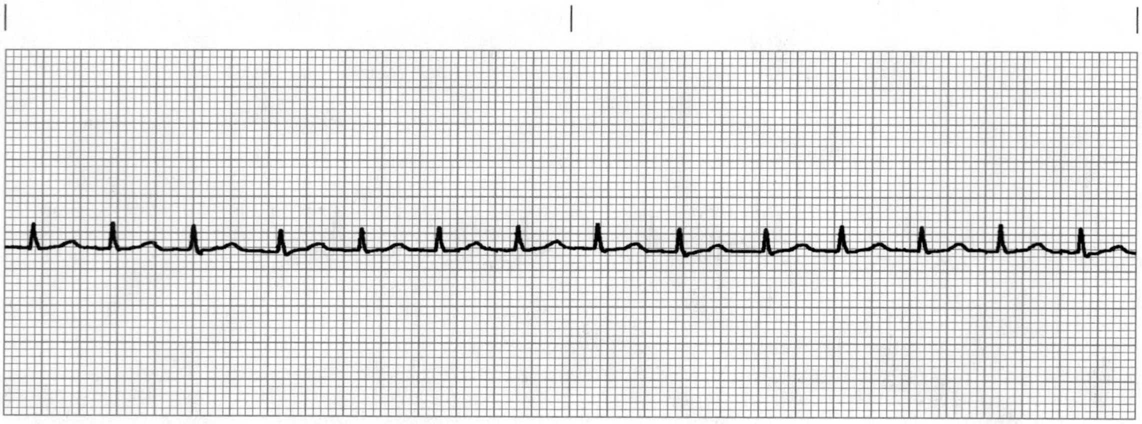

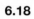

Regularity: _____	PRI: _____
Rate: _____	QRS: _____
P Waves: _____	Interp: _____

6.18

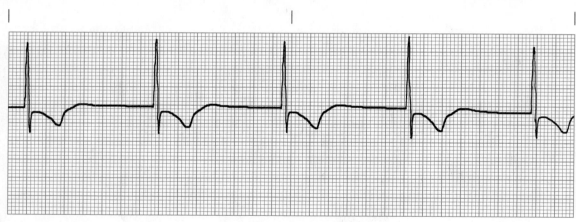

Regularity: _____	PRI: _____
Rate: _____	QRS: _____
P Waves: _____	Interp: _____

6.19

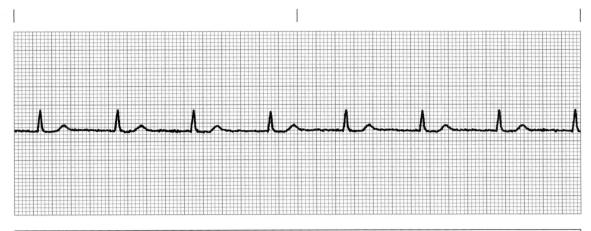

Regularity: _____	PRI: _____
Rate: _____	QRS: _____
P Waves: _____	Interp: _____

6.20

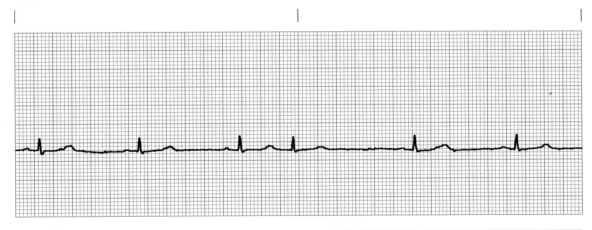

Regularity: _____	PRI: _____
Rate: _____	QRS: _____
P Waves: _____	Interp: _____

6.21

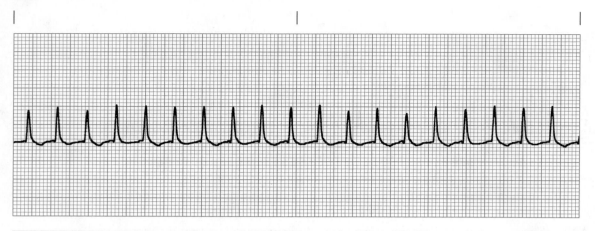

Regularity: _____	PRI: _____
Rate: _____	QRS: _____
P Waves: _____	Interp: _____

6.22

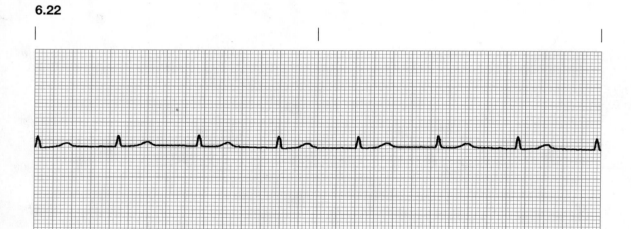

Regularity: _____	PRI: _____
Rate: _____	QRS: _____
P Waves: _____	Interp: _____

6.23

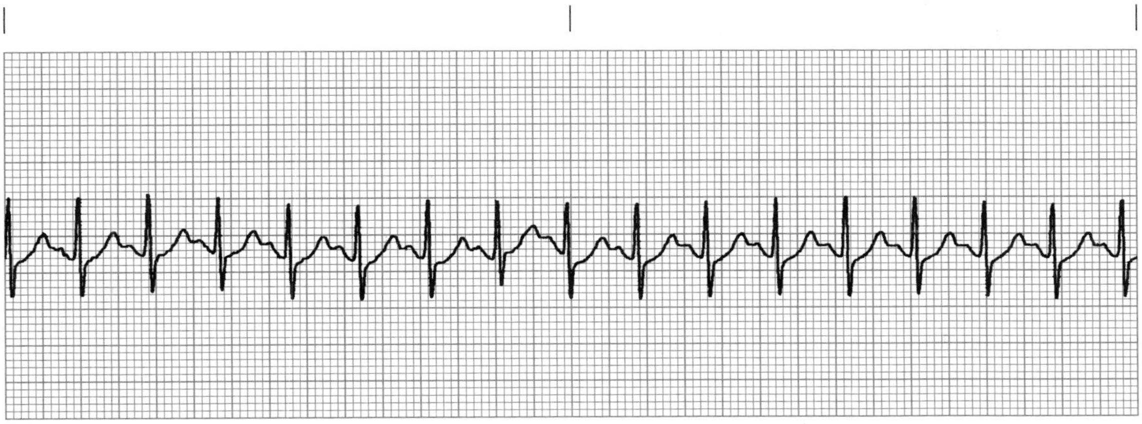

Regularity: _____	PRI: _____
Rate: _____	QRS: _____
P Waves: _____	Interp: _____

6.24

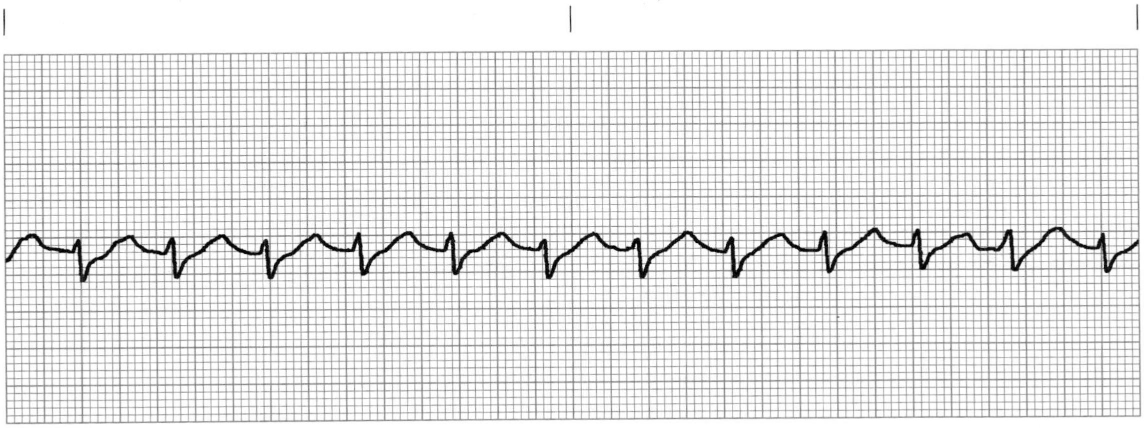

Regularity: _____	PRI: _____
Rate: _____	QRS: _____
P Waves: _____	Interp: _____

6.25

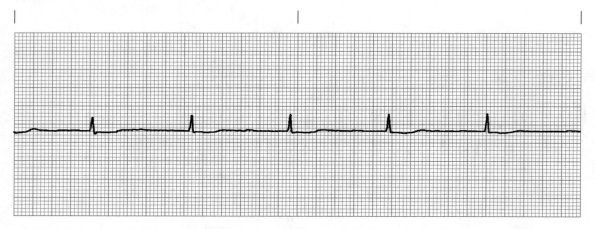

Regularity: _____	PRI: _____
Rate: _____	QRS: _____
P Waves: _____	Interp: _____

6.26

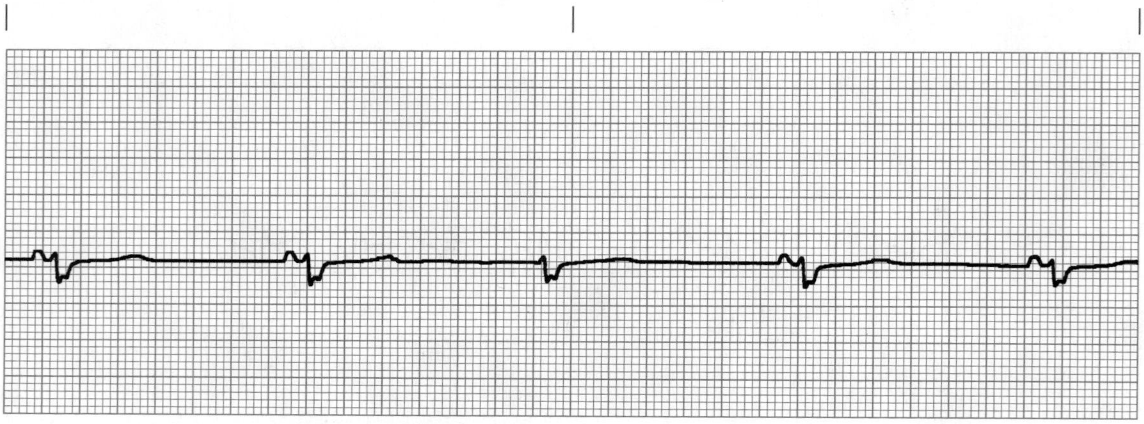

Regularity: _____	PRI: _____
Rate: _____	QRS: _____
P Waves: _____	Interp: _____

6.27

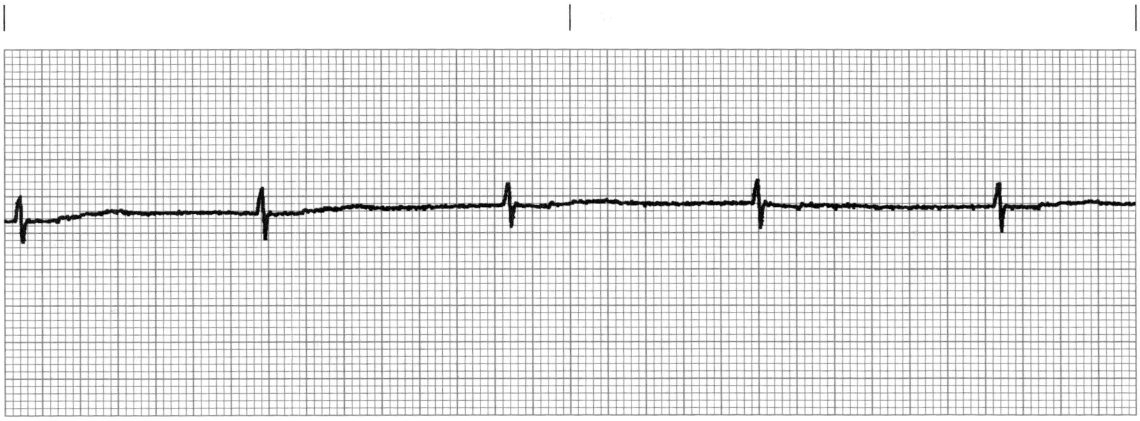

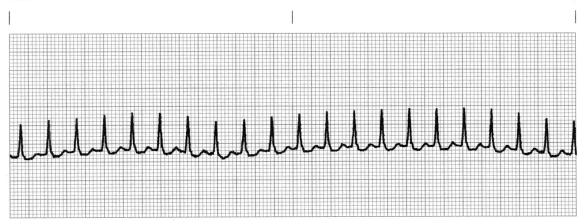

Regularity: _____	**PRI:** _____
Rate: _____	**QRS:** _____
P Waves: _____	**Interp:** _____

6.28

Regularity: _____	**PRI:** _____
Rate: _____	**QRS:** _____
P Waves: _____	**Interp:** _____

6.29

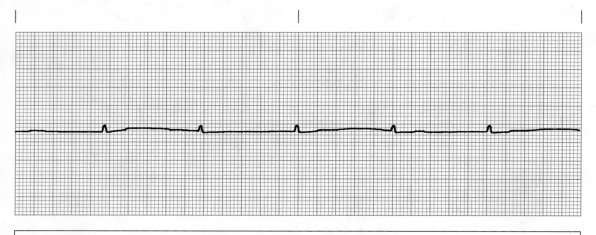

Regularity: _____	**PRI:** _____
Rate: _____	**QRS:** _____
P Waves: _____	**Interp:** _____

6.30

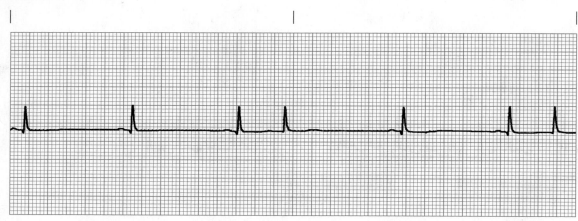

Regularity: _____	**PRI:** _____
Rate: _____	**QRS:** _____
P Waves: _____	**Interp:** _____

6.31

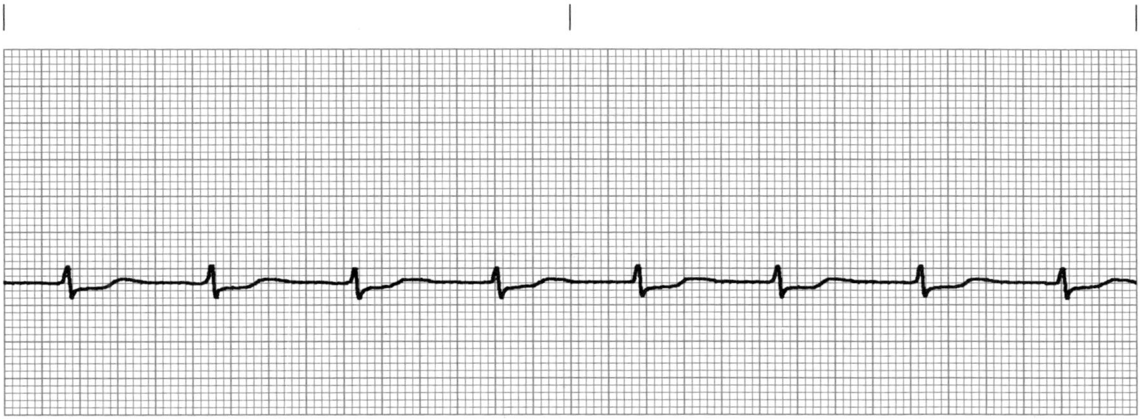

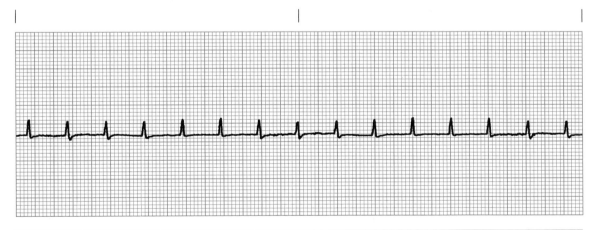

Regularity: _____	PRI: _____
Rate: _____	QRS: _____
P Waves: _____	Interp: _____

6.32

Regularity: _____	PRI: _____
Rate: _____	QRS: _____
P Waves: _____	Interp: _____

6.33

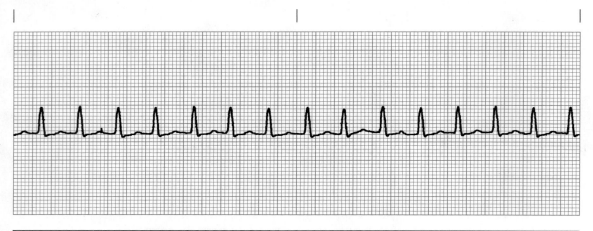

Regularity: _____	**PRI:** _____	
Rate: _____	**QRS:** _____	
P Waves: _____	**Interp:** _____	

6.34

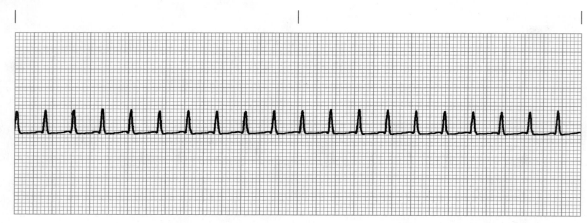

Regularity: _____	**PRI:** _____	
Rate: _____	**QRS:** _____	
P Waves: _____	**Interp:** _____	

6.35

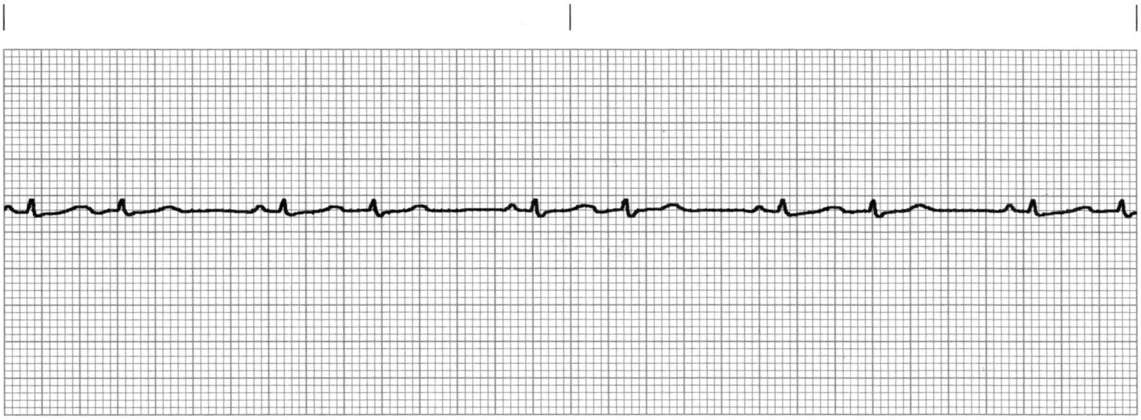

Regularity: _____	PRI: _____
Rate: _____	QRS: _____
P Waves: _____	Interp: _____

6.36

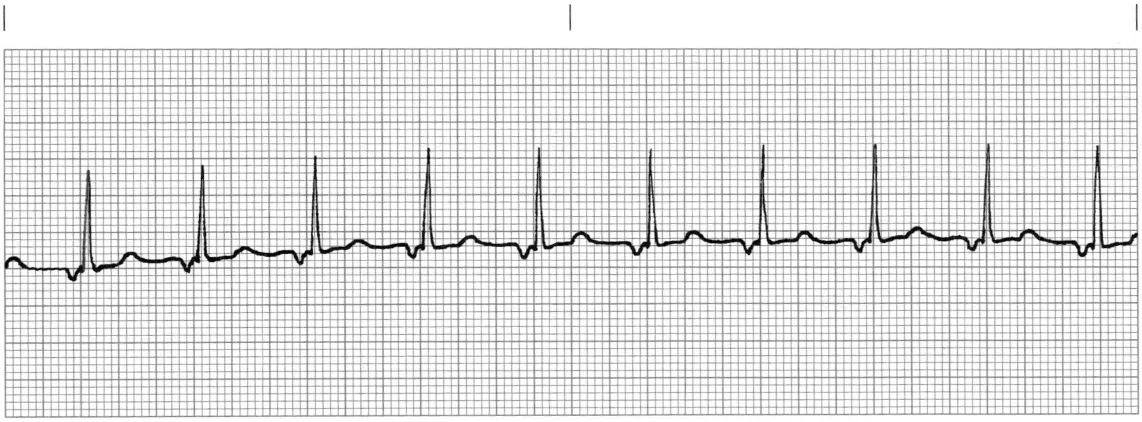

Regularity: _____	PRI: _____
Rate: _____	QRS: _____
P Waves: _____	Interp: _____

6.37

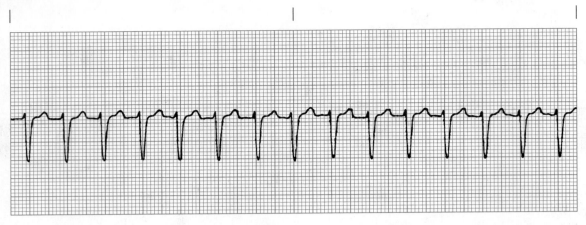

Regularity: _____	PRI: _____	
Rate: _____	QRS: _____	
P Waves: _____	Interp: _____	

6.38

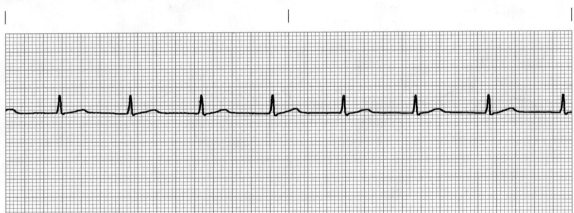

Regularity: _____	PRI: _____	
Rate: _____	QRS: _____	
P Waves: _____	Interp: _____	

6.39

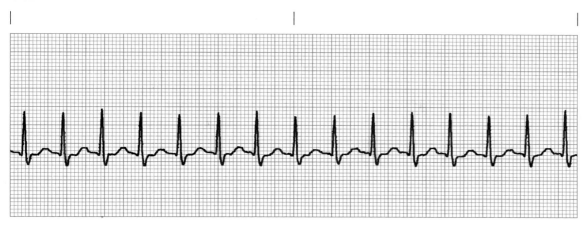

Regularity: _____	PRI: _____
Rate: _____	QRS: _____
P Waves: _____	Interp: _____

6.40

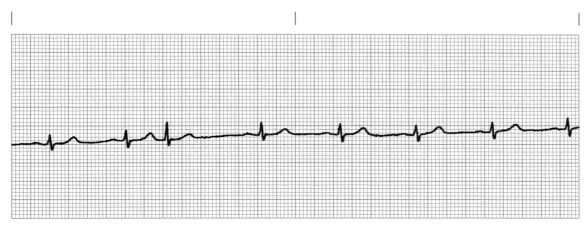

Regularity: _____	PRI: _____
Rate: _____	QRS: _____
P Waves: _____	Interp: _____

6.41

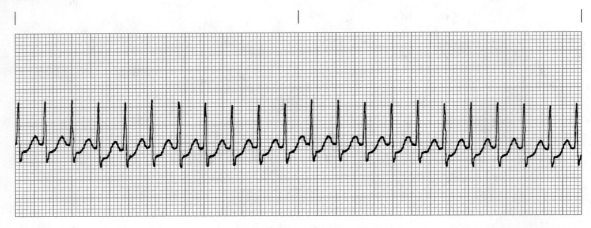

Regularity: _____   PRI: _____

Rate: _____   QRS: _____

P Waves: _____   Interp: _____

Chapter 7
Heart Blocks

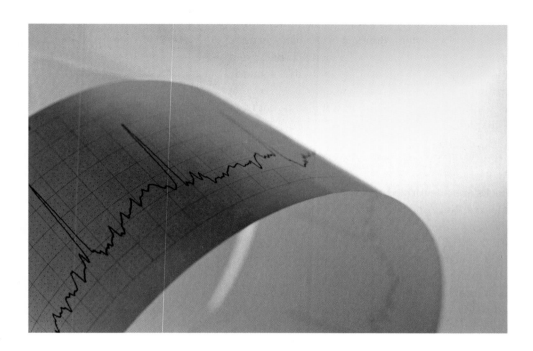

Overview

IN THIS CHAPTER, you will learn to recognize arrhythmias that are manifestations of conduction defects (blocks) at the AV node, and you will learn to describe characteristics that are common to this category of arrhythmia. You will then learn the names and features of four different arrhythmias that are in this category called Heart Blocks. For each of these arrhythmias, you will learn about the etiology, conduction, and resulting EKG features (regularity, rate, P waves, PR intervals, and QRS complexes).

Conduction Through the AV Node

1. In the preceding chapter you learned about four arrhythmias that originate in the AV junction. You will next learn about four different arrhythmias that don't actually *originate* in the AV junction but are the result of conduction disturbances at the AV node (or sometimes just below it, within or below the Bundle of His). Each of these arrhythmias is caused when an impulse that originates above the AV node, usually in the sinus node, has trouble getting through the AV node to the ventricles. This category of arrhythmias is most commonly called **heart block** because conduction fails to make it through the AV node to depolarize the ventricles normally. Heart blocks are

arrhythmias caused when a supraventricular impulse is unable to be conducted normally through to the ventricles because of a conduction disturbance at or below the _____ . Because this is a basic book, we will not explore the different | **AV node**
pathology sites around the AV node. Instead, we are going to cluster these areas of pathology by calling them all conduction problems *at the AV node.* You will know that when we say the block is "at the node," we include the entire area of the node. This means that the block might be in the node, below the node, and even lower in the Bundle of _____ . | **His**

Note: You may hear people refer to another type of block, called *bundle branch block.* This is a condition caused by a conduction defect below the area of the node, within one of the branches of the *ventricular* conduction system. Bundle branch block is not a rhythm itself, but it does cause a rhythm to have an abnormally wide QRS. Because it is not an arrhythmia, and because it is analyzed using a 12-lead EKG rather than the single-lead rhythm strips we are learning about here, we will not learn about bundle branch block now. It is mentioned here only so you will realize that it is different from the AV heart blocks discussed in this chapter.

Heart Blocks

2. The different types of AV heart blocks are categorized according to the severity of obstruction at the AV node. A **First-Degree Block** indicates that the obstruction at the _____ is not complete; all impulses are conducted but each under- | **AV node**
goes a delay before being transmitted to the _____ . A **Second-** | **ventricles**
Degree Heart Block means that there is an actual block, but it is intermittent; some of the impulses will be conducted through to the ventricles, but others will not. A **Third-Degree Block** means that the block is complete; that is, none of the impulses will be conducted through to the ventricles. First-Degree Block is the mildest because it is a delay rather than an actual block. In a First-Degree Block, each impulse is delayed but all are conducted through to the _____ . A Second-Degree Block is | **ventricles**
more serious because some impulses are actually _____ , whereas | **blocked**
others are allowed to be conducted through to the ventricles. Third--Degree is the most serious because _____ of the impulses reach the ventricles; | **none**
Third-Degree Block is also called a **Complete Heart Block** (CHB).

3. This is an easy way to divide the blocks:

When **all** beats are conducted, it's _____ -Degree Heart Block. | **First**

When **some** beats are conducted, it's _____ -Degree Heart Block. | **Second**

And if **no** beats are conducted, it's _____ -Degree Heart Block. | **Third**

First-and Third-Degree Blocks are easy—each has only one arrhythmia to learn. The Second-Degree group gets a little more complicated. As Figure 46 shows, Second-Degree Block can be subdivided into several more categories because there are a number of different conditions that can cause intermittent block. It would be very confusing to try learning them all at one time, so we're going to simplify your job: We'll cluster all the Second-Degree Blocks into two groups, Type I and Type II. In this chapter you will learn these four types of heart block:

- First Degree
- Second Degree—Type I (Wenckebach) (pronounced wink´-ee-bok)
- Second Degree—Type II (combining Type II, 2:1, and High Grade)
- Third Degree (Complete Heart Block)

Figure 46 AV Heart Blocks

MECHANISM OF BLOCK

FIRST-DEGREE

- Not a true block
- Delay at the AV node
- Each impulse is eventually conducted

SECOND-DEGREE

TYPE I
  - Wenckebach
TYPE II
  - Type II
  - 2:1 AV Block
  - High-Grade AV Block

- Intermittent block: some beats are conducted, others are blocked
- Pathology can be within the AV node or below it in the Bundle of His
- Pathology is often blended with other types of block

THIRD-DEGREE
Complete Heart Block

- Atria and ventricles are completely dissociated
- There is a total block at the AV node

Each of these is considered a heart block because there is a disturbance in conduction through the AV _____ .

node

4. A First-Degree Heart Block is not really a true block at all, because each impulse *is* conducted through to the ventricles. But it is included with the blocks because a partial block exists, which causes a _____ in transmission of each impulse to the ventricles.

delay

5. Both types of Second-Degree Heart Block exhibit some type of intermittent block at the AV node. Both types allow some impulses through to the ventricles, whereas others are _____ .

blocked

6. There are two types of Second-Degree Heart Block: Type I and Type II. Both types of Second-Degree Heart Block allow some impulses through to the ventricles while intermittently _____ others.

blocking

7. Third-Degree Block is called _____ Heart Block (CHB) because all impulses are completely _____ at the AV node; no impulses are allowed through to the ventricles.

Complete
blocked

First-Degree Heart Block

8. Now that you have a general idea of the types of heart blocks and the mechanisms of each, let's take each one individually and examine it in more detail. We'll start with First-Degree Heart Block (Figure 47) because it is the least serious. First-Degree Heart Block is the least _____ of all the heart blocks because, even though it does cause a _____ in conduction, it still allows _____ impulses through to the ventricles.

serious
delay
all

9. As you recall, atrial depolarization is depicted on the EKG by the _____ , and the delay in the AV node is shown by the

P wave

Figure 47 Mechanism of First-Degree Heart Block

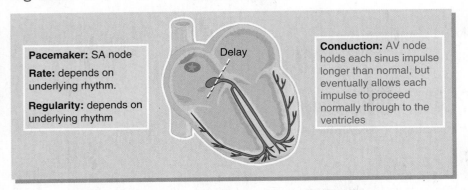

Pacemaker: SA node

Rate: depends on underlying rhythm.

Regularity: depends on underlying rhythm

Delay

Conduction: AV node holds each sinus impulse longer than normal, but eventually allows each impulse to proceed normally through to the ventricles

The AV node holds each impulse longer than normal before conducting it through to the ventricles. Each impulse is eventually conducted. Once into the ventricles, conduction proceeds normally. *This is not a rhythm itself, but a conduction problem affecting an underlying rhythm, which also must be identified.*

_____ segment. Together, these make up the PR   PR _____ . Thus, if a heart block causes an increased delay in the AV   interval node, you would expect the PRI to become prolonged. This is one of the foremost clues to a First-Degree Heart Block. In First-Degree Heart Block, the PRI is _____ than usual.   longer

10. It's important to keep in mind with First-Degree Heart Block that each sinus impulse, even though delayed in the AV node, does eventually reach the ventricles to depolarize them. The PRI will be _____ but will be the same dura-   prolonged tion from one beat to the next. This is because each pacemaker impulse is coming from the same site (usually the SA node) and is being conducted in the same manner through the AV node. So each impulse takes the same amount of time to pass through the atria and is delayed the same amount of time in the AV node. Even though the PRI is _____ in First-Degree Heart Block, all of the PRIs will be the same   prolonged length because they all come from the same site and are conducted in the same manner.

11. Thus, by definition, the PRI in First-Degree Heart Block must be longer than 0.20 second and must be constant from one beat to the next. This is the only abnormality in this arrhythmia. Ventricular conduction is normal, producing a QRS complex of less than _____ second. Because the SA node is the usual pace-   0.12 maker, the rhythm is usually regular, although this can change if the underlying rhythm is something other than NSR. First-Degree Heart Block is usually regular, has a PRI greater than _____ second, and each PRI is the same as all   0.20 other _____ across the strip. Because ventricular conduction is nor-   PRIs mal, the QRS will be less than _____ second.   0.12

12. At this point it should be apparent that First-Degree Heart Block is not really a rhythm itself but is actually a condition that is superimposed on another arrhythmia. This is an important distinction to keep in mind because you will also need to identify the underlying arrhythmia. For example, if you have a rhythm that fits all of the rules for Sinus Tachycardia except that the PRI is prolonged, you would call the rhythm Sinus Tachycardia with _____ -Degree Heart Block. In the same   First way, if the underlying rhythm fits the definition for NSR except that the PRI was greater than 0.20 second, you would call the arrhythmia a Sinus Rhythm with _____ Block.   First-Degree

Figure 48 Rules for First-Degree Heart Block

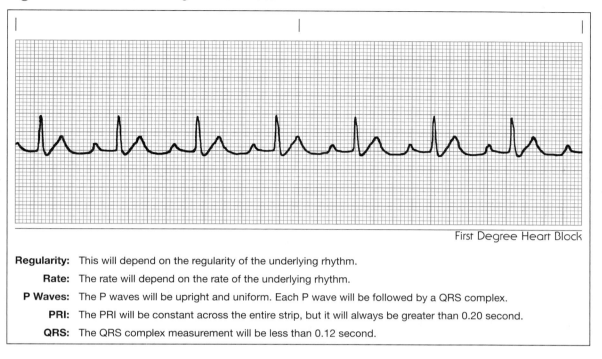

First Degree Heart Block

Regularity:	This will depend on the regularity of the underlying rhythm.
Rate:	The rate will depend on the rate of the underlying rhythm.
P Waves:	The P waves will be upright and uniform. Each P wave will be followed by a QRS complex.
PRI:	The PRI will be constant across the entire strip, but it will always be greater than 0.20 second.
QRS:	The QRS complex measurement will be less than 0.12 second.

13. First-Degree Heart Block is not a rhythm in itself. It is a prolonged PRI in an otherwise normal rhythm. Thus, in addition to recognizing that a First-Degree Heart Block exists, you must also identify the _____ rhythm.

underlying

14. Here are the rules for First-Degree Heart Block (Figure 48):

Regularity:	depends on underlying rhythm
Rate:	depends on underlying rhythm
P Waves:	upright and uniform; each P wave will be followed by a QRS complex
PRI:	greater than 0.20 second; constant across the strip
QRS:	less than 0.12 second

Second-Degree Heart Blocks

15. There are two types of Second-Degree Heart Block. Both occur when the AV node begins selectively blocking impulses that are being initiated in the SA node. On the EKG this will be seen as normal P waves, but not every one will be followed by a QRS complex. This indicates that the atria are being depolarized normally but that not every impulse is being conducted through to the ventricles. Hence, you will see more _____ depolarizations than _____ depolarizations. In Second-Degree Heart Block, you will always see more _____ waves than _____ complexes.

atrial; ventricular

P

QRS

16. With all heart blocks, the problem is the way pacemaker impulses are conducted through to the ventricles. Because there is no pathology in the sinus node itself, you would expect the P waves to be _____ in all the blocks, and the P–P interval should be regular. Where you will see evidence of block is in the EKG features that show the relationship between atrial and ventricular activity, namely, the _____ intervals and the ratio of P waves to _____ complexes. The PRIs might change, and there can be more P waves than

normal

PR; QRS

Figure 49   Blocked P Waves

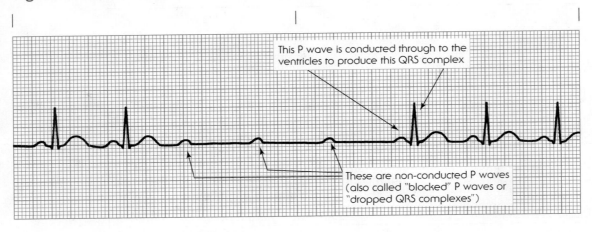

This P wave is conducted through to the ventricles to produce this QRS complex

These are non-conducted P waves (also called "blocked" P waves or "dropped QRS complexes")

_____ complexes, but you would expect the P–P intervals to be _____ across the strip.

QRS

regular

17. A key feature of Second-Degree Heart Blocks is that not every P wave is followed by a QRS complex. Sometimes you will see P waves without an associated ventricular depolarization (Figure 49). The appearance of P waves without a subsequent QRS complex indicates that the atria were depolarized by a pacemaker impulse, but that impulse was not conducted through to the _____ because it was blocked at the _____ .

ventricles

AV node

18. An important distinction is that some of the impulses *are* being conducted to the ventricles. Therefore, the QRS complexes you do see were conducted from the same impulse that produced the immediately preceding P wave. When a sinus impulse passes through the AV node and depolarizes the ventricles normally, the QRS measurement will be _____ . On those complexes that are preceded by a P wave with a normal PRI, you would expect the QRS to measure less than _____ second. However, we know that this isn't always the case with Second-Degree Block. Conduction is often delayed below the node, causing the QRS to be greater than _____ second. When this happens, you can simply identify the rhythm and note that it has a "wide QRS."

normal

0.12

0.12

19. Regardless of the QRS measurement, both types of Second-Degree Block will have some P waves that are followed by QRS complexes and some that are not. Even though some pacemaker impulses are blocked at the AV node, some *do* get through to depolarize the _____ .

ventricles

20. There are two categories of Second-Degree Heart Block. One is called Wenckebach (Type I), and the other is called Type II. In both types, the impulse originates in the sinus node but is conducted through the AV node in an intermittent fashion. That is, not every P wave will be followed by a QRS complex. These arrhythmias are classified as Second-Degree Heart Block because some of the impulses *are* conducted through the AV node, but others are not. In Second-Degree Heart Block the AV node is unreliable in conducting impulses. Conduction to the ventricles is accomplished only on an _____ basis.

intermittent

21. The difference between Wenckebach and Type II Second-Degree Block is the *pattern* in which the P waves are blocked. Because the activity of the AV node is depicted

by the _____ interval, the PRI is the most important clue to distin-   PR
guishing between these two arrhythmias. When attempting to distinguish between
Wenckebach and a Type II Second-Degree Heart Block, you should concentrate on the
_____ intervals.   PR

Type II Second-Degree Heart Block

22. Let's skip Wenckebach for the moment and look first at Type II -Second-Degree
Heart Block. Type II Heart Block is really a grouping of several types of blocks with
similar mechanisms. We're not going to learn each of them separately; we'll just look
at them as a single rhythm. In Type II Second-Degree Heart Block (Figure 50), the AV
node selectively chooses either to conduct or block individual impulses from the SA
node. This results in a pattern of _____ P waves than QRS com-   more
plexes. Sometimes the AV node will allow every other P wave to be conducted, resulting in a ratio of two P waves for one QRS, called a 2:1 conduction ratio. When every
third P is conducted, the pattern is 3:1. You might also see 4:3, 5:4, or other ratios, but
there will always be more _____ waves than _____   P; QRS
complexes.

23. Sometimes the ratio will vary within one strip. That is, rather than maintaining a
constant ratio across the strip, the ratio will change: for example, 4:3, 3:2, 4:3, 3:2, all
within one strip (Figure 51). This is called variable conduction. Conduction ratios refer
to the number of P waves to QRS complexes and can be constant across the strip or
can _____ within a single strip.   vary

24. Regardless of the conduction ratio, there will always be more
_____ waves than QRS complexes. However, when you do see QRS   P
complexes, the PR intervals preceding them will all have the same measurement
because conduction through the node proceeds uniformly on conducted beats. Hence,
the PRI in a Type II Second-Degree Block will always be *constant* from one complex to
the next across the entire strip. This is probably the most important feature about a
Type II Second-Degree Heart Block. The PRI will always be _____   constant
on those complexes that were conducted.

25. It is also possible for a Type II Second-Degree Heart Block to have a prolonged
PRI. That is, the PRI will be constant across the strip, there will be more than one
P wave for every QRS complex, and the PRI will be greater than 0.20 second on the

Figure 50 Mechanism of Type II Second-Degree Heart Block

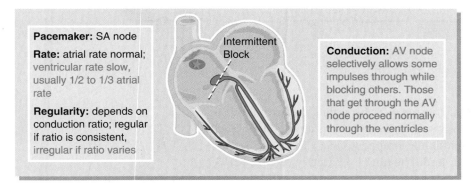

Pacemaker: SA node

Rate: atrial rate normal; ventricular rate slow, usually 1/2 to 1/3 atrial rate

Regularity: depends on conduction ratio; regular if ratio is consistent, irregular if ratio varies

Intermittent Block

Conduction: AV node selectively allows some impulses through while blocking others. Those that get through the AV node proceed normally through the ventricles

The AV node selectively conducts some beats while blocking others. Those that are not blocked are conducted through to the ventricles, although they may encounter a slight delay in the node. Once in the ventricles, conduction proceeds normally.

Figure 51 Examples of Conduction Ratios in Type II Second-Degree Heart Block

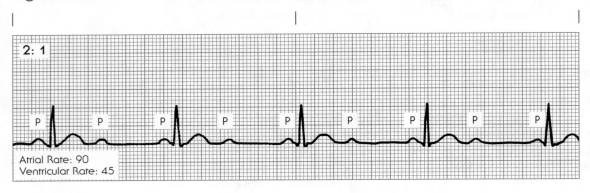

2: 1

Atrial Rate: 90
Ventricular Rate: 45

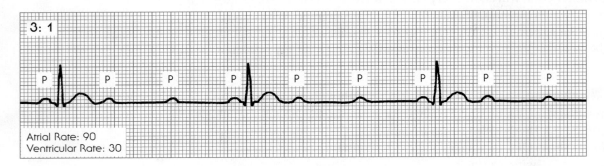

3: 1

Atrial Rate: 90
Ventricular Rate: 30

4:1

Atrial Rate: 90
Ventricular Rate: 22

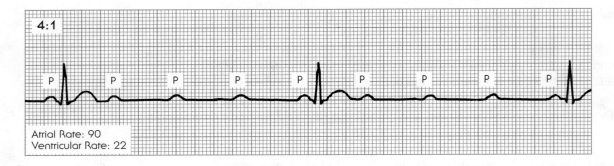

Variable

Atrial Rate: 90
Ventricular Varies

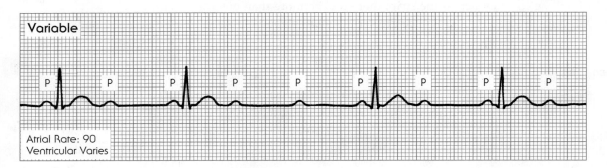

conducted beats. However, even though this fits the rules for calling the arrhythmia a Second-Degree Heart Block with a First-Degree Heart Block, this is a redundant label and should not be used. Such an arrhythmia should simply be called a Type II Second-Degree Heart Block, and the PRI duration should be noted separately (Figure 52). A Type II Second-Degree Heart Block must have a _____ PRI on conducted beats, and the PRI may even be _____ . Regardless, it is not called a First-Degree Heart Block but simply a Type II _____ -Degree Heart Block.

constant

prolonged

Second

Figure 52 Type II Second-Degree Heart Block with a Prolonged PRI

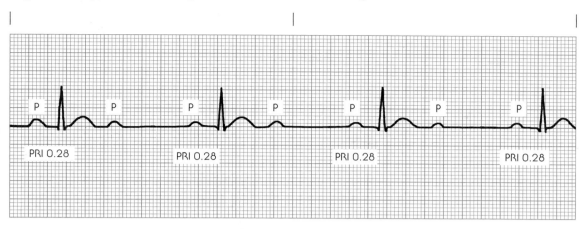

When a Type II Second-Degree Heart Block has a prolonged PRI on the conducted beats, it is still called a Second-Degree Heart Block, *not* a Second-Degree Heart Block with a First-Degree Heart Block.

26. Because the normal rate for the sinus node is _____ bpm, and a   60–100
Type II Second-Degree Heart Block conducts only some of the sinus impulses, the ventricular rate for Type II Second-Degree Heart Block will generally be in the bradycardia range. Often the rate will be one-half to one-third the normal rate, depending on the ratio of conduction. In Type II Second-Degree Heart Block, the ventricular rate will be _____ than normal because many of the impulses are blocked at   slower
the AV node.

27. The regularity of the R–R intervals will depend on the manner in which the AV node is blocking the impulses. If it is a regular ratio of block (e.g., always 2:1, or always 4:3, etc.), the ventricular rhythm will be regular. However, if the ratio is variable (e.g., 3:2, 4:3, 3:2, 5:4, etc.), the ventricular rhythm will be irregular. Type II Second-Degree Heart Block can be regular or irregular, depending on the conduction _____ .   ratio

28. Here are the rules for Type II Second-Degree Heart Block (Figure 53):

Regularity:	R–R interval can be regular or irregular; P–P interval is regular
Rate:	usually in the bradycardia range (< 60 bpm); can be one-half to one-third the normal rate
P Waves:	upright and uniform; more than one P wave for every QRS complex
PRI:	always constant across the strip; can be greater than 0.20 second
QRS:	less than 0.12 second

Wenckebach (Type I Second-Degree Heart Block)

29. Now that we've looked at Type II Second-Degree Heart Block, let's go back to Type I. This rhythm is called Wenckebach (Figure 54), after the man who first defined it. Wenckebach is a _____ -Degree Heart Block, but its conduction   Second
pattern is distinctly different than Type II Second-Degree Heart Block, even though they both result in some "blocked" (non-conducted) beats.

Figure 53   Rules for Type II Second-Degree Heart Block

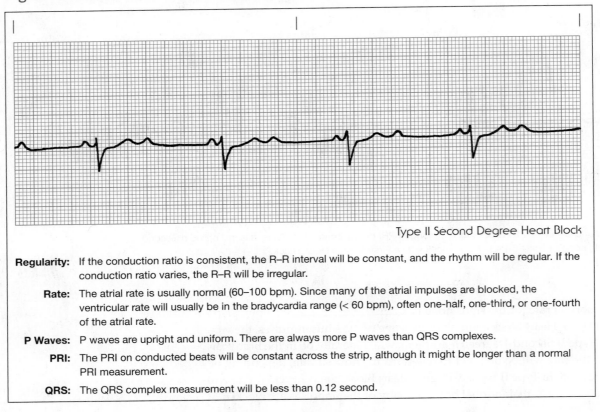

Type II Second Degree Heart Block

Regularity: If the conduction ratio is consistent, the R–R interval will be constant, and the rhythm will be regular. If the conduction ratio varies, the R–R will be irregular.

Rate: The atrial rate is usually normal (60–100 bpm). Since many of the atrial impulses are blocked, the ventricular rate will usually be in the bradycardia range (< 60 bpm), often one-half, one-third, or one-fourth of the atrial rate.

P Waves: P waves are upright and uniform. There are always more P waves than QRS complexes.

PRI: The PRI on conducted beats will be constant across the strip, although it might be longer than a normal PRI measurement.

QRS: The QRS complex measurement will be less than 0.12 second.

30.   As with Type II Second-Degree Heart Block, the key to recognizing a Wenckebach is in the PR intervals. Each PRI will get progressively longer until you see a P wave without a resultant QRS complex. Then the cycle starts again with the shortest PRI. As you measure the PRIs across the strip, you will notice a pattern of "long PRI, longer PRI, longer PRI, longer PRI, blocked P wave." This conduction cycle runs continuously across the strip. Wenckebach is characterized by increasingly long PRIs followed by a _____ P wave.

blocked

31.   The classic cycle seen with Wenckebach does not have to adhere to the 5:4 conduction ratio described in the previous frame. It can have any variety of conduction ratios:

Figure 54   Mechanism of Wenckebach (Type I Second-Degree Heart Block)

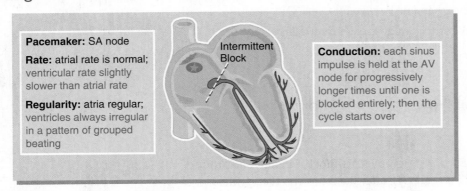

Pacemaker: SA node

Rate: atrial rate is normal; ventricular rate slightly slower than atrial rate

Regularity: atria regular; ventricles always irregular in a pattern of grouped beating

Intermittent Block

Conduction: each sinus impulse is held at the AV node for progressively longer times until one is blocked entirely; then the cycle starts over

As the sinus node initiates impulses, each one is delayed in the AV node a little longer than the preceding one, until one impulse is eventually blocked completely. Those impulses that are conducted travel normally through the ventricles.

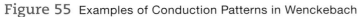

Figure 55 Examples of Conduction Patterns in Wenckebach

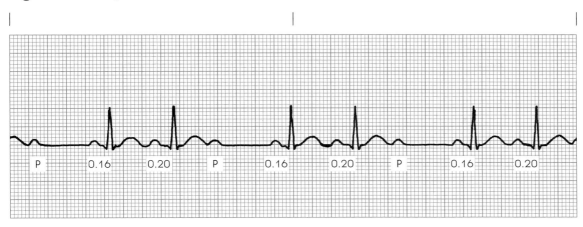

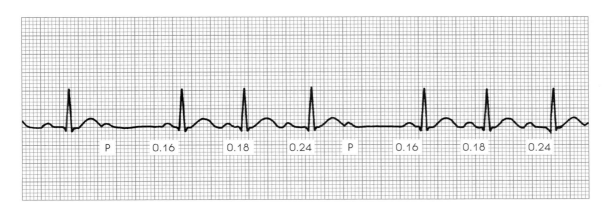

4:3 (long, longer, longer, blocked), 3:2 (long, longer, blocked), or even variable (Figure 55). However, it will consistently follow a pattern of increasing PRIs until one P wave is not followed by a QRS complex. Regardless of the conduction ratio, a Wenckebach will always have progressively longer _____ intervals   PR with blocked P waves.

32. As with Type II Second-Degree Heart Block, those P waves that are conducted are expected to produce normal QRS complexes, meaning that the QRS measurements in Wenckebach should be less than _____ second. *(Of course, we know*   0.12 *that all the blocks frequently have wide QRS complexes because they so often have associated conduction disturbances lower in the conduction system. However, Wenckebach alone would have a normal QRS measurement.)*

33. Because the PR intervals are changing in Wenckebach and some of the QRS complexes are being dropped, the R–R intervals will be irregular. The changing PRI creates a cyclic pattern to the irregularity. Wenckebach has an _____ R–R   irregular interval that reflects the changes in the PR intervals.

34. However, Wenckebach does not usually block out as many P waves as does Type II Second-Degree Heart Block. Therefore, the rate of a Wenckebach is generally faster than Type II block but probably in the low/normal range. Because Wenckebach usually conducts two out of three, or three out of four, impulses, the ventricular rate will be somewhat slower than normal but still _____ than a Type II Sec-   faster ond-Degree Heart Block.

Figure 56 Rules for Wenckebach

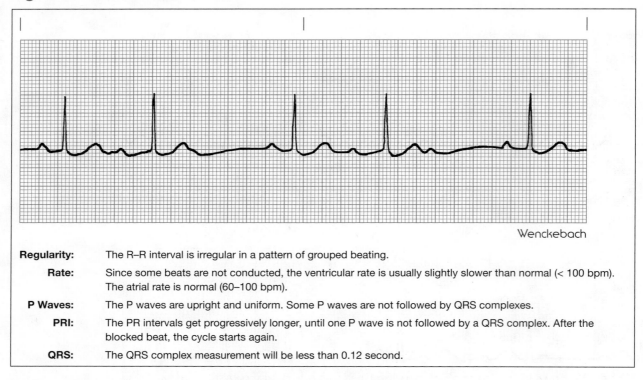

Wenckebach

Regularity:	The R–R interval is irregular in a pattern of grouped beating.
Rate:	Since some beats are not conducted, the ventricular rate is usually slightly slower than normal (< 100 bpm). The atrial rate is normal (60–100 bpm).
P Waves:	The P waves are upright and uniform. Some P waves are not followed by QRS complexes.
PRI:	The PR intervals get progressively longer, until one P wave is not followed by a QRS complex. After the blocked beat, the cycle starts again.
QRS:	The QRS complex measurement will be less than 0.12 second.

35. Here are the rules for Wenckebach Type I Second-Degree Heart Block (Figure 56):

Regularity:	irregular in a pattern of grouped beating
Rate:	usually slightly slower than normal
P Waves:	upright and uniform; some P waves are not followed by QRS complexes
PRI:	progressively lengthens until one P wave is blocked
QRS:	less than 0.12 second

Third-Degree Heart Block (Complete Heart Block)

36. You now know that First-Degree Heart Block is simply a _____ in conduction of impulses from the SA node through the AV node, but each of the impulses *is* conducted. Both types of Second-Degree Heart Block have intermittent AV conduction, where some impulses are conducted but others are _____ . We'll now look at Third-Degree Heart Block, where *none* of the impulses is conducted because of a total block at the AV node. Third-Degree Heart Block is also called Complete Heart Block (CHB) (Figure 57) because the block at the _____ is complete.

delay

blocked

AV node

37. The pathology of CHB is at the AV node; the higher pacemaker in the SA node is not affected. Therefore, the P waves will be normal, and atrial activity will be within a normal rate range. However, all of the P waves are blocked at the node. This means that the ventricles won't be _____ , and, unless one of the heart's fail-safe mechanisms comes into play, they won't be able to _____ to pump blood. Because CHB involves a total block at the AV node, a lower escape mechanism will have to take over to _____ the ventricles.

depolarized

contract

depolarize

Figure 57 Mechanism of Complete Heart Block (CHB)

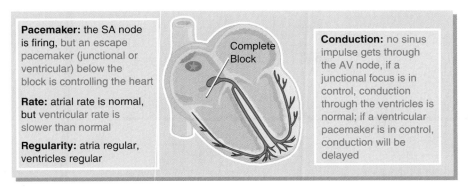

Pacemaker: the SA node is firing, but an escape pacemaker (junctional or ventricular) below the block is controlling the heart

Rate: atrial rate is normal, but ventricular rate is slower than normal

Regularity: atria regular, ventricles regular

Complete Block

Conduction: no sinus impulse gets through the AV node, if a junctional focus is in control, conduction through the ventricles is normal; if a ventricular pacemaker is in control, conduction will be delayed

The block at the AV node is complete. The sinus beats cannot penetrate the node and thus are not conducted through to the ventricles. An escape mechanism from either the junction or the ventricles will take over to pace the -ventricles. The atria and ventricles function in a totally dissociated fashion.

38. If possible, a junctional focus below the block site will take over pacemaking responsibilities by initiating a junctional _____ rhythm to depolar-   escape
ize the ventricles. However, if damage to the node extends into the junction, a ventricular focus may have to assume pacemaking responsibility. In either case, the ventricles are controlled by a lower escape focus. In CHB, the SA node functions normally but cannot get past the block at the AV node, so a lower escape focus in either the AV junction or the _____ takes over to control ventricular   ventricles
activity.

39. This means that ventricular activity will fall into one of two categories. If it originates in the AV junction, the rate will be in the range of _____ bpm,   40–60
and the QRS complex will measure less than 0.12 second. But if a ventricular focus initiates the escape rhythm, the rate will be _____ bpm, and the   20–40
QRS will be wider than 0.12 second because of longer conduction time within the ventricles. This information can help you determine the source of the ventricular pacemaker. If the rate is 20–40 and the QRS complex is greater than 0.12 second, you assume that the impulse is _____ in origin. But if the junction initi-   ventricular
ated the rhythm, the QRS complex is usually less than 0.12 second and the rate will be _____ bpm. Remember, though, that because lower sites are less   40–60
reliable than higher sites, and because the blocks often involve more than one type of conduction pathology, both the rate and QRS ranges are guidelines rather than concrete rules.

40. While all this takes place, the SA node continues to control the atria. When you have two pacemakers controlling the upper and lower chambers of the heart without regard to each other, the situation is called atrioventricular (A–V) dissociation—the atria and the ventricles are *dissociated* (Figure 58). A–V dissociation is not a rhythm in itself. It is a description of the condition that exists in CHB (and some other arrhythmias) when the atria and ventricles function totally _____ of each   independently
other. On the EKG you will see normal P waves marching regularly across the strip. You will also see QRS complexes at regular intervals. But the two wave forms will not have any _____ to each other. The PRIs will be totally inconsistent,   relation
and you may even see P waves superimposed in the middle of QRS complexes. There will be more P waves than QRS complexes because the intrinsic rate of the sinus node is _____ than either the junctional or ventricular rate. In CHB, the   faster
_____ waves will have absolutely no relation to the QRS complexes,   P
and you may even see P waves superimposed on QRS complexes.

Figure 58 A–V Dissociation in CHB

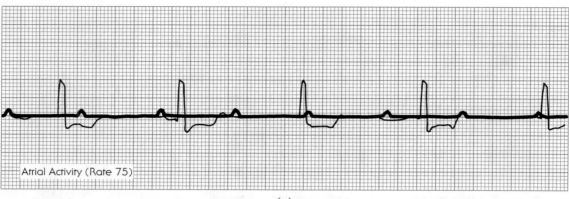

Atrial Activity (Rate 75)

(a)

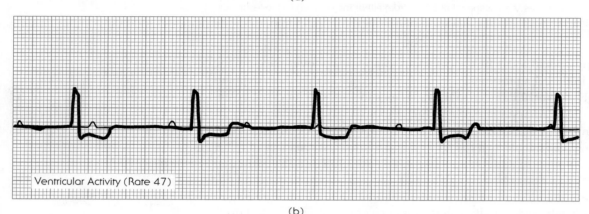

Ventricular Activity (Rate 47)

(b)

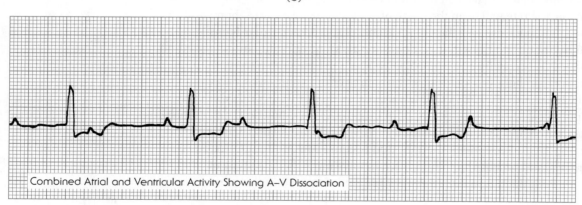

Combined Atrial and Ventricular Activity Showing A–V Dissociation

(c)

41. As with other forms of AV block, the PRI is one of your most important clues to interpreting CHB. In CHB, the PRIs are totally inconsistent across the strip. The P waves have no relation to the QRS complexes; thus, the PR intervals will *not* be

_____ .

constant

42. Another important feature about CHB is that the R–R interval is regular. This is an important item to remember because the PRIs can occasionally appear to be progressively lengthening and can be confused with Wenckebach. This is purely coincidental, however, because the atria and ventricles are completely _____ in Third-Degree Heart Block. If you are trying to distinguish a Wenckebach from a CHB, you should recall that the R–R interval in CHB is _____ , whereas in Wenckebach the R–R interval is _____ .

dissociated

regular

irregular

Figure 59 Rules for Complete Heart Block

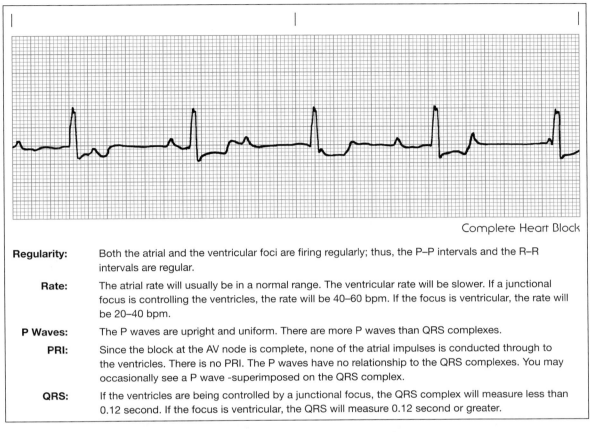

Complete Heart Block

Regularity:	Both the atrial and the ventricular foci are firing regularly; thus, the P–P intervals and the R–R intervals are regular.
Rate:	The atrial rate will usually be in a normal range. The ventricular rate will be slower. If a junctional focus is controlling the ventricles, the rate will be 40–60 bpm. If the focus is ventricular, the rate will be 20–40 bpm.
P Waves:	The P waves are upright and uniform. There are more P waves than QRS complexes.
PRI:	Since the block at the AV node is complete, none of the atrial impulses is conducted through to the ventricles. There is no PRI. The P waves have no relationship to the QRS complexes. You may occasionally see a P wave -superimposed on the QRS complex.
QRS:	If the ventricles are being controlled by a junctional focus, the QRS complex will measure less than 0.12 second. If the focus is ventricular, the QRS will measure 0.12 second or greater.

43. Here are the rules for Third-Degree Heart Block (CHB) (Figure 59):

Regularity:	regular
Rate:	AR—usually normal (60–100 bpm);
	VR—40–60 if focus is junctional; 20–40 if focus is ventricular
P Waves:	upright and uniform; more P waves than QRS complexes
PRI:	no relationship between P waves and QRS complexes; P waves can occasionally be found superimposed on the QRS complex
QRS:	less than 0.12 second if focus is junctional; 0.12 second or greater if focus is ventricular

44. Third-Degree Heart Block (CHB) is a *total* block at the AV node, resulting in A–V dissociation. On the EKG, this is seen as P waves and QRS complexes that have no _____ to each other.

relation

45. In both types of Second-Degree Heart Block, some P waves will initiate QRS complexes, whereas others will be _____ at the AV node. There will be some P waves that are not followed by QRS complexes, but the QRS complexes that do exist were initiated by the preceding P waves (Figure 60).

blocked

46. In First-Degree Heart Block there is no real block. Instead, there is a delay in conduction at the AV _____ , resulting in a _____ PR interval. But all P waves are conducted through to the ventricles.

node; prolonged

47. In Wenckebach, the delay at the AV node gets increasingly longer, resulting in progressively longer _____ intervals. Those impulses that are conducted through produce normal QRS complexes.

PR

Figure 60 The Heart Blocks

	P–P	R–R	PRI	CONDUCTION
FIRST-DEGREE	Regular	Usually regular (depending on underlying rhythm)	Greater than 0.20 second, constant	One P wave for every QRS complex
SECOND-DEGREE Type I Wenckebach	Regular	Irregular	Increasingly longer until one P wave is blocked	More P waves than QRS complexes
SECOND-DEGREE Type II	Regular	Usually regular (can be irregular if conduction ratio varies)	Constant on conducted beats (can be greater than 0.20 second)	More P waves than QRS complexes
THIRD-DEGREE (CHB)	Regular	Regular	PRI not constant; no relation of P waves to QRS complexes (P waves march through)	More P waves than QRS complexes

48. Type II Second-Degree Heart Block intermittently conducts some impulses through the AV node, whereas others are blocked. This means that some P waves will not produce a QRS complex. However, those that do will have a PR interval that is _____ across the strip.

constant

49. First-Degree Heart Block is actually a feature within a rhythm rather than an arrhythmia itself. Therefore, a rhythm with First-Degree Heart Block can be regular or irregular, depending on the regularity of the _____ rhythm.

underlying

50. Wenckebach always has an _____ R–R interval due to the progressively lengthening PRIs and the dropped QRS complexes. This type of Second-Degree Heart Block often has a visible pattern of "grouping" of the QRS complexes, emphasized by the missing QRS complex. This is frequently the feature that separates Wenckebach from CHB because CHB has _____ R–R intervals.

irregular

regular

51. You now have a very good foundation for approaching the heart blocks. As you go over the arrhythmias in the Practice Strips at the end of this chapter, remember to use your systematic approach for gathering all of the data available for each strip. To make the distinctions, pay particular attention to the PR intervals, because this will give you the most information about AV nodal activity.

Practice Strips

KEY POINTS

- The arrhythmias categorized as heart blocks are caused by conduction disturbances at the AV node.

- The four types of heart block we learned in this chapter are:

  First-Degree: not actually a block; merely a delay in conduction

  Second-Degree Type I (Wenckebach): an intermittent block; each beat is progressively delayed until one is blocked

  Second-Degree Type II: an intermittent block; the node selectively lets some beats through and blocks others

  Third-Degree (CHB): a complete block; none of the supraventricular pacemaker impulses is conducted through the node to the ventricles; the ventricles are depolarized by a dissociated pacemaker from below the site of the block

- A First-Degree Heart Block is not a rhythm itself but is a condition that is superimposed on another rhythm. Therefore, when identifying a First-Degree Heart Block, you must also identify the underlying rhythm.

- Here are the rules for *First-Degree Heart Block*:

Regularity:	depends on underlying rhythm
Rate:	depends on underlying rhythm
P Waves:	upright and uniform; each P wave will be followed by a QRS complex
PRI:	greater than 0.20 second; constant across the strip
QRS:	less than 0.12 second

- Wenckebach is a characteristic cyclic pattern in which the PRIs get longer and longer until one P wave does not produce a QRS complex. This cycle repeats itself, producing grouping of the R waves.

- The rules for *Wenckebach* are:

Regularity:	irregular in a pattern of grouped beating
Rate:	usually slightly slower than normal
P Waves:	upright and uniform; some P waves are not followed by QRS complexes
PRI:	progressively lengthens until one P wave is blocked
QRS:	less than 0.12 second

- In Type II Second-Degree Heart Block, there can be two, three, four, or more P waves for every QRS complex because the AV node blocks out many of the impulses.

- The rules for *Type II Second-Degree Heart Block* are:

Regularity:	R–R interval can be regular or irregular; P–P interval is regular
Rate:	usually in the bradycardia range; can be one-half to one-third the normal rate
P Waves:	upright and uniform; more than one P wave for every QRS complex
PRI:	always constant across the strip; can be greater than 0.20 second
QRS:	less than 0.12 second

- In Third-Degree Heart Block (CHB), there is a total obstruction at the AV node, resulting in A–V dissociation. The atria and ventricles are totally dissociated from each other.

- In CHB, the ventricles can be controlled by either a junctional or a ventricular escape rhythm. The lower pacemaker site can be identified by looking at the ventricular rate and the width of the QRS.

- The rules for *Complete Heart Block* are:

Regularity:	regular
Rate:	AR—usually normal (60–100 bpm);VR—40–60 if focus is junctional;20–40 if focus is ventricular
P Waves:	upright and uniform; more P waves than QRS complexes
PRI:	no relationship between P waves and QRS complexes; P waves can occasionally be found superimposed on the QRS complex
QRS:	less than 0.12 second if focus is junctional; 0.12 second or greater if focus is ventricular

SELF-TEST

Directions: Complete this self-evaluation of the information you have learned from this chapter. If your answers are all correct and you feel comfortable with your understanding of the material, proceed to the next chapter. However, if you miss any of the questions, you should review the referenced frames before proceeding. If you feel unsure of any of the underlying principles, invest the time now to go back over the entire chapter. **Do not proceed with the next chapter until you are very comfortable with the material in this chapter.**

Questions	Referenced Frames	Answers
1. What kind of disturbance causes the arrhythmias you learned in this chapter?	1	conduction disturbances in the AV node
2. Which of the arrhythmias you learned in this chapter is not a true block?	2, 3, 4, 46	First-Degree Heart Block is not a true block; it is a delay in conduction.
3. Which of the wave patterns on the EKG will yield information about the AV node?	9	the PR interval (specifically, the PR segment), since it will tell you the relationship between the atria and the ventricles
4. What will the PRI be like in a First-Degree Heart Block?	4, 9, 10, 11, 14, 46	It will be longer than normal, greater than 0.20 second.
5. What is the rate of a First-Degree Heart Block?	12, 14	First-Degree Heart Block is not a rhythm in itself; thus, it cannot have a rate. The rate of the rhythm will depend on the underlying rhythm.
6. Is a First-Degree Heart Block regular or irregular?	11, 14, 49	Again, this will depend on the regularity of the underlying rhythm.
7. In addition to identifying a First-Degree Heart Block, what other information must you provide in order for your interpretation to be complete?	12, 13	the identity of the underlying rhythm
8. Does the PRI in First-Degree Heart Block vary from one beat to the next?	10, 11, 14	No, it remains constant across the strip.
9. In First-Degree Heart Block, how many P waves will you see for every complex?	14	One; all beats are eventually conducted QRS through to the ventricles, even though each one encounters a delay at the AV node.
10. Is the QRS measurement also prolonged in First-Degree Heart Block?	11, 35	No; once the impulse passes through the AV node, conduction through the ventricles is normal.
11. In Wenckebach, do any of the sinus impulses get through the AV node to depolarize the ventricles?	2, 5, 15, 18, 19, 20, 29, 32, 45, 47	Yes, most of them do; but the AV node holds each one a little longer than the preceding one, until one is blocked completely. Then the cycle starts over.
12. What is the ventricular rate of a Wenckebach?	34, 35	It's usually just a little bit slower than normal, since most of the impulses are conducted.
13. Is the R–R interval regular in a Wenckebach?	33, 35, 50	No; it is irregular in a pattern of grouped beating.
14. Does a Wenckebach have a regular P–P interval?	29, 35	Yes; even though the PRIs and the R–Rs change, the P–P remains regular.
15. Is the R–R interval grossly irregular in a Wenckebach?	33, 35, 50	No; it has a distinctive cyclic pattern of grouped beating.
16. Does a Wenckebach produce one P wave for every QRS complex?	5, 15, 20, 29, 30, 31, 35, 45	No; most P waves are followed by QRS complexes, but some P waves are not conducted through to the ventricles.

Questions	Referenced Frames	Answers
17. What is the key feature of a Wenckebach?	21, 30	progressively lengthening PRIs with eventual blocked impulses
18. Does Type II Second-Degree Heart Block have an equal number of P waves and QRS complexes?	17, 20, 21, 22, 23, 24, 28, 45, 48	No; a Type II Second-Degree Heart Block will always have more P waves than QRS complexes.
19. Is the PRI of a Type II Second-Degree Heart Block constant, or does it vary between beats?	24, 25, 28, 48	It's constant. This is a key diagnostic feature that helps distinguish it from Wenckebach and CHB.
20. Is the PRI measurement normal in Type II Second-Degree Heart Block?	25, 28	It can be normal or it can be prolonged. Whatever the measurement, however, it will always be constant.
21. What is the usual rate range for a Type II Second-Degree Heart Block?	26, 28	Because most of the P waves are being blocked, it will be in the bradycardia range; usually one-half to one-third the normal rate.
22. What is meant by a variable conduction ratio?	27	It means that the AV node is varying the pattern in which sinus impulses are being conducted to the ventricles. It changes from one beat to the next (e.g., 4:3, 5:4, 4:3, 5:4, etc.).
23. Is the R–R interval regular or irregular in a Type II Second-Degree Heart Block?	27, 28	It will be regular unless the conduction ratio is variable, in which case the rhythm will be irregular.
24. Is the QRS measurement normal or abnormal in a Type II Second-Degree Heart Block?	18, 19, 28	It should be normal because those impulses that are allowed to pass through the AV node are expected to continue on through the ventricles in a normal way.
25. In Third-Degree Heart Block (CHB), do any of the impulses from the SA node penetrate the AV node to depolarize the ventricles?	36, 37, 40, 44	No. In CHB, the block at the AV node is complete. None of the sinus impulses passes through to the ventricles.
26. In CHB, will there be more P waves or more QRS complexes on the EKG?	37, 43	There will be more P waves.
27. If none of the sinus impulses is able to depolarize the ventricles, what focus is producing the QRS complexes?	38, 40	A lower site will take over at an escape rate. This rhythm can be either junctional or ventricular in origin.
28. How would you differentiate between a junctional focus and a ventricular focus in a CHB?	39, 40, 43	Junctional focus—QRS complex is less than 0.12 second; rate 40–60 bpm. With ven-tricular focus, QRS is 0.12 second or more and rate 20–40 bpm.
29. Is CHB regular or irregular?	42, 43	Regular; this will help you distinguish it from Wenckebach.
30. What will the PRI be in a CHB?	40, 43, 44	There is no PRI, as atria and ventricles are dissociated. The P waves have no relationship to the QRS complexes.

PRACTICE STRIPS (answers can be found in the Answer Key on page 558)

7.1

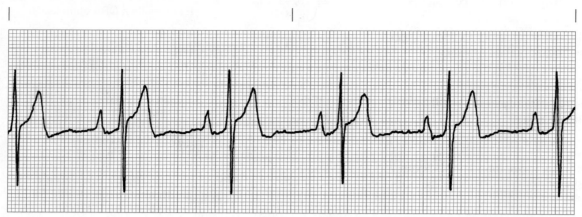

Regularity: _____   PRI: _____

Rate: _____   QRS: _____

P Waves: _____   Interp: _____

7.2

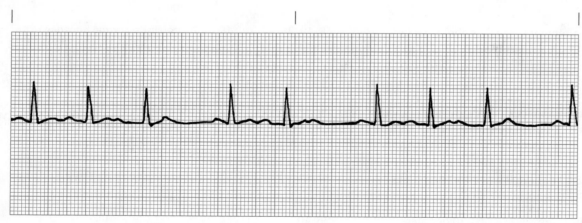

Regularity: _____   PRI: _____

Rate: _____   QRS: _____

P Waves: _____   Interp: _____

7.3

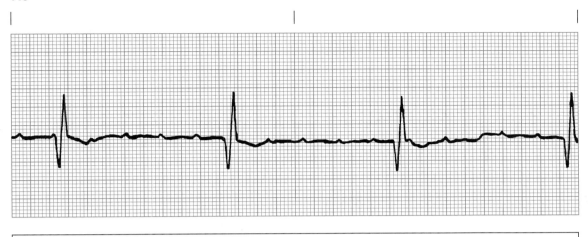

Regularity: _____	PRI: _____
Rate: _____	QRS: _____
P Waves: _____	Interp: _____

7.4

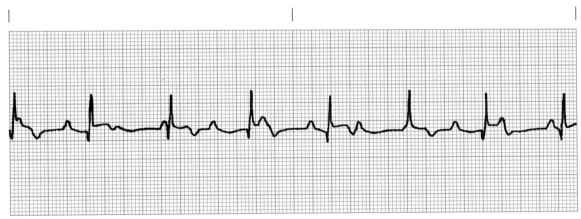

Regularity: _____	PRI: _____
Rate: _____	QRS: _____
P Waves: _____	Interp: _____

7.5

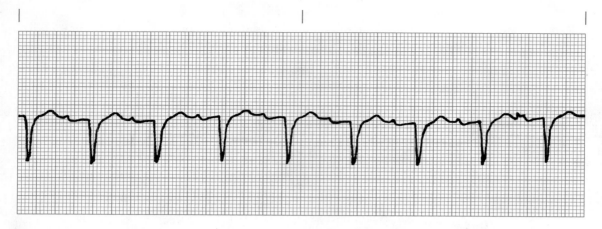

Regularity: _____ PRI: _____

Rate: _____ QRS: _____

P Waves: _____ Interp: _____

7.6

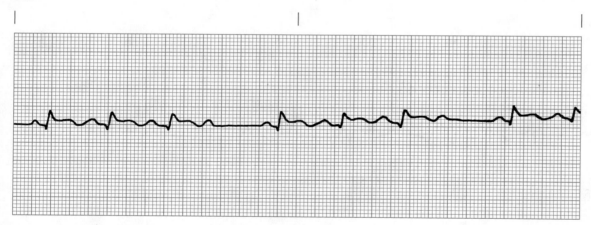

Regularity: _____ PRI: _____

Rate: _____ QRS: _____

P Waves: _____ Interp: _____

7.7

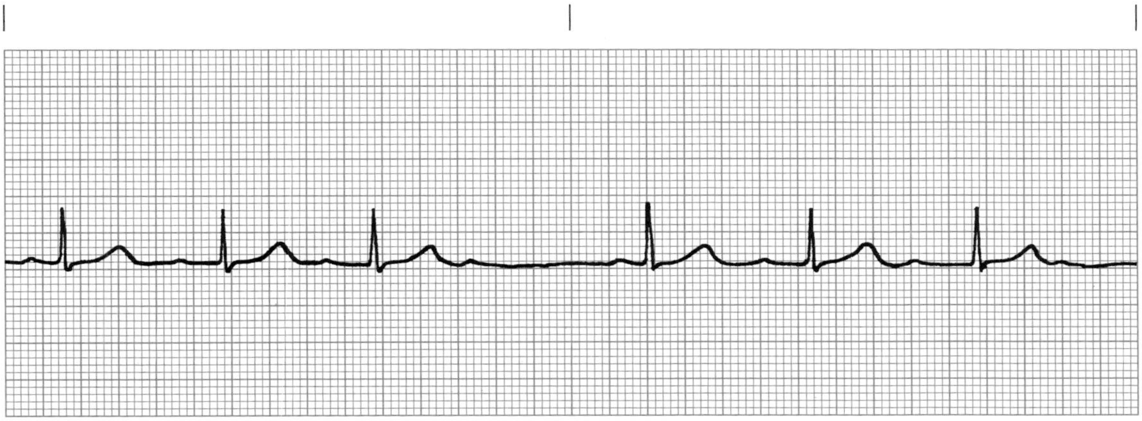

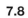

Regularity: _____	PRI: _____
Rate: _____	QRS: _____
P Waves: _____	Interp: _____

7.8

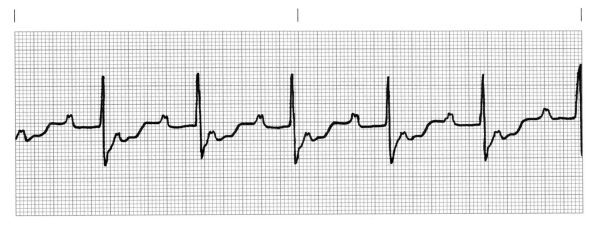

Regularity: _____	PRI: _____
Rate: _____	QRS: _____
P Waves: _____	Interp: _____

7.9

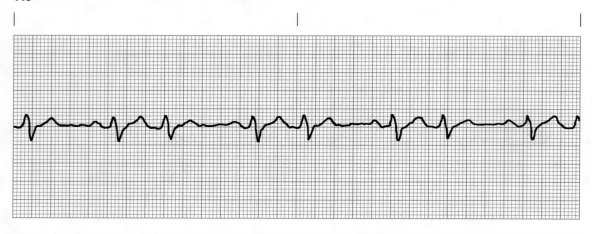

Regularity: _____	PRI: _____
Rate: _____	QRS: _____
P Waves: _____	Interp: _____

7.10

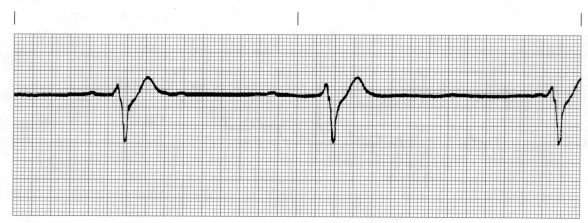

Regularity: _____	PRI: _____
Rate: _____	QRS: _____
P Waves: _____	Interp: _____

7.11

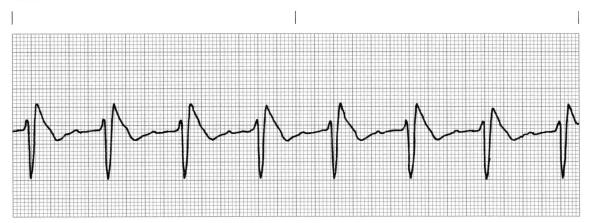

Regularity: _____	PRI: _____
Rate: _____	QRS: _____
P Waves: _____	Interp: _____

7.12

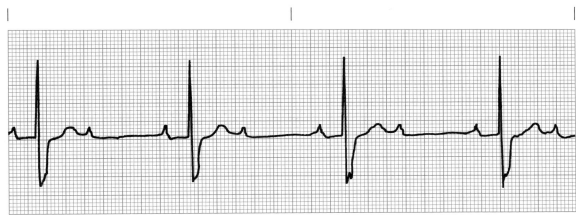

Regularity: _____	PRI: _____
Rate: _____	QRS: _____
P Waves: _____	Interp: _____

7.13

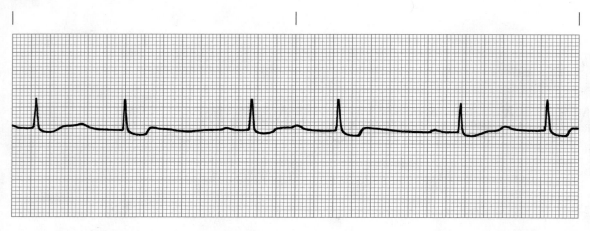

Regularity: _____	PRI: _____
Rate: _____	QRS: _____
P Waves: _____	Interp: _____

7.14

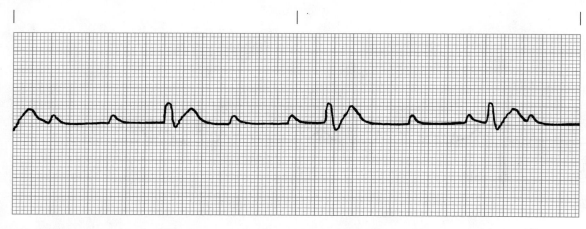

Regularity: _____	PRI: _____
Rate: _____	QRS: _____
P Waves: _____	Interp: _____

7.15

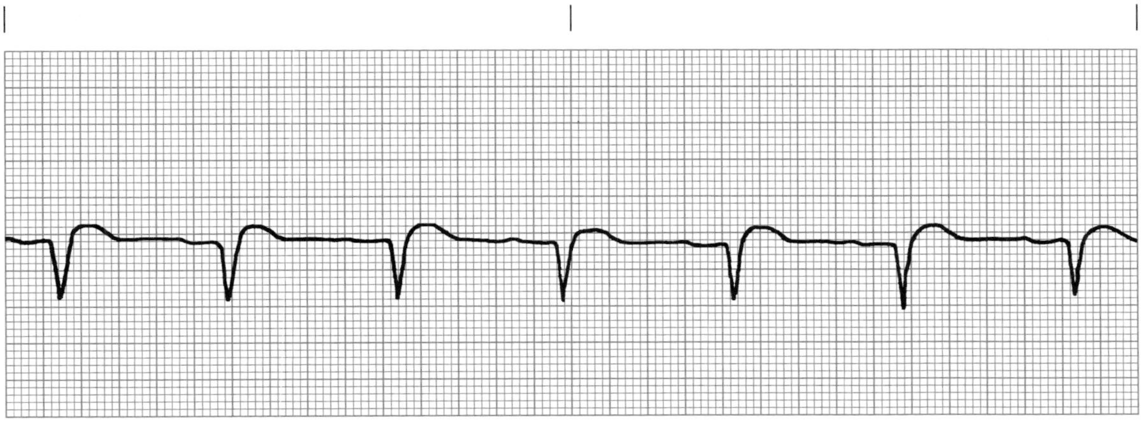

Regularity: _____	PRI: _____
Rate: _____	QRS: _____
P Waves: _____	Interp: _____

7.16

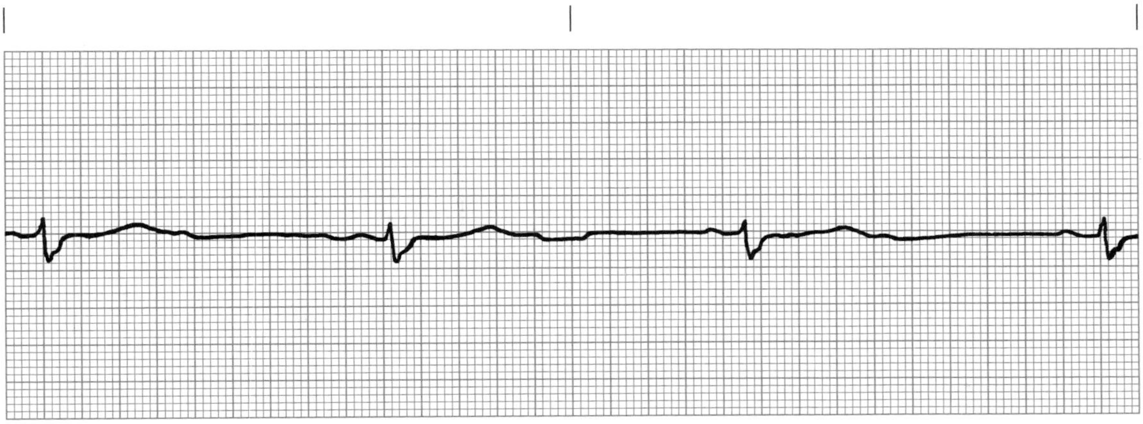

Regularity: _____	PRI: _____
Rate: _____	QRS: _____
P Waves: _____	Interp: _____

7.17

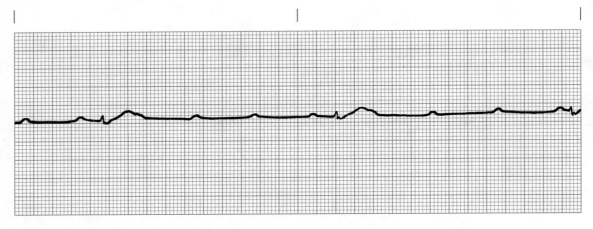

Regularity: _____	PRI: _____
Rate: _____	QRS: _____
P Waves: _____	Interp: _____

7.18

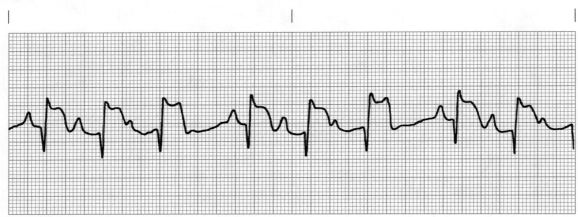

Regularity: _____	PRI: _____
Rate: _____	QRS: _____
P Waves: _____	Interp: _____

7.19

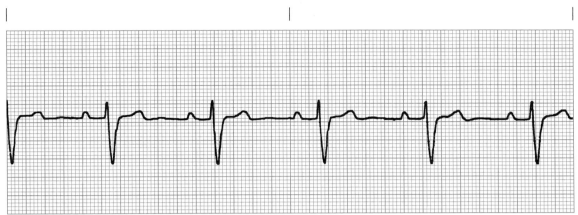

Regularity: _____	PRI: _____	
Rate: _____	QRS: _____	
P Waves: _____	Interp: _____	

7.20

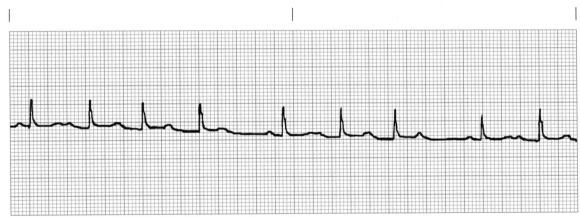

Regularity: _____	PRI: _____	
Rate: _____	QRS: _____	
P Waves: _____	Interp: _____	

7.21

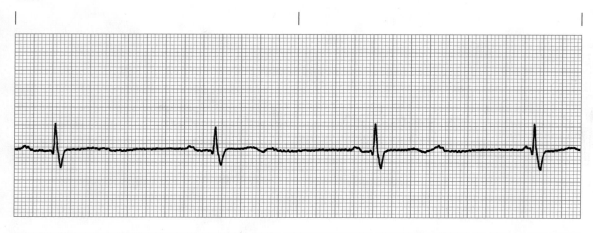

Regularity: _____	PRI: _____
Rate: _____	QRS: _____
P Waves: _____	Interp: _____

7.22

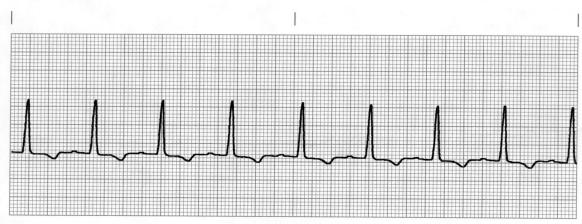

Regularity: _____	PRI: _____
Rate: _____	QRS: _____
P Waves: _____	Interp: _____

7.23

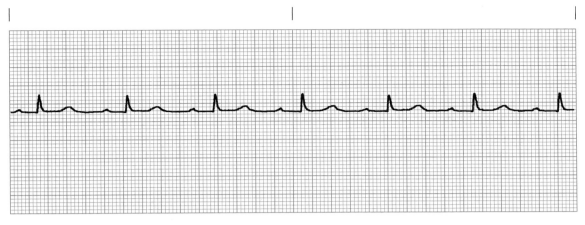

Regularity: _____   PRI: _____

Rate: _____   QRS: _____

P Waves: _____   Interp: _____

7.24

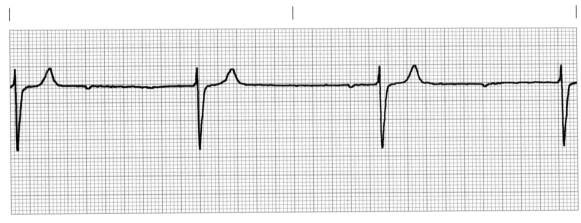

Regularity: _____   PRI: _____

Rate: _____   QRS: _____

P Waves: _____   Interp: _____

7.25

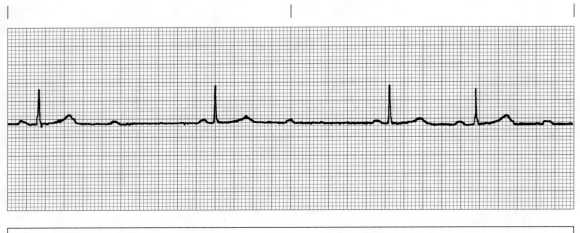

Regularity: _____	PRI: _____
Rate: _____	QRS: _____
P Waves: _____	Interp: _____

7.26

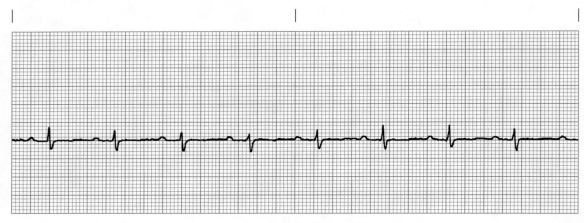

Regularity: _____	PRI: _____
Rate: _____	QRS: _____
P Waves: _____	Interp: _____

7.27

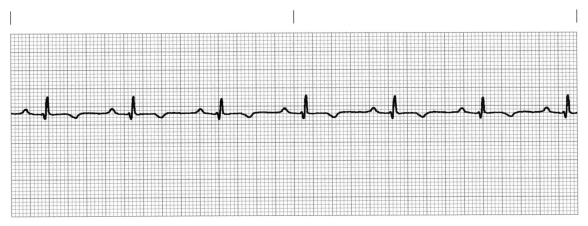

Regularity: _____	**PRI:** _____
Rate: _____	**QRS:** _____
P Waves: _____	**Interp:** _____

7.28

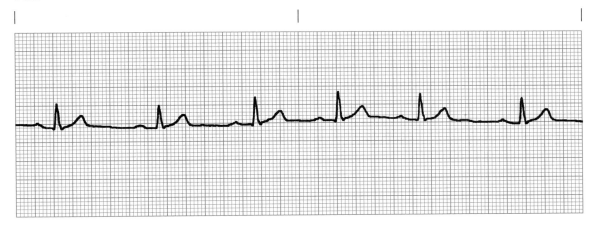

Regularity: _____	**PRI:** _____
Rate: _____	**QRS:** _____
P Waves: _____	**Interp:** _____

7.29

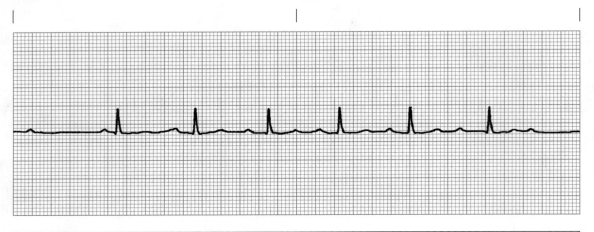

Regularity: _____	PRI: _____
Rate: _____	QRS: _____
P Waves: _____	Interp: _____

7.30

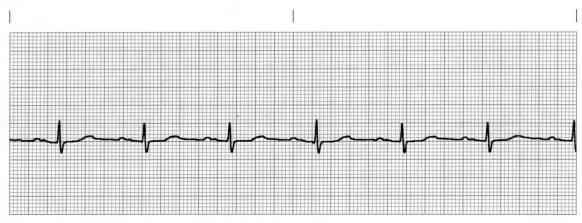

Regularity: _____	PRI: _____
Rate: _____	QRS: _____
P Waves: _____	Interp: _____

7.31

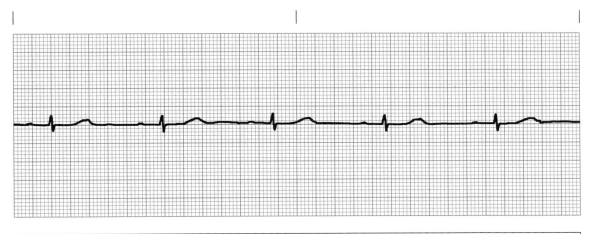

Regularity: _____	PRI: _____
Rate: _____	QRS: _____
P Waves: _____	Interp: _____

7.32

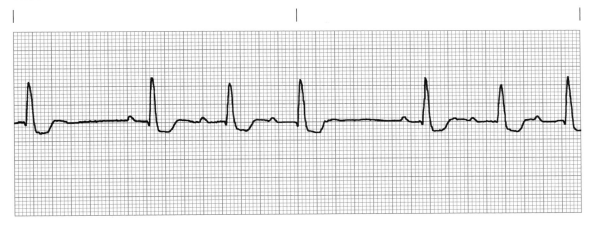

Regularity: _____	PRI: _____
Rate: _____	QRS: _____
P Waves: _____	Interp: _____

7.33

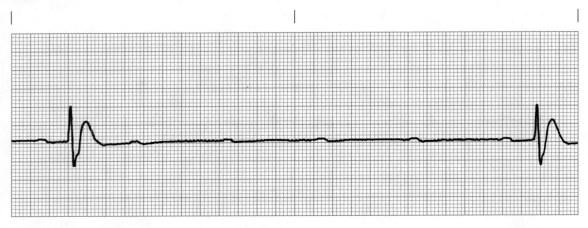

Regularity: _____	PRI: _____
Rate: _____	QRS: _____
P Waves: _____	Interp: _____

7.34

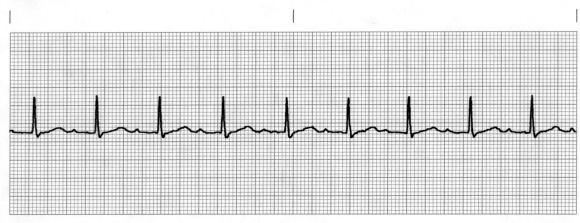

Regularity: _____	PRI: _____
Rate: _____	QRS: _____
P Waves: _____	Interp: _____

7.35

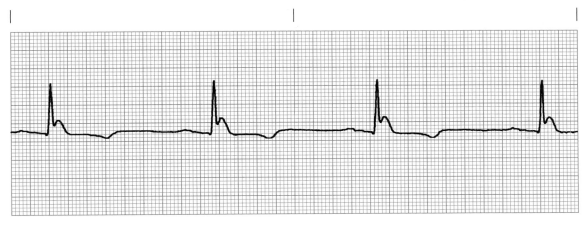

Regularity: _____	PRI: _____
Rate: _____	QRS: _____
P Waves: _____	Interp: _____

7.36

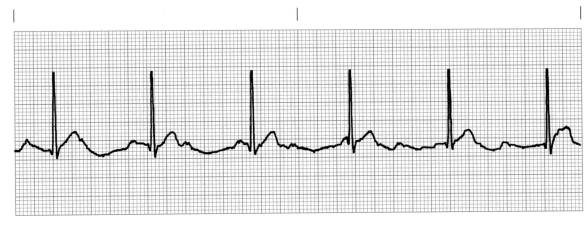

Regularity: _____	PRI: _____
Rate: _____	QRS: _____
P Waves: _____	Interp: _____

7.37

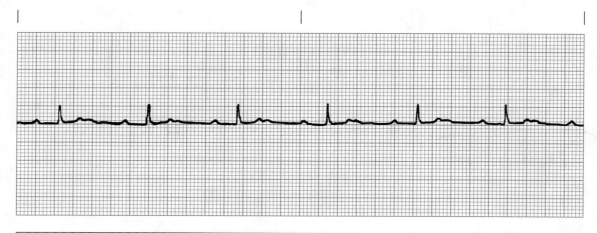

Regularity: _____ PRI: _____

Rate: _____ QRS: _____

P Waves: _____ Interp: _____

7.38

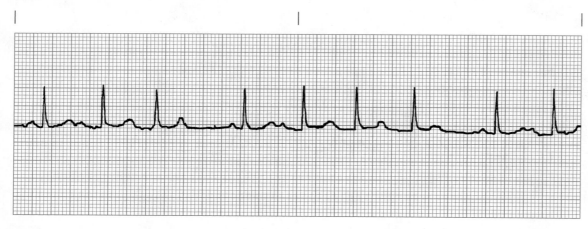

Regularity: _____ PRI: _____

Rate: _____ QRS: _____

P Waves: _____ Interp: _____

7.39

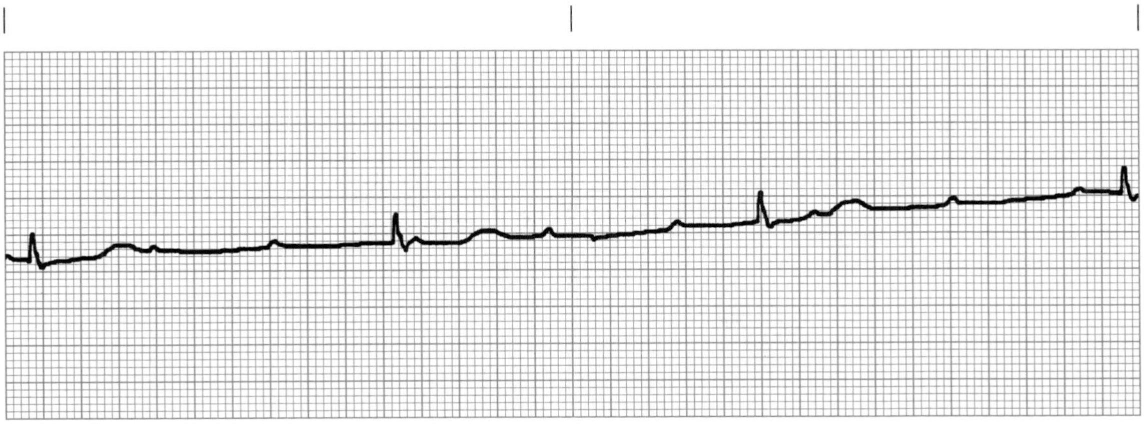

Regularity: _____   PRI: _____

Rate: _____   QRS: _____

P Waves: _____   Interp: _____

7.40

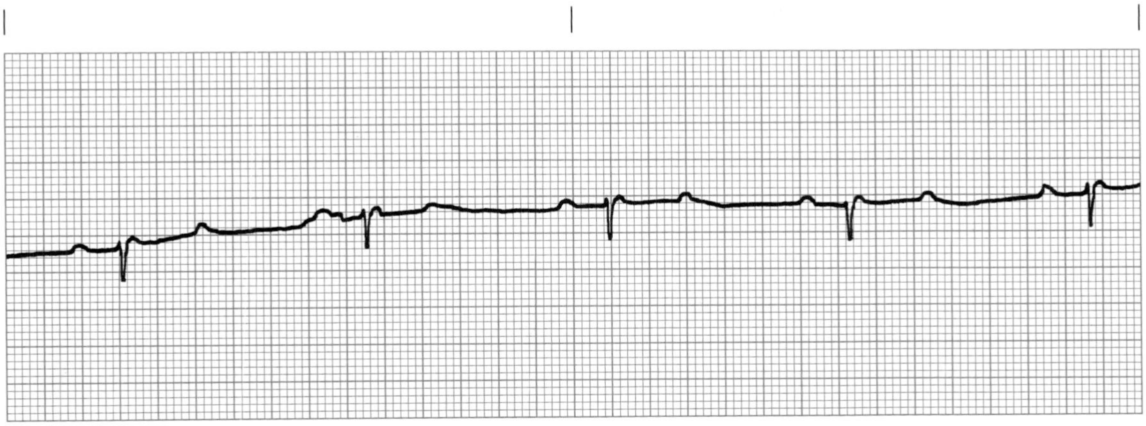

Regularity: _____   PRI: _____

Rate: _____   QRS: _____

P Waves: _____   Interp: _____

7.41

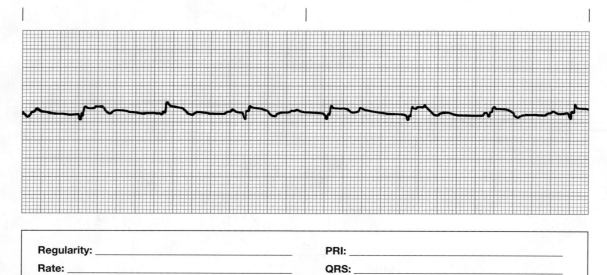

Regularity: _____	**PRI:** _____	
Rate: _____	**QRS:** _____	
P Waves: _____	**Interp:** _____	

Chapter 8
Ventricular Rhythms

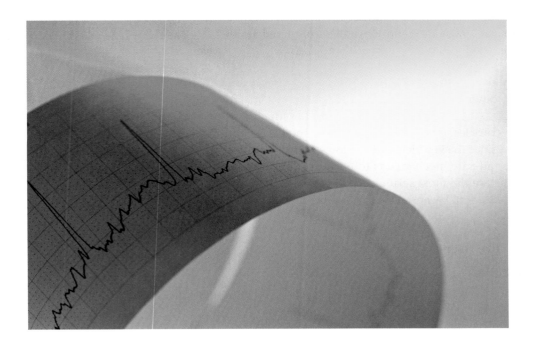

Overview

IN THIS CHAPTER, you will learn the characteristics of rhythms that originate within the ventricles, and you will find out what things are common to all ventricular arrhythmias. You will then learn the names and features of five different arrhythmias that originate in the ventricles. For each of these arrhythmias, you will learn about the etiology, conduction, and resulting EKG features (regularity, rate, P waves, PR intervals, and QRS complexes).

Ventricular Rhythms

1. All of the arrhythmias you have learned so far are classified as supraventricular arrhythmias, because they originate above the ventricles. All supraventricular arrhythmias have one thing in common: they all have QRS complexes of less than _____ second duration. This classification has a very scientific basis. We know from physiological measurements that an impulse originating above the ventricles and that follows the normal conduction pathways can depolarize the ventricles in less than 0.12 second. We also learned that it is possible for a supraventricular impulse to produce a QRS that is wider than 0.12 second, but that this would indicate some kind of delay in _____ through the ventricles and

0.12

conduction

thus would be considered an abnormality to be noted. Generally speaking, a normal supraventricular complex will have a _____ measurement of less than _____ second.

QRS
0.12

2. We say that a supraventricular arrhythmia should have a QRS complex of less than 0.12 second, but we also acknowledge that an abnormality could cause the QRS to be wider than that. However, we can say with certainty that an impulse that originated in the ventricles cannot depolarize the ventricles in less than 0.12 second. Hence, a basic rule for ventricular arrhythmias is that the QRS measurement will be 0.12 second or greater. If a complex measures less than 0.12 second, we know that it must have been initiated by a _____ impulse. But if it is 0.12 second or greater, it could either have originated above the ventricles and encountered a conduction disturbance, or it must have originated in the _____ .

supraventricular

ventricles

3. Ventricular arrhythmias are very serious for several reasons. First, the heart was intended to depolarize from the top down. The _____ were meant to contract before the _____ in order to pump blood effectively. When an impulse originates in the ventricles, this process is reversed, and the heart's efficiency is greatly reduced. Further, since the ventricles are the lowest site in the conduction system, there are no more fail-safe mechanisms to back up a ventricular arrhythmia. Ventricular arrhythmias are the most serious arrhythmias because the heart has lost its _____ and because it is functioning on its last level of backup support.

atria
ventricles

effectiveness

4. In this section we will be learning five ventricular arrhythmias:

- Premature Ventricular Complex (PVC)
- Ventricular Tachycardia
- Ventricular Fibrillation
- Idioventricular Rhythm
- Asystole

Although their mechanisms differ, each of these arrhythmias originates in the _____ and thus will have a QRS measurement of _____ second or more.

ventricles
0.12

Premature Ventricular Complex (PVC)

5. The first arrhythmia is not a rhythm but instead a single ectopic beat originating from an irritable ventricular focus. Since it arises from an irritable focus, the complex will come _____ than expected in the cardiac cycle and will interrupt the regularity of the underlying rhythm. PVCs (Figure 61) are single _____ that come earlier than expected and interrupt the underlying _____ .

earlier

ectopics
rhythm

6. Because PVCs originate in the ventricles, the QRS will be _____ than normal. But a second feature of a ventricular focus is that there is no P wave preceding the QRS complex. This is logical, since the SA node did not precipitate the ventricular depolarization. On the EKG you will see a very wide, bizarre QRS complex that is *not* preceded by a _____ wave.

wider

P

7. One of the things that gives a PVC such a bizarre appearance, in addition to the width of the QRS complex, is the tendency for PVCs to produce a T wave that extends

Figure 61 Mechanism of Premature Ventricular Complex

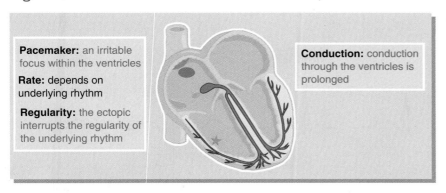

Pacemaker: an irritable focus within the ventricles

Rate: depends on underlying rhythm

Regularity: the ectopic interrupts the regularity of the underlying rhythm

Conduction: conduction through the ventricles is prolonged

A single irritable focus within the ventricles that fires prematurely to initiate an ectopic complex. *This is a single beat, not an entire rhythm; the underlying rhythm also must be identified.*

in the opposite direction of the QRS complex (Figure 62). That is, if the QRS is negative, the T wave will be _____ . This is not a hard-and-fast rule, but is a very frequent finding that contributes to an overall _____ appearance of a PVC.

upright
bizarre

8. PVCs are usually easy to spot because they are wide and bizarre, with a QRS complex measurement of _____ second or more, and they are not preceded by a _____ wave (Figure 63). Another feature common to many PVCs is that the T wave is in the opposite direction of the _____ complex.

0.12
P
QRS

9. Another frequent feature that may be helpful in identifying a PVC is the compensatory pause that usually follows a ventricular ectopic. A **compensatory pause** is created when a PVC comes early, but since it doesn't conduct the impulse retrograde through the AV node, the atria are not depolarized. This leaves the sinus node undisturbed and able to discharge again at its next expected time. The result is that the distance between the complex preceding the PVC and the complex following the PVC is exactly twice the distance of one R–R interval (Figure 64). If an ectopic is followed by a _____ pause, it is a good indication that the ectopic was a _____ .

compensatory
PVC

Figure 62 T Wave Configuration in PVCs

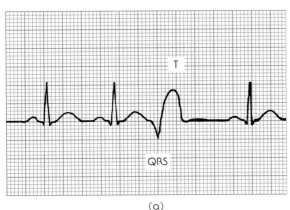

(a)

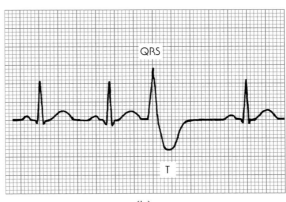

(b)

Figure 63 Typical Examples of PVC Configuration

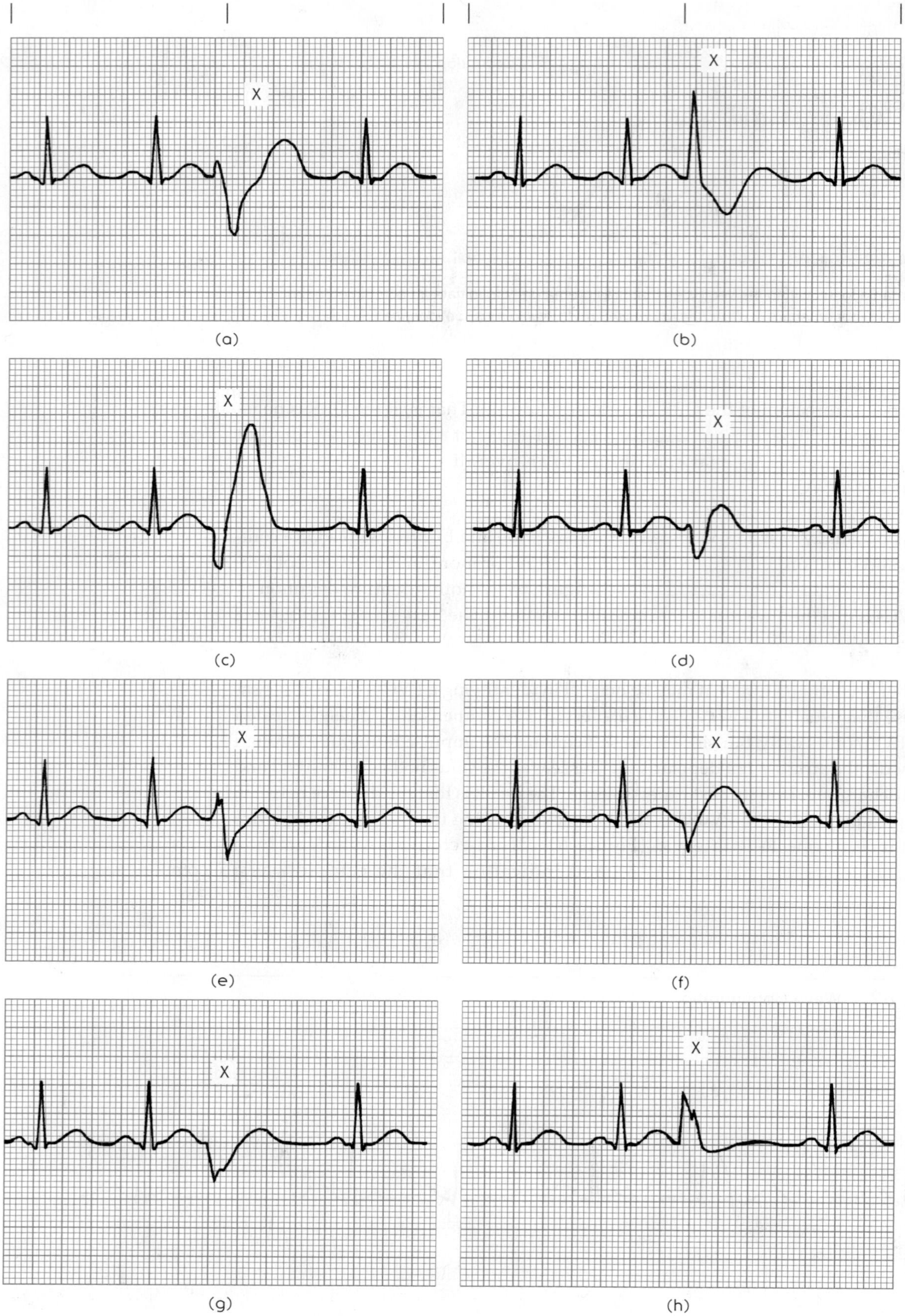

(a)

(b)

(c)

(d)

(e)

(f)

(g)

(h)

Figure 64 Compensatory Pause

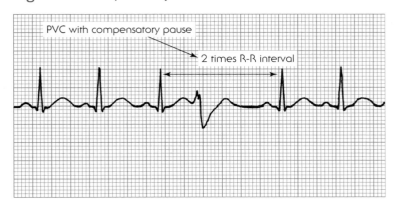

10. Although it is most common for PVCs to be followed by compensatory pauses, this is not a rigid requirement. Another configuration possibility is that the PVC be followed by no pause whatsoever. This occurs when the PVC squeezes itself in between two regular complexes and does not disturb the regular pattern of the sinus node. This phenomenon is called an **interpolated** PVC, because the PVC inserts itself between two regular beats (Figure 65). With an interpolated PVC, the R–R interval remains _____ , since the PVC does not interrupt the sinus rhythm.   regular

11. If a PVC is followed by a pause before the next sinus beat, leaving a distance between the sinus beat preceding the PVC and the sinus beat following the PVC, which measures exactly twice the normal R–R interval, you would call this a _____ pause. However, if the PVC falls directly between two sinus   compensatory
beats, without interrupting the regularity of the underlying rhythm, you would call this an _____ PVC.   interpolated

12. As with other types of ectopics, a PVC will interrupt the underlying rhythm. In interpreting the rhythm strip, it is important to identify both the ectopic and the underlying arrhythmia. For example, the arrhythmia might be Sinus Tachycardia with a PVC. When you are reporting a PVC, you should convey as much information about the disorder as possible, including the _____ rhythm.   underlying

13. Several other items are important information about a PVC. Since PVCs are an indication of myocardial irritability, it is important to note how frequently they are occurring. If the patient is having only an occasional PVC, this may be a normal rhythm

Figure 65 Interpolated PVC

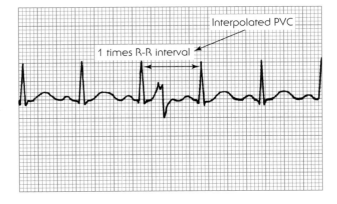

for that person. But if the frequency picks up so that you are seeing 5–10 per minute, you would suspect that the ectopics were an indication of increasing _____ . If the patient is experiencing chest pain of any sort, even a single PVC could be considered ominous. It is important that you not only note the presence of PVCs but also that you indicate the _____ of occurrence.

irritability

frequency

Unifocal vs. Multifocal

14. If a single focus within the ventricles has become irritable and is the source of the PVCs, all of these ectopics will have an identical appearance. That is, if one first has a positive deflection, and then a wide negative deflection, all other PVCs from that single focus will have the same configuration. These are called **unifocal** PVCs (Figure 66), because they come from a _____ focus and are all uniform in configuration. If all the PVCs on a rhythm strip had similar appearances, you would assume that they all originated from a _____ ectopic focus and would call them _____ PVCs.

single

single

unifocal

15. In cases of greater irritability, several ventricular foci might begin to initiate ectopics. In such an instance, the PVCs would have a variety of configurations (Figure 67). If two foci were initiating PVCs, all of the PVCs would have one of two configurations. If more sites were irritable, there would be a greater variety of _____ . In this situation, the PVCs are called **multifocal** because the

configurations

Figure 66 Unifocal PVCs

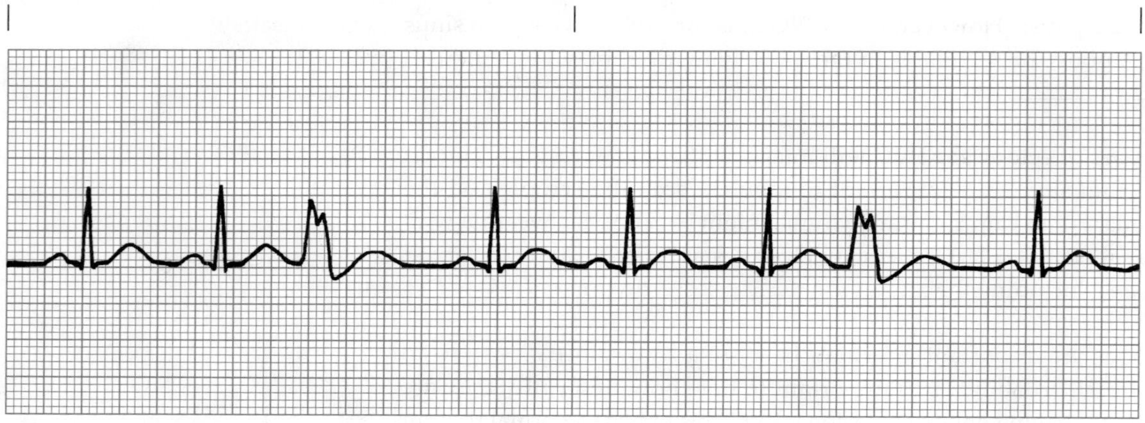

Figure 67 Multifocal PVCs

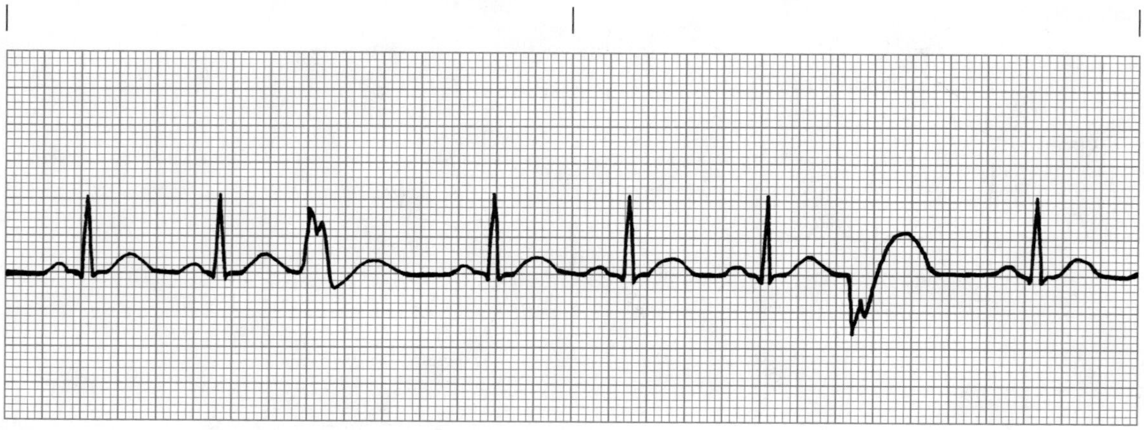

heart is so irritable that many foci are initiating the ectopics. Since they originate from many foci, _____ PVCs are more serious than unifocal PVCs because they are associated with a more irritable myocardium.

multifocal

16. If the PVCs on a rhythm strip all had the same basic configuration, they would be considered _____ . If the PVCs had differing configurations, they would be considered _____ .

unifocal
multifocal

The terms *unifocal* and *multifocal* are used to describe whether ectopics have a consistent configuration or varying morphologies. These terms are based on the presumption that uniform shapes result from a single irritable focus, whereas varying configurations are caused by multiple irritable foci. You may hear other terms used for the same purpose: *uniformed* for ectopics with one shape and *multiformed* for ectopics with varying shapes. For our purposes, you may consider *unifocal* and *uniformed* to be synonymous. Consider *multifocal* and *multiformed* synonymous as well.

R on T Phenomenon

17. PVCs represent a major electrical force, since they are a depiction of a premature depolarization of the ventricles. Because they come prematurely, they often fall near the end of the preceding QRS complex. If you recall, in Chapter 2 we learned that a portion of the T wave is considered a vulnerable area, because an electrical impulse could cause an aberrant depolarization of the heart if it should occur during that phase. If a PVC occurs during the _____ phase, it could throw the heart into an uncontrolled repetitive pattern. For this reason, it is important to note any PVC that is falling on or near the _____ wave of the preceding beat. This phenomenon is called *R on T* because the R wave of the PVC is hitting on the T wave (Figure 68). If you see PVCs creeping up on the preceding T wave, you would call this an _____ phenomenon and know that it represents a very serious situation.

vulnerable

T

R on T

18. The R on T phenomenon exists when the R wave of a _____ falls on or near the vulnerable phase of the cardiac cycle. The vulnerable phase, or relative refractory period, is located on the downslope of the _____ wave. (*Note:* If you have forgotten this material, turn back to Chapter 2, Frames 51–57, for a quick review.)

PVC

T

Figure 68 R on T Phenomenon: Ectopic A exhibits R on T phenomenon; Ectopic B does not

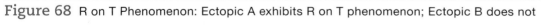
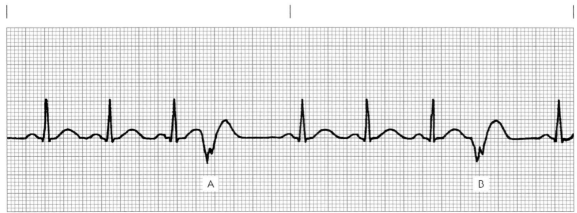

Runs and Couplets

19. Another sign of increasing myocardial irritability is when PVCs occur in immediate succession, without a normal beat intervening. If only two PVCs occur before the normal pattern resumes, you would see two PVCs attached to each other. This is called a **couplet** (Figure 69), but if you see three or more PVCs occurring in succession, this would be called a **run of PVCs** (Figure 70). The important distinction here is that several PVCs have fired without allowing the normal pacemaker to resume pacemaking responsibility. This is an indication of significant _____. Regardless of whether you call this pattern a couplet or a run of PVCs, you should note that the PVCs are occurring in immediate succession and indicate the number of PVCs observed. Technically, two successive PVCs would be called a _____, but it is sufficient to call any number of successive PVCs a _____ of PVCs and then indicate the number of PVCs involved.

irritability

couplet

run

20. A pair of PVCs in immediate succession could be called either a _____ or a _____ of two PVCs. But if there were three or more PVCs in a row, it should be called a _____ of three (or more) _____.

couplet; run

run

PVCs

Figure 69 PVCs Occurring as a Couplet (Pair)

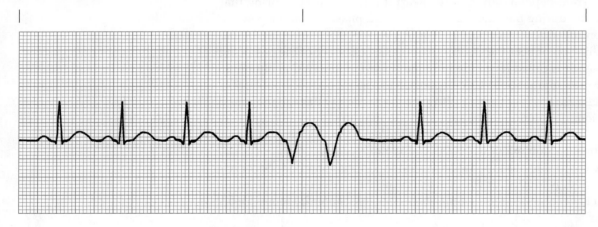

Figure 70 PVCs Occurring in a Run

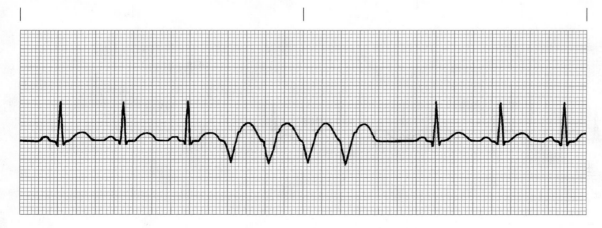

Grouped Beating

21. Sometimes, frequently occurring PVCs will fall into a pattern with the surrounding normal beats. This is called **grouped beating**. For example, you may see a PVC, then a normal beat, then a PVC, then a normal beat, and so on. When the PVCs are falling in a pattern of "every other beat" (Figure 71) with the normal beats, this is called **bigeminy** (pronounced *bī-jem'-eny*). Bigeminy refers to a repetitive pattern of grouped beating (e.g., one normal and one PVC) across the entire strip. When you see a pattern of one PVC, then one normal beat, then one PVC, then one normal beat, and this pattern continues across the strip, you would call the rhythm _____ of PVCs.

bigeminy

Figure 71 Patterns of Grouped Beating

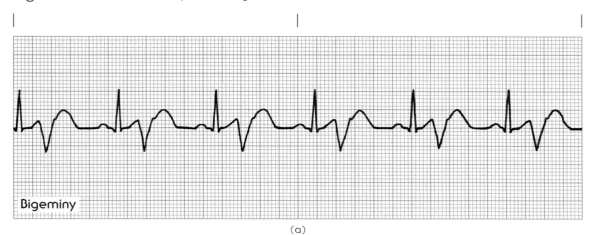

Bigeminy

(a)

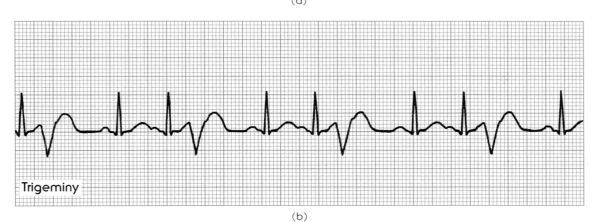

Trigeminy

(b)

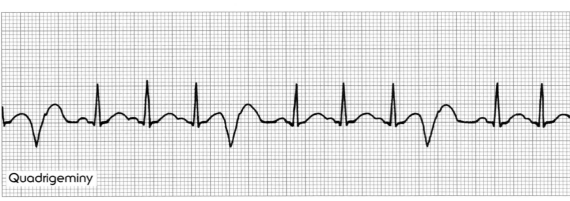

Quadrigeminy

(c)

22. Don't forget, though, to include the identification of the underlying rhythm. For example, if you saw a sinus beat, then a PVC, then a sinus beat, then a PVC, across the strip, you would call this Sinus Rhythm with bigeminy of _____ .

PVCs

23. Several other patterns of grouped beating that are very similar to bigeminy result from PVCs falling into a rhythm with normal beats. For example, if you saw a PVC followed by two sinus beats, then another PVC followed by two sinus beats, you would have a repetitive cycle of three beats: one PVC, and two sinus beats. This pattern is called **trigeminy**, since the cycle contains three beats. Such a rhythm would be called Sinus Rhythm with _____ of PVCs.

trigeminy

24. Another such pattern is **quadrigeminy**, where a pattern of four beats consists of one PVC and three normal beats. If you had a long enough rhythm strip, you could probably map out patterns of as many as eight, nine, or more beats to a cycle. However, the most common are bigeminy, a cycle consisting of one PVC and one normal beat; trigeminy, a cycle including one PVC and two normal beats; and _____ , where there are four complexes to the cycle: one PVC, and three normal beats.

quadrigeminy

25. Patterns such as bigeminy, trigeminy, and quadrigeminy can be found with other ectopics as well as PVCs. For example, you can have bigeminy of PACs or quadrigeminy of PJCs. But to qualify as a true patterned beat, the grouping should continue across the entire strip. Just because you happen to have two PACs on the strip with a single normal beat between them, you could not necessarily call this bigeminy. But if the pattern continued regularly across the strip, you would call it Sinus Rhythm with bigeminy of _____ .

PACs

26. You now know quite a few things about PVCs. They are wide and bizarre, with a QRS measurement of _____ . Frequently, the T wave will be in the opposite direction of the _____ . PVCs are a sign of myocardial _____ , so you should note how frequently they are occurring. You should also note if they are all coming from a single focus, in which case you would call them _____ . If they are coming from more than one focus, you would call them _____ .

0.12 second or more
QRS complex
irritability

unifocal
multifocal

27. You should be very cautious with a PVC that is falling near the downslope of the _____ wave, since this is the vulnerable phase of the cardiac cycle. This is called the _____ phenomenon and is dangerous because it could throw the heart into an ineffective repetitive pattern.

T
R on T

28. If the myocardial irritability is sufficient, you may notice PVCs falling in succession, without an intervening normal beat. If there were several PVCs connected in this manner, you would call it a _____ of PVCs and would note how many ectopics were involved. If there were only two PVCs paired, you might call this a _____ .

run

couplet

29. Finally, you know that PVCs can fall into patterns with the underlying normal beats. If it is a pattern of twos (i.e., one normal, one PVC), you would call this _____ . If it is a pattern of threes, it is called _____ , and it is called quadrigeminy if there are _____ complexes in the pattern.

bigeminy; trigeminy
four

Figure 72 Rules for Premature Ventricular Complex

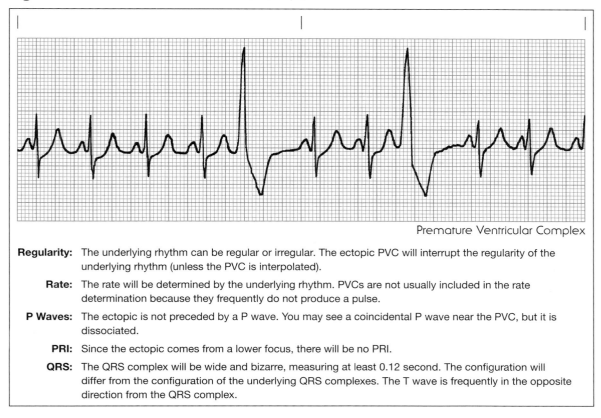

Premature Ventricular Complex

Regularity: The underlying rhythm can be regular or irregular. The ectopic PVC will interrupt the regularity of the underlying rhythm (unless the PVC is interpolated).

Rate: The rate will be determined by the underlying rhythm. PVCs are not usually included in the rate determination because they frequently do not produce a pulse.

P Waves: The ectopic is not preceded by a P wave. You may see a coincidental P wave near the PVC, but it is dissociated.

PRI: Since the ectopic comes from a lower focus, there will be no PRI.

QRS: The QRS complex will be wide and bizarre, measuring at least 0.12 second. The configuration will differ from the configuration of the underlying QRS complexes. The T wave is frequently in the opposite direction from the QRS complex.

30. Here are the rules for PVCs (Figure 72):

Regularity: ectopics will disrupt regularity of underlying rhythm

Rate: depends on underlying rhythm and number of ectopics

P Waves: will not be preceded by a P wave; dissociated P wave may be seen near PVC

PRI: since the ectopic comes from a lower focus, there will be no PRI

QRS: wide and bizarre; 0.12 second or greater; T wave is usually in opposite direction from R wave

Ventricular Tachycardia (VT)

31. If the myocardium is extremely irritable, the ventricular focus could speed up and override higher pacemaker sites. This would create what is essentially a sustained run of PVCs. This rhythm is called **Ventricular Tachycardia (VT)** (Figure 73). In fact, a run of PVCs is often called a short burst of VT. They both result from myocardial _____ , and they both fit the same rules. However, PVCs are _____ ectopics, whereas VT is an actual arrhythmia. In VT you will see a succession of PVCs across the strip at a rate of about 150–250 bpm. This arrhythmia usually has a very uniform appearance, even though the R–R interval may be *slightly* irregular. It is possible for VT to occur at slower rates, but when it does, it is qualified by calling it a slow VT. A true VT has a ventricular rate of _____ bpm.

irritability

single

150–250

32. Each of the other rules for a PVC also applies to VT. The QRS complex will be 0.12 second or greater, and the complex will be _____ and bizarre,

wide

Figure 73   Mechanism of Ventricular Tachycardia

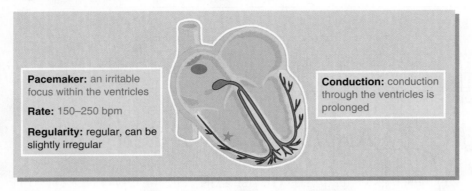

Pacemaker: an irritable focus within the ventricles

Rate: 150–250 bpm

Regularity: regular, can be slightly irregular

Conduction: conduction through the ventricles is prolonged

An irritable focus within the ventricles fires regularly at a rapid rate to override higher sites for control of the heart.

with the T wave usually in the opposite direction of the _____   R
wave. Since this rhythm originates from a _____ focus, you will not   ventricular
see a P wave in front of the QRS complex. However, this is another form of AV dissociation, so you may see an occasional P wave coincidentally occurring near the QRS
complex. As with PVCs, VT will have a QRS measurement of _____   0.12
second or greater, with a bizarre configuration of the _____ com-   QRS
plex and T wave, and there will be no _____ waves preceding the   P
QRS complexes.

33. Ventricular Tachycardia is caused by a _____ focus in the ven-   single
tricles that fires at a tachycardia rate to override the higher pacemaker sites and take
over control of the heart. It is also possible for the ventricular focus to change to a flutter mechanism, which would result in an arrhythmia very similar to VT but with a
ventricular rate of more than 300. When the ventricles depolarize at such a rapid rate,
the resultant EKG pattern becomes a very uniform, regular tracing and looks almost
like a coiled spring. There is very little difference between VT and Ventricular Flutter,
except for the rate. Most clinicians choose to consider Ventricular Flutter in with VT
and eliminate this academic distinction. For our purposes, we will consider Ventricular Flutter a rapid form of VT. We will not make a distinction between the two, since
the only real difference is in the ventricular _____ .   rate

34. Here are the rules of Ventricular Tachycardia (Figure 74):

Regularity: usually regular; can be slightly irregular

Rate: 150–250 bpm; can exceed 250 bpm if the rhythm progresses to Ventricular Flutter; may occasionally be slower than 150 bpm, in which case it
is called slow VT

P Waves: will not be preceded by P waves; dissociated P waves may be seen

PRI: since the focus is in the ventricles, there will be no PRI

QRS: wide and bizarre; 0.12 second or greater; T wave is usually in opposite
direction from R wave

Ventricular Fibrillation

35. In extremely severe cases of ventricular irritability, the electrical foci in the ventricles can begin fibrillating. This means that many foci are firing in a chaotic, ineffective

Figure 74 Rules for Ventricular Tachycardia

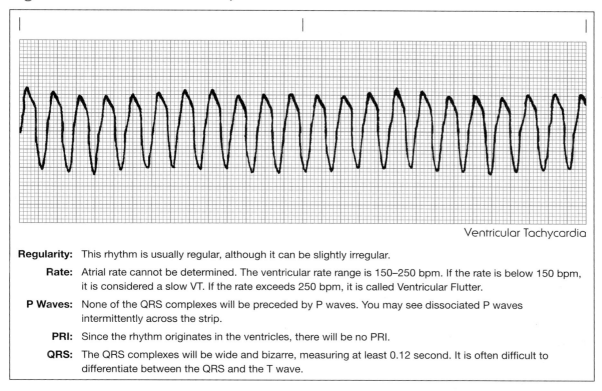

Ventricular Tachycardia

Regularity:	This rhythm is usually regular, although it can be slightly irregular.
Rate:	Atrial rate cannot be determined. The ventricular rate range is 150–250 bpm. If the rate is below 150 bpm, it is considered a slow VT. If the rate exceeds 250 bpm, it is called Ventricular Flutter.
P Waves:	None of the QRS complexes will be preceded by P waves. You may see dissociated P waves intermittently across the strip.
PRI:	Since the rhythm originates in the ventricles, there will be no PRI.
QRS:	The QRS complexes will be wide and bizarre, measuring at least 0.12 second. It is often difficult to differentiate between the QRS and the T wave.

manner, and the heart muscle is unable to contract in response. **Ventricular Fibrillation** (Figure 75) is a lethal arrhythmia, since the rhythm is very chaotic and
_____ .

ineffective

36. Ventricular Fibrillation (VF) is probably the easiest of all the arrhythmias to recognize. This is because there are no discernible complexes or intervals and the entire rhythm consists of chaotic, irregular activity. Since there are no identifiable complexes or wave forms, the EKG pattern of VF is simply a grossly _____ fibrillatory pattern.

chaotic

37. VT is distinguishable from VF because Ventricular Tachycardia has wide, bizarre complexes, but they are uniform and measurable. VF has no measurable waves or _____ .

complexes

Figure 75 Mechanism of Ventricular Fibrillation

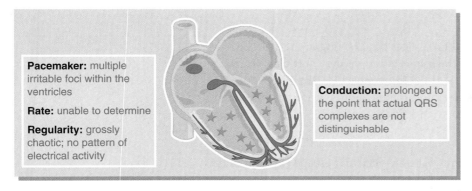

Pacemaker: multiple irritable foci within the ventricles

Rate: unable to determine

Regularity: grossly chaotic; no pattern of electrical activity

Conduction: prolonged to the point that actual QRS complexes are not distinguishable

Multiple foci within the ventricles become irritable and generate uncoordinated, chaotic impulses that cause the heart to fibrillate rather than contract.

Figure 76 Rules for Ventricular Fibrillation

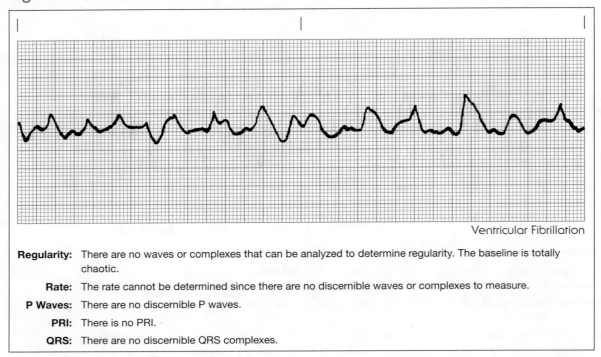

Ventricular Fibrillation

Regularity: There are no waves or complexes that can be analyzed to determine regularity. The baseline is totally chaotic.

Rate: The rate cannot be determined since there are no discernible waves or complexes to measure.

P Waves: There are no discernible P waves.

PRI: There is no PRI.

QRS: There are no discernible QRS complexes.

38. Here are the rules for Ventricular Fibrillation (Figure 76):

Regularity:
Rate:
P Wave: } totally chaotic with no discernible waves or complexes
PRI:
QRS:

Idioventricular Rhythm

39. So far, you have learned three ventricular arrhythmias, all of which are the result of ventricular irritability. These are PVCs, Ventricular Tachycardia, and Ventricular Fibrillation. It is also possible for a ventricular rhythm to be produced by an escape mechanism. If a higher pacemaker site fails, a ventricular focus can step in to take over pacemaking responsibility. There are two ways a ventricular focus can assume control of the heart. One is irritability and the other is _____ escape mechanism.

40. A ventricular escape rhythm is one that takes over pacemaking in the absence of a higher focus and depolarizes the heart of the inherent rate of the ventricles, which is _____ bpm. This rhythm is called **Idioventricular Rhythm** (Figure 77) 20–40 because the ventricles are initiating the rhythm on their own, without a conducted stimulus from a higher focus. The rate for Idioventricular Rhythm would be _____ bpm. 20–40

41. You can consider Idioventricular Rhythm to be a ventricular escape rhythm, since it is a fail-safe rhythm that takes over when _____ pacemaker sites higher fail. A ventricular focus firing within the inherent rate range of the ventricles would produce a rhythm called _____ Rhythm. Idioventricular

Figure 77 Mechanism of Idioventricular Rhythm

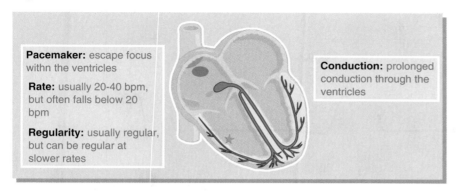

Pacemaker: escape focus
withn the ventricles

Rate: usually 20-40 bpm,
but often falls below 20
bpm

Regularity: usually regular,
but can be regular at
slower rates

Conduction: prolonged
conduction through the
ventricles

In the absence of a higher pacemaker, the ventricles initiate a regular impulse at their inherent rate to take control of the heart.

42. You should not see P waves in an Idioventricular Rhythm, since the escape mechanism would take over only if the atrial pacemaker sites had failed. What you will see is a rhythm of very slow ventricular complexes, usually in a regular rhythm, although it is possible for such an unreliable pacemaker to discharge irregularly. An Idioventricular Rhythm will not have _____ waves. Instead, you will see ventricular complexes measuring at least _____ second, firing at a rate below 40 bpm.

P

0.12

43. Idioventricular Rhythm is initiated by the very last possible fail-safe mechanism within the heart. This means that it is frequently an unreliable focus. It may fire a little irregularly, and the rate may be less than 20 bpm, even though the intrinsic ventricular rate is supposed to be 20–40 bpm. When the rhythm is in its terminal stages—that is, as the patient is dying—the complexes can lose some of their form and be quite irregular. In this stage, the arrhythmia is said to be **agonal**, or a dying heart. The word *agonal* is used to describe a terminal, lethal arrhythmia, especially when it has stopped beating in a reliable pattern. Idioventricular Rhythm is an _____ rhythm, especially when the rate drops below 20 bpm and the pattern loses its uniformity.

agonal

44. Here are the rules for Idioventricular Rhythm (Figure 78):

Regularity: usually regular

Rate: 20–40 bpm; can drop below 20 bpm

P Waves: none

PRI: none

QRS: wide and bizarre; 0.12 second or more

Asystole

45. The last stage of a dying heart is when all electrical activity ceases. This results in a straight line on the EKG, an arrhythmia called **Asystole** (pronounced *ā · siś-toe-lee*) (Figure 79). Asystole is a period of absent electrical activity, seen on the EKG as a _____ line. Asystole is a lethal arrhythmia that is very resistant to resuscitation efforts.

straight

46. The absence of cardiac electrical activity will cause a straight line on the EKG. This rhythm is called _____ . To be certain there is no electrical activity, you should view the rhythm in more than one lead and, of course, make sure the machine is functioning correctly.

Asystole

Figure 78 Rules for Idioventricular Rhythm

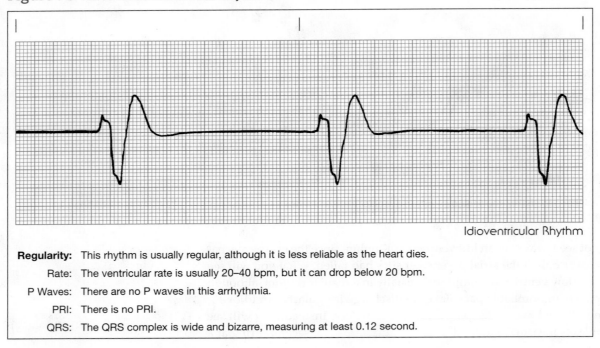

Idioventricular Rhythm

Regularity: This rhythm is usually regular, although it is less reliable as the heart dies.

Rate: The ventricular rate is usually 20–40 bpm, but it can drop below 20 bpm.

P Waves: There are no P waves in this arrhythmia.

PRI: There is no PRI.

QRS: The QRS complex is wide and bizarre, measuring at least 0.12 second.

Here are the rules for Asystole (Figure 80):

Regularity:
Rate:
P Wave: } straight line indicates no electrical activity
PRI:
QRS:

47. A straight line on the EKG would suggest that there is no electrical activity left in the heart. This rhythm would be called _____ .

Asystole

48. If the EKG only has ventricular complexes at a rate between 20 and 40 bpm, with no P waves, you would call the arrhythmia _____ Rhythm.

Idioventricular

49. An EKG that is totally chaotic, with no discernible waves or complexes, and nothing but a lot of irregular undulations, would fit the rules of _____ .

Ventricular Fibrillation

Figure 79 Mechanism of Asystole

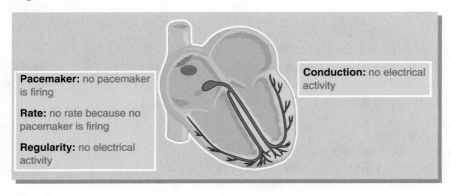

Pacemaker: no pacemaker is firing

Rate: no rate because no pacemaker is firing

Regularity: no electrical activity

Conduction: no electrical activity

The heart has lost its electrical activity. There is no electrical pacemaker to initiate electrical flow.

Figure 80 Rules for Asystole

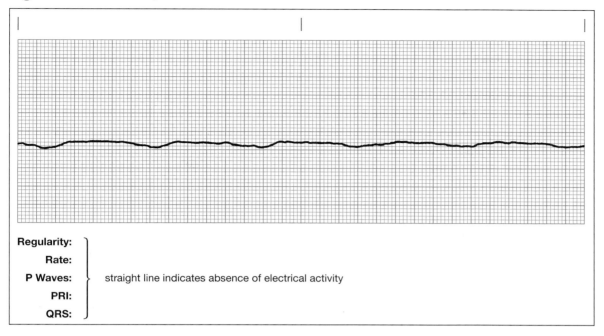

Regularity:
Rate:
P Waves: } straight line indicates absence of electrical activity
PRI:
QRS:

50. Ventricular Tachycardia is a very rapid rhythm with no _____ P
waves and wide, bizarre QRS complexes.

51. A single ectopic with a QRS greater than 0.12 second, with a T wave in the opposite direction of the R wave and having no P wave preceding it, would be called a
Premature _____ Complex. Ventricular

52. You now have all the information you need to approach ventricular rhythms. Turn Practice Strips
to the Practice Strips at the end of this chapter and apply your new knowledge until
you feel very comfortable in this area.

Pulseless Electrical Activity (PEA)

53. There is a condition in which the EKG shows electrical activity that should produce a pulse, but no pulse is detected in the patient. This is not a rhythm itself; it is
a condition called Pulseless Electrical Activity. PEA can be seen in many rhythms,
including NSR, tachycardias, and bradycardias. PEA occurs when a heart rhythm
on the EKG does not produce the expected _____ . The key to a pulse
quick diagnosis is to take the patient's pulse to see if the electrical activity is generating a mechanical response.

54. PEA cannot be detected by looking at the EKG alone. It is necessary to take the
patient's _____ before the diagnosis can be made. pulse

55. PEA often has a treatable underlying cause. One of the most common causes,
and most treatable, is hypovolemia. In order to diagnose PEA, it is necessary to
look at the _____ while checking the patient for a corresponding EKG
_____ . pulse

56. If no cause for PEA can be found, it should be treated as Asystole.

KEY POINTS

- A QRS measurement of less than 0.12 second indicates a supraventricular pacemaker. If the QRS is 0.12 second or greater, it could be ventricular, or it could be supraventricular with a ventricular conduction defect.

- All ventricular impulses will have a QRS measurement of 0.12 second or greater.

- Ventricular arrhythmias are the most serious arrhythmias because the heart is less effective than usual and because the heart is functioning on its last level of backup support.

- A PVC is a single ectopic beat arising from an irritable focus in the ventricles. It comes earlier than expected and interrupts the regularity of the underlying rhythm.

- PVCs are usually wide and bizarre and usually have a T wave in the opposite direction of the QRS complex. They are not preceded by a P wave.

- A compensatory pause usually follows a PVC. This means that the distance between the R wave of the complex preceding the PVC and the R wave of the complex following the PVC is exactly twice the R–R interval of the underlying rhythm.

- A PVC does not have to have a compensatory pause. It can be "interpolated" between two sinus beats without interrupting the underlying rhythm.

- PVCs are an indication of myocardial irritability. The frequency of PVCs should be noted because this suggests the degree of myocardial irritability.

- PVCs are considered unifocal if they all originate from a single ventricular focus and thus have similar configurations.

- PVCs are considered multifocal if they arise from many foci and assume a variety of configurations.

- If a PVC lands during the vulnerable (relative refractory) phase of the cardiac cycle it can produce a lethal, repetitive arrhythmia. Thus, a PVC that falls on the downslope of the T wave is referred to as the "R on T" phenomenon and is considered very dangerous.

- With increasing irritability, the PVCs can occur in pairs, called couplets, or in runs of three or more consecutive ectopics.

- PVCs frequently occur in patterns of grouped beating. If every other beat is a PVC, it is called bigeminy. If every third beat is a PVC, it is called trigeminy. If every fourth beat is a PVC, it is called a quadrigeminy. Bigeminy, trigeminy, and quadrigeminy can also describe patterns of PACs or PJCs.

- The rules for *Premature Ventricular Complexes* are:

  Regularity: ectopics will disrupt regularity of underlying rhythm

  Rate: depends on underlying rhythm and number of ectopics

  P Waves: will not be preceded by a P wave; dissociated P waves may be seen near PVC

  PRI: since the ectopic comes from a lower focus, there will be no PRI

  QRS: wide and bizarre; 0.12 second or greater; T wave is usually in opposite direction from R wave.

- Ventricular Tachycardia is a rhythm originating from a single irritable focus within the ventricles. It looks very much like an uninterrupted series of PVCs.

- You may see some P waves in a VT, but they are dissociated from the QRS complexes.

- The rules for *Ventricular Tachycardia* are:

  Regularity: usually regular; can be slightly irregular

  Rate: 150–250 bpm; can exceed 250 bpm if the rhythm progresses to Ventricular Flutter; may occasionally be slower than 150 bpm, in which case it is called a slow VT

  P Waves: will not be preceded by P waves; dissociated P waves may be seen

  PRI: since the focus is in the ventricles, there will be no PRI

  QRS: wide and bizarre; 0.12 second or greater; T wave is usually in opposite direction from R wave

- Ventricular Fibrillation is an indication of extreme myocardial irritability. Many ventricular foci initiate impulses in a chaotic fashion, causing the ventricles to fibrillate in an ineffective manner.

- In Ventricular Fibrillation, no waves or complexes are identifiable. All that is visible is a grossly chaotic baseline.

- The rules for *Ventricular Fibrillation* are:

  Regularity:
  Rate:
  P Waves: } totally chaotic with no discernible waves or complexes
  PRI:
  QRS:

- Idioventricular Rhythm is an escape rhythm that takes over pacemaking responsibility when higher centers fail.

- The rules for *Idioventricular Rhythm* are:

Regularity:	usually regular (it can be unreliable since it is such a low site)
Rate:	20–40 bpm; can drop below 20 bpm
P Waves:	none
PRI:	none
QRS	wide and bizarre; 0.12 second or greater

- Agonal is the term used to describe a terminal, lethal arrhythmia, especially when it has stopped beating in a reliable pattern; also called a dying heart.

- When all electrical activity within the heart ceases, it is seen on the EKG as a straight line, possibly with some undulations in it. This arrhythmia is called Asystole.

- The rules for *Asystole* are:

Regularity:	
Rate:	
P Waves:	straight line indicates absence of electrical activity
PRI:	
QRS:	

- Pulseless Electrical Activity (PEA) is a condition in which the EKG shows activity that should produce a pulse, but no pulse is detectable in the patient.

- PEA is not a rhythm itself. It occurs in many rhythms including NSR, tachycardias, and bradycardias.

- PEA often has a treatable cause. It is important to correlate the patient's pulse with the EKG tracing to identify the condition.

- If an underlying cause cannot be determined, PEA should be treated as Asystole.

SELF-TEST

Directions: Complete this self-evaluation of the information you have learned from this chapter. If your answers are all correct and you feel comfortable with your understanding of the material, proceed to the next chapter. However, if you miss any of the questions, you should review the referenced frames before proceeding. If you feel unsure of any of the underlying principles, invest the time now to go back over the entire chapter. **Do not proceed with the next chapter until you are very comfortable with the material in this chapter.**

Questions	Referenced Frames	Answers
1. What is the minimum QRS measurement for a ventricular complex?	1, 4	0.12 second
2. Are all wide QRS complexes ventricular in origin?	2	Not necessarily; they might also be supraventricular with a ventricular conduction defect.
3. Why are ventricular arrhythmias so serious?	3	It is because the heart can't pump effectively if the ventricles contract first. Also, the heart is relying on its final fail-safe mechanism.
4. What is a PVC?	5, 6, 7, 8, 26, 30, 51	It is a single premature ectopic arising from an irritable focus within the ventricles.
5. How can you tell whether a PVC is unifocal or multifocal?	14, 15, 16, 26	Unifocal PVCs will all have similar configurations; if they have a variety of shapes, they are multifocal.
6. Are PVCs preceded by P waves?	6, 30, 51	No, these ectopics originate in the ventricles. They are not initiated by a sinus impulse.
7. What do you call two PVCs that are connected to each other without a normal beat in between?	19, 20, 28	a couplet, or a pair
8. What is a "run" of PVCs?	19, 20, 28	It is three or more PVCs occurring in rapid succession without an intervening normal beat. This might also be called a short burst of VT.

Questions	Referenced Frames	Answers
9. What is a compensatory pause?	9, 11	It is the pause that usually follows a PVC. It means that the distance between the R wave of the beat preceding the PVC and the R wave following the PVC is exactly twice the R–R interval of the underlying rhythm.
10. What is an interpolated PVC?	10, 11	It is a PVC that squeezes itself in between two normal beats without interrupting the underlying rhythm.
11. How can you tell if the myocardium is irritable?	13, 19, 26, 28	The frequency of ventricular activity (PVCs, ventricular tachyarrhythmias) will increase with an increase in myocardial irritability.
12. What do you call the grouping of PVCs so that every other beat is an ectopic?	21, 23, 24, 29	bigeminy
13. Do patterns of grouped beats such as trigeminy occur only with ventricular ectopics, or can they occur with ectopics from other areas of the heart?	25	Bigeminy, trigeminy, and quadrigeminy can all occur with PACs, PJCs, and PVCs.
14. What is meant by "R on T"?	17, 18, 27	It means that a PVC is falling on the downslope of the preceding T wave and thus is causing a stimulus during the vulnerable relative refractory phase. This is very dangerous, since it can cause the rhythm to change to VT or VF.
15. In addition to identifying a PVC, what other information must you provide in order for your interpretation of the rhythm to be complete?	12, 13, 22	the identity of the underlying rhythm
16. A PVC shouldn't have a P wave, but don't you sometimes see a P wave somewhere near the PVC?	32, 30	You may, but it is dissociated. It did not initiate the ventricular depolarization.
17. Will a PVC have a PRI?	6, 8, 30	No, it will not, since it originates in the ventricles.
18. What will the rate be for a PVC?	30	That will depend on the rate of the underlying rhythm.
19. Are PVCs included when you calculate the heart rate?	3, 30	Not usually, since PVCs frequently do not produce a pulse.
20. What rhythm is produced if the irritable ventricular focus that produced a single PVC suddenly continued firing to produce a rapid succession of ventricular complexes at a rate of 150–250 bpm?	31, 34	Ventricular Tachycardia
21. Does Ventricular Tachycardia have P waves?	32, 34, 50	In VT, a P wave does not appear in front of every QRS complex. However, you may see dissociated P waves since the sinus node can still be firing.
22. Is VT regular or irregular?	31, 34	It is usually regular, although it can be slightly irregular.

Questions	Referenced Frames	Answers
23. Does VT ever occur at a rate below 150 bpm?	31, 34	Yes, it can, but it is then identified as a slow VT.
24. Can VT exceed 250 bpm?	33, 34	Yes, it can. To be technically accurate, this rhythm is then called Ventricular Flutter. However, Ventricular Flutter is clinically identical to VT and differs only in rate. Thus, both rhythms are frequently grouped in the category of VT.
25. What does the QRS complex look like in VT?	32, 34, 50	As in all ventricular rhythms, the QRS in VT is wide and bizarre, and the T wave goes in the opposite direction from the QRS complex. The measurement is 0.12 second or greater.
26. What is the PRI in a VT?	32, 34	VT does not have a PRI, since it originates in the ventricles.
27. What do the QRS complexes look like in Ventricular Fibrillation?	36, 37, 38, 49	VF does not have any identifiable waves or complexes. The QRS complex cannot be distinguished from other undulations.
28. Why is VF such an ominous rhythm?	35	The ventricles are not pumping; they are merely quivering. No blood is being pumped. The patient is clinically dead.
29. Is VF an irritable rhythm or an escape mechanism?	35	VF is a sign of extreme irritability.
30. Is VF regular or irregular?	35, 36, 37, 38	Again, VF is grossly chaotic, with no discernible waves or complexes.
31. Can the ventricles produce an escape rhythm?	39	Yes. If higher pacemaker sites fail, the ventricles can initiate an Idioventricular Rhythm as a fail-safe escape mechanism.
32. What does Idioventricular Rhythm look like?	40, 41, 42, 44, 48	wide ventricular complexes at a rate of 20–40 bpm, with no P waves
33. What is the QRS measurement in an Idioventricular Rhythm?	44	at least 0.12 second
34. Is Idioventricular Rhythm regular or irregular?	42, 44	Idioventricular Rhythm is usually regular, but it can be slightly irregular since it is a relatively unreliable pacemaker site.
35. What is the PRI in an Idioventricular Rhythm?	42, 44	Idioventricular Rhythm has no P waves, thus it has no PRI.
36. Can Idioventricular Rhythm be slower than 20 bpm?	43, 44	Yes, it can. As the heart dies, the rate slows, and the rate can drop below the inherent rate of the ventricular pacemaker. At this point, the rhythm becomes less formed and is described as being agonal, or a dying heart.

Questions	Referenced Frames	Answers
37. What does a straight line on the EKG indicate?	45, 47	Assuming that the machine is turned on and is functioning correctly, a straight line indicates that the heart is producing no electrical activity. This arrhythmia is called Asystole.
38. What is the QRS measurement for Asystole?	46	Asystole has no waves or complexes. It has no P waves, no QRS complexes, and no PRIs.
39. Is Pulseless Electrical Activity (PEA) a rhythm in itself?	53, 54, 55, 56	No. PEA is a condition associated with many other rhythms.
40. How can you diagnose PEA?	53, 54, 55, 56	The only way to diagnose PEA is to take the patient's pulse while looking at the EKG. If the EKG would be expected to produce a pulse but the patient does not have a pulse, the diagnosis is PEA.
41. Is PEA treatable?	53, 54, 55, 56	Yes, it is often treatable. That's why you want to diagnose it quickly.
42. How do you treat PEA if there is no apparent cause?	53, 54, 55, 56	If no cause can be determined, PEA should be treated as Asystole.
43. Can you tell if any of the rhythm strips in this book are PEA?	53, 54, 55, 56	No, because PEA can only be diagnosed by correlating the EKG with the patient's pulse.

PRACTICE STRIPS (answers can be found in the Answer Key on page 561)

8.1

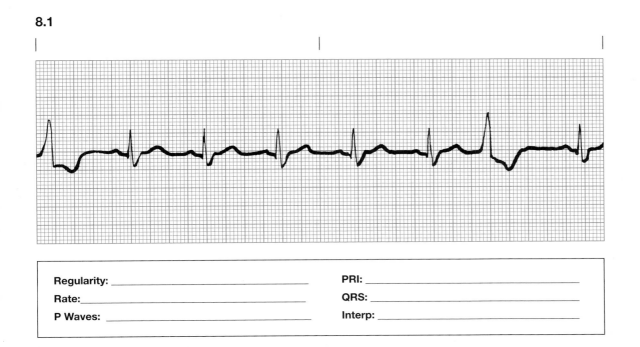

Regularity: _____   PRI: _____

Rate: _____   QRS: _____

P Waves: _____   Interp: _____

8.2

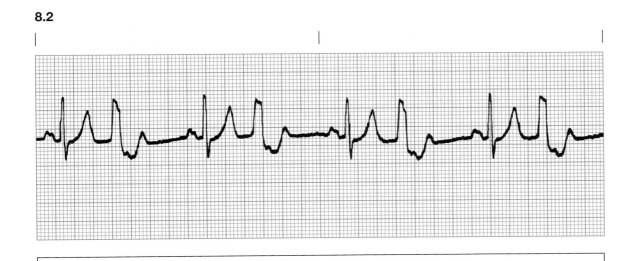

Regularity: _____   PRI: _____

Rate: _____   QRS: _____

P Waves: _____   Interp: _____

8.3

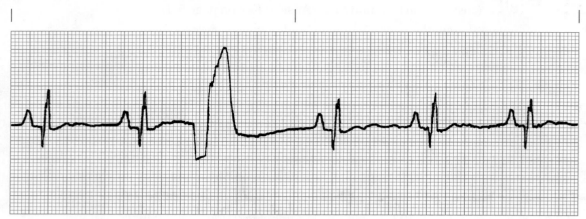

Regularity: _____   PRI: _____

Rate: _____   QRS: _____

P Waves: _____   Interp: _____

8.4

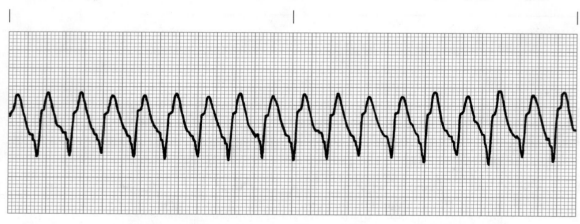

Regularity: _____   PRI: _____

Rate: _____   QRS: _____

P Waves: _____   Interp: _____

8.5

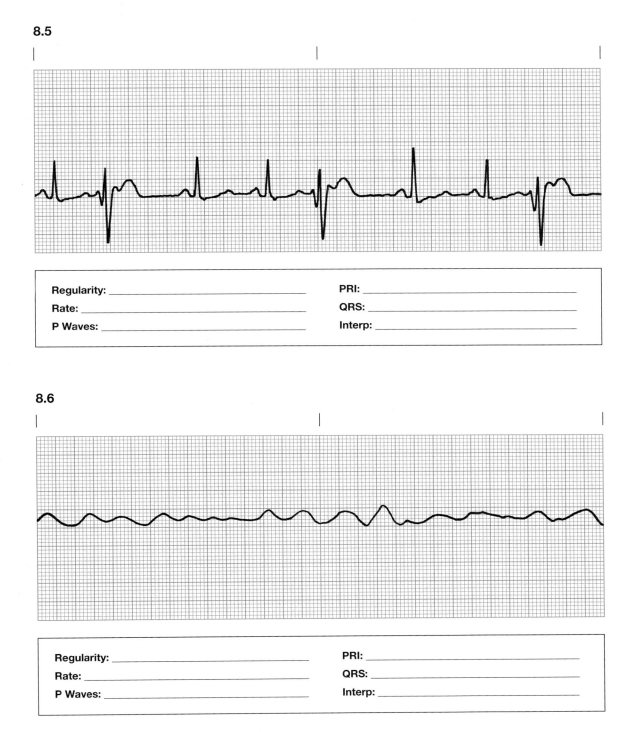

Regularity: _____	PRI: _____
Rate: _____	QRS: _____
P Waves: _____	Interp: _____

8.6

Regularity: _____	PRI: _____
Rate: _____	QRS: _____
P Waves: _____	Interp: _____

8.7

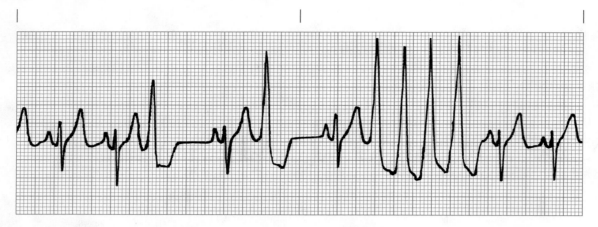

Regularity: _____   PRI: _____

Rate: _____   QRS: _____

P Waves: _____   Interp: _____

8.8

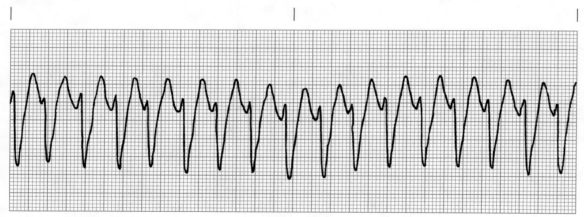

Regularity: _____   PRI: _____

Rate: _____   QRS: _____

P Waves: _____   Interp: _____

8.9

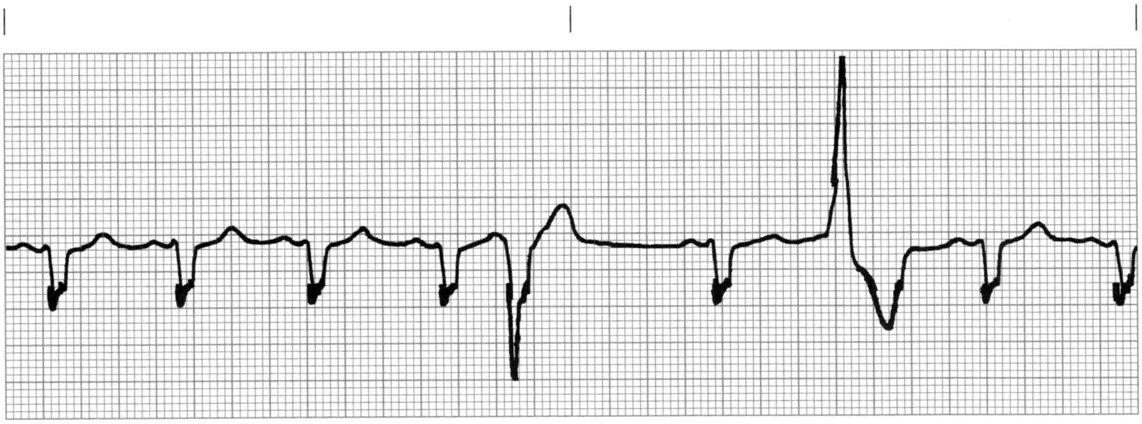

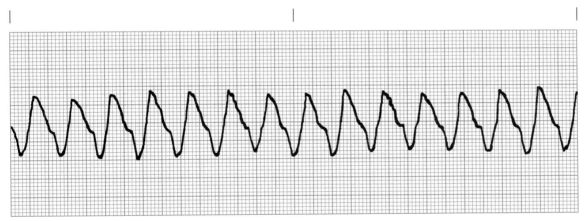

Regularity: _____	**PRI:** _____
Rate: _____	**QRS:** _____
P Waves: _____	**Interp:** _____

8.10

Regularity: _____	**PRI:** _____
Rate: _____	**QRS:** _____
P Waves: _____	**Interp:** _____

8.11

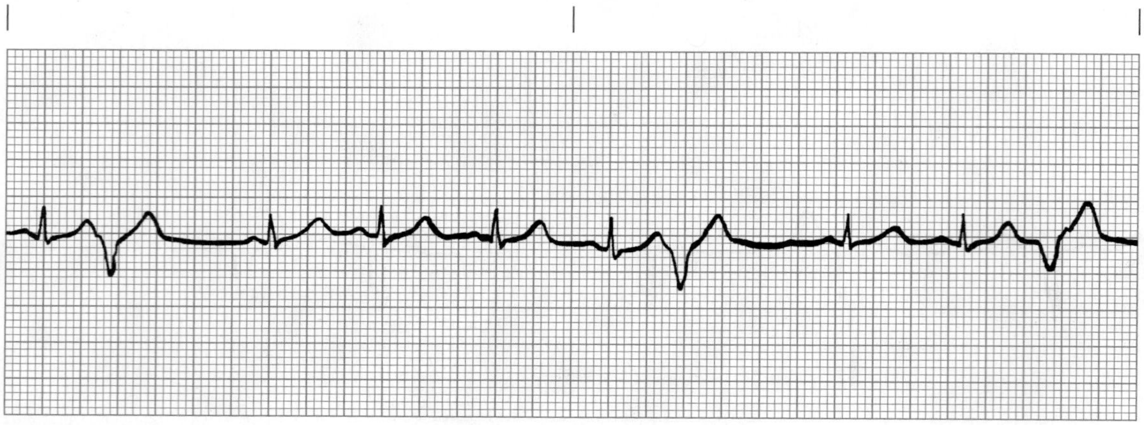

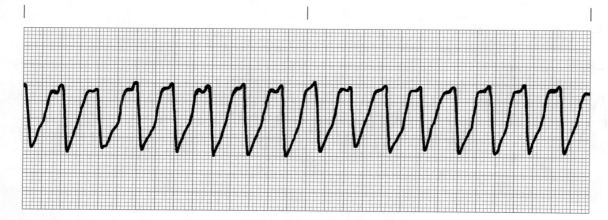

Regularity: _____   PRI: _____

Rate: _____   QRS: _____

P Waves: _____   Interp: _____

8.12

Regularity: _____   PRI: _____

Rate: _____   QRS: _____

P Waves: _____   Interp: _____

8.13

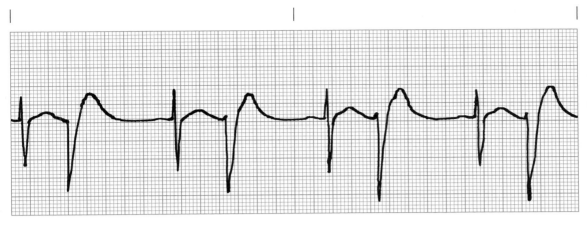

Regularity: _____	PRI: _____
Rate: _____	QRS: _____
P Waves: _____	Interp: _____

8.14

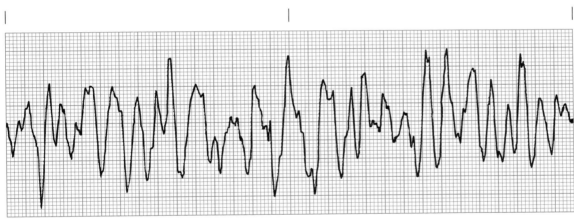

Regularity: _____	PRI: _____
Rate: _____	QRS: _____
P Waves: _____	Interp: _____

8.15

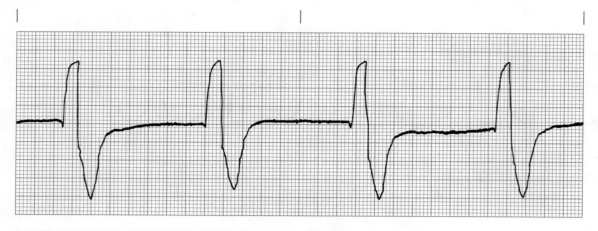

Regularity: _____	PRI: _____	
Rate: _____	QRS: _____	
P Waves: _____	Interp: _____	

8.16

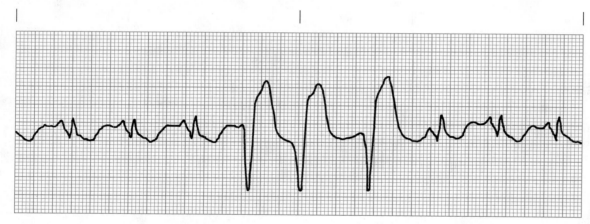

Regularity: _____	PRI: _____	
Rate: _____	QRS: _____	
P Waves: _____	Interp: _____	

8.17

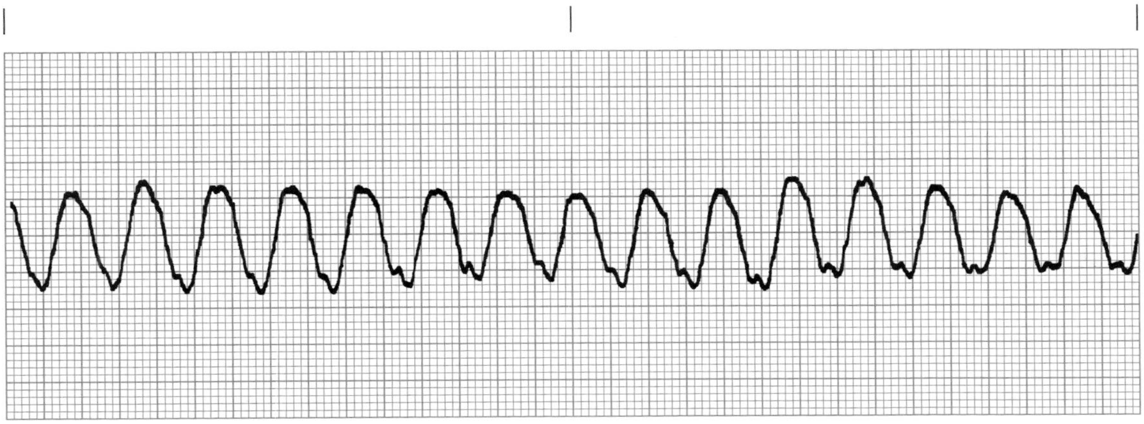

Regularity: _____	PRI: _____
Rate: _____	QRS: _____
P Waves: _____	Interp: _____

8.18

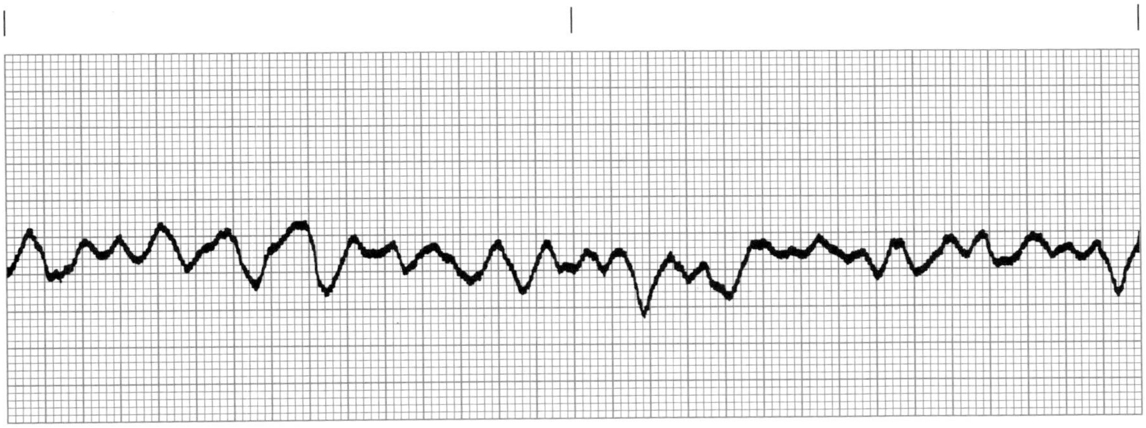

Regularity: _____	PRI: _____
Rate: _____	QRS: _____
P Waves: _____	Interp: _____

8.19

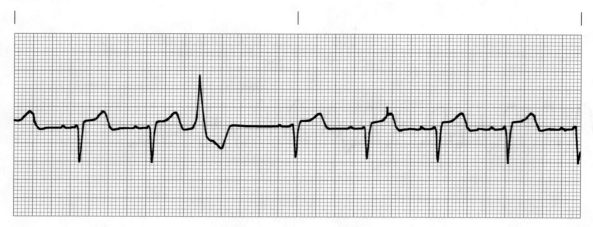

Regularity: _____	PRI: _____
Rate: _____	QRS: _____
P Waves: _____	Interp: _____

8.20

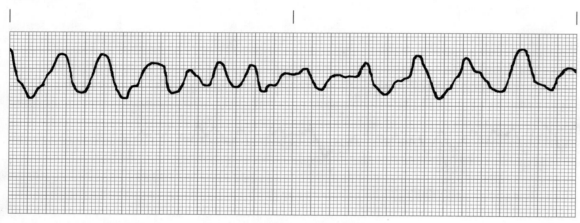

Regularity: _____	PRI: _____
Rate: _____	QRS: _____
P Waves: _____	Interp: _____

8.21

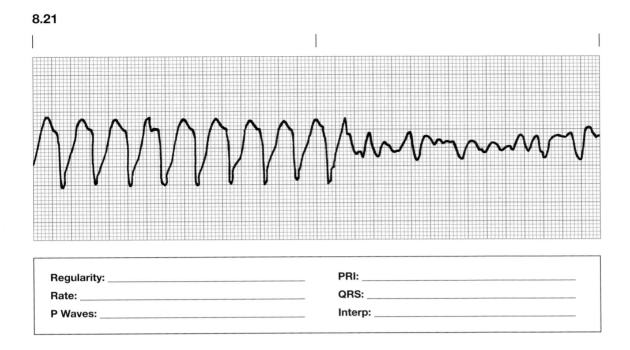

Regularity: _____   PRI: _____

Rate: _____   QRS: _____

P Waves: _____   Interp: _____

8.22

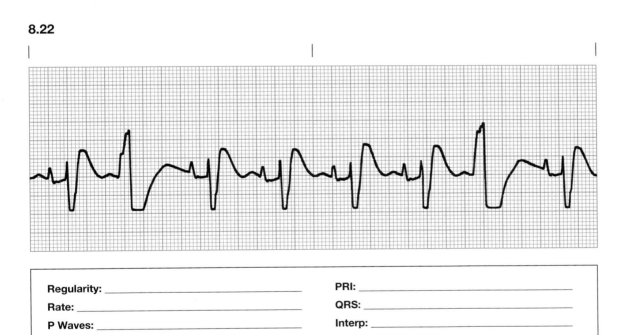

Regularity: _____   PRI: _____

Rate: _____   QRS: _____

P Waves: _____   Interp: _____

8.23

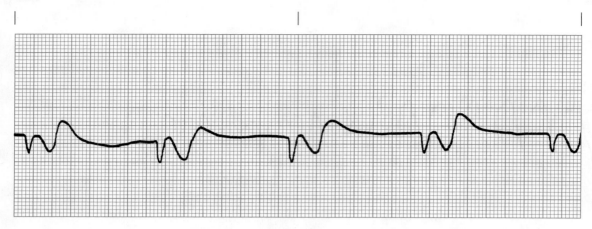

Regularity: _____	PRI: _____
Rate: _____	QRS: _____
P Waves: _____	Interp: _____

8.24

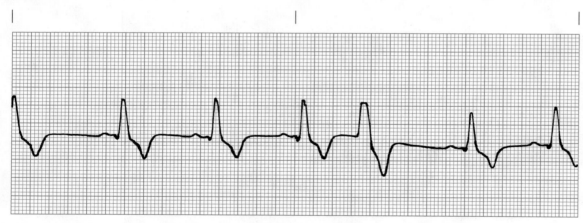

Regularity: _____	PRI: _____
Rate: _____	QRS: _____
P Waves: _____	Interp: _____

8.25

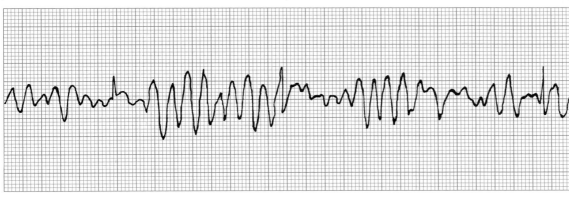

Regularity: _____	PRI: _____
Rate: _____	QRS: _____
P Waves: _____	Interp: _____

8.26

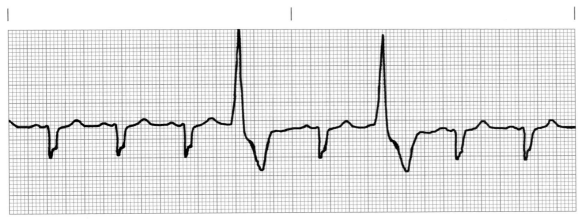

Regularity: _____	PRI: _____
Rate: _____	QRS: _____
P Waves: _____	Interp: _____

8.27

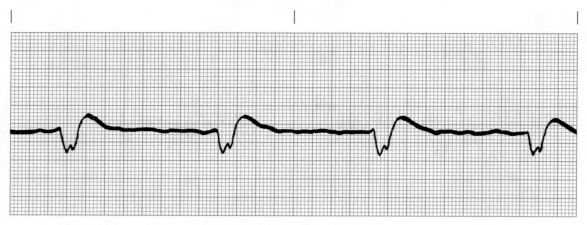

Regularity: _____	PRI: _____
Rate: _____	QRS: _____
P Waves: _____	Interp: _____

8.28

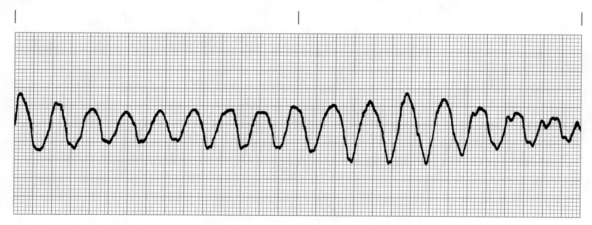

Regularity: _____	PRI: _____
Rate: _____	QRS: _____
P Waves: _____	Interp: _____

8.29

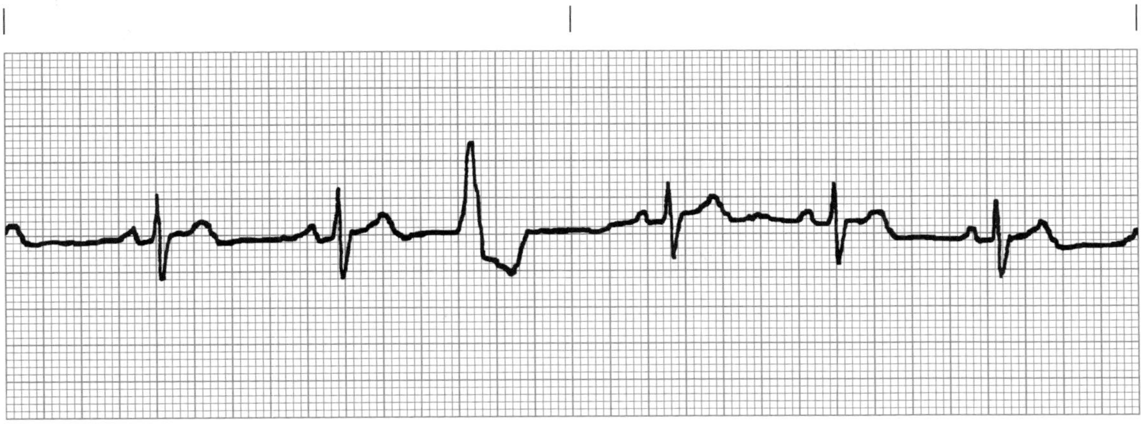

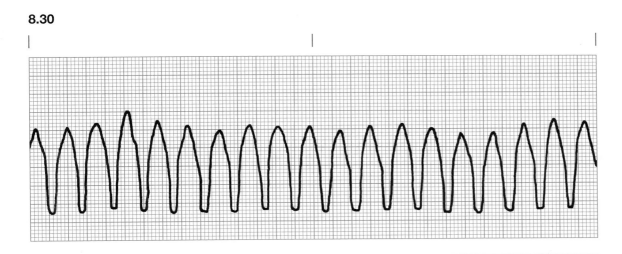

Regularity: _____   PRI: _____

Rate: _____   QRS: _____

P Waves: _____   Interp: _____

8.30

Regularity: _____   PRI: _____

Rate: _____   QRS: _____

P Waves: _____   Interp: _____

8.31

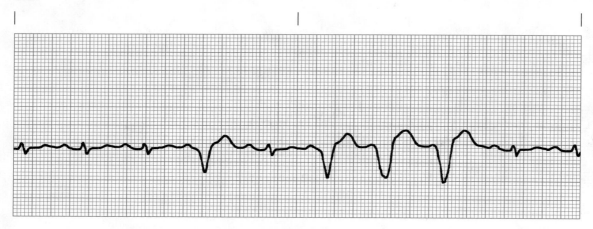

Regularity: _____ PRI: _____

Rate: _____ QRS: _____

P Waves: _____ Interp: _____

8.32

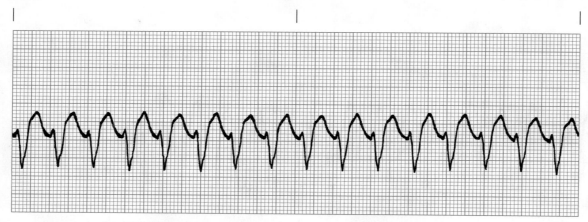

Regularity: _____ PRI: _____

Rate: _____ QRS: _____

P Waves: _____ Interp: _____

8.33

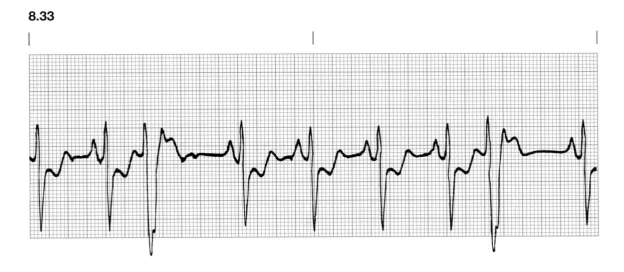

Regularity: _____	PRI: _____
Rate: _____	QRS: _____
P Waves: _____	Interp: _____

8.34

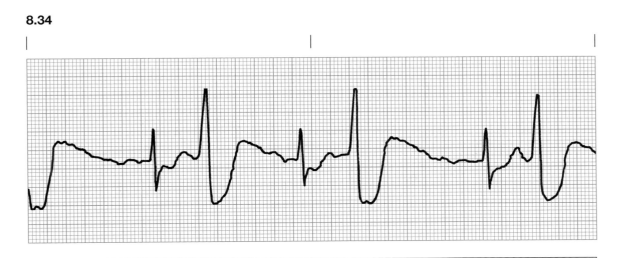

Regularity: _____	PRI: _____
Rate: _____	QRS: _____
P Waves: _____	Interp: _____

8.35

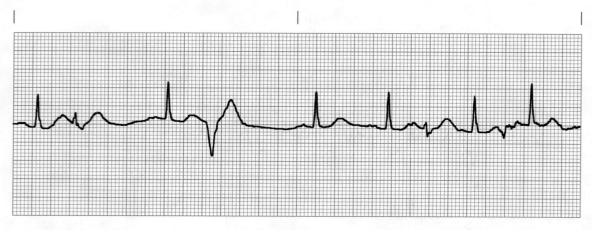

Regularity: _____   PRI: _____

Rate: _____   QRS: _____

P Waves: _____   Interp: _____

8.36

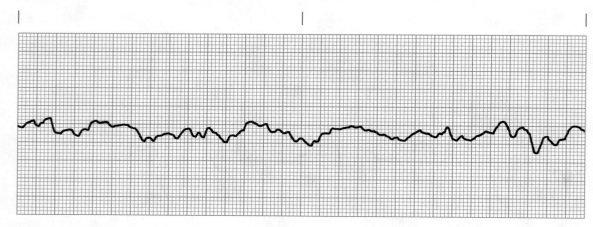

Regularity: _____   PRI: _____

Rate: _____   QRS: _____

P Waves: _____   Interp: _____

8.37

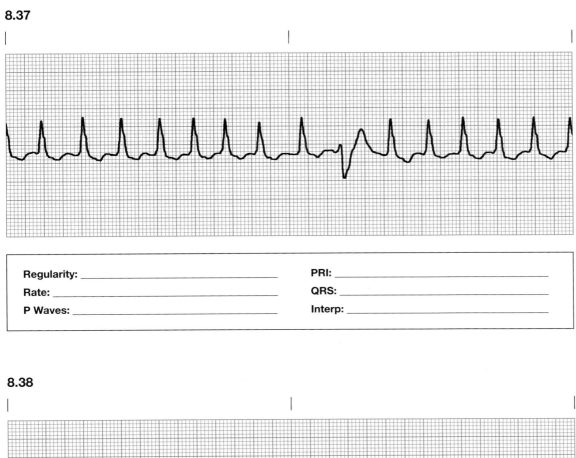

Regularity: _____	PRI: _____
Rate: _____	QRS: _____
P Waves: _____	Interp: _____

8.38

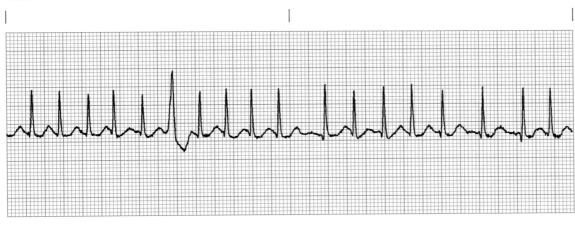

Regularity: _____	PRI: _____
Rate: _____	QRS: _____
P Waves: _____	Interp: _____

8.39

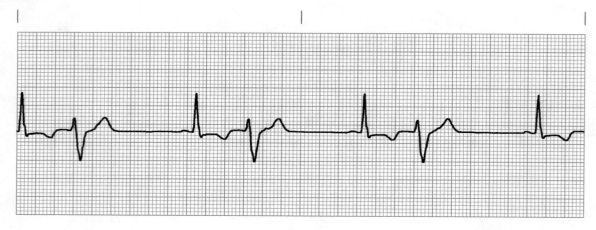

Regularity: _____	PRI: _____
Rate: _____	QRS: _____
P Waves: _____	Interp: _____

8.40

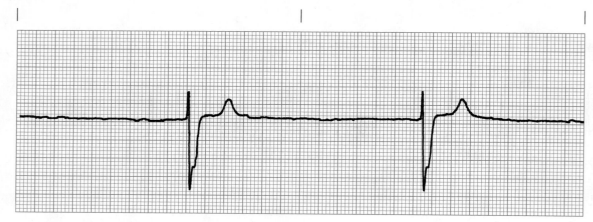

Regularity: _____	PRI: _____
Rate: _____	QRS: _____
P Waves: _____	Interp: _____

8.41

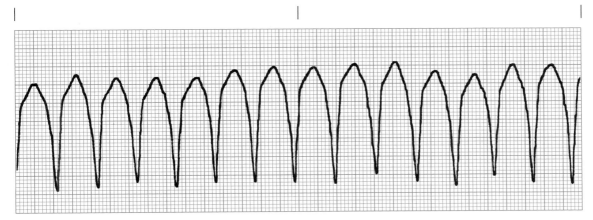

Regularity: _____	PRI: _____
Rate: _____	QRS: _____
P Waves: _____	Interp: _____

8.42

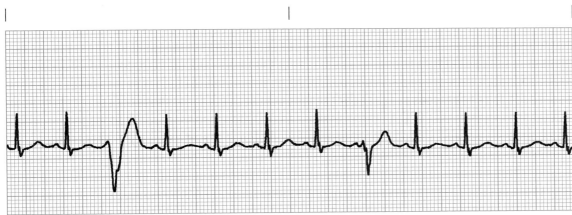

Regularity: _____	PRI: _____
Rate: _____	QRS: _____
P Waves: _____	Interp: _____

8.43

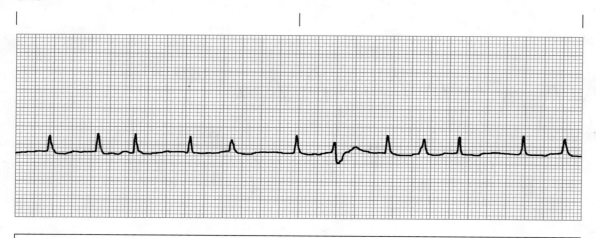

Regularity: _____	PRI: _____
Rate: _____	QRS: _____
P Waves: _____	Interp: _____

8.44

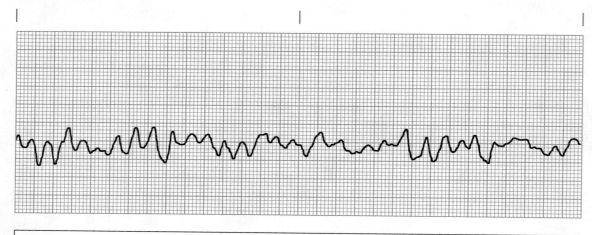

Regularity: _____	PRI: _____
Rate: _____	QRS: _____
P Waves: _____	Interp: _____

8.45

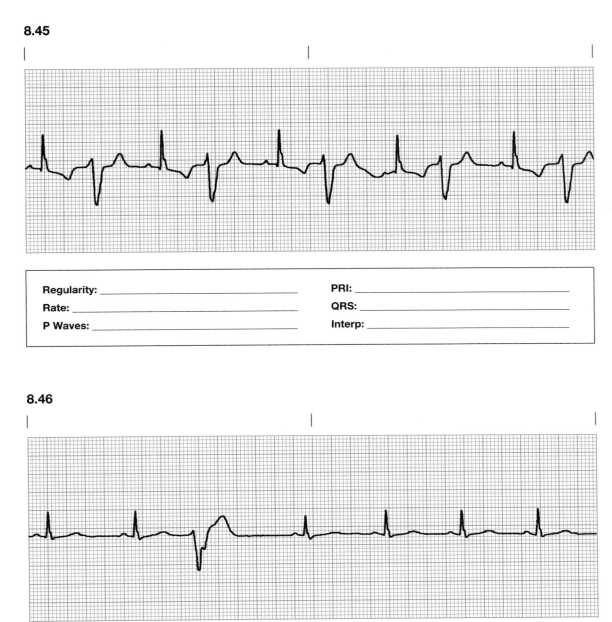

Regularity: _____   PRI: _____

Rate: _____   QRS: _____

P Waves: _____   Interp: _____

8.46

Regularity: _____   PRI: _____

Rate: _____   QRS: _____

P Waves: _____   Interp: _____

8.47

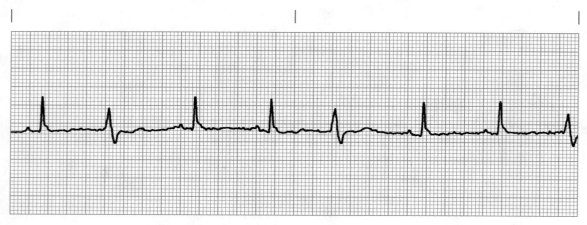

Regularity: _____		PRI: _____	
Rate: _____		QRS: _____	
P Waves: _____		Interp: _____	

8.48

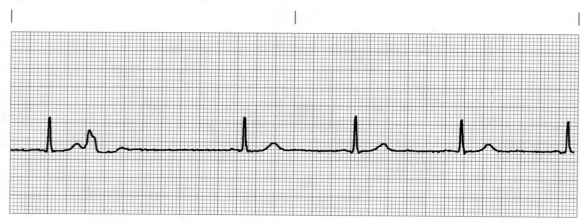

Regularity: _____		PRI: _____	
Rate: _____		QRS: _____	
P Waves: _____		Interp: _____	

8.49

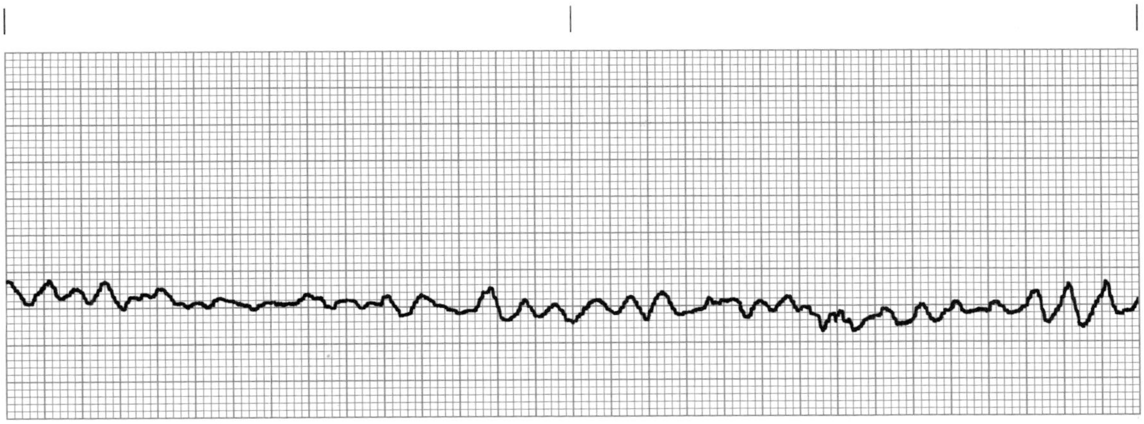

Regularity: _____   PRI: _____

Rate: _____   QRS: _____

P Waves: _____   Interp: _____

8.50

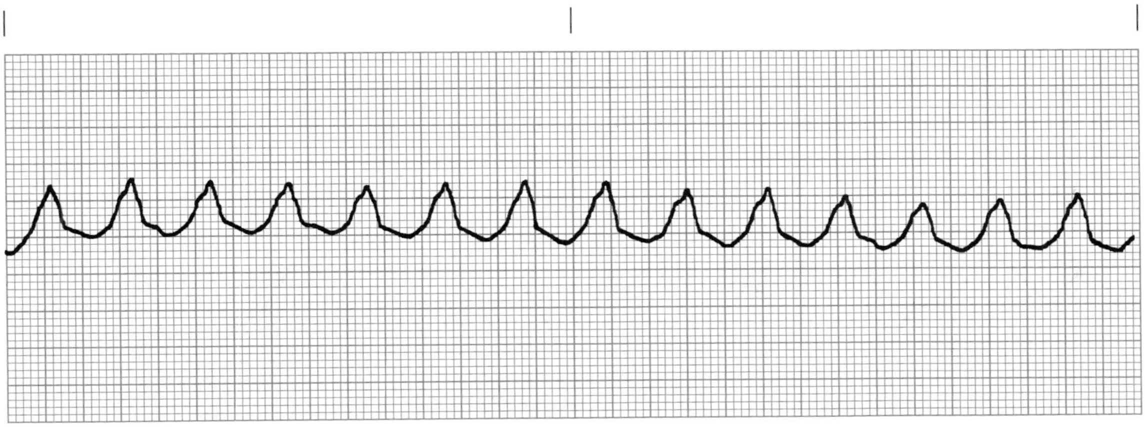

Regularity: _____   PRI: _____

Rate: _____   QRS: _____

P Waves: _____   Interp: _____

8.51

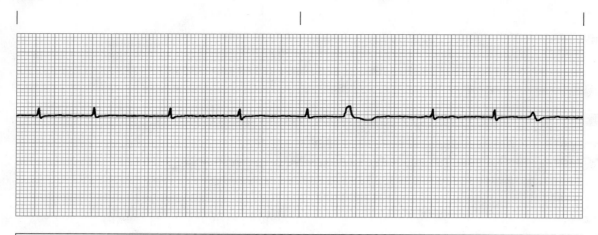

Regularity: _____		PRI: _____
Rate: _____		QRS: _____
P Waves: _____		Interp: _____

8.52

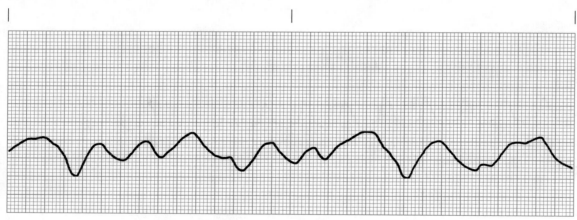

Regularity: _____		PRI: _____
Rate: _____		QRS: _____
P Waves: _____		Interp: _____

8.53

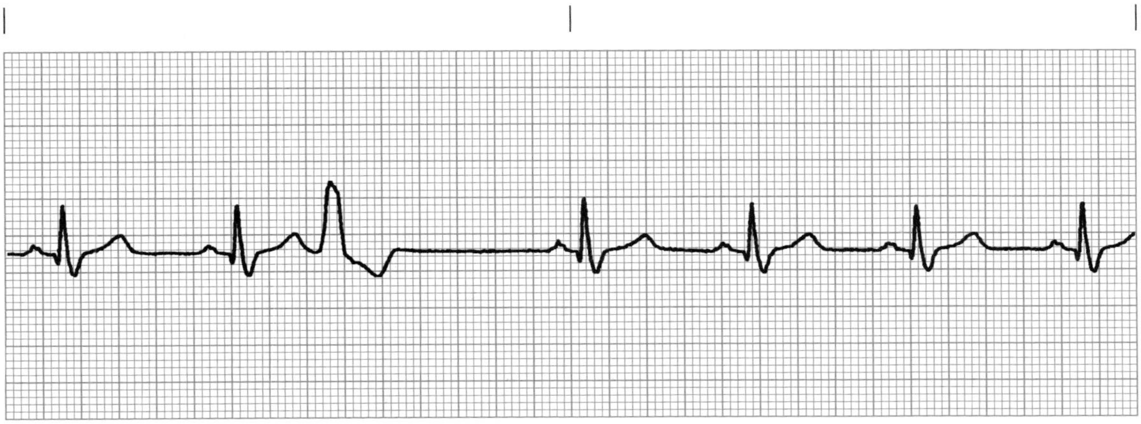

Regularity: _____   PRI: _____

Rate: _____   QRS: _____

P Waves: _____   Interp: _____

8.54

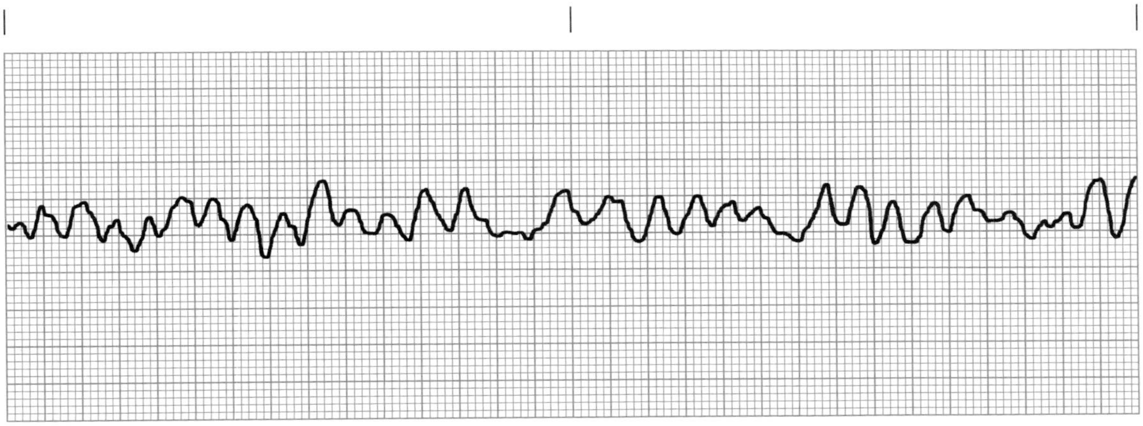

Regularity: _____   PRI: _____

Rate: _____   QRS: _____

P Waves: _____   Interp: _____

8.55

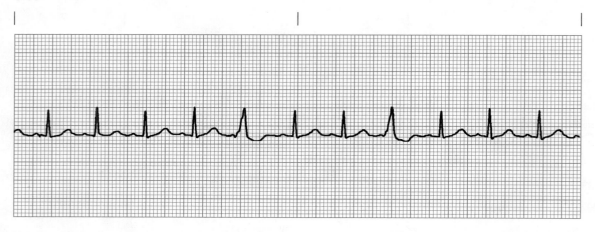

Regularity: _____	PRI: _____	
Rate: _____	QRS: _____	
P Waves: _____	Interp: _____	

8.56

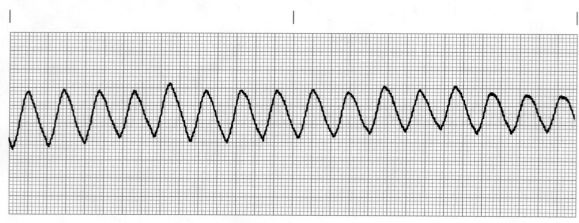

Regularity: _____	PRI: _____	
Rate: _____	QRS: _____	
P Waves: _____	Interp: _____	

8.57

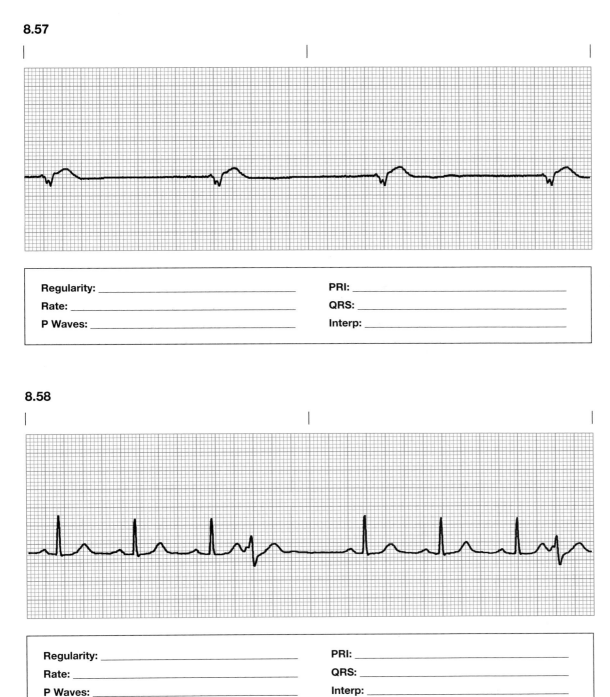

Regularity: _____ PRI: _____

Rate: _____ QRS: _____

P Waves: _____ Interp: _____

8.58

Regularity: _____ PRI: _____

Rate: _____ QRS: _____

P Waves: _____ Interp: _____

8.59

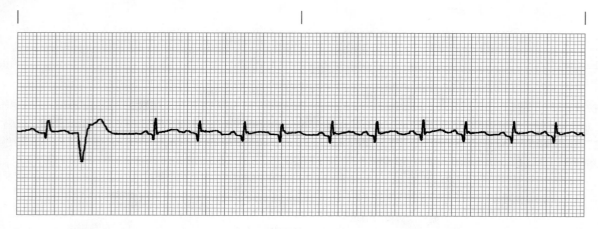

Regularity: _____   PRI: _____

Rate: _____   QRS: _____

P Waves: _____   Interp: _____

8.60

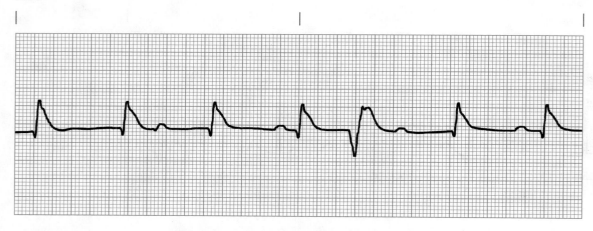

Regularity: _____   PRI: _____

Rate: _____   QRS: _____

P Waves: _____   Interp: _____

8.61

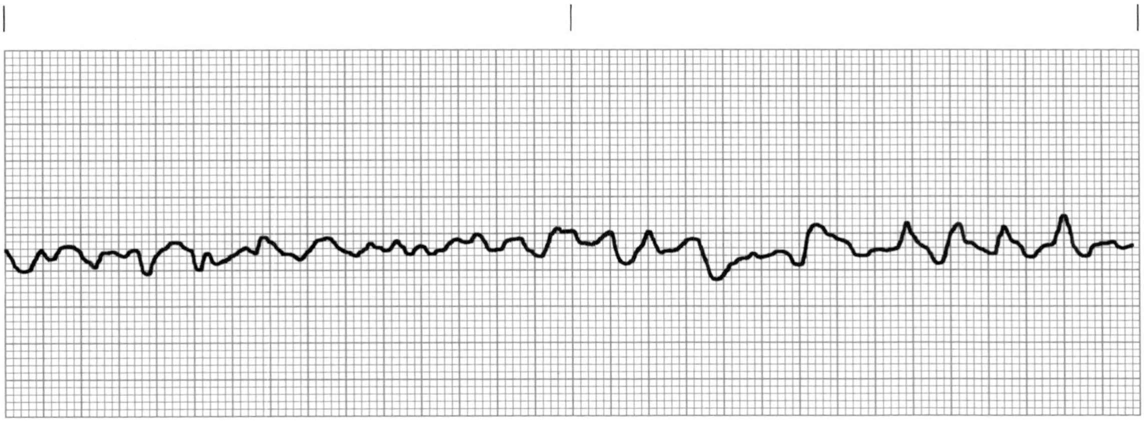

Regularity: _____   PRI: _____

Rate: _____   QRS: _____

P Waves: _____   Interp: _____

8.62

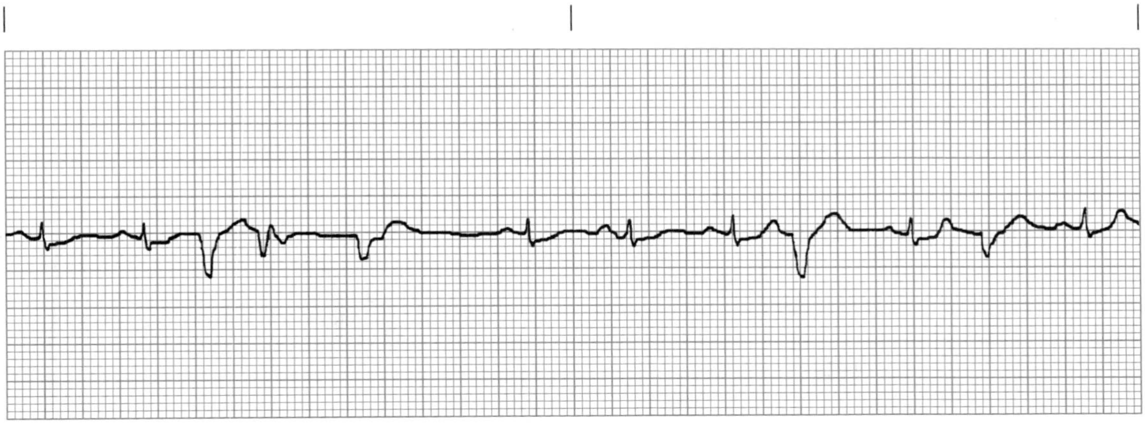

Regularity: _____   PRI: _____

Rate: _____   QRS: _____

P Waves: _____   Interp: _____

8.63

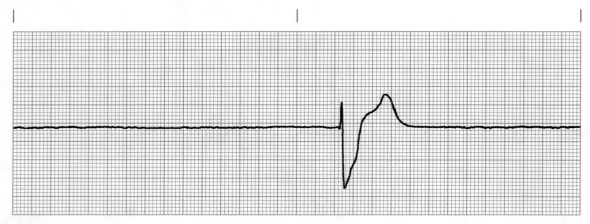

Regularity: _____	PRI: _____
Rate: _____	QRS: _____
P Waves: _____	Interp: _____

8.64

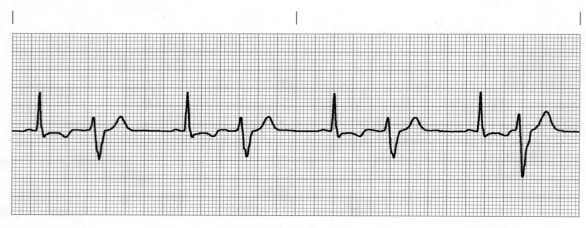

Regularity: _____	PRI: _____
Rate: _____	QRS: _____
P Waves: _____	Interp: _____

8.65

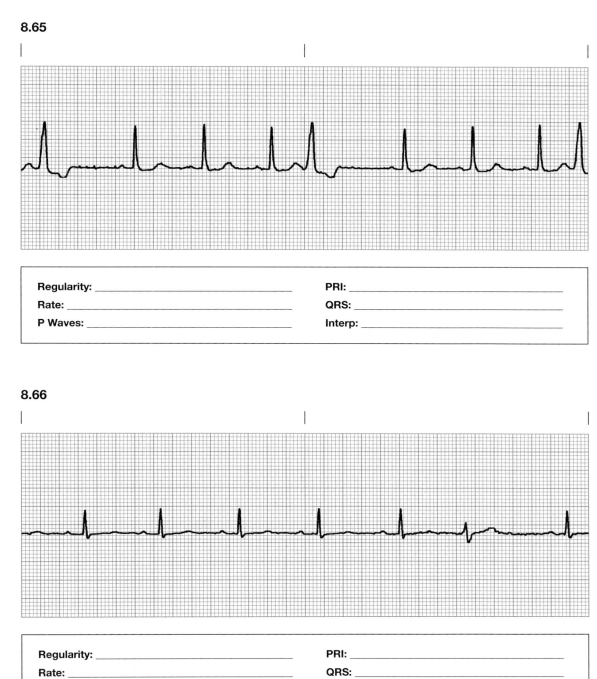

Regularity: _____	**PRI:** _____
Rate: _____	**QRS:** _____
P Waves: _____	**Interp:** _____

8.66

Regularity: _____	**PRI:** _____
Rate: _____	**QRS:** _____
P Waves: _____	**Interp:** _____

8.67

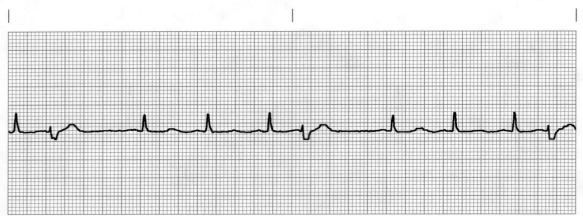

Regularity: _____	PRI: _____
Rate: _____	QRS: _____
P Waves: _____	Interp: _____

8.68

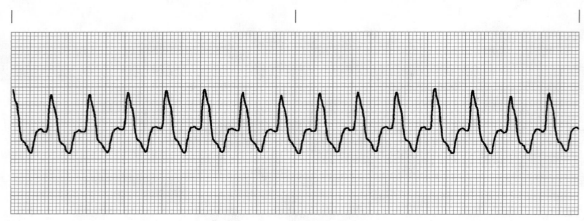

Regularity: _____	PRI: _____
Rate: _____	QRS: _____
P Waves: _____	Interp: _____

8.69

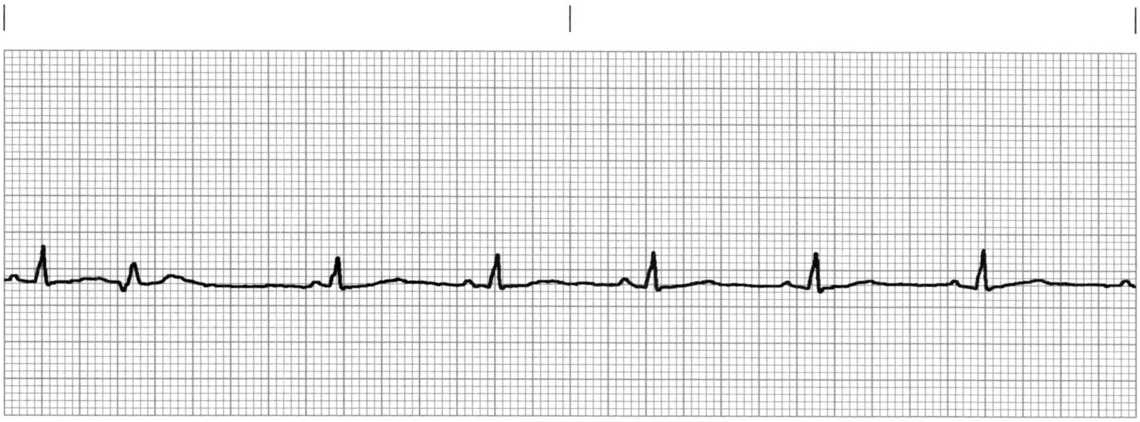

Regularity: _____	**PRI:** _____
Rate: _____	**QRS:** _____
P Waves: _____	**Interp:** _____

8.70

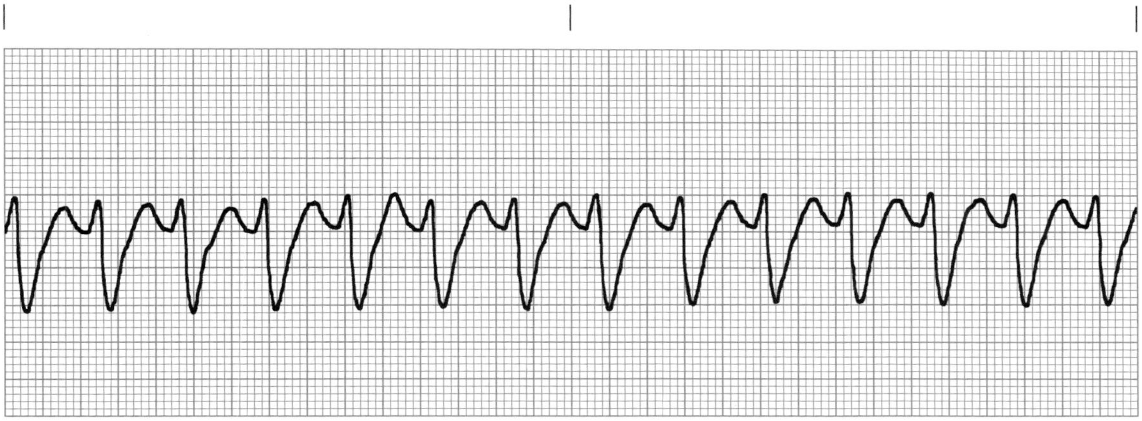

Regularity: _____	**PRI:** _____
Rate: _____	**QRS:** _____
P Waves: _____	**Interp:** _____

8.71

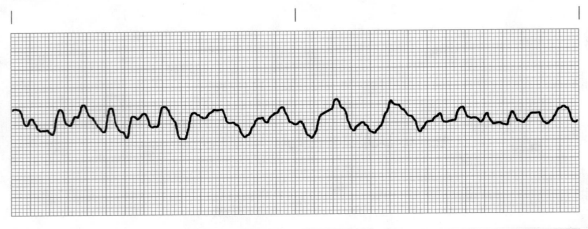

Regularity: _____	PRI: _____
Rate: _____	QRS: _____
P Waves: _____	Interp: _____

8.72

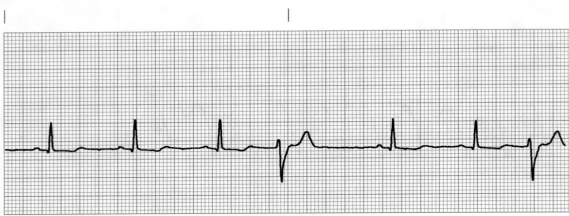

Regularity: _____	PRI: _____
Rate: _____	QRS: _____
P Waves: _____	Interp: _____

8.73

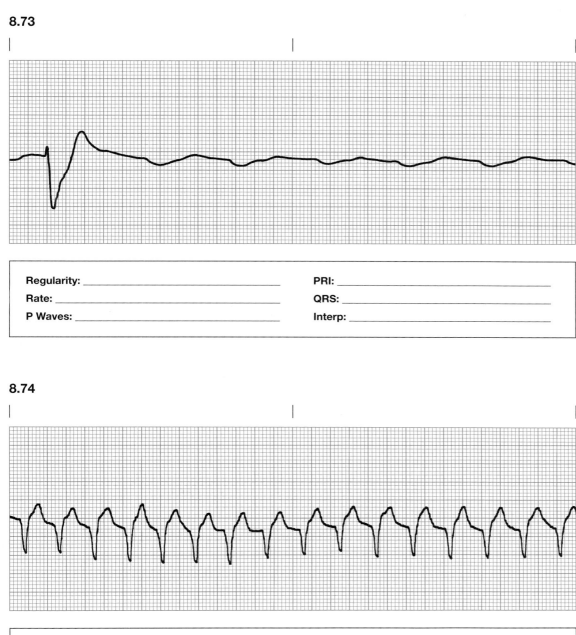

Regularity: _____	**PRI:** _____
Rate: _____	**QRS:** _____
P Waves: _____	**Interp:** _____

8.74

Regularity: _____	**PRI:** _____
Rate: _____	**QRS:** _____
P Waves: _____	**Interp:** _____

8.75

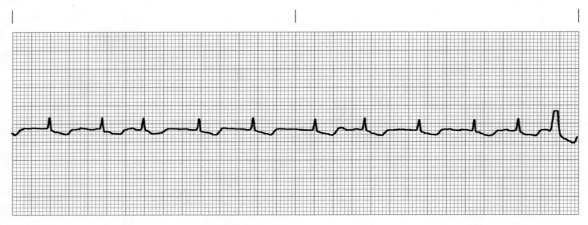

Regularity: _____	PRI: _____
Rate: _____	QRS: _____
P Waves: _____	Interp: _____

8.76

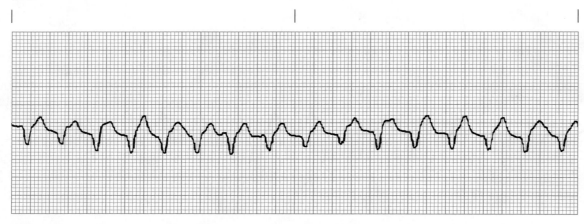

Regularity: _____	PRI: _____
Rate: _____	QRS: _____
P Waves: _____	Interp: _____

8.77

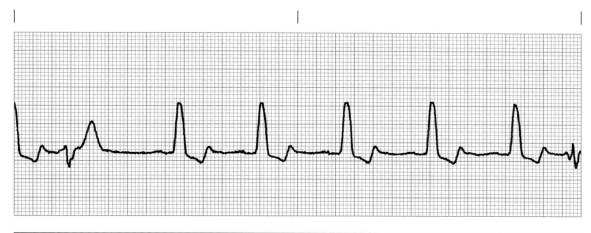

Regularity: _____	PRI: _____
Rate: _____	QRS: _____
P Waves: _____	Interp: _____

Chapter 9
Practice Makes Perfect

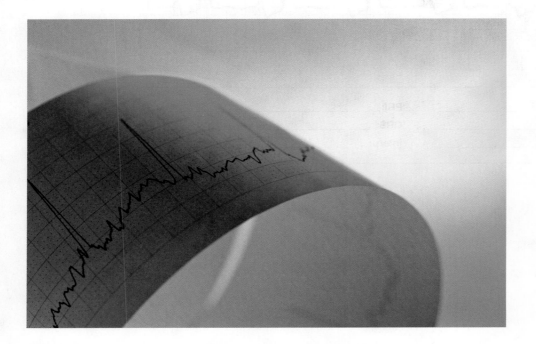

Introduction

In this program you learned the basic principles of arrhythmia interpretation. You also learned the rules for twenty-two of the most common arrhythmias. This book has provided you with a format for analyzing any arrhythmia so that you can compare it to the rules and identify it. The format directs you to systematically inspect the regularity, rate, P waves, PR intervals, and QRS complexes, and to use all of that information to help you identify the arrhythmia.

As you practice on more and more rhythm strips, you will develop your interpretation skill. The more you practice, the easier this process will become, and you will find that you are conducting many of the format steps without really thinking about them. It will become almost second nature to you. At that point, you might begin to think that the format is no longer useful, or that it no longer applies. In fact, you have simply learned to perform the process quickly. The important issue is that you know the format, and if you ever need to interpret a very complex arrhythmia, you can always revert to the five-step process. Once you are comfortable using this format, it will always be available to help you identify even the most intimidating arrhythmia.

For you to be truly comfortable in arrhythmia identification, you must practice. That is what this chapter is for. As you go through the practice strips, remember the analysis format, even if you only use it mentally most of the time. When you check your answers with the key, look to see how the answers were reached. If you repeatedly make errors in the same area, go back to the related chapter and review the key points. If possible, have an instructor or other knowledgeable person assist you.

This book was designed to provide you with a solid foundation of knowledge and skill in arrhythmia interpretation. As you complete the program, you should be very capable of recognizing and understanding the most common uncomplicated arrhythmias. But this is only the tip of the iceberg in the field of electrocardiography. If you are interested in continuing to learn more about this field, you can add to the core of information you already have by attending higher-level EKG classes, reading the many books that are available, or talking to people who work with EKGs every day. This is a fascinating area of study. Researchers are discovering new things daily that add to our understanding of electrocardiography. The most difficult step in the learning process is the very first phase of learning the basics, and now you have completed that phase. Now there is nothing to prevent you from becoming an expert in this field. Nothing but practice, that is. And practice begins here.

PRACTICE STRIPS (answers can be found in the Answer Key on page 565)

9.1

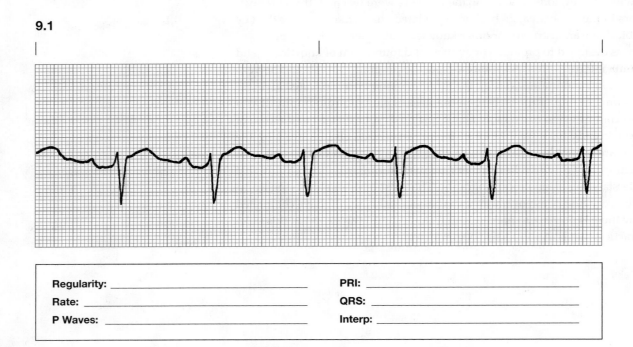

Regularity: _____	PRI: _____
Rate: _____	QRS: _____
P Waves: _____	Interp: _____

9.2

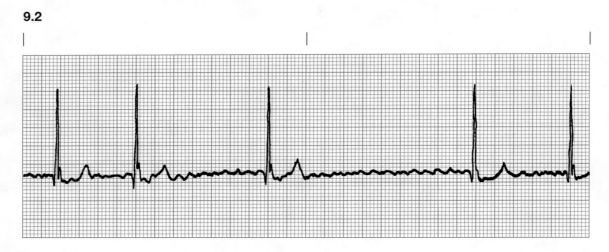

Regularity: _____	PRI: _____
Rate: _____	QRS: _____
P Waves: _____	Interp: _____

9.3

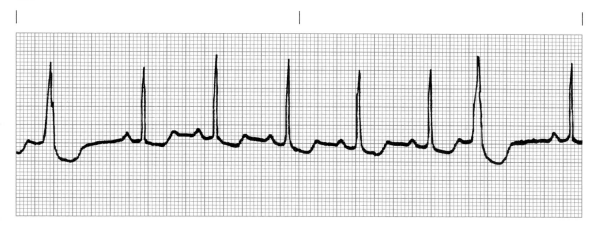

Regularity: _____	PRI: _____
Rate: _____	QRS: _____
P Waves: _____	Interp: _____

9.4.

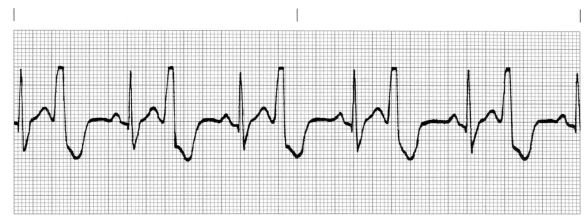

Regularity: _____	PRI: _____
Rate: _____	QRS: _____
P Waves: _____	Interp: _____

9.5

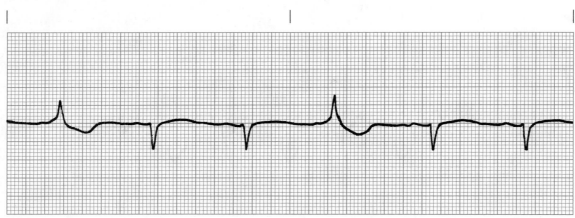

Regularity: _____		**PRI:** _____
Rate: _____		**QRS:** _____
P Waves: _____		**Interp:** _____

9.6

Regularity: _____		**PRI:** _____
Rate: _____		**QRS:** _____
P Waves: _____		**Interp:** _____

9.7

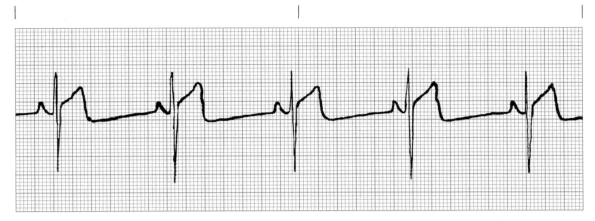

Regularity: _____	**PRI:** _____
Rate: _____	**QRS:** _____
P Waves: _____	**Interp:** _____

9.8

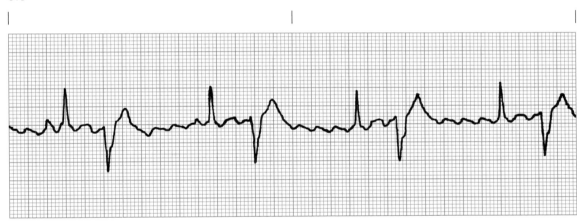

Regularity: _____	**PRI:** _____
Rate: _____	**QRS:** _____
P Waves: _____	**Interp:** _____

9.9

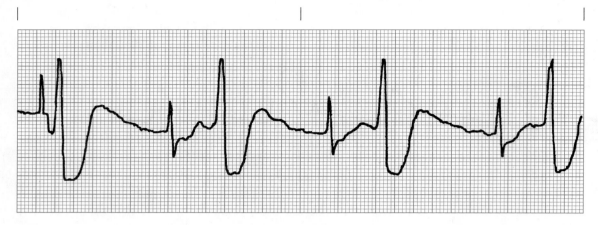

Regularity: _____   PRI: _____

Rate: _____   QRS: _____

P Waves: _____   Interp: _____

9.10

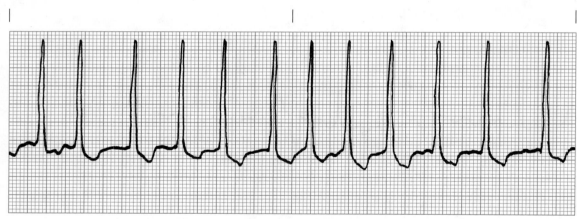

Regularity: _____   PRI: _____

Rate: _____   QRS: _____

P Waves: _____   Interp: _____

9.11

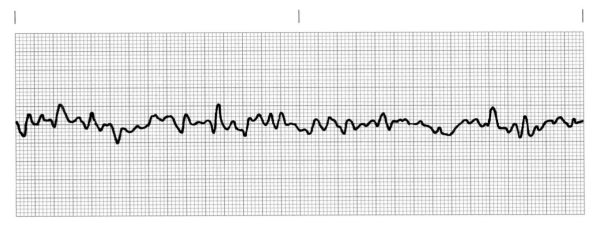

Regularity: _____   PRI: _____

Rate: _____   QRS: _____

P Waves: _____   Interp: _____

9.12

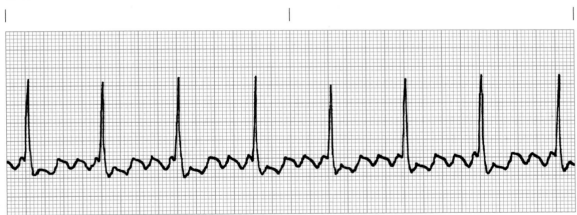

Regularity: _____   PRI: _____

Rate: _____   QRS: _____

P Waves: _____   Interp: _____

9.13

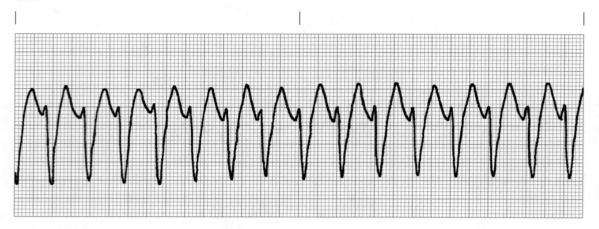

Regularity: _____   PRI: _____

Rate: _____   QRS: _____

P Waves: _____   Interp: _____

9.14

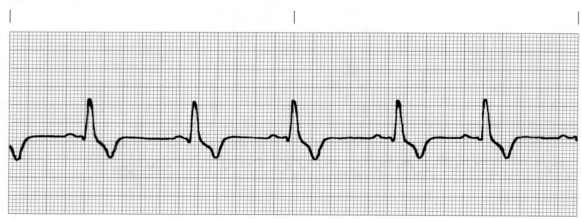

Regularity: _____   PRI: _____

Rate: _____   QRS: _____

P Waves: _____   Interp: _____

9.15

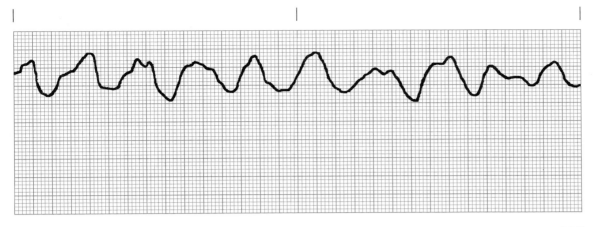

Regularity: _____	PRI: _____
Rate: _____	QRS: _____
P Waves: _____	Interp: _____

9.16

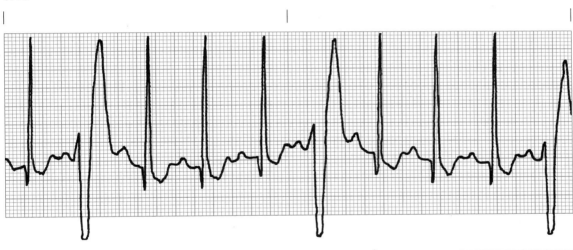

Regularity: _____	PRI: _____
Rate: _____	QRS: _____
P Waves: _____	Interp: _____

9.17

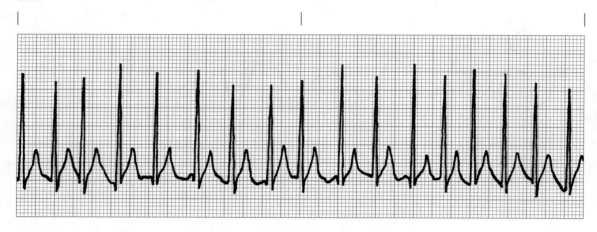

Regularity: _____	PRI: _____
Rate: _____	QRS: _____
P Waves: _____	Interp: _____

9.18

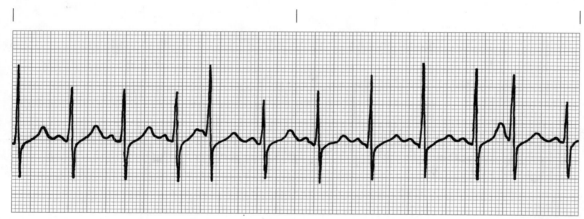

Regularity: _____	PRI: _____
Rate: _____	QRS: _____
P Waves: _____	Interp: _____

9.19

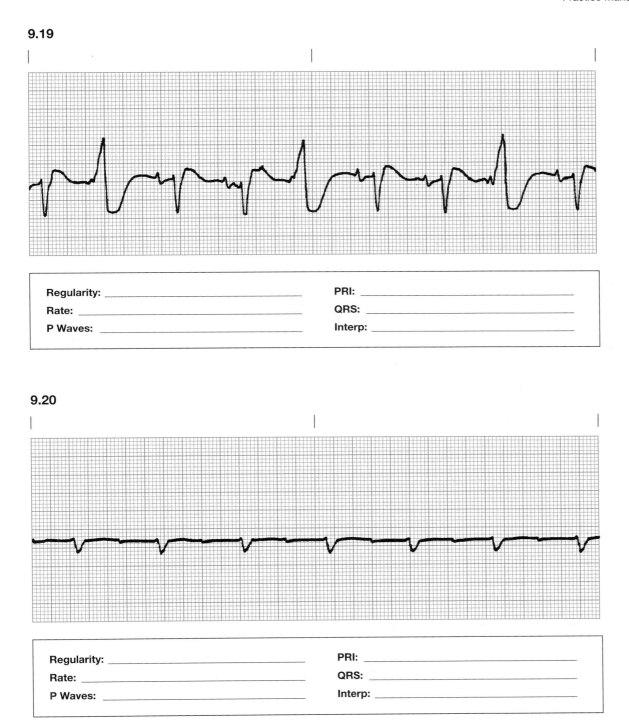

Regularity: _____	PRI: _____
Rate: _____	QRS: _____
P Waves: _____	Interp: _____

9.20

Regularity: _____	PRI: _____
Rate: _____	QRS: _____
P Waves: _____	Interp: _____

9.21

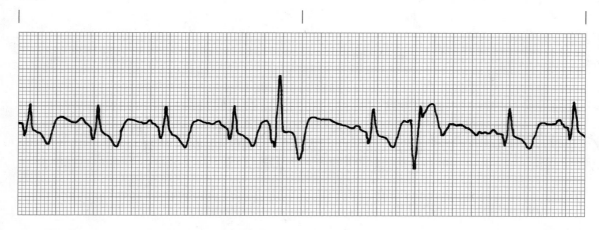

Regularity: _____   PRI: _____

Rate: _____   QRS: _____

P Waves: _____   Interp: _____

9.22

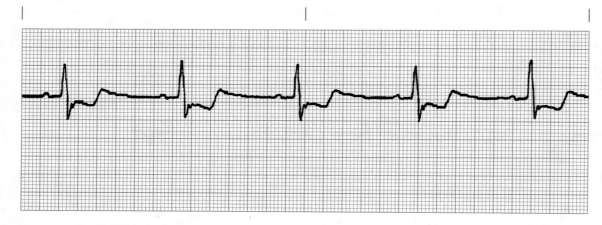

Regularity: _____   PRI: _____

Rate: _____   QRS: _____

P Waves: _____   Interp: _____

9.23

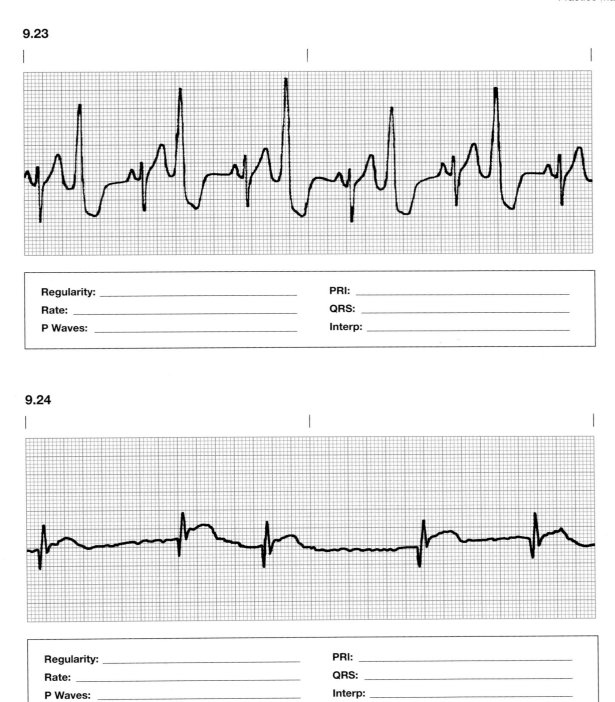

Regularity: _____   PRI: _____

Rate: _____   QRS: _____

P Waves: _____   Interp: _____

9.24

Regularity: _____   PRI: _____

Rate: _____   QRS: _____

P Waves: _____   Interp: _____

9.25

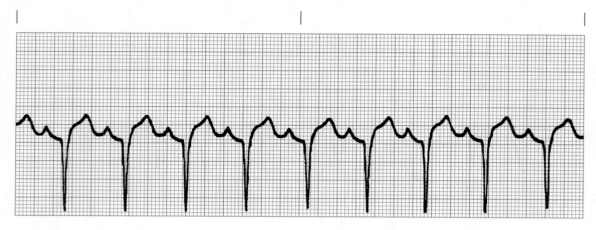

Regularity: _____   PRI: _____

Rate: _____   QRS: _____

P Waves: _____   Interp: _____

9.26

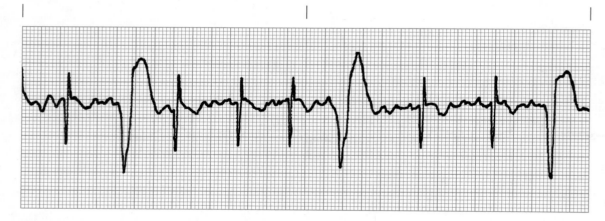

Regularity: _____   PRI: _____

Rate: _____   QRS: _____

P Waves: _____   Interp: _____

9.27

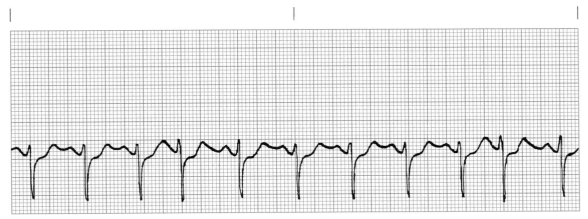

Regularity: _____   PRI: _____

Rate: _____   QRS: _____

P Waves: _____   Interp: _____

9.28

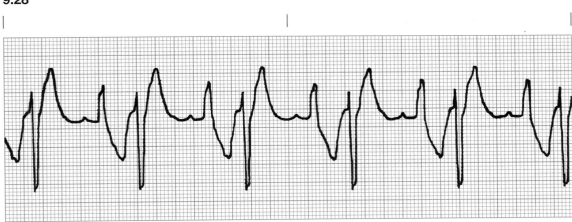

Regularity: _____   PRI: _____

Rate: _____   QRS: _____

P Waves: _____   Interp: _____

9.29

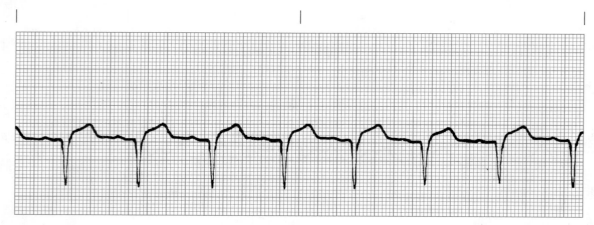

Regularity: _____		PRI: _____	
Rate: _____		QRS: _____	
P Waves: _____		Interp: _____	

9.30

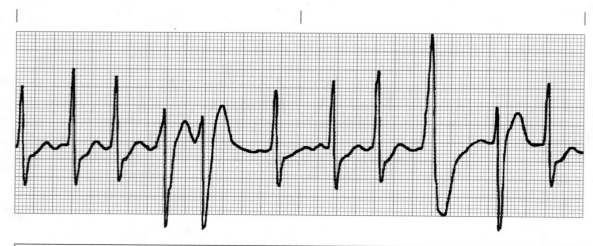

Regularity: _____		PRI: _____	
Rate: _____		QRS: _____	
P Waves: _____		Interp: _____	

9.31

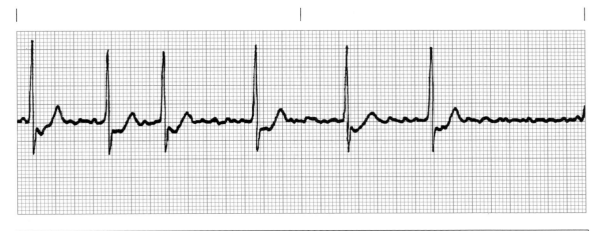

Regularity: _____	PRI: _____
Rate: _____	QRS: _____
P Waves: _____	Interp: _____

9.32

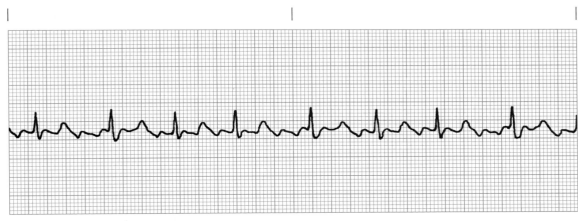

Regularity: _____	PRI: _____
Rate: _____	QRS: _____
P Waves: _____	Interp: _____

9.33

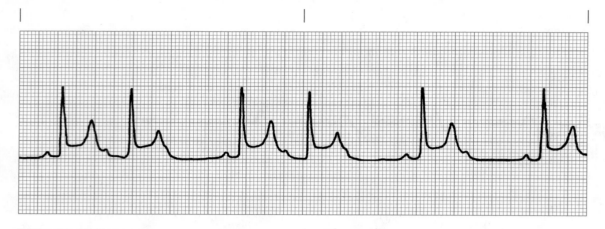

Regularity: _____	PRI: _____
Rate: _____	QRS: _____
P Waves: _____	Interp: _____

9.34

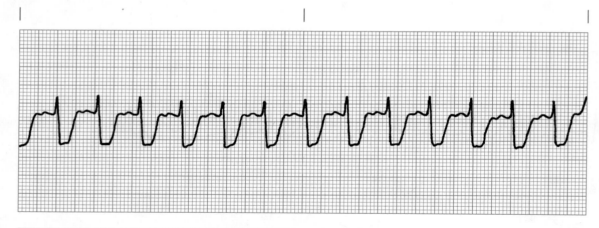

Regularity: _____	PRI: _____
Rate: _____	QRS: _____
P Waves: _____	Interp: _____

9.35

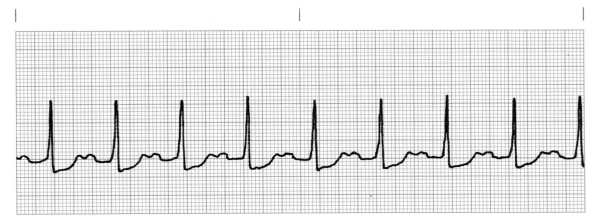

Regularity: _____	**PRI:** _____	
Rate: _____	**QRS:** _____	
P Waves: _____	**Interp:** _____	

9.36

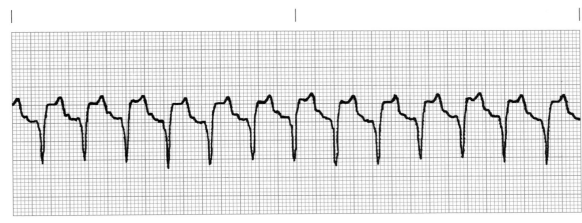

Regularity: _____	**PRI:** _____	
Rate: _____	**QRS:** _____	
P Waves: _____	**Interp:** _____	

9.37

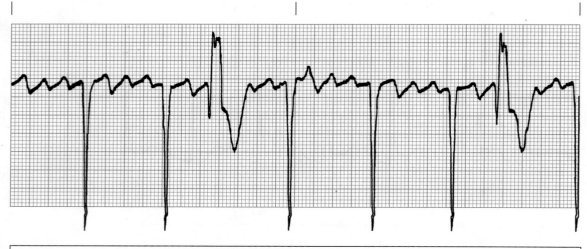

Regularity: _____	**PRI:** _____	
Rate: _____	**QRS:** _____	
P Waves: _____	**Interp:** _____	

9.38

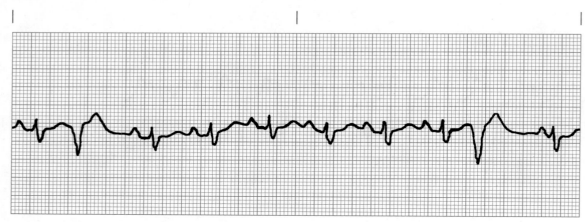

Regularity: _____	**PRI:** _____	
Rate: _____	**QRS:** _____	
P Waves: _____	**Interp:** _____	

9.39

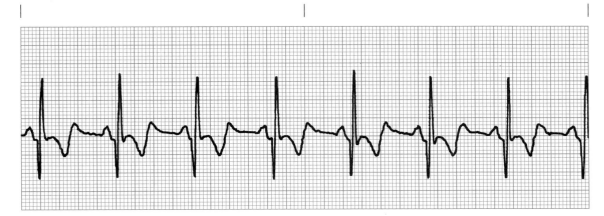

Regularity: _____   PRI: _____

Rate: _____   QRS: _____

P Waves: _____   Interp: _____

9.40

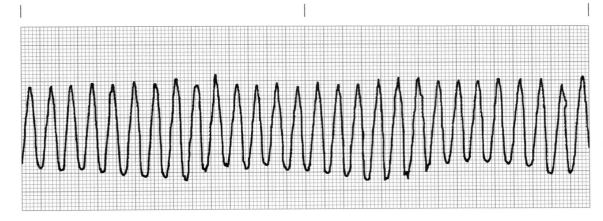

Regularity: _____   PRI: _____

Rate: _____   QRS: _____

P Waves: _____   Interp: _____

9.41

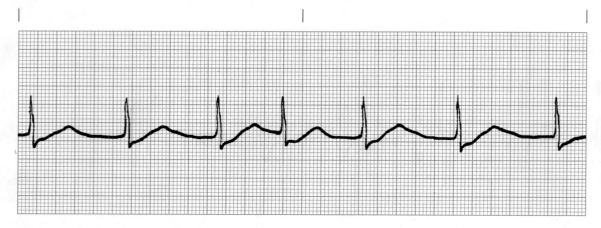

Regularity: _____	PRI: _____
Rate: _____	QRS: _____
P Waves: _____	Interp: _____

9.42

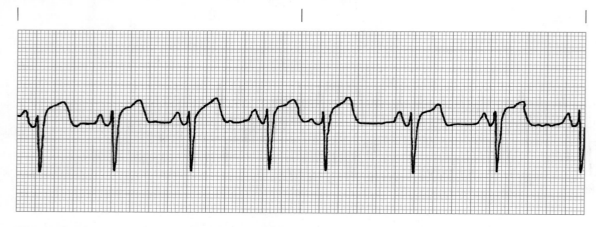

Regularity: _____	PRI: _____
Rate: _____	QRS: _____
P Waves: _____	Interp: _____

9.43

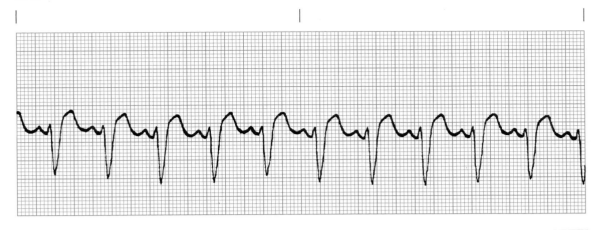

Regularity: _____	PRI: _____
Rate: _____	QRS: _____
P Waves: _____	Interp: _____

9.44

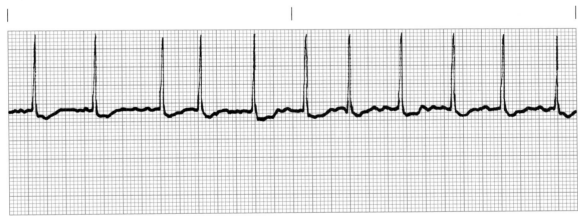

Regularity: _____	PRI: _____
Rate: _____	QRS: _____
P Waves: _____	Interp: _____

9.45

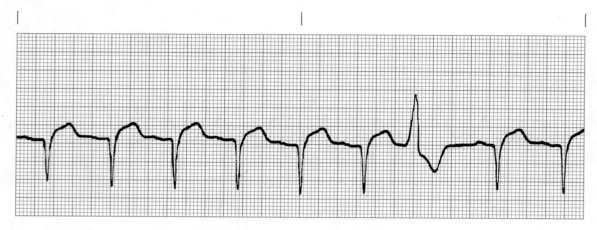

Regularity: _____	**PRI:** _____	
Rate: _____	**QRS:** _____	
P Waves: _____	**Interp:** _____	

9.46

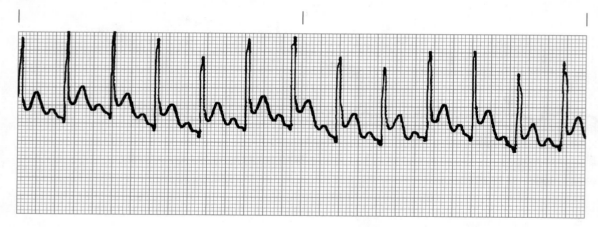

Regularity: _____	**PRI:** _____	
Rate: _____	**QRS:** _____	
P Waves: _____	**Interp:** _____	

9.47

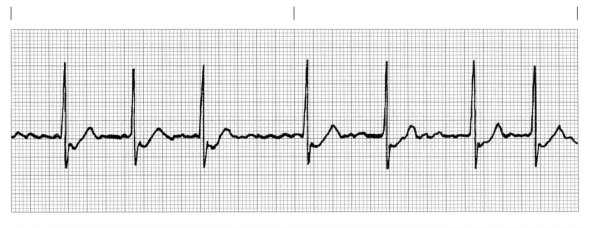

Regularity: _____	PRI: _____
Rate: _____	QRS: _____
P Waves: _____	Interp: _____

9.48

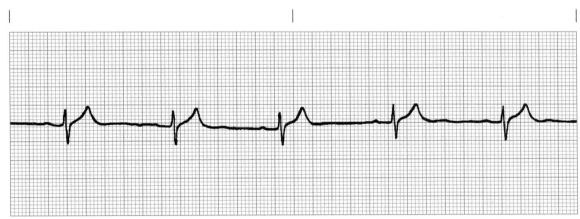

Regularity: _____	PRI: _____
Rate: _____	QRS: _____
P Waves: _____	Interp: _____

9.49

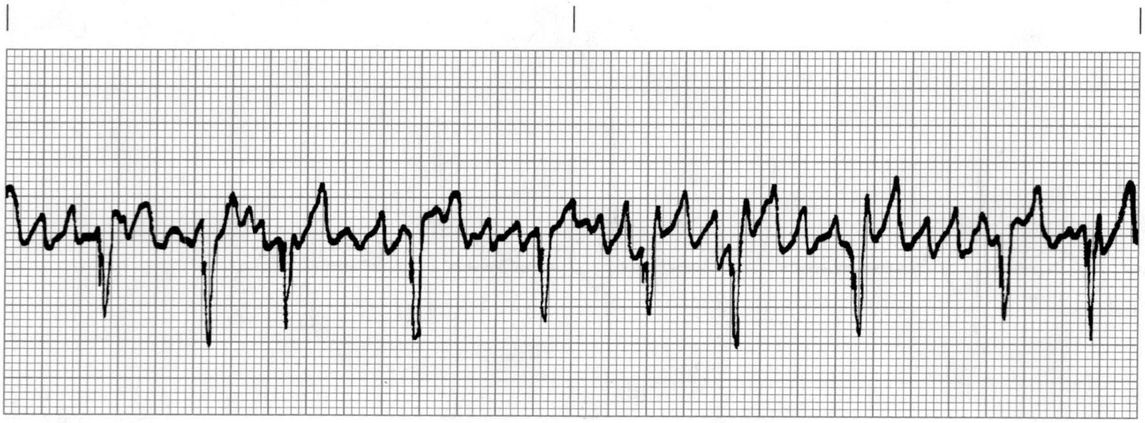

Regularity: _____   PRI: _____

Rate: _____   QRS: _____

P Waves: _____   Interp: _____

9.50

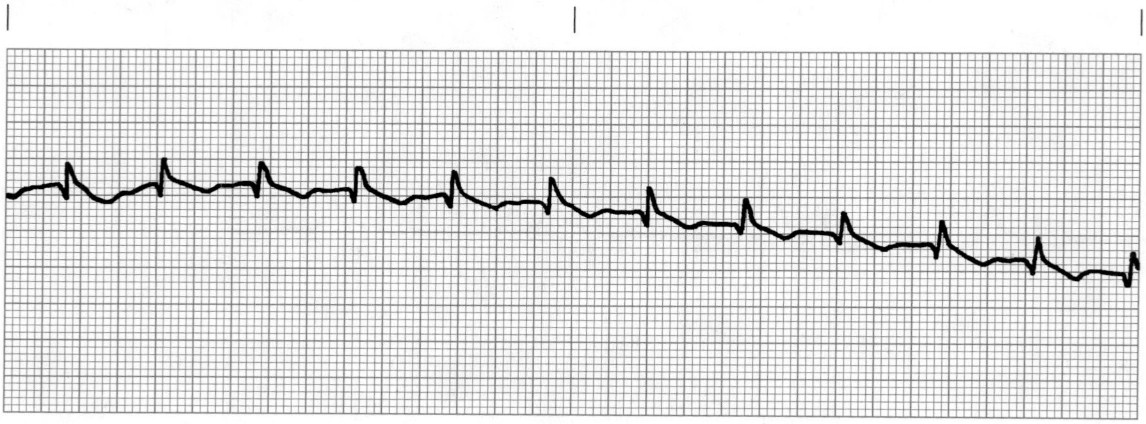

Regularity: _____   PRI: _____

Rate: _____   QRS: _____

P Waves: _____   Interp: _____

9.51

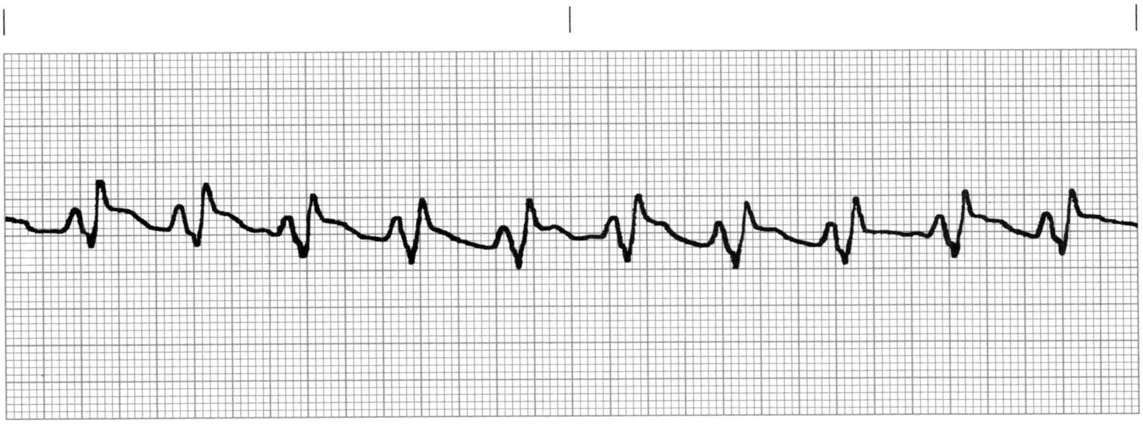

Regularity: _____	PRI: _____
Rate: _____	QRS: _____
P Waves: _____	Interp: _____

9.52

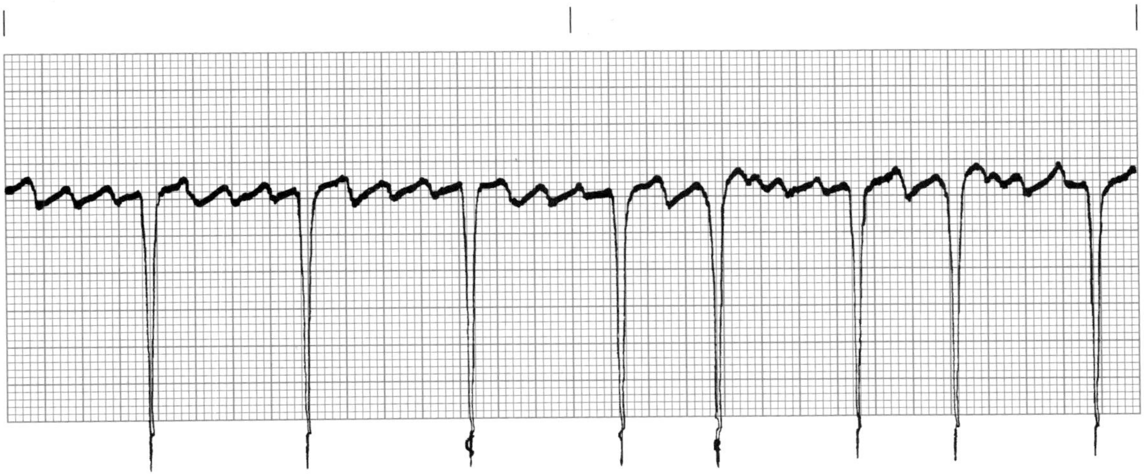

Regularity: _____	PRI: _____
Rate: _____	QRS: _____
P Waves: _____	Interp: _____

9.53

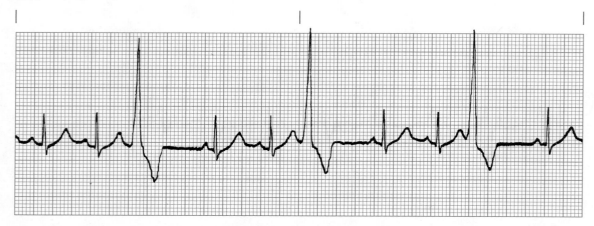

Regularity: _____   PRI: _____

Rate: _____   QRS: _____

P Waves: _____   Interp: _____

9.54

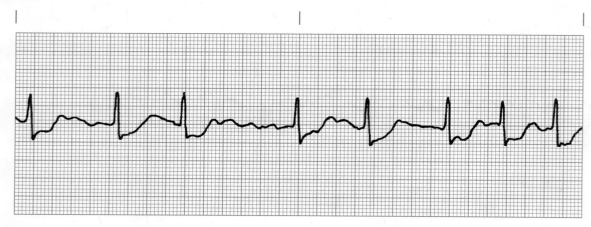

Regularity: _____   PRI: _____

Rate: _____   QRS: _____

P Waves: _____   Interp: _____

9.55

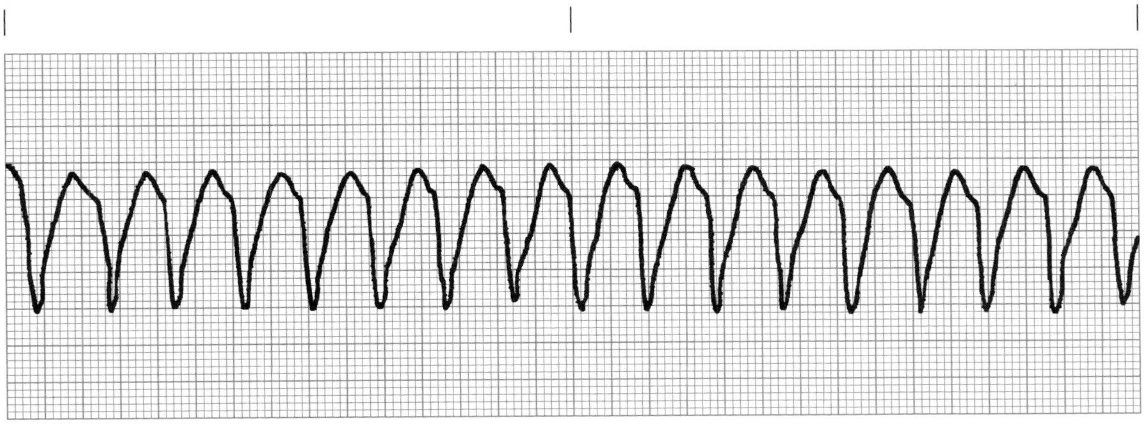

Regularity: _____	PRI: _____
Rate: _____	QRS: _____
P Waves: _____	Interp: _____

9.56

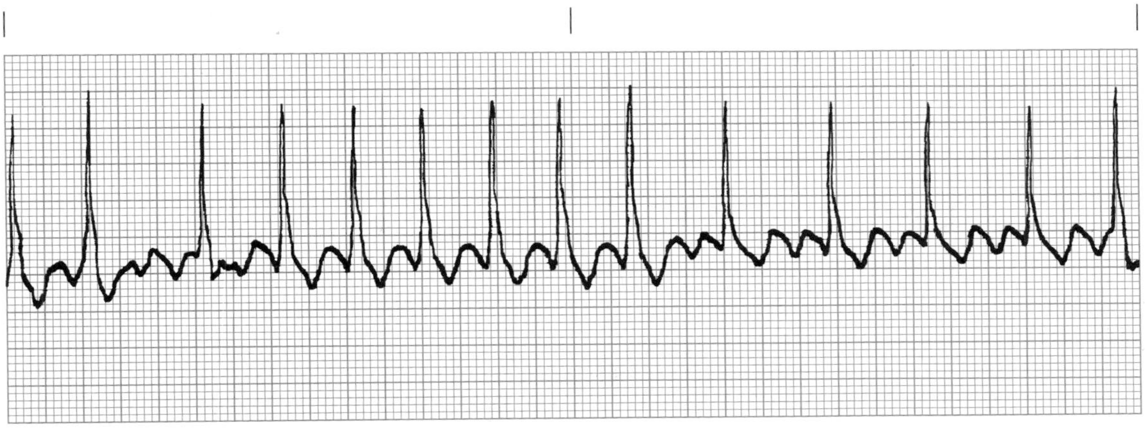

Regularity: _____	PRI: _____
Rate: _____	QRS: _____
P Waves: _____	Interp: _____

9.57

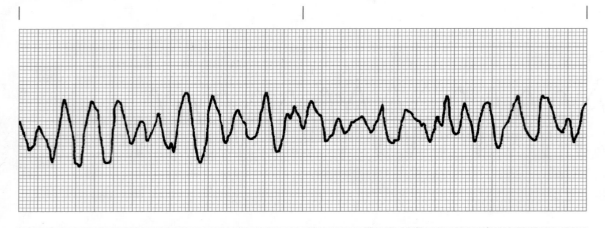

Regularity: _____	PRI: _____
Rate: _____	QRS: _____
P Waves: _____	Interp: _____

9.58

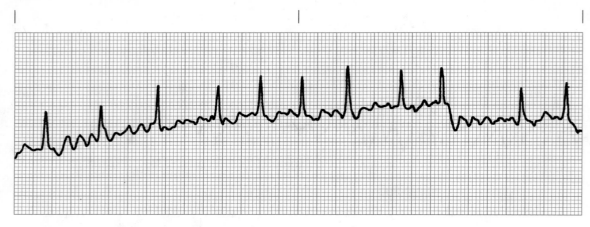

Regularity: _____	PRI: _____
Rate: _____	QRS: _____
P Waves: _____	Interp: _____

9.59

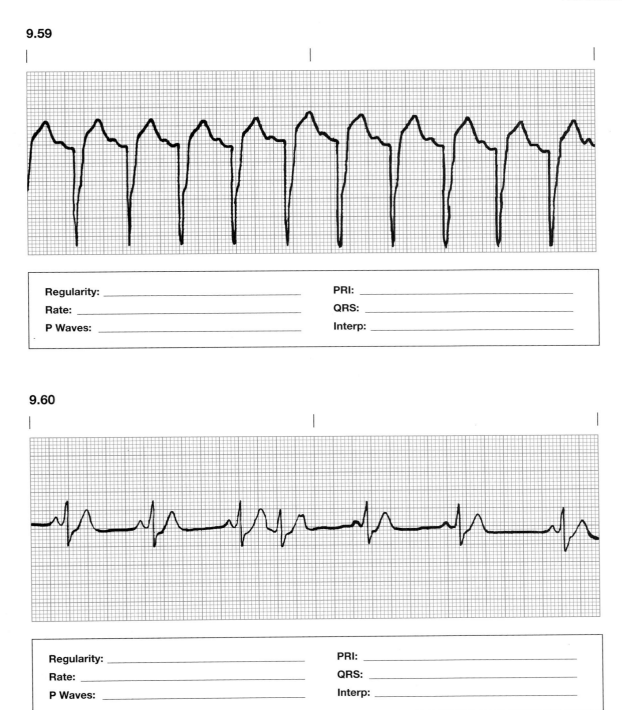

Regularity: _____   PRI: _____

Rate: _____   QRS: _____

P Waves: _____   Interp: _____

9.60

Regularity: _____   PRI: _____

Rate: _____   QRS: _____

P Waves: _____   Interp: _____

9.61

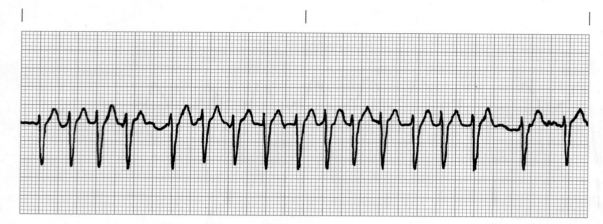

Regularity: _____	PRI: _____
Rate: _____	QRS: _____
P Waves: _____	Interp: _____

9.62

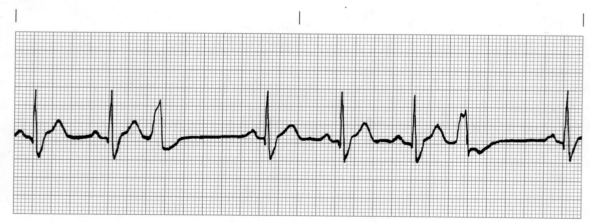

Regularity: _____	PRI: _____
Rate: _____	QRS: _____
P Waves: _____	Interp: _____

9.63

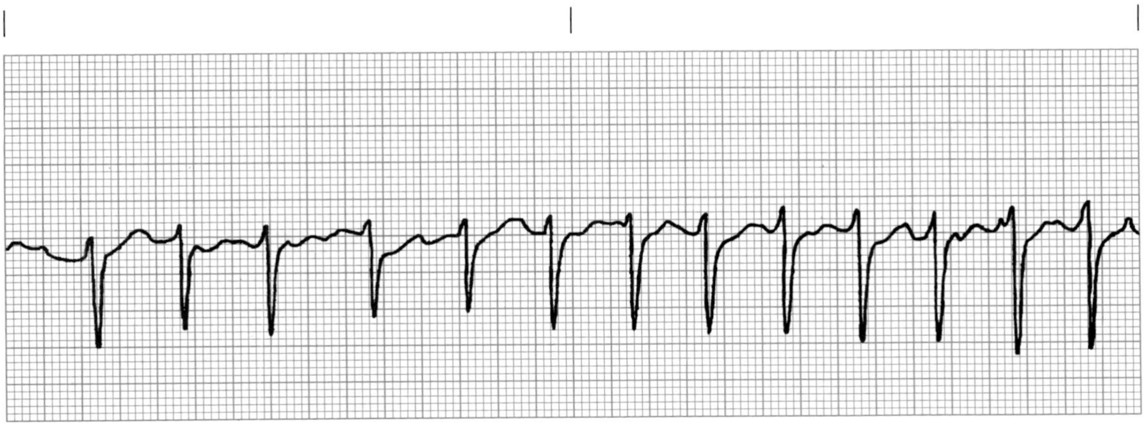

Regularity: _____	PRI: _____
Rate: _____	QRS: _____
P Waves: _____	Interp: _____

9.64

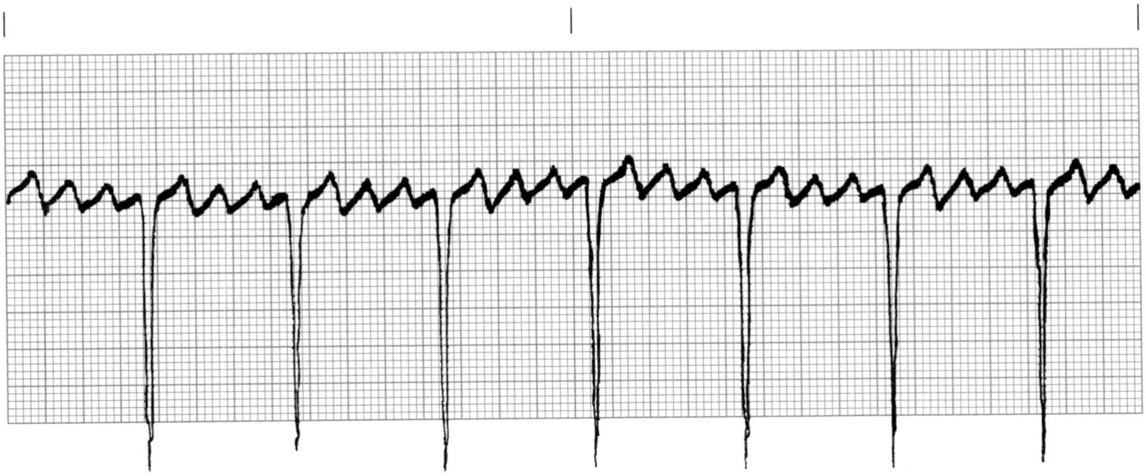

Regularity: _____	PRI: _____
Rate: _____	QRS: _____
P Waves: _____	Interp: _____

9.65

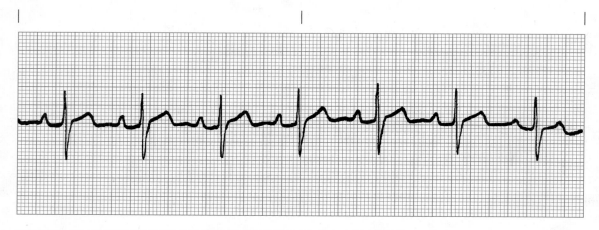

Regularity: _____   PRI: _____

Rate: _____   QRS: _____

P Waves: _____   Interp: _____

9.66

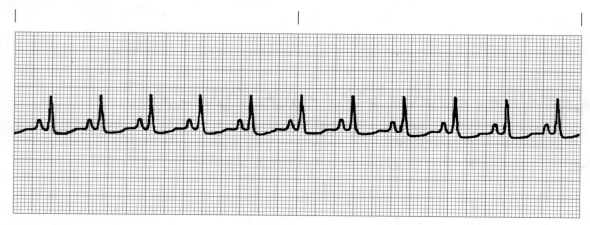

Regularity: _____   PRI: _____

Rate: _____   QRS: _____

P Waves: _____   Interp: _____

9.67

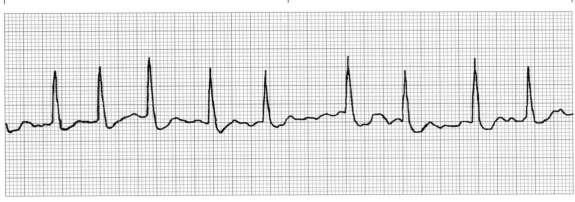

Regularity: _____	**PRI:** _____	
Rate: _____	**QRS:** _____	
P Waves: _____	**Interp:** _____	

9.68

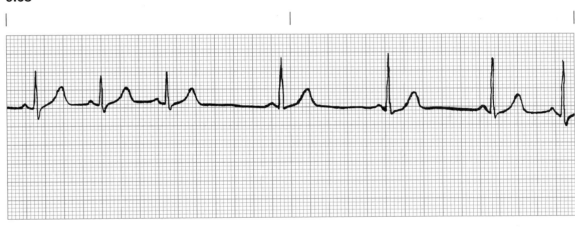

Regularity: _____	**PRI:** _____	
Rate: _____	**QRS:** _____	
P Waves: _____	**Interp:** _____	

9.69

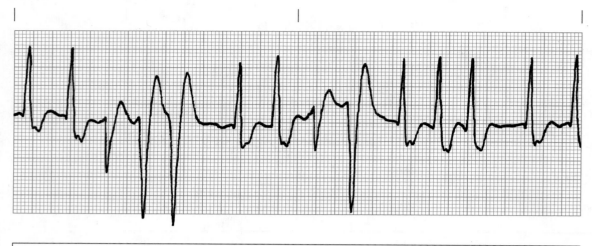

Regularity: _____	PRI: _____	
Rate: _____	QRS: _____	
P Waves: _____	Interp: _____	

9.70

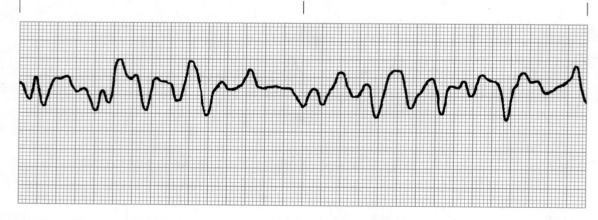

Regularity: _____	PRI: _____	
Rate: _____	QRS: _____	
P Waves: _____	Interp: _____	

9.71

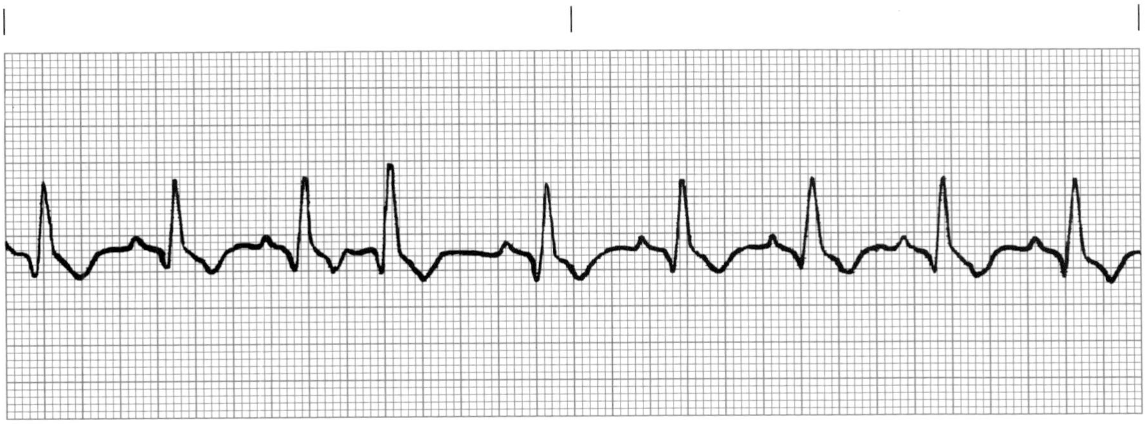

Regularity: _____	**PRI:** _____
Rate: _____	**QRS:** _____
P Waves: _____	**Interp:** _____

9.72

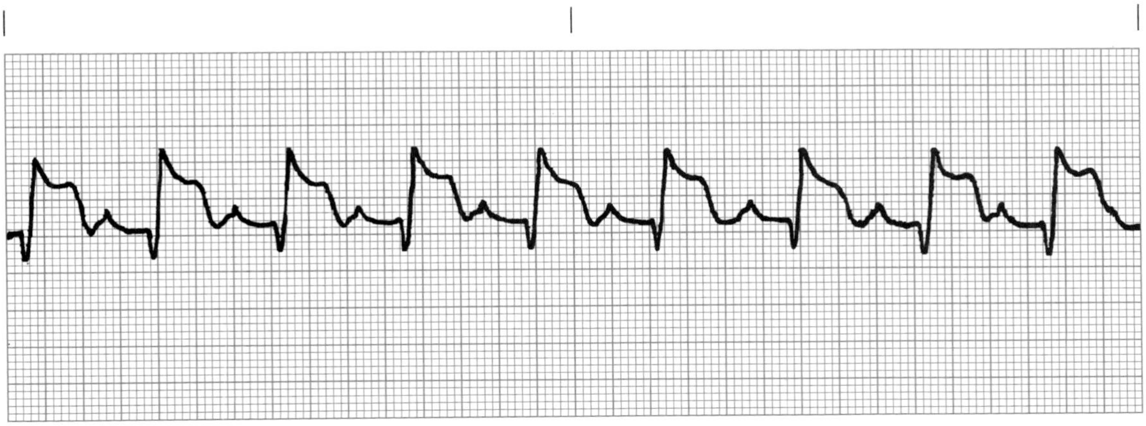

Regularity: _____	**PRI:** _____
Rate: _____	**QRS:** _____
P Waves: _____	**Interp:** _____

9.73

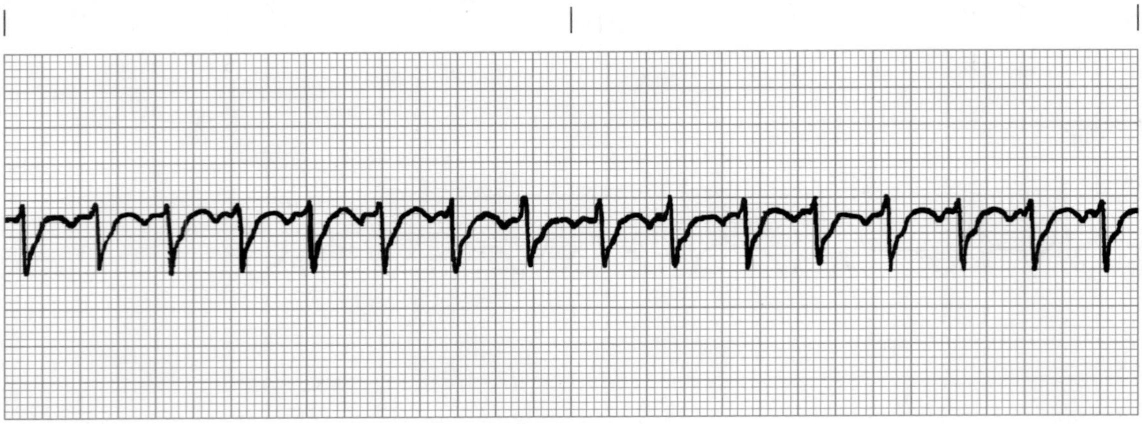

Regularity: _____		PRI: _____	
Rate: _____		QRS: _____	
P Waves: _____		Interp: _____	

9.74

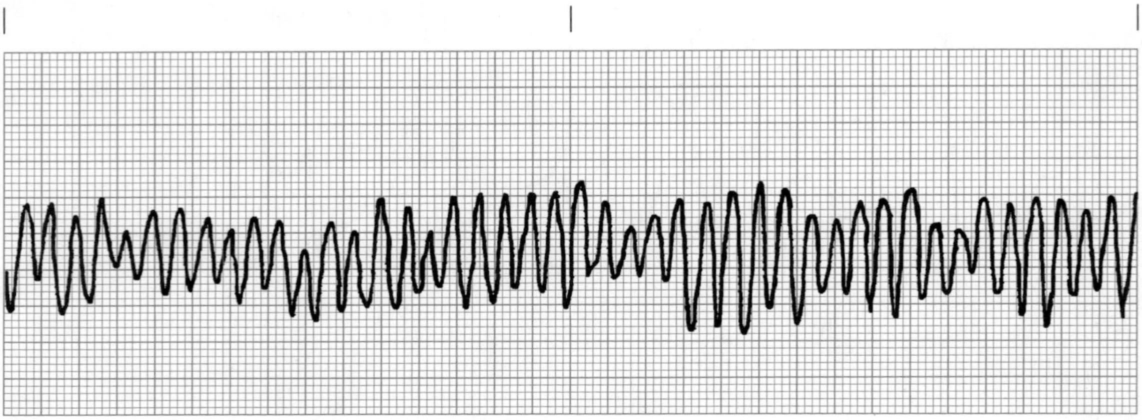

Regularity: _____		PRI: _____	
Rate: _____		QRS: _____	
P Waves: _____		Interp: _____	

9.75

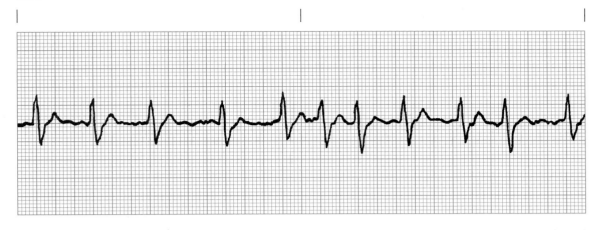

Regularity: _____		PRI: _____
Rate: _____		QRS: _____
P Waves: _____		Interp: _____

9.76

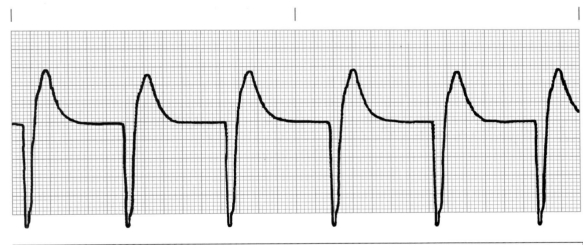

Regularity: _____		PRI: _____
Rate: _____		QRS: _____
P Waves: _____		Interp: _____

9.77

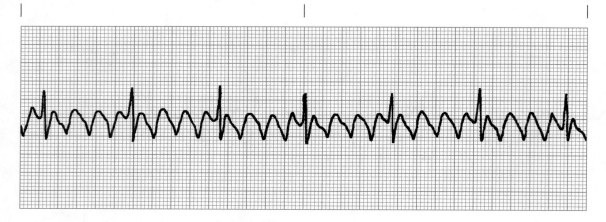

Regularity: _____	PRI: _____
Rate: _____	QRS: _____
P Waves: _____	Interp: _____

9.78

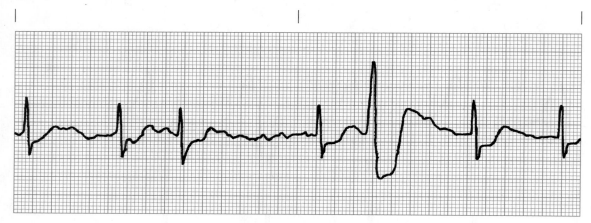

Regularity: _____	PRI: _____
Rate: _____	QRS: _____
P Waves: _____	Interp: _____

9.79

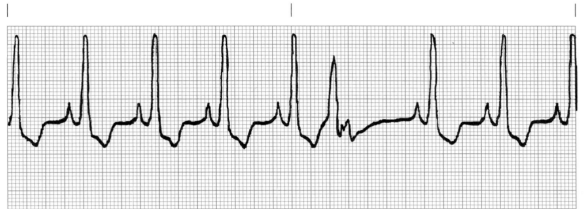

Regularity: _____	PRI: _____
Rate: _____	QRS: _____
P Waves: _____	Interp: _____

9.80

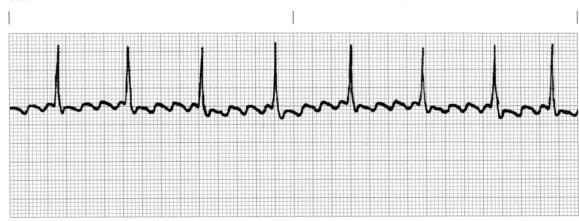

Regularity: _____	PRI: _____
Rate: _____	QRS: _____
P Waves: _____	Interp: _____

9.81

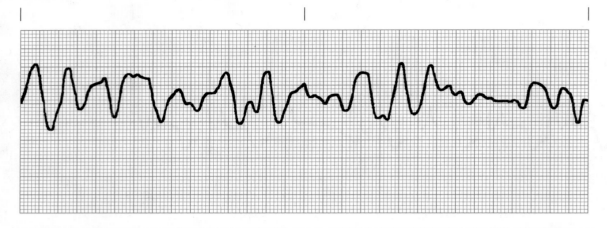

Regularity: _____	PRI: _____
Rate: _____	QRS: _____
P Waves: _____	Interp: _____

9.82

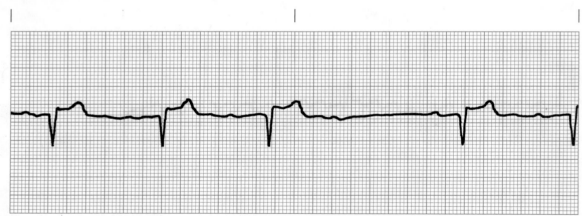

Regularity: _____	PRI: _____
Rate: _____	QRS: _____
P Waves: _____	Interp: _____

9.83

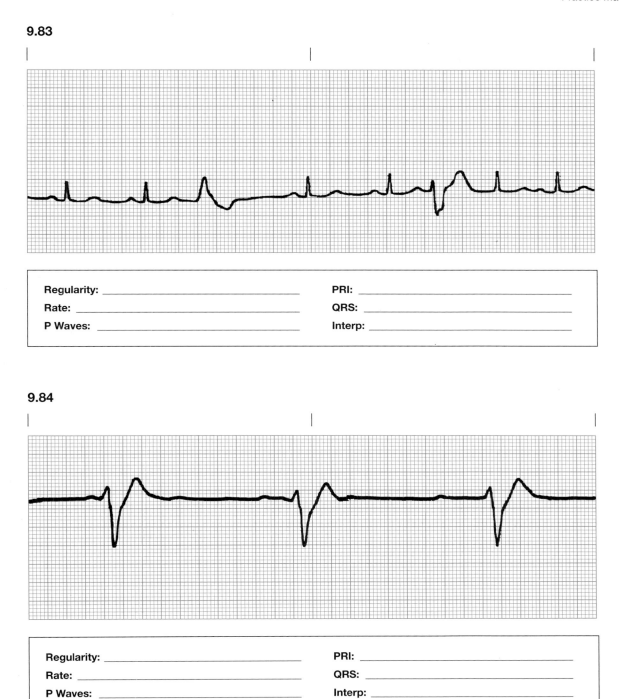

Regularity: _____	PRI: _____
Rate: _____	QRS: _____
P Waves: _____	Interp: _____

9.84

Regularity: _____	PRI: _____
Rate: _____	QRS: _____
P Waves: _____	Interp: _____

9.85

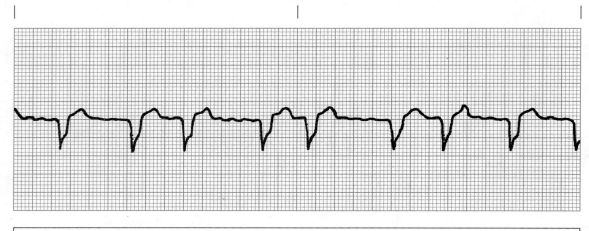

Regularity: _____	**PRI:** _____
Rate: _____	**QRS:** _____
P Waves: _____	**Interp:** _____

9.86

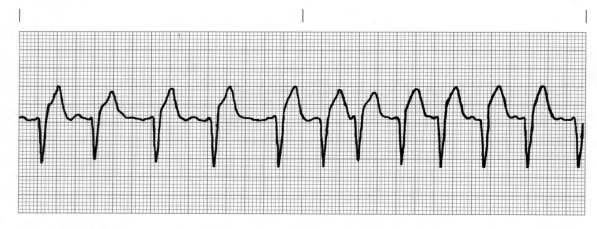

Regularity: _____	**PRI:** _____
Rate: _____	**QRS:** _____
P Waves: _____	**Interp:** _____

9.87

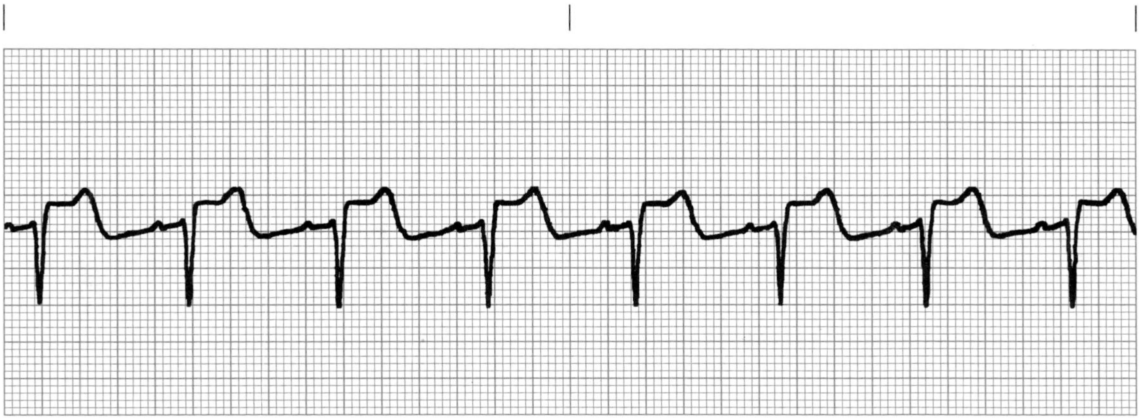

Regularity: _____   PRI: _____

Rate: _____   QRS: _____

P Waves: _____   Inter: _____

9.88

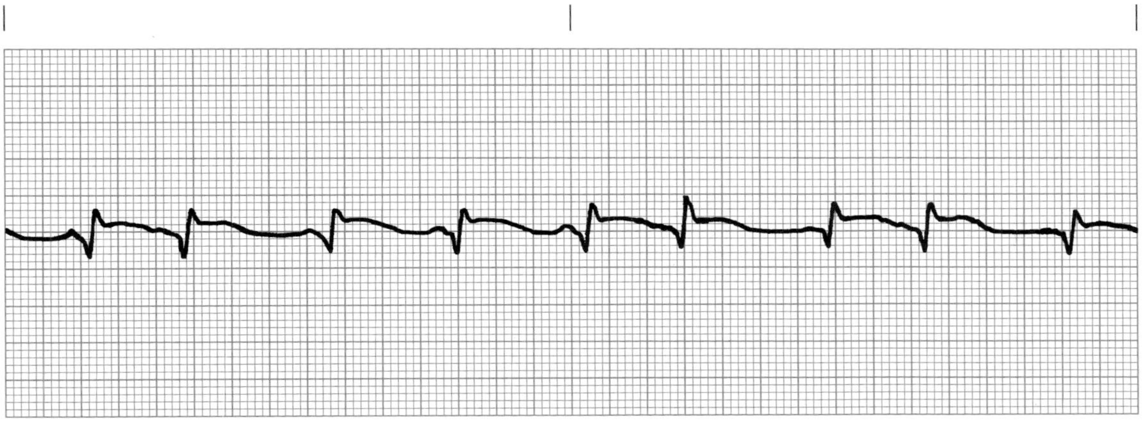

Regularity: _____   PRI: _____

Rate: _____   QRS: _____

P Waves: _____   Interp: _____

9.89

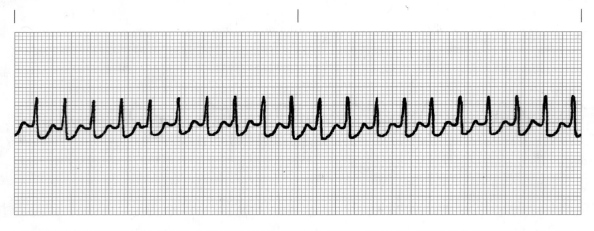

Regularity: _____   PRI: _____

Rate: _____   QRS: _____

P Waves: _____   Interp: _____

9.90

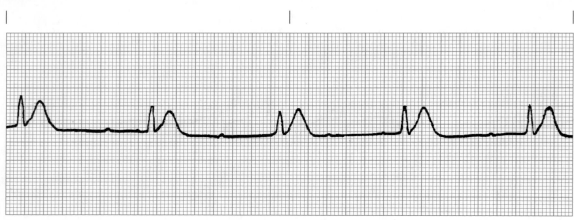

Regularity: _____   PRI: _____

Rate: _____   QRS: _____

P Waves: _____   Interp: _____

9.91

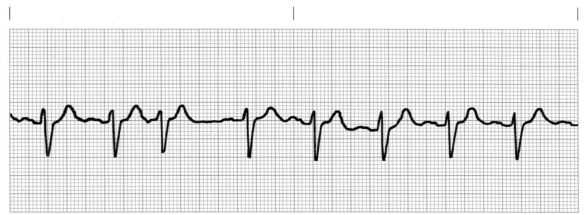

Regularity: _____   PRI: _____

Rate: _____   QRS: _____

P Waves: _____   Interp: _____

9.92

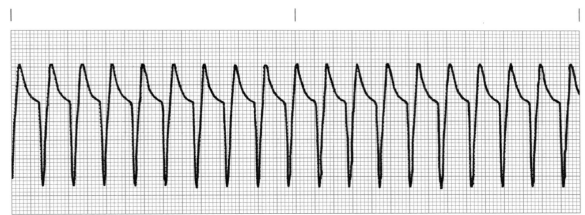

Regularity: _____   PRI: _____

Rate: _____   QRS: _____

P Waves: _____   Interp: _____

9.93

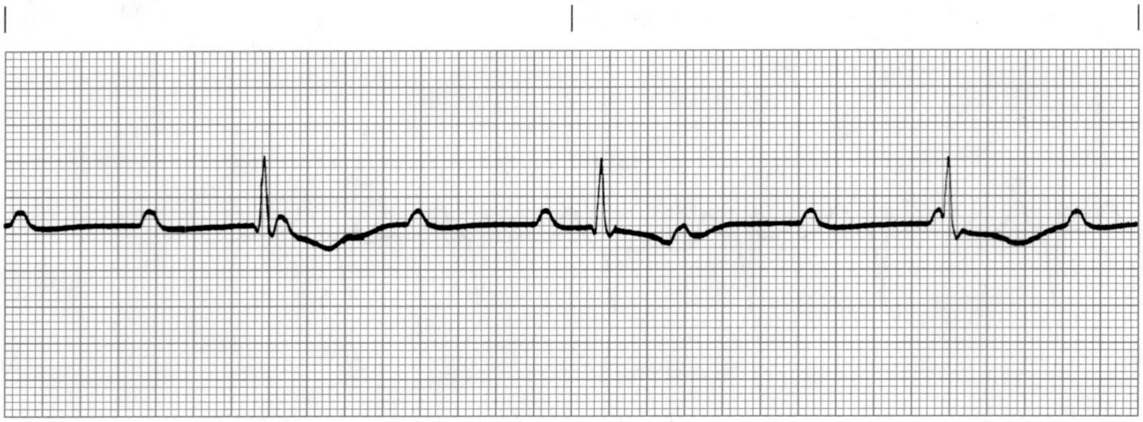

Regularity: _____ PRI: _____

Rate: _____ QRS: _____

P Waves: _____ Interp: _____

9.94

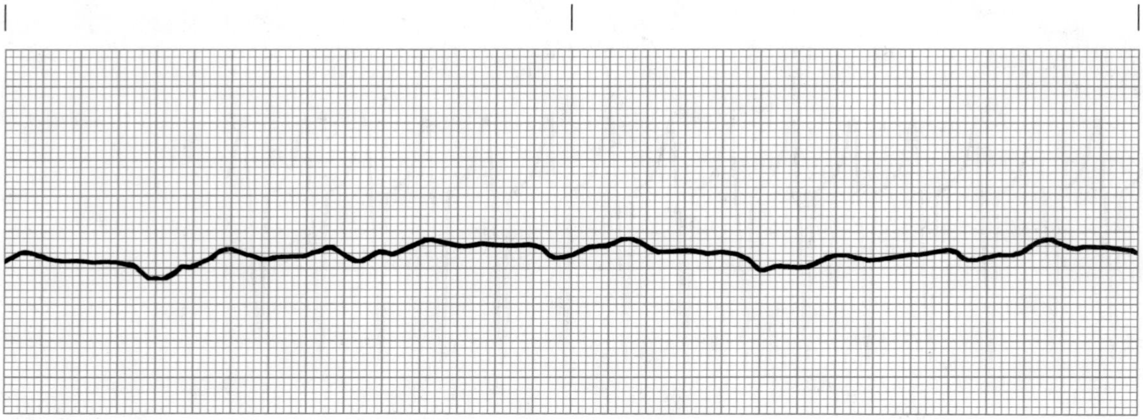

Regularity: _____ PRI: _____

Rate: _____ QRS: _____

P Waves: _____ Interp: _____

9.95

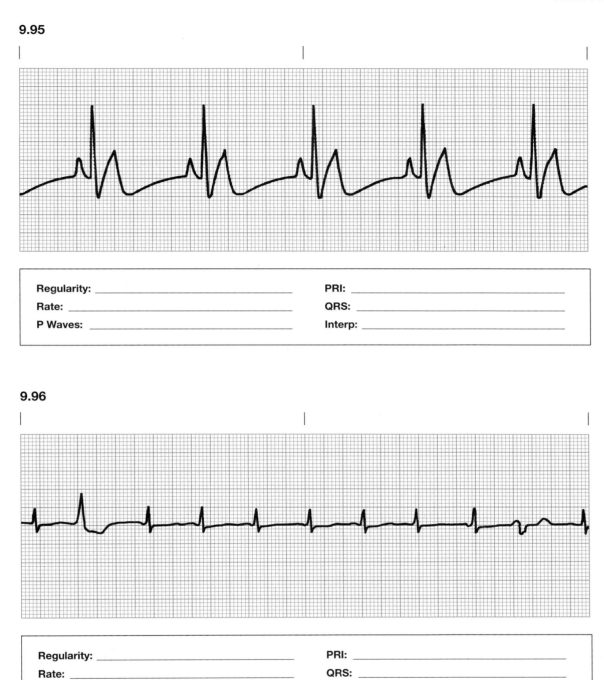

Regularity: _____

Rate: _____

P Waves: _____

PRI: _____

QRS: _____

Interp: _____

9.96

Regularity: _____

Rate: _____

P Waves: _____

PRI: _____

QRS: _____

Interp: _____

9.97

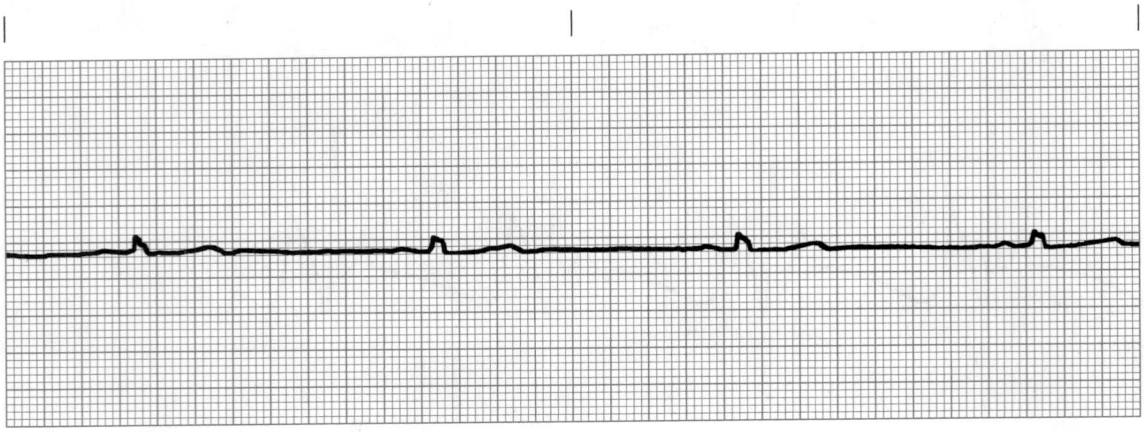

Regularity: _____	PRI: _____
Rate: _____	QRS: _____
P Waves: _____	Interp: _____

9.98

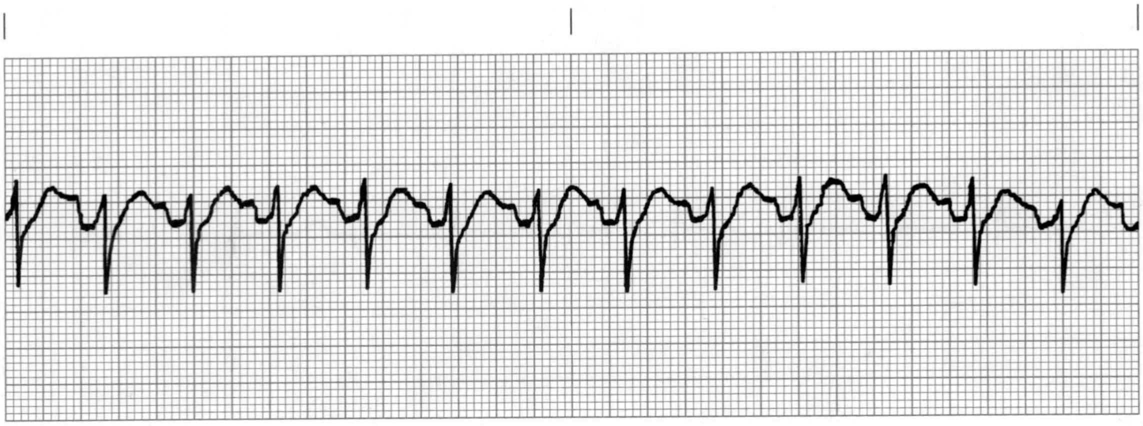

Regularity: _____	PRI: _____
Rate: _____	QRS: _____
P Waves: _____	Interp: _____

9.99

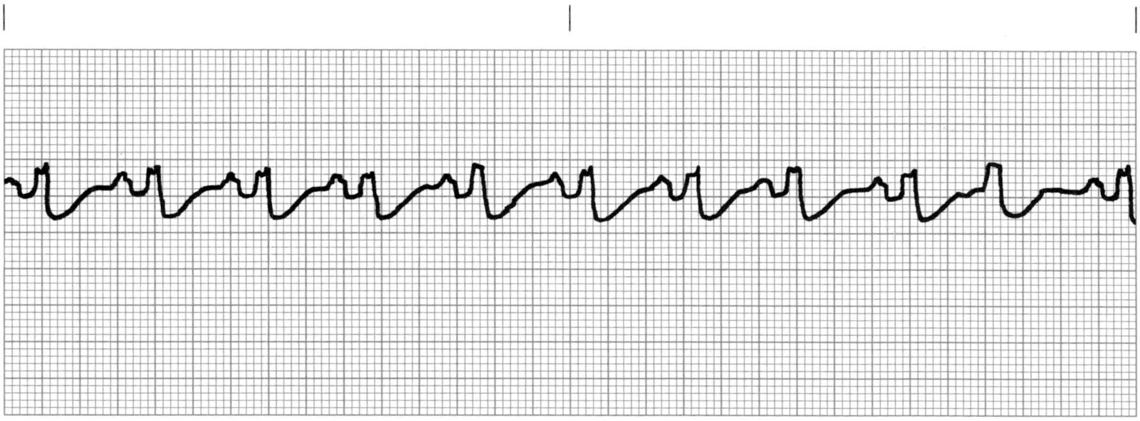

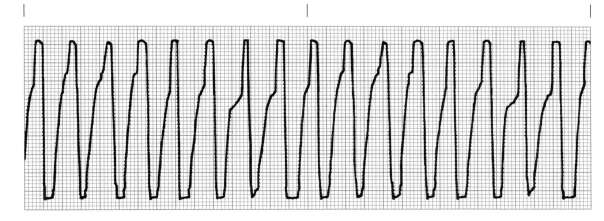

Regularity: _____	PRI: _____
Rate: _____	QRS: _____
P Waves: _____	Interp: _____

9.100

Regularity: _____	PRI: _____
Rate: _____	QRS: _____
P Waves: _____	Interp: _____

9.101

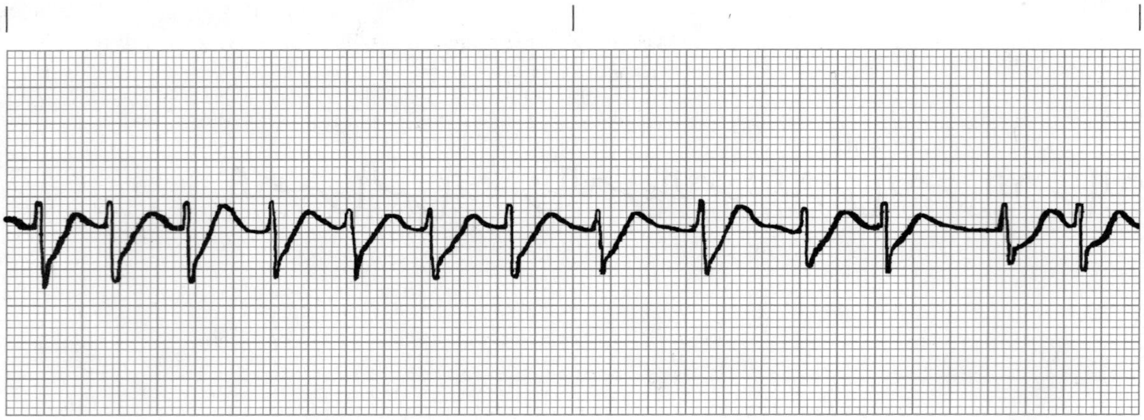

Regularity: _____	PRI: _____
Rate: _____	QRS: _____
P Waves: _____	Interp: _____

9.102

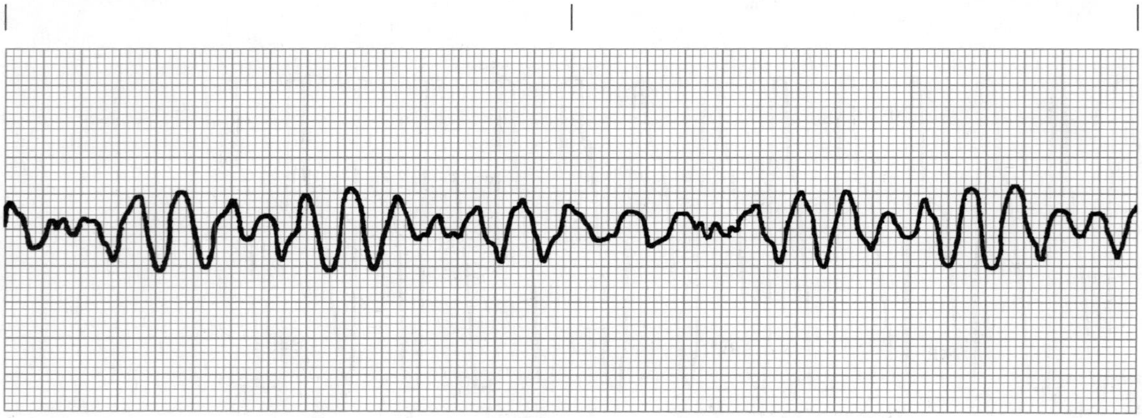

Regularity: _____	PRI: _____
Rate: _____	QRS: _____
P Waves: _____	Interp: _____

9.103

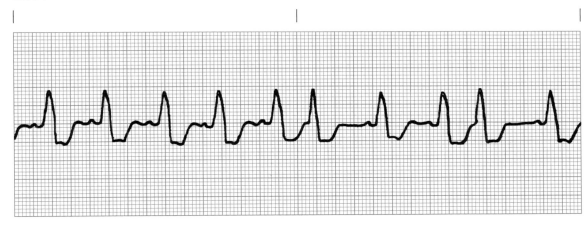

Regularity: _____	**PRI:** _____	
Rate: _____	**QRS:** _____	
P Waves: _____	**Interp:** _____	

9.104

Regularity: _____	**PRI:** _____	
Rate: _____	**QRS:** _____	
P Waves: _____	**Interp:** _____	

9.105

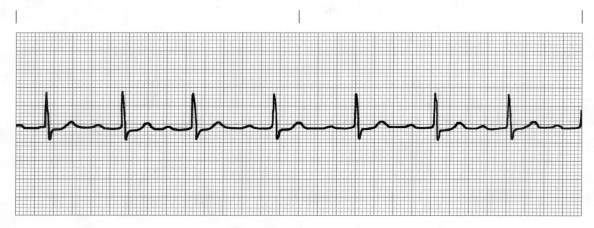

Regularity: _____	PRI: _____
Rate: _____	QRS: _____
P Waves: _____	Interp: _____

9.106

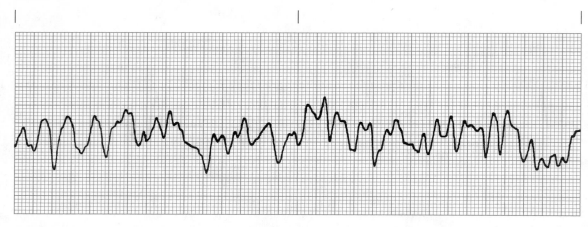

Regularity: _____	PRI: _____
Rate: _____	QRS: _____
P Waves: _____	Interp: _____

9.107

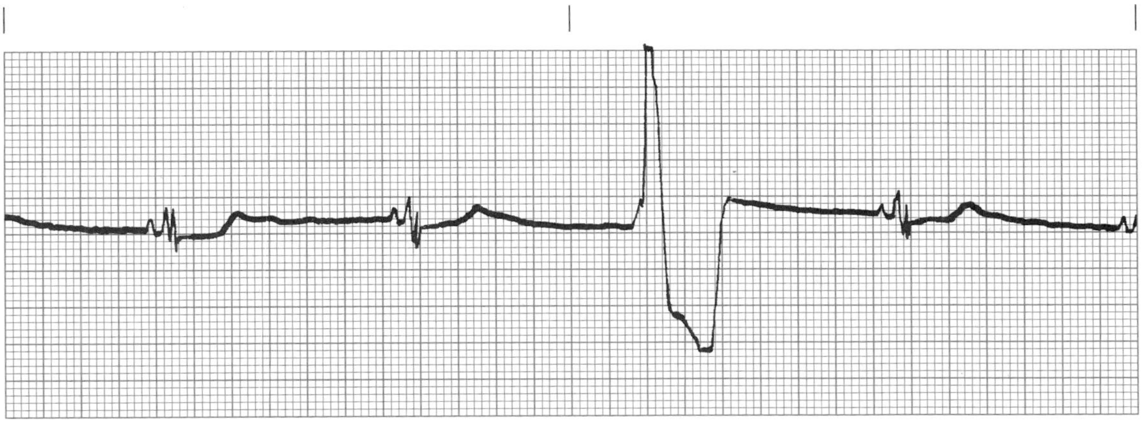

Regularity: _____	PRI: _____
Rate: _____	QRS: _____
P Waves: _____	Interp: _____

9.108

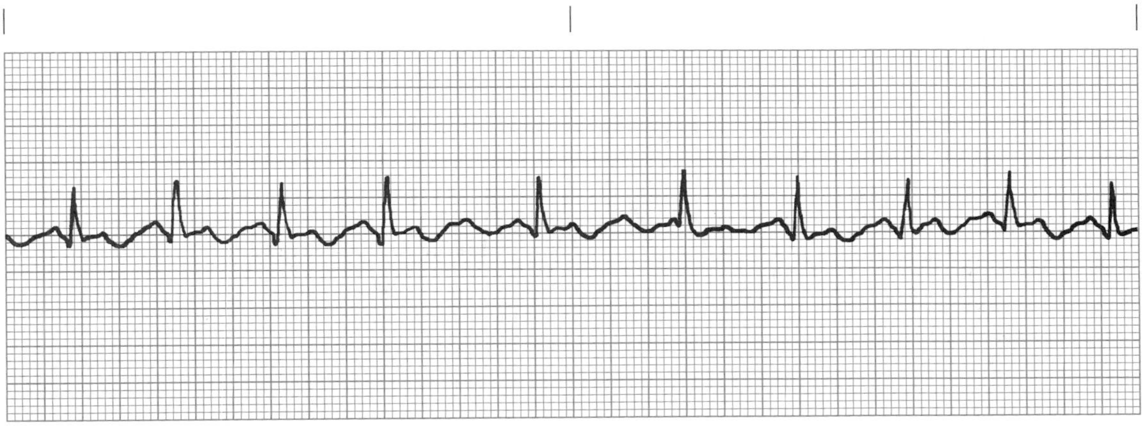

Regularity: _____	PRI: _____
Rate: _____	QRS: _____
P Waves: _____	Interp: _____

9.109

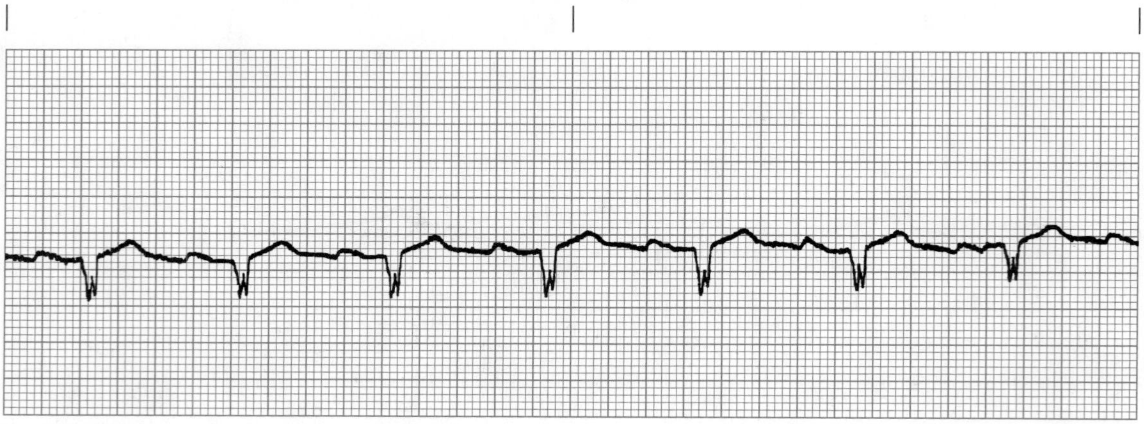

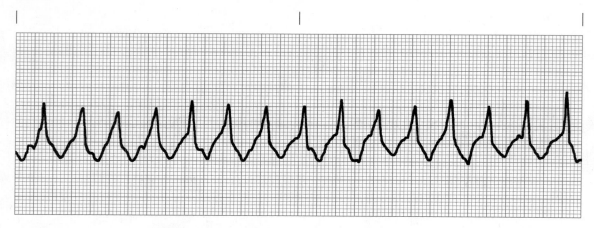

Regularity: _____	PRI: _____
Rate: _____	QRS: _____
P Waves: _____	Interp: _____

9.110

Regularity: _____	PRI: _____
Rate: _____	QRS: _____
P Waves: _____	Interp: _____

9.111

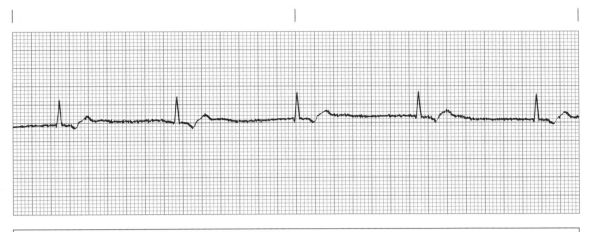

Regularity: _____   PRI: _____

Rate: _____   QRS: _____

P Waves: _____   Interp: _____

9.112

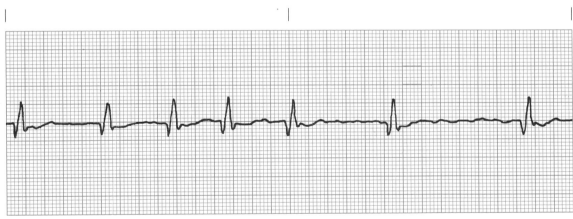

Regularity: _____   PRI: _____

Rate: _____   QRS: _____

P Waves: _____   Interp: _____

9.113

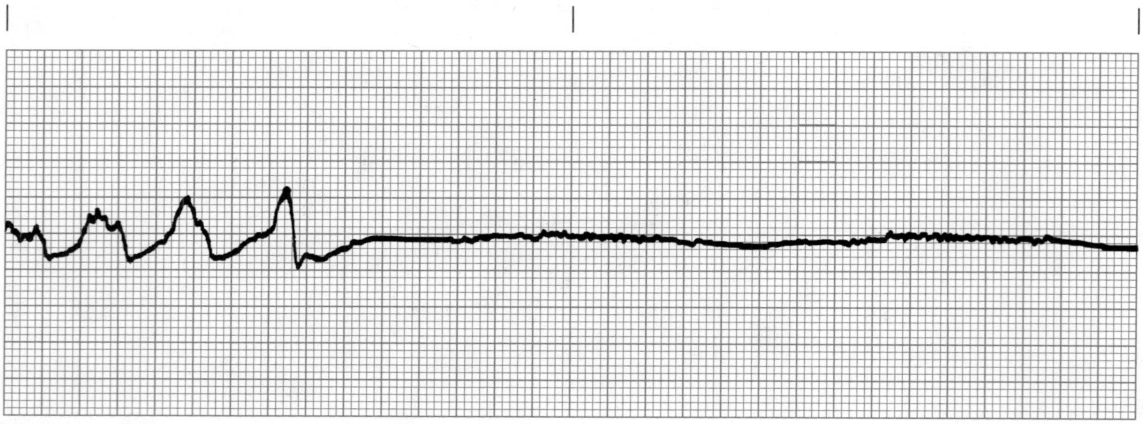

Regularity: _____   PRI: _____

Rate: _____   QRS: _____

P Waves: _____   Interp: _____

9.114

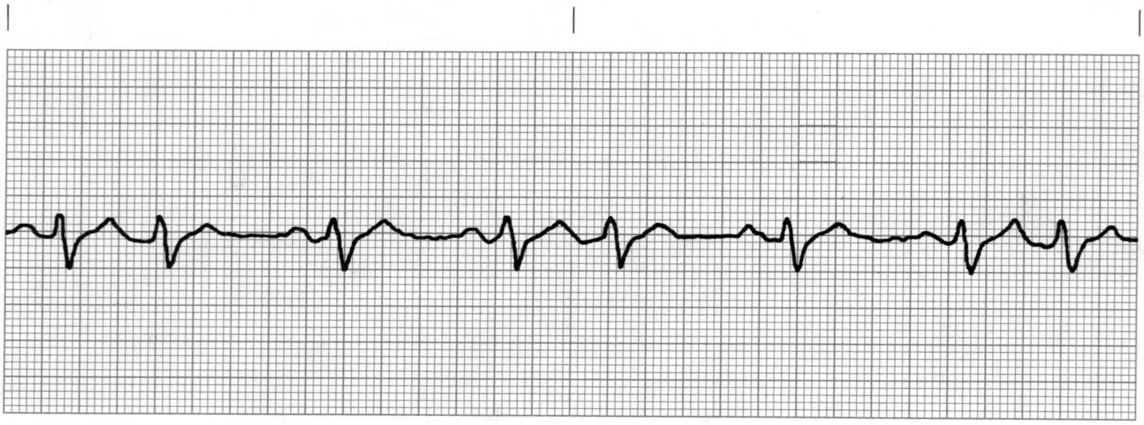

Regularity: _____   PRI: _____

Rate: _____   QRS: _____

P Waves: _____   Interp: _____

9.115

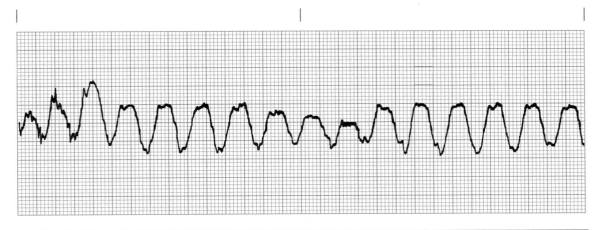

Regularity: _____	**PRI:** _____
Rate: _____	**QRS:** _____
P Waves: _____	**Interp:** _____

9.116

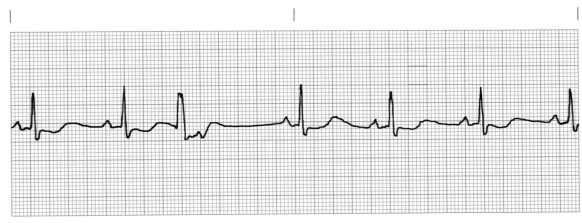

Regularity: _____	**PRI:** _____
Rate: _____	**QRS:** _____
P Waves: _____	**Interp:** _____

9.117

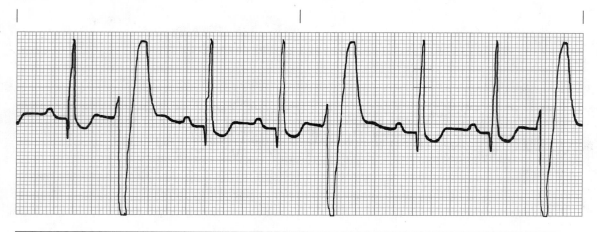

Regularity: _____	PRI: _____
Rate: _____	QRS: _____
P Waves: _____	Interp: _____

9.118

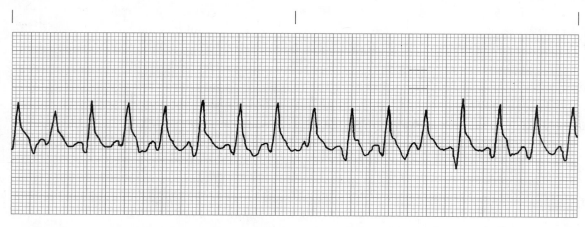

Regularity: _____	PRI: _____
Rate: _____	QRS: _____
P Waves: _____	Interp: _____

9.119

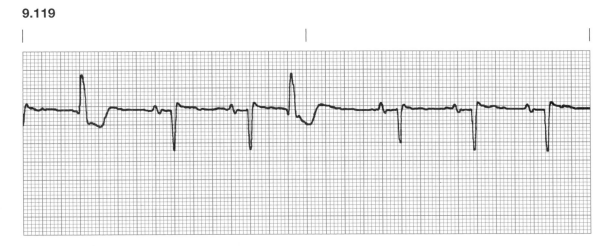

Regularity: _____   PRI: _____

Rate: _____   QRS: _____

P Waves: _____   Interp: _____

9.120

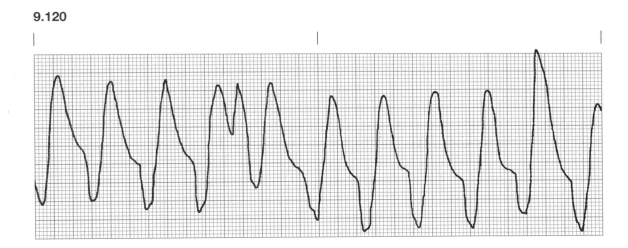

Regularity: _____   PRI: _____

Rate: _____   QRS: _____

P Waves: _____   Interp: _____

9.121

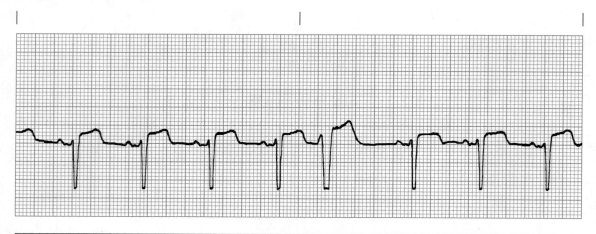

Regularity: _____ PRI: _____

Rate: _____ QRS: _____

P Waves: _____ Interp: _____

9.122

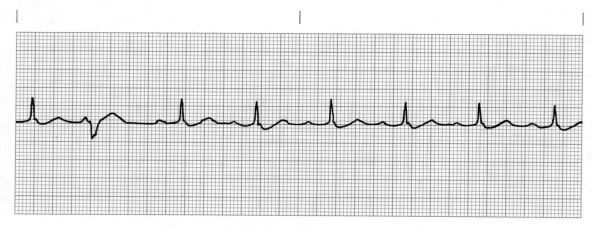

Regularity: _____ PRI: _____

Rate: _____ QRS: _____

P Waves: _____ Interp: _____

9.123

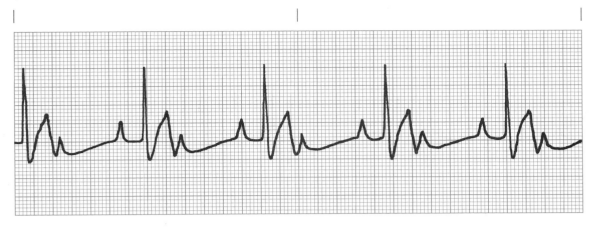

Regularity: _____	PRI: _____	
Rate: _____	QRS: _____	
P Waves: _____	Interp: _____	

9.124

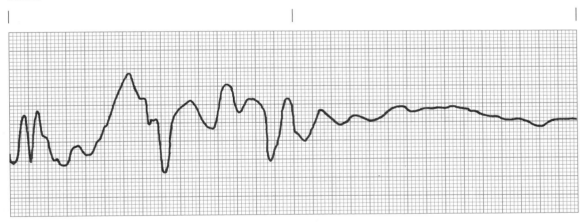

Regularity: _____	PRI: _____	
Rate: _____	QRS: _____	
P Waves: _____	Interp: _____	

9.125

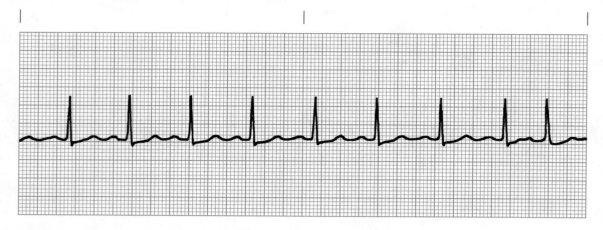

Regularity: _____	PRI: _____	
Rate: _____	QRS: _____	
P Waves: _____	Interp: _____	

9.126

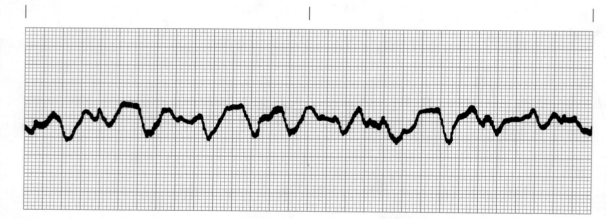

Regularity: _____	PRI: _____	
Rate: _____	QRS: _____	
P Waves: _____	Interp: _____	

9.127

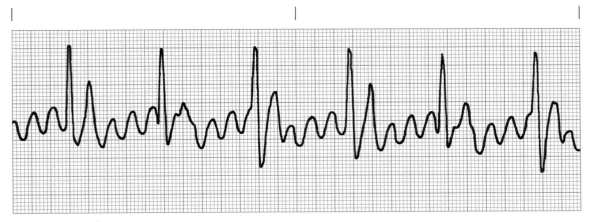

Regularity: _____	PRI: _____
Rate: _____	QRS: _____
P Waves: _____	Interp: _____

9.128

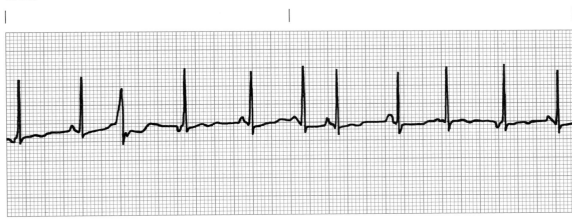

Regularity: _____	PRI: _____
Rate: _____	QRS: _____
P Waves: _____	Interp: _____

9.129

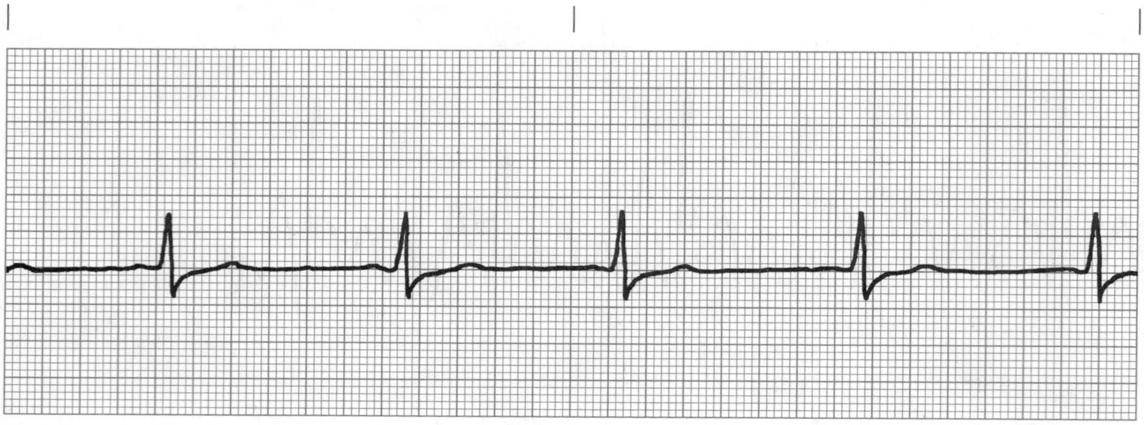

Regularity: _____	PRI: _____
Rate: _____	QRS: _____
P Waves: _____	Interp: _____

9.130

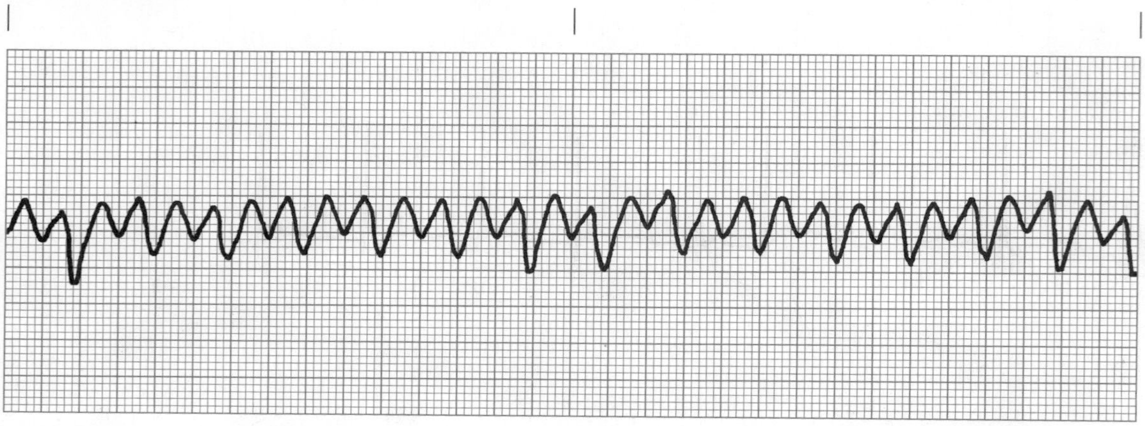

Regularity: _____	PRI: _____
Rate: _____	QRS: _____
P Waves: _____	Interp: _____

9.131

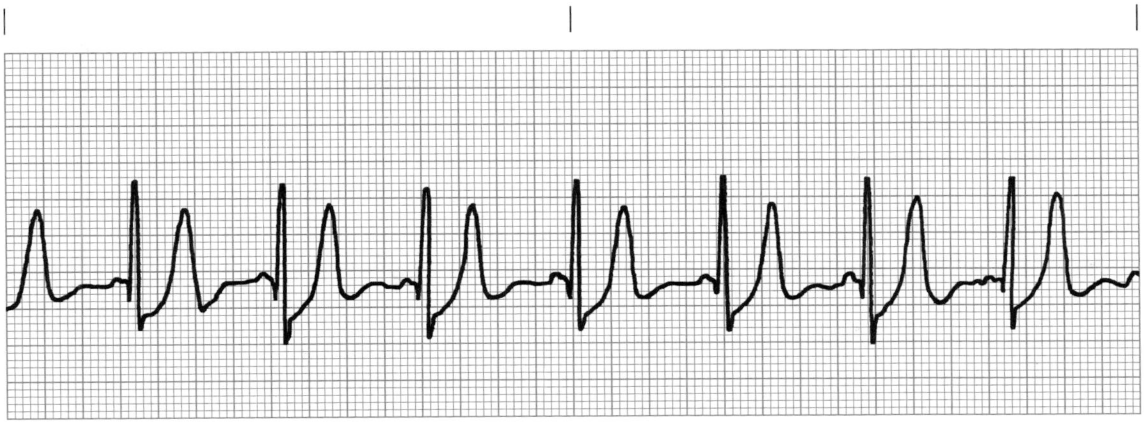

Regularity: _____	PRI: _____
Rate: _____	QRS: _____
P Waves: _____	Interp: _____

9.132

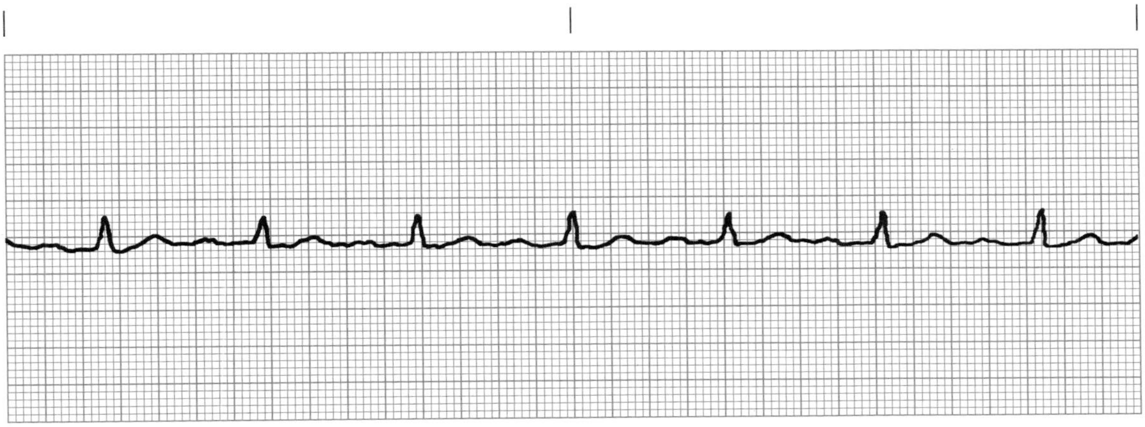

Regularity: _____	PRI: _____
Rate: _____	QRS: _____
P Waves: _____	Interp: _____

9.133

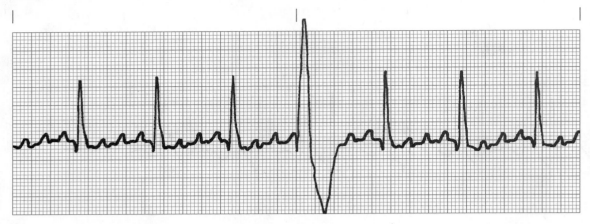

Regularity: _____	PRI: _____
Rate: _____	QRS: _____
P Waves: _____	Interp: _____

9.134

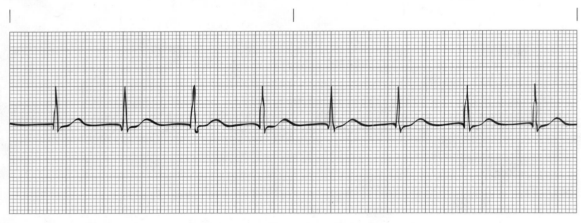

Regularity: _____	PRI: _____
Rate: _____	QRS: _____
P Waves: _____	Interp: _____

9.135

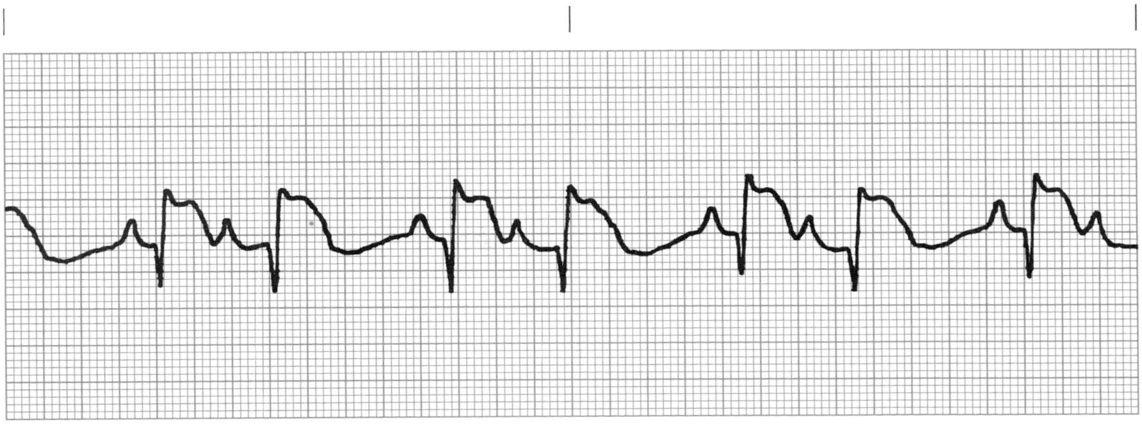

Regularity: _____	PRI: _____
Rate: _____	QRS: _____
P Waves: _____	Interp: _____

9.136

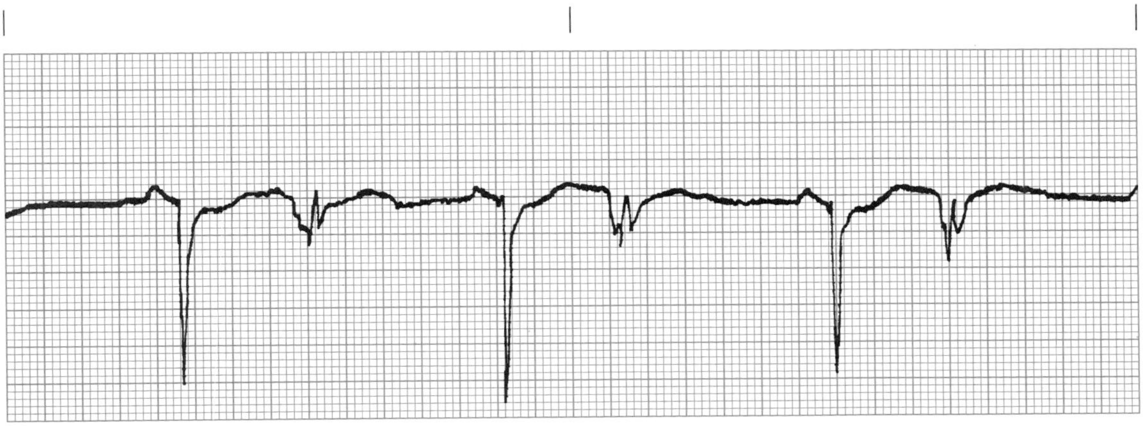

Regularity: _____	PRI: _____
Rate: _____	QRS: _____
P Waves: _____	Interp: _____

9.137

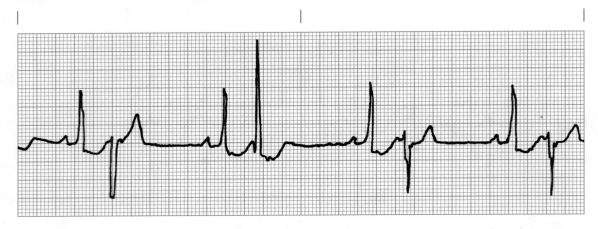

Regularity: _____   PRI: _____

Rate: _____   QRS: _____

P Waves: _____   Interp: _____

9.138

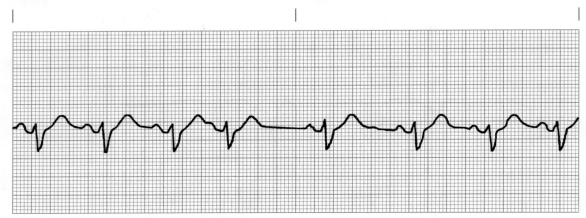

Regularity: _____   PRI: _____

Rate: _____   QRS: _____

P Waves: _____   Interp: _____

9.139

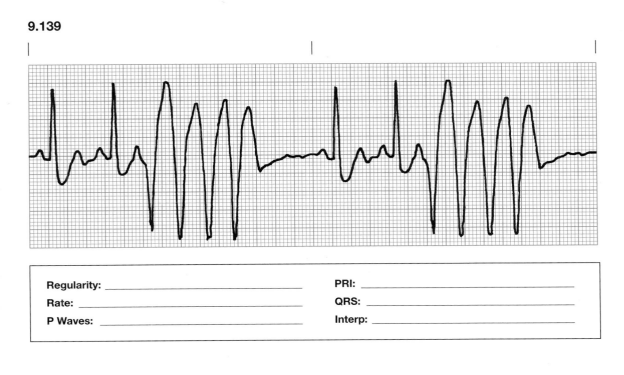

Regularity: _____ PRI: _____

Rate: _____ QRS: _____

P Waves: _____ Interp: _____

9.140

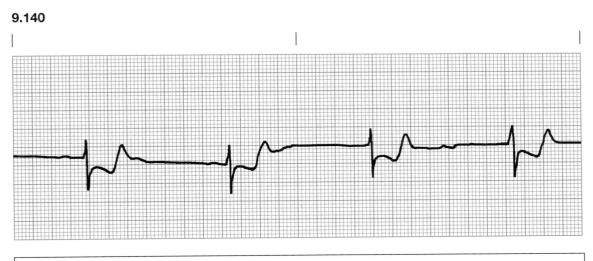

Regularity: _____ PRI: _____

Rate: _____ QRS: _____

P Waves: _____ Interp: _____

9.141

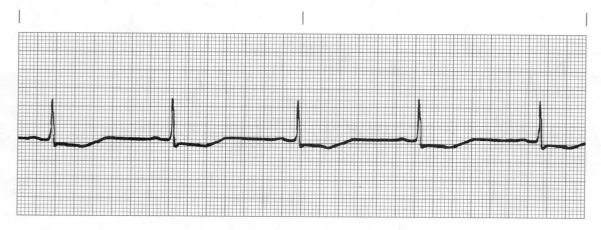

Regularity: _____   PRI: _____

Rate: _____   QRS: _____

P Waves: _____   Interp: _____

9.142

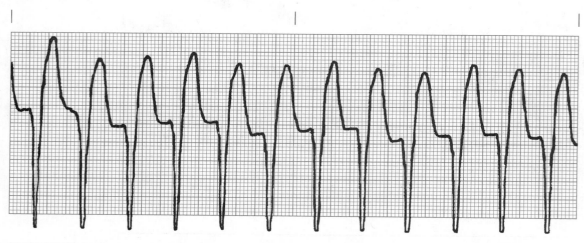

Regularity: _____   PRI: _____

Rate: _____   QRS: _____

P Waves: _____   Interp: _____

9.143

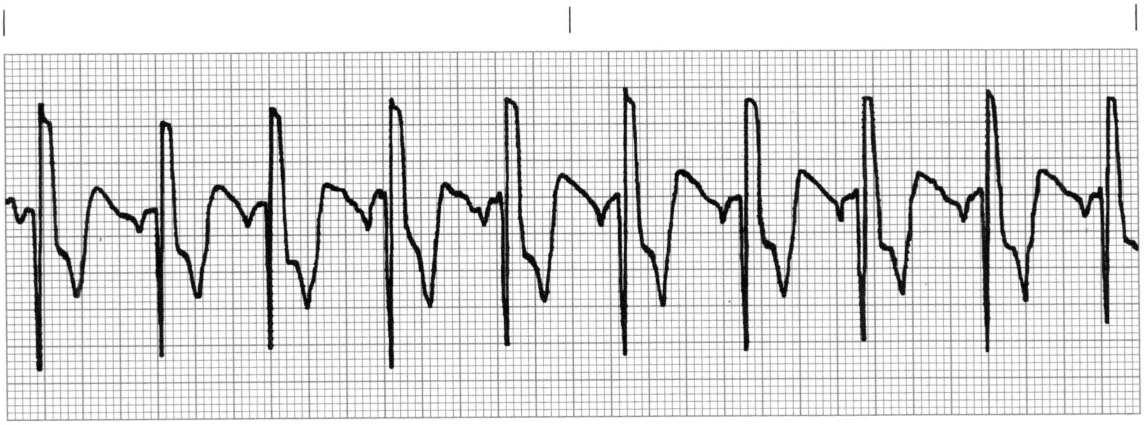

Regularity: _____	PRI: _____
Rate: _____	QRS: _____
P Waves: _____	Interp: _____

9.144

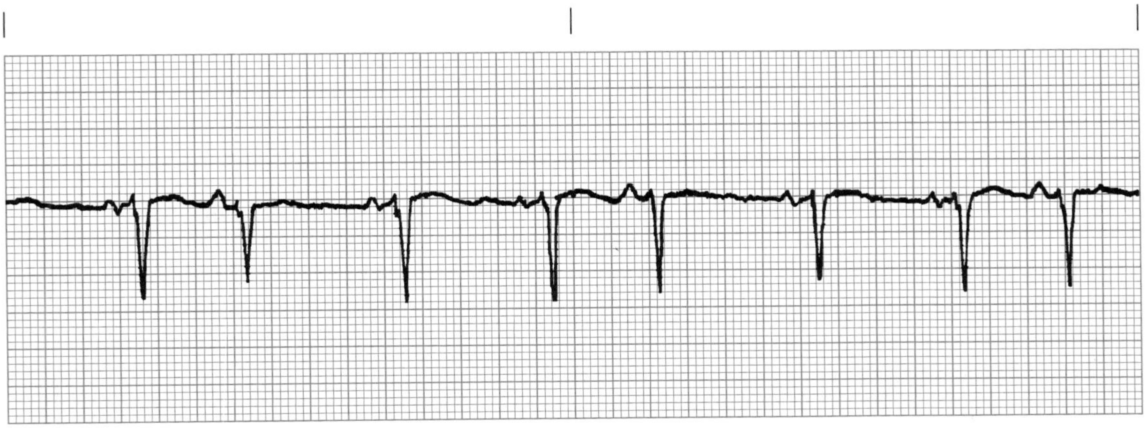

Regularity: _____	PRI: _____
Rate: _____	QRS: _____
P Waves: _____	Interp: _____

9.145

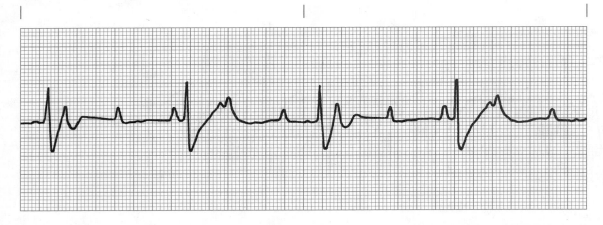

Regularity: _____	PRI: _____
Rate: _____	QRS: _____
P Waves: _____	Interp: _____

9.146

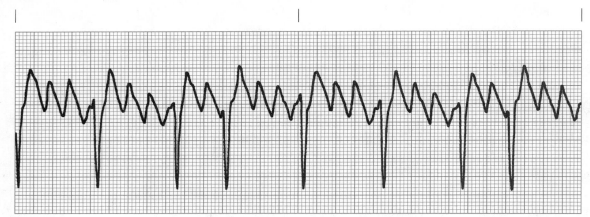

Regularity: _____	PRI: _____
Rate: _____	QRS: _____
P Waves: _____	Interp: _____

9.147

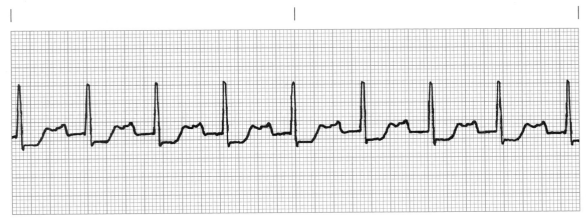

Regularity: _____   PRI: _____

Rate: _____   QRS: _____

P Waves: _____   Interp: _____

9.148

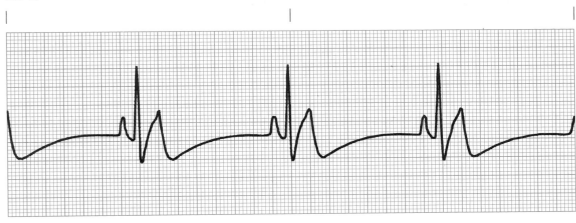

Regularity: _____   PRI: _____

Rate: _____   QRS: _____

P Waves: _____   Interp: _____

9.149

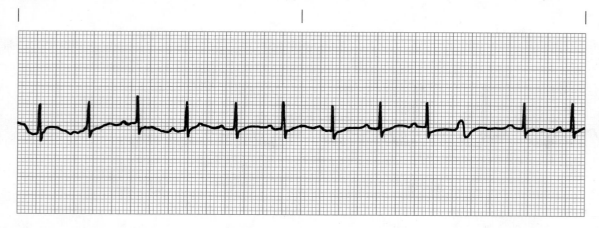

Regularity: _____	PRI: _____
Rate: _____	QRS: _____
P Waves: _____	Interp: _____

9.150

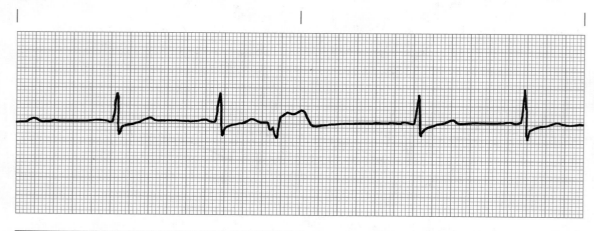

Regularity: _____	PRI: _____
Rate: _____	QRS: _____
P Waves: _____	Interp: _____

9.151

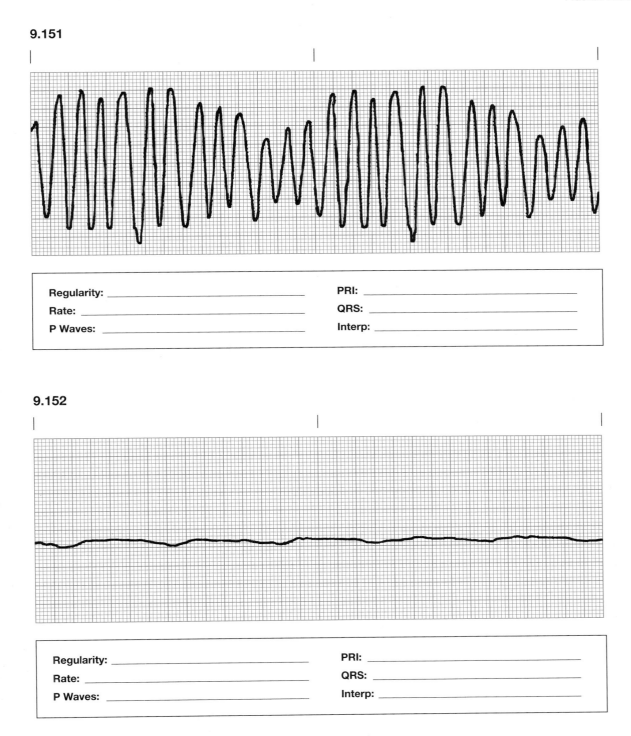

Regularity: _____	PRI: _____
Rate: _____	QRS: _____
P Waves: _____	Interp: _____

9.152

Regularity: _____	PRI: _____
Rate: _____	QRS: _____
P Waves: _____	Interp: _____

9.153

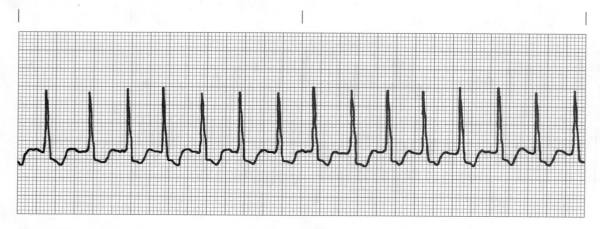

Regularity: _____ PRI: _____

Rate: _____ QRS: _____

P Waves: _____ Interp: _____

9.154

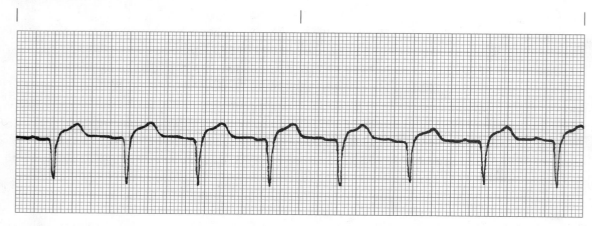

Regularity: _____ PRI: _____

Rate: _____ QRS: _____

P Waves: _____ Interp: _____

9.155

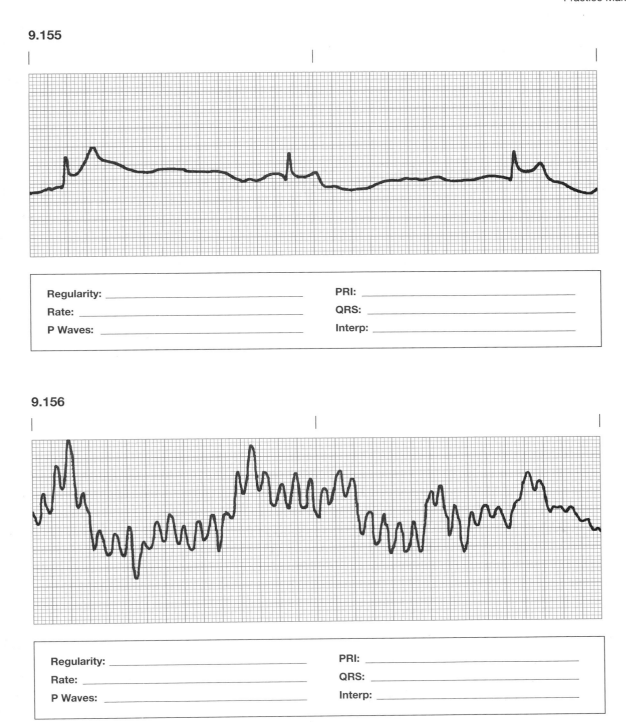

Regularity: _____		PRI: _____	
Rate: _____		QRS: _____	
P Waves: _____		Interp: _____	

9.156

Regularity: _____		PRI: _____	
Rate: _____		QRS: _____	
P Waves: _____		Interp: _____	

9.157

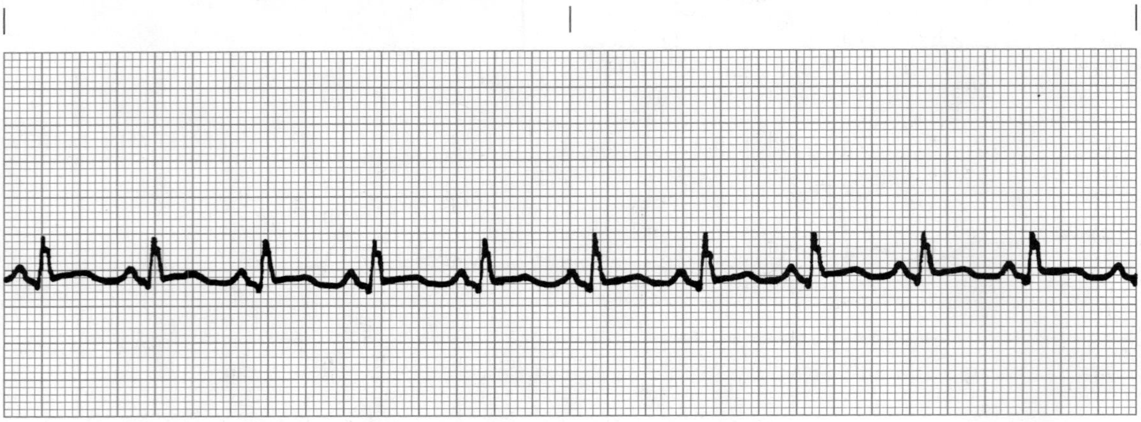

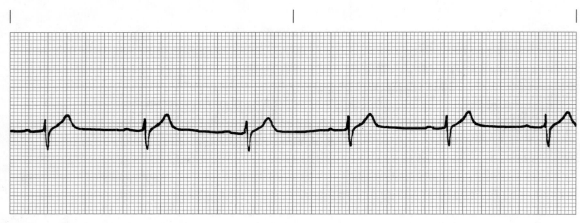

Regularity: _____	**PRI:** _____
Rate: _____	**QRS:** _____
P Waves: _____	**Interp:** _____

9.158

Regularity: _____	**PRI:** _____
Rate: _____	**QRS:** _____
P Waves: _____	**Interp:** _____

9.159

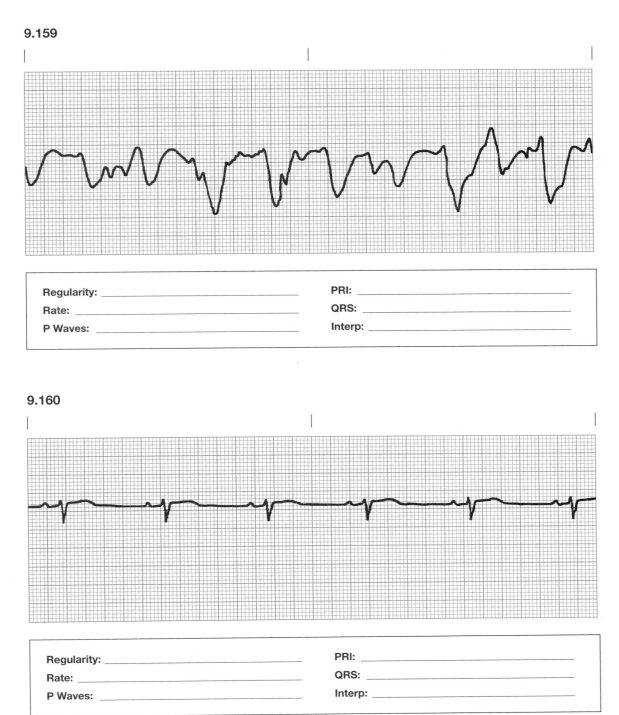

Regularity: _____	PRI: _____
Rate: _____	QRS: _____
P Waves: _____	Interp: _____

9.160

Regularity: _____	PRI: _____
Rate: _____	QRS: _____
P Waves: _____	Interp: _____

9.161

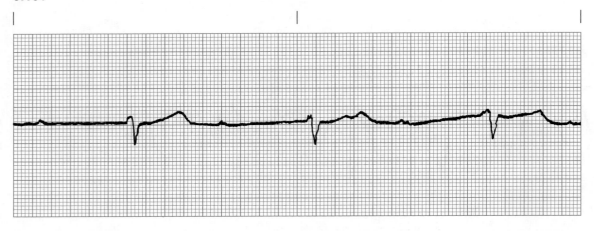

Regularity: _____ PRI: _____

Rate: _____ QRS: _____

P Waves: _____ Interp: _____

9.162

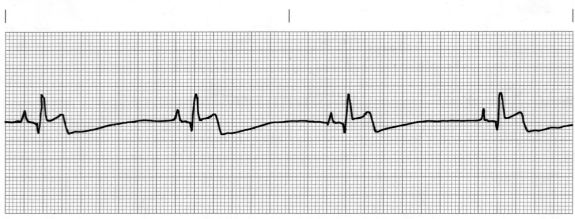

Regularity: _____ PRI: _____

Rate: _____ QRS: _____

P Waves: _____ Interp: _____

9.163

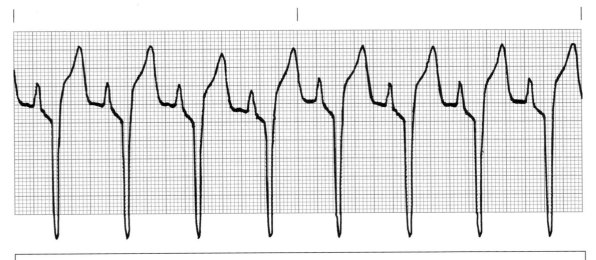

Regularity: _____	PRI: _____
Rate: _____	QRS: _____
P Waves: _____	Interp: _____

9.164

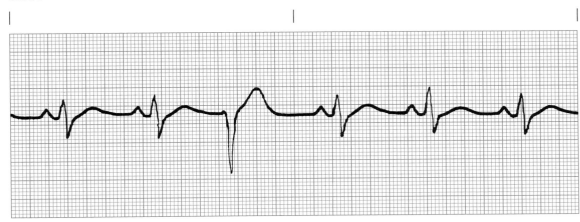

Regularity: _____	PRI: _____
Rate: _____	QRS: _____
P Waves: _____	Interp: _____

9.165

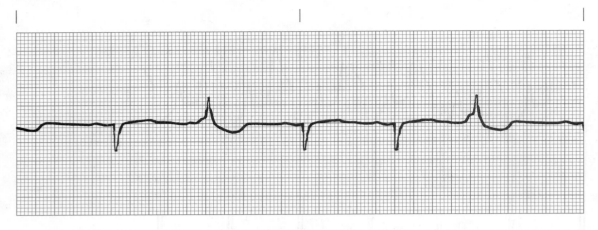

Regularity: _____	PRI: _____
Rate: _____	QRS: _____
P Waves: _____	Interp: _____

9.166

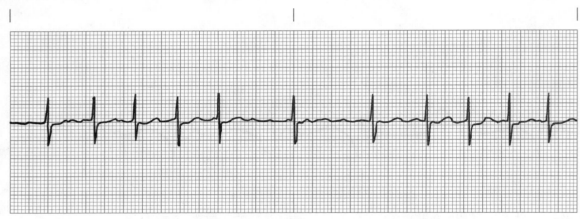

Regularity: _____	PRI: _____
Rate: _____	QRS: _____
P Waves: _____	Interp: _____

9.167

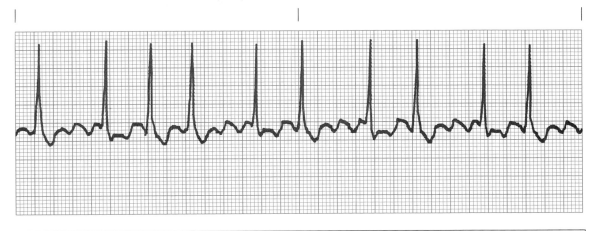

Regularity: _____   PRI: _____

Rate: _____   QRS: _____

P Waves: _____   Interp: _____

9.168

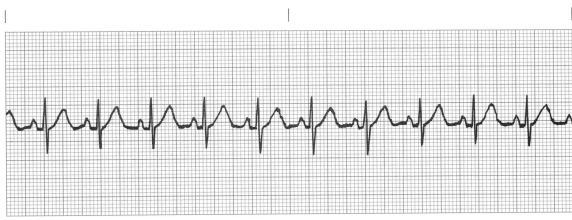

Regularity: _____   PRI: _____

Rate: _____   QRS: _____

P Waves: _____   Interp: _____

9.169

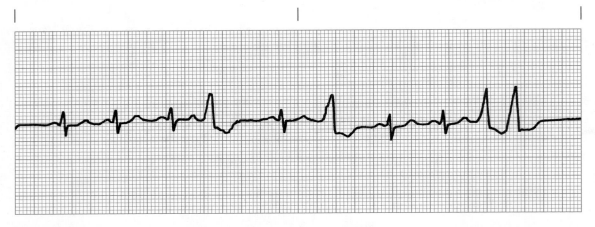

Regularity: _____	PRI: _____
Rate: _____	QRS: _____
P Waves: _____	Interp: _____

9.170

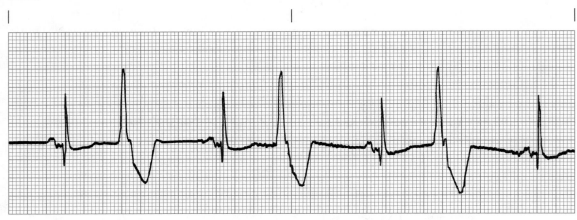

Regularity: _____	PRI: _____
Rate: _____	QRS: _____
P Waves: _____	Interp: _____

9.171

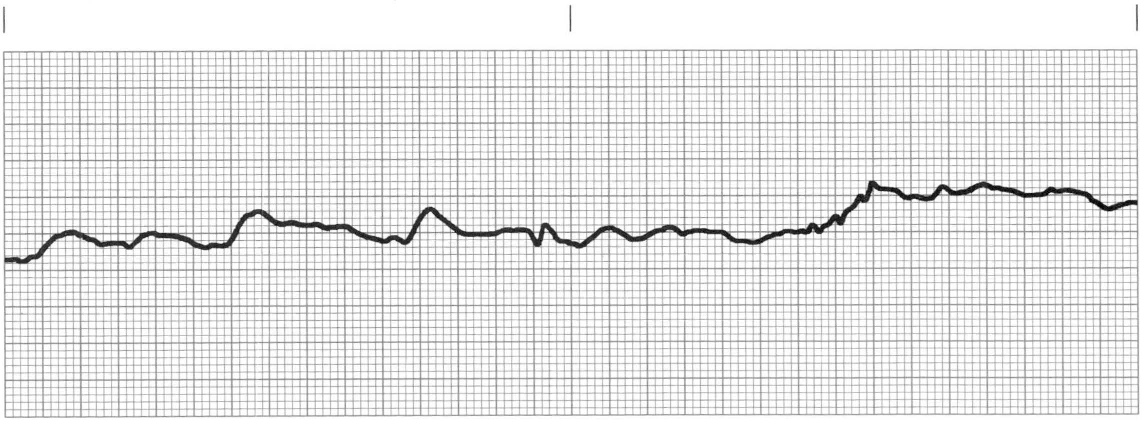

Regularity: _____	PRI: _____
Rate: _____	QRS: _____
P Waves: _____	Interp: _____

9.172

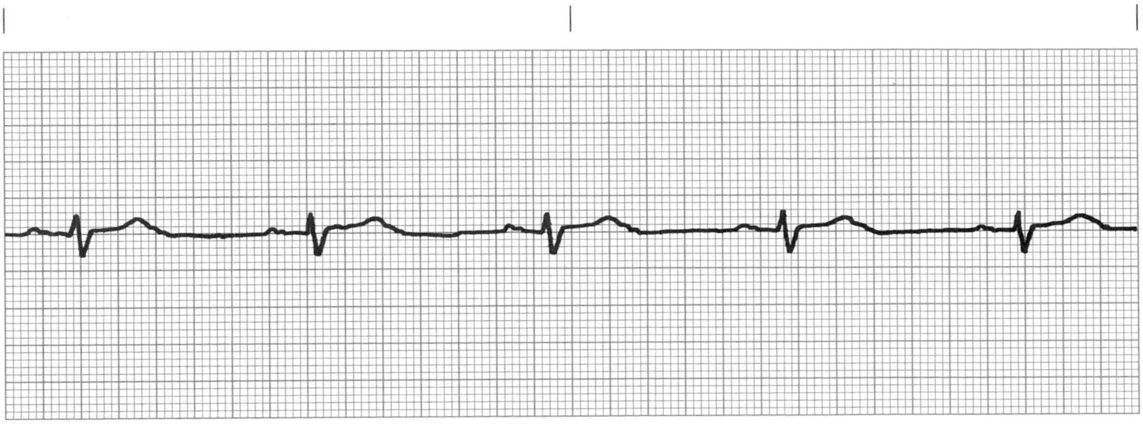

Regularity: _____	PRI: _____
Rate: _____	QRS: _____
P Waves: _____	Interp: _____

9.173

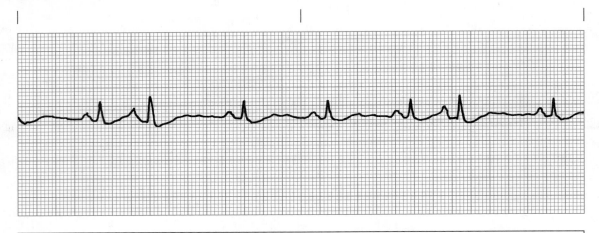

Regularity: _____ PRI: _____

Rate: _____ QRS: _____

P Waves: _____ Interp: _____

9.174

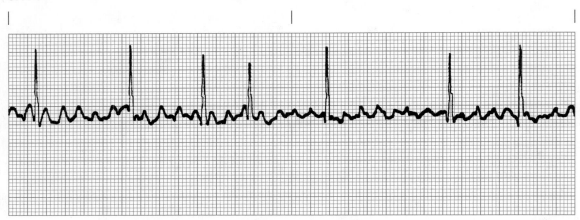

Regularity: _____ PRI: _____

Rate: _____ QRS: _____

P Waves: _____ Interp: _____

9.175

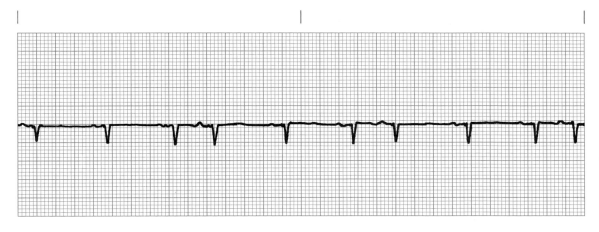

Regularity: _____	PRI: _____
Rate: _____	QRS: _____
P Waves: _____	Interp: _____

9.176

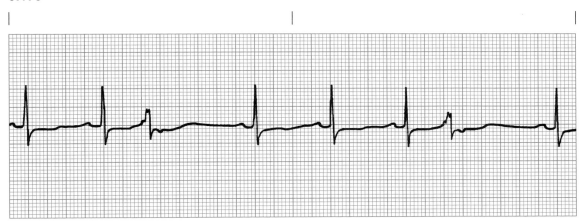

Regularity: _____	PRI: _____
Rate: _____	QRS: _____
P Waves: _____	Interp: _____

9.177

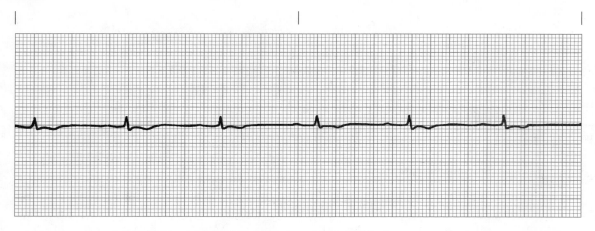

Regularity: _____	PRI: _____
Rate: _____	QRS: _____
P Waves: _____	Interp: _____

9.178

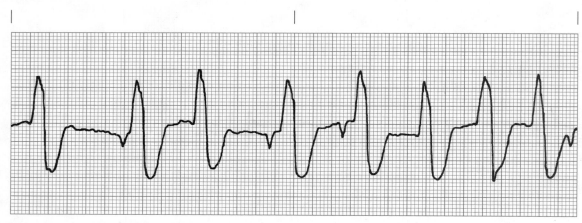

Regularity: _____	PRI: _____
Rate: _____	QRS: _____
P Waves: _____	Interp: _____

9.179

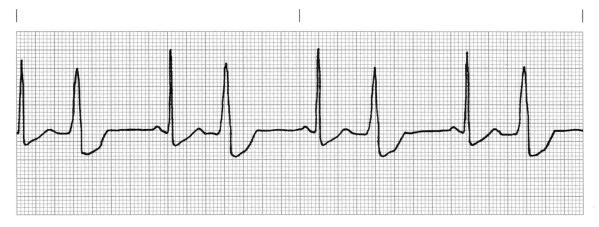

Regularity: _____	**PRI:** _____
Rate: _____	**QRS:** _____
P Waves: _____	**Interp:** _____

9.180

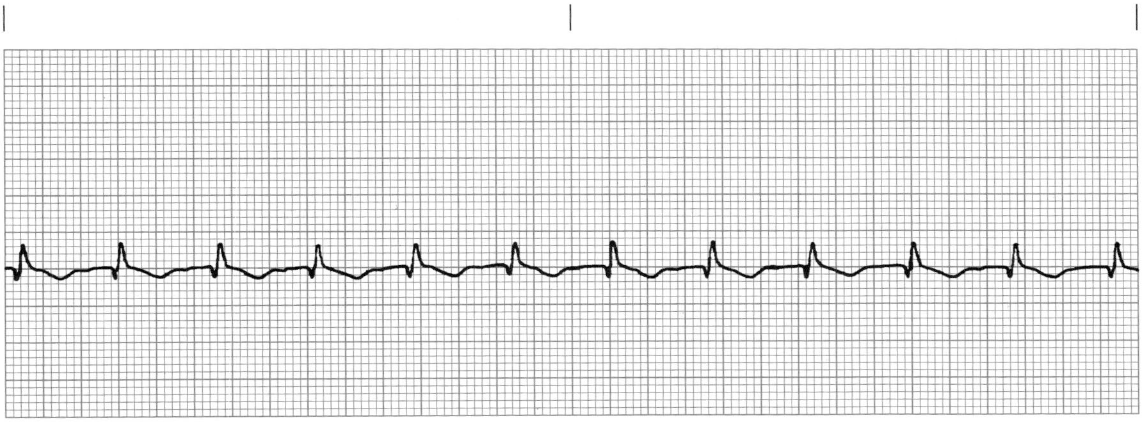

Regularity: _____	**PRI:** _____
Rate: _____	**QRS:** _____
P Waves: _____	**Interp:** _____

9.181

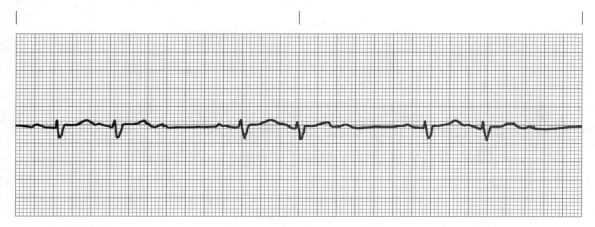

Regularity: _____	PRI: _____
Rate: _____	QRS: _____
P Waves: _____	Interp: _____

9.182

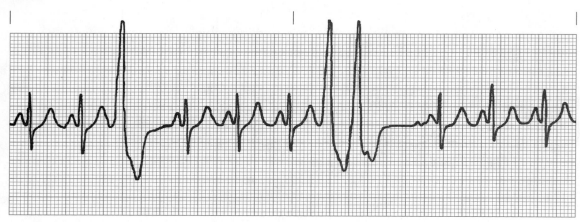

Regularity: _____	PRI: _____
Rate: _____	QRS: _____
P Waves: _____	Interp: _____

9.183

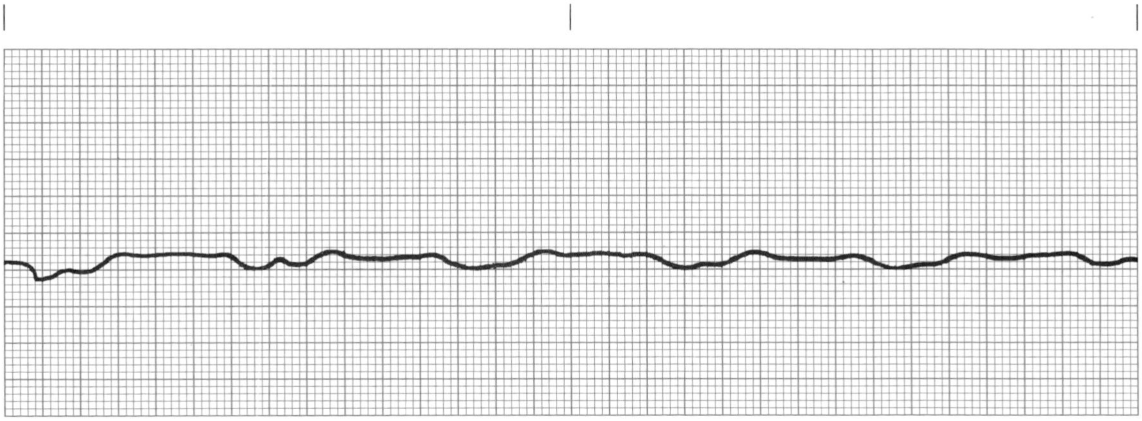

Regularity: _____	PRI: _____
Rate: _____	QRS: _____
P Waves: _____	Interp: _____

9.184

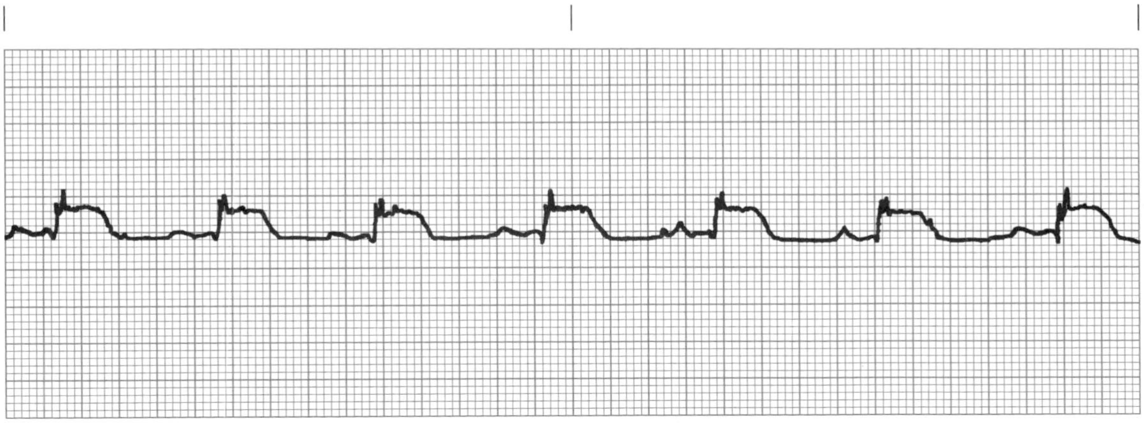

Regularity: _____	PRI: _____
Rate: _____	QRS: _____
P Waves: _____	Interp: _____

9.185

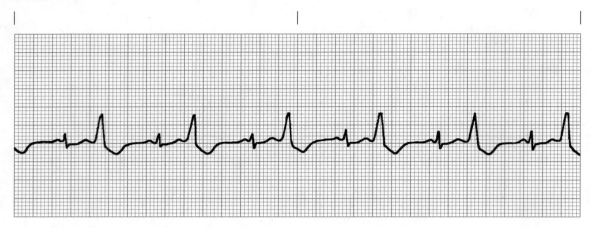

Regularity: _____	PRI: _____
Rate: _____	QRS: _____
P Waves: _____	Interp: _____

9.186

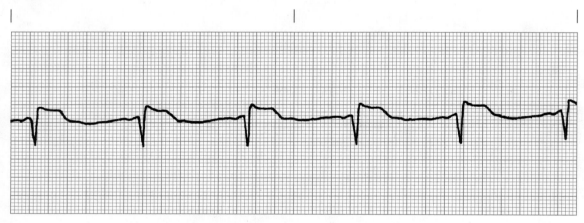

Regularity: _____	PRI: _____
Rate: _____	QRS: _____
P Waves: _____	Interp: _____

9.187

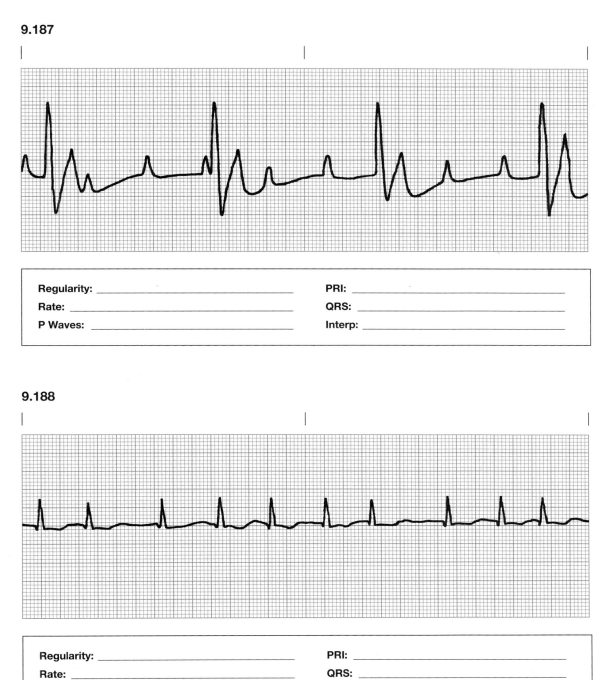

Regularity: _____   PRI: _____
Rate: _____   QRS: _____
P Waves: _____   Interp: _____

9.188

Regularity: _____   PRI: _____
Rate: _____   QRS: _____
P Waves: _____   Interp: _____

9.189

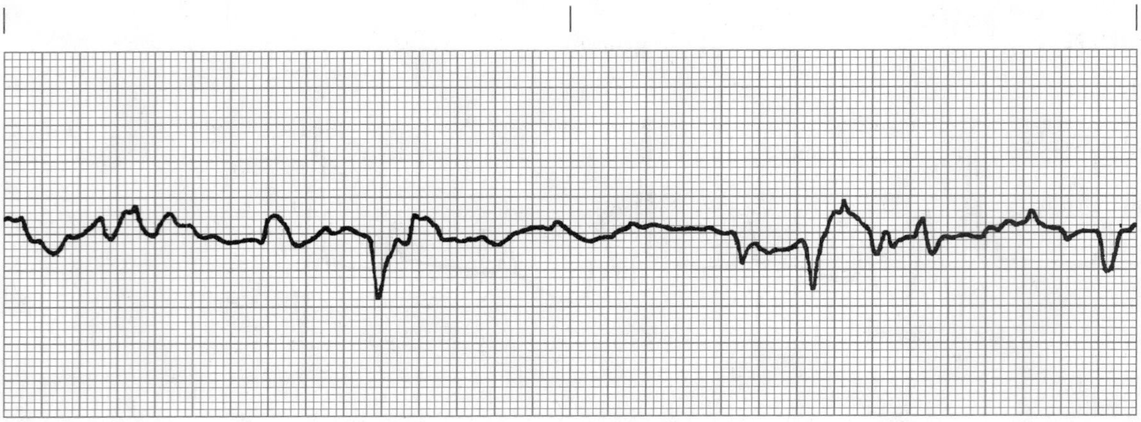

Regularity: _____	PRI: _____
Rate: _____	QRS: _____
P Waves: _____	Interp: _____

9.190

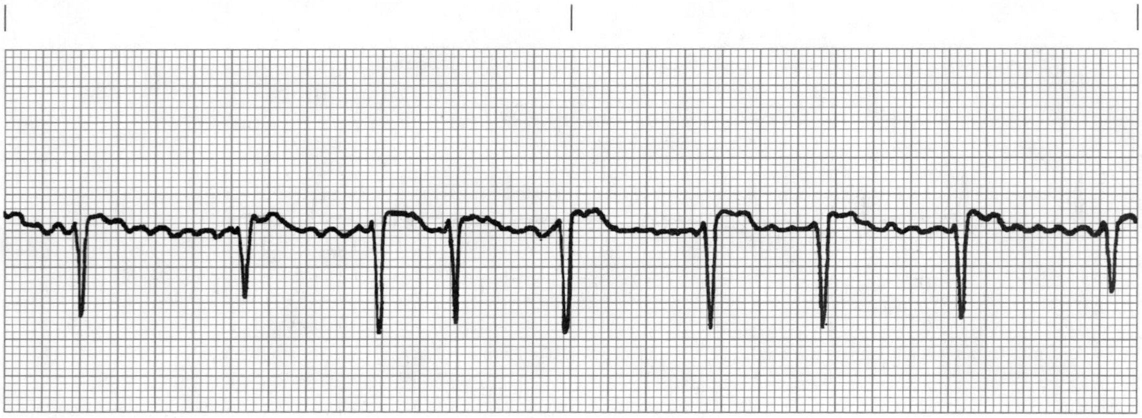

Regularity: _____	PRI: _____
Rate: _____	QRS: _____
P Waves: _____	Interp: _____

9.191

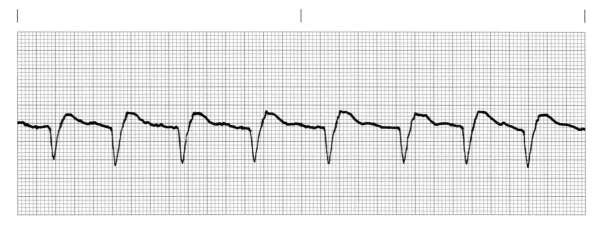

Regularity: _____	PRI: _____
Rate: _____	QRS: _____
P Waves: _____	Interp: _____

9.192

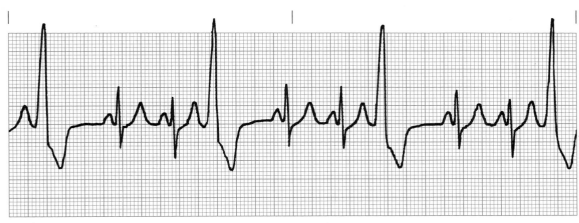

Regularity: _____	PRI: _____
Rate: _____	QRS: _____
P Waves: _____	Interp: _____

9.193

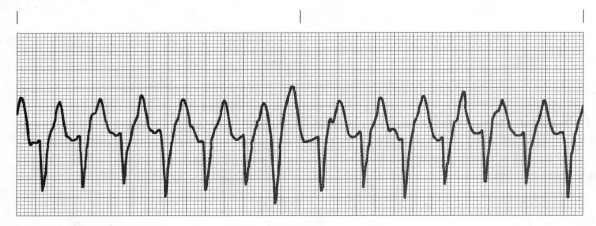

Regularity: _____	PRI: _____
Rate: _____	QRS: _____
P Waves: _____	Interp: _____

9.194

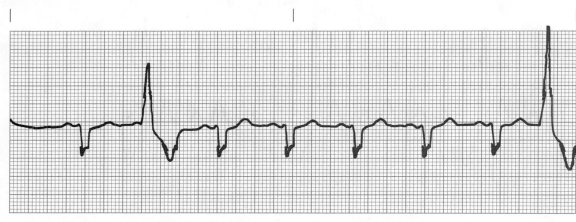

Regularity: _____	PRI: _____
Rate: _____	QRS: _____
P Waves: _____	Interp: _____

9.195

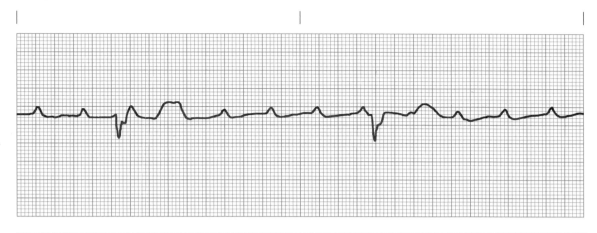

Regularity: _____

Rate: _____

P Waves: _____

PRI: _____

QRS: _____

Interp: _____

9.196

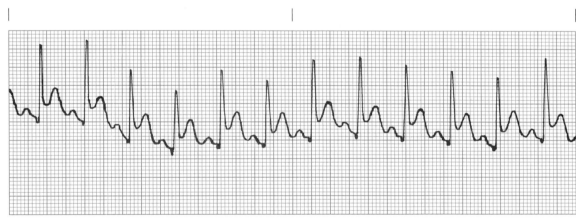

Regularity: _____

Rate: _____

P Waves: _____

PRI: _____

QRS: _____

Interp: _____

9.197

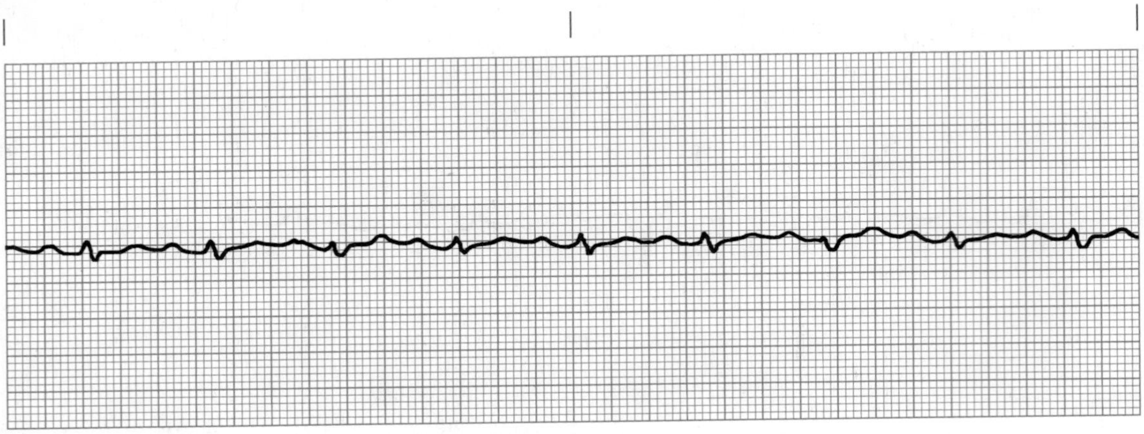

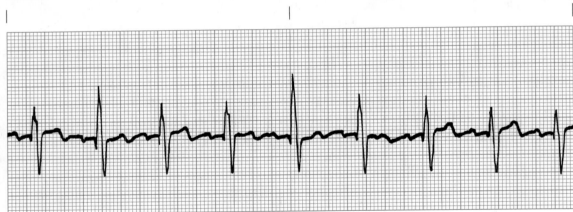

Regularity: _____	PRI: _____
Rate: _____	QRS: _____
P Waves: _____	Interp: _____

9.198

Regularity: _____	PRI: _____
Rate: _____	QRS: _____
P Waves: _____	Interp: _____

9.199

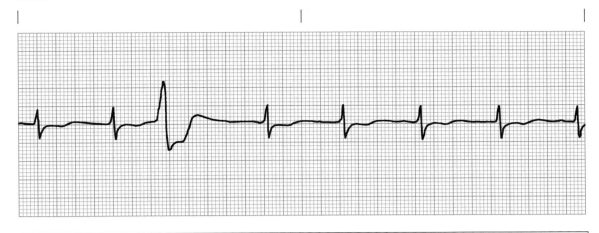

Regularity: _____   PRI: _____

Rate: _____   QRS: _____

P Waves: _____   Interp: _____

9.200

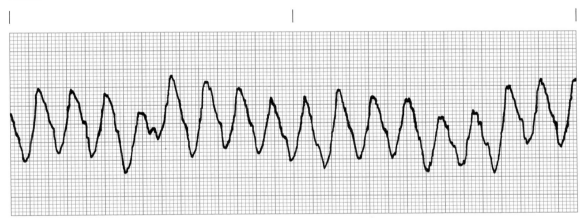

Regularity: _____   PRI: _____

Rate: _____   QRS: _____

P Waves: _____   Interp: _____

9.201

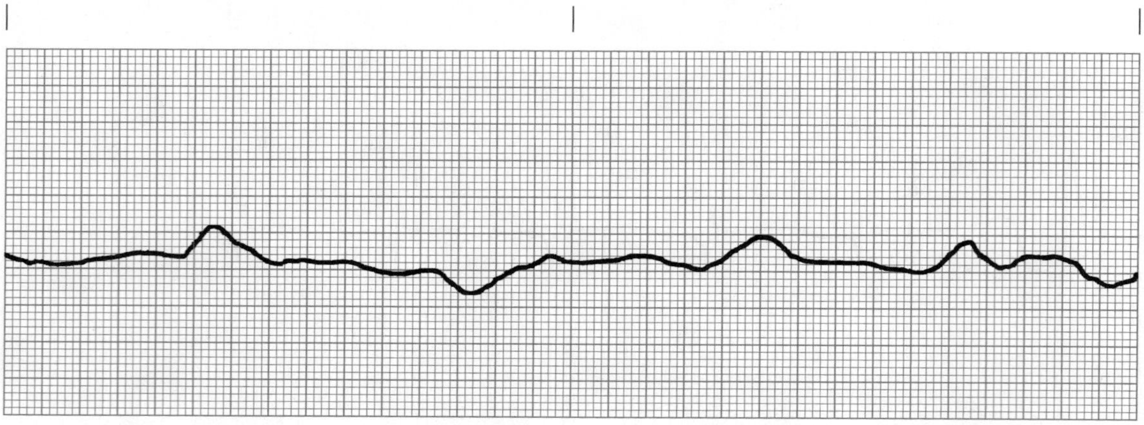

Regularity: _____   PRI: _____

Rate: _____   QRS: _____

P Waves: _____   Interp: _____

9.202

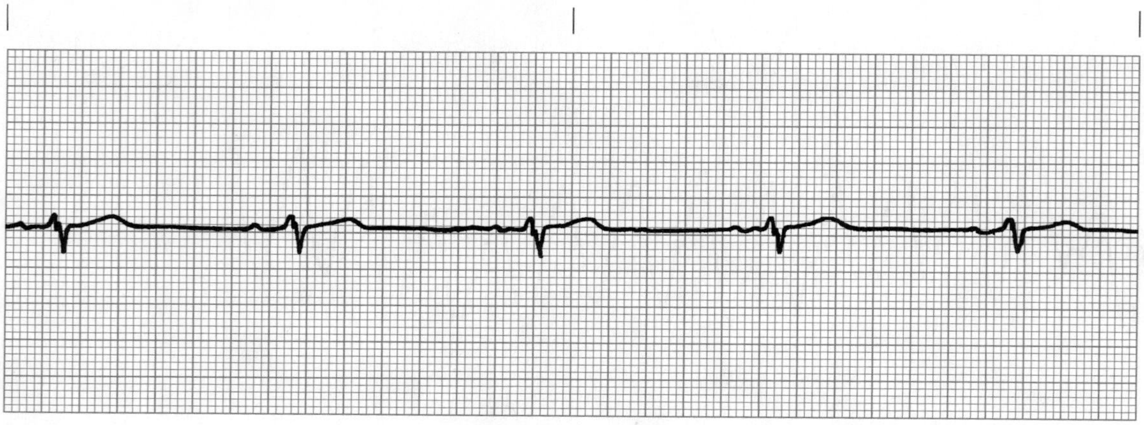

Regularity: _____   PRI: _____

Rate: _____   QRS: _____

P Waves: _____   Interp: _____

9.203

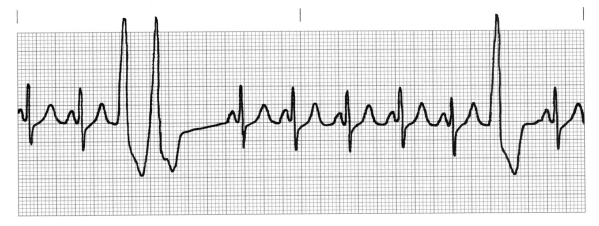

Regularity: _____   PRI: _____

Rate: _____   QRS: _____

P Waves: _____   Interp: _____

9.204

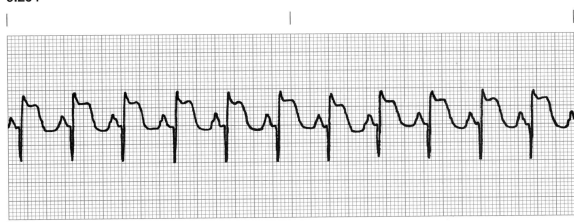

Regularity: _____   PRI: _____

Rate: _____   QRS: _____

P Waves: _____   Interp: _____

9.205

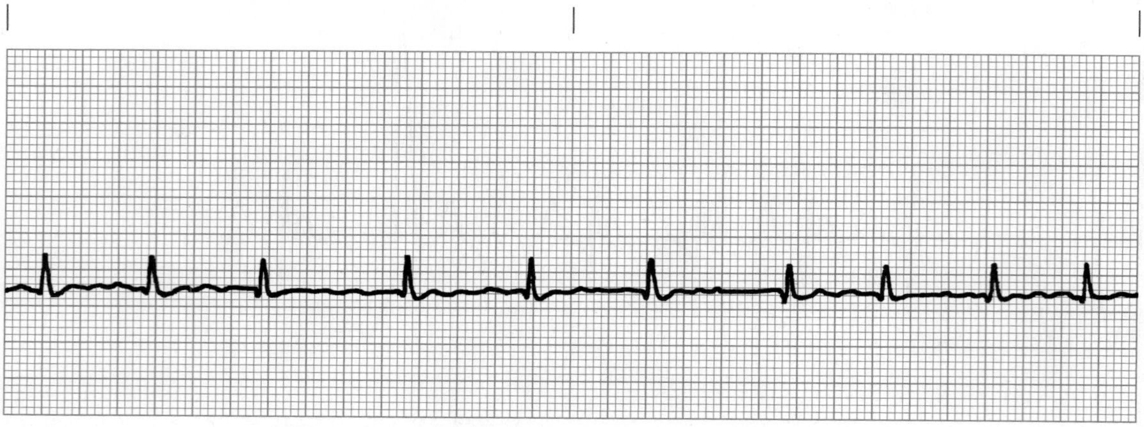

Regularity: _____	PRI: _____
Rate: _____	QRS: _____
P Waves: _____	Interp: _____

9.206

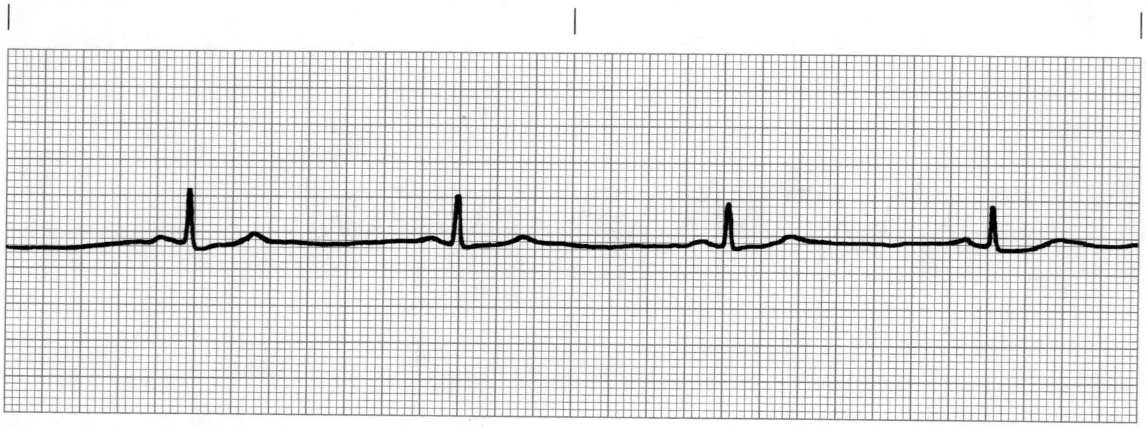

Regularity: _____	PRI: _____
Rate: _____	QRS: _____
P Waves: _____	Interp: _____

9.207

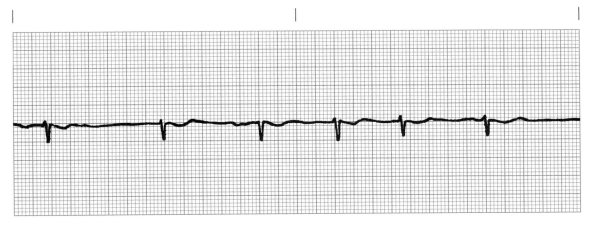

Regularity: _____ PRI: _____

Rate: _____ QRS: _____

P Waves: _____ Interp: _____

9.208

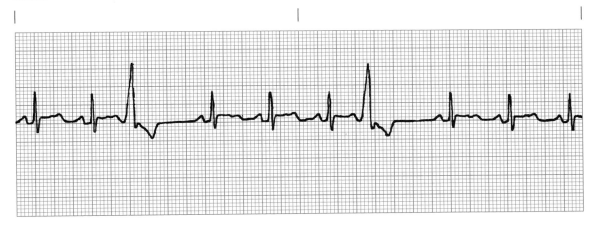

Regularity: _____ PRI: _____

Rate: _____ QRS: _____

P Waves: _____ Interp: _____

9.209

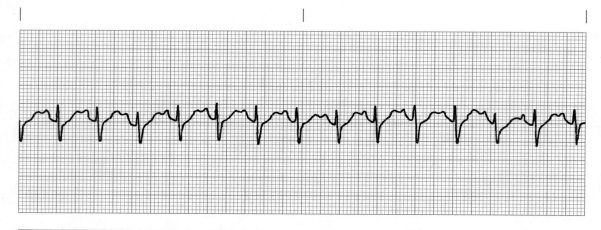

Regularity:		PRI:	
Rate:		QRS:	
P Waves:		Interp:	

9.210

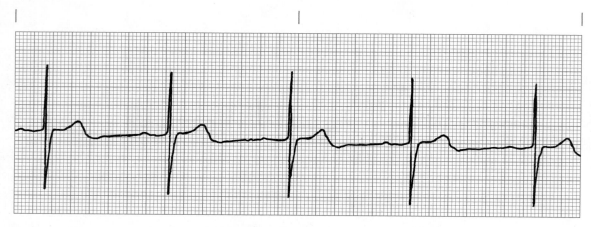

Regularity:		PRI:	
Rate:		QRS:	
P Waves:		Interp:	

9.211

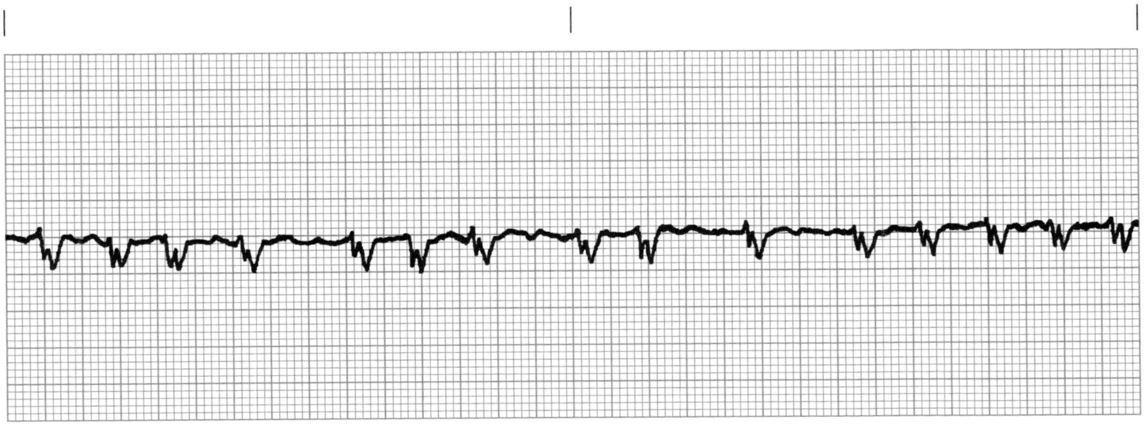

Regularity: _____   PRI: _____

Rate: _____   QRS: _____

P Waves: _____   Interp: _____

9.212

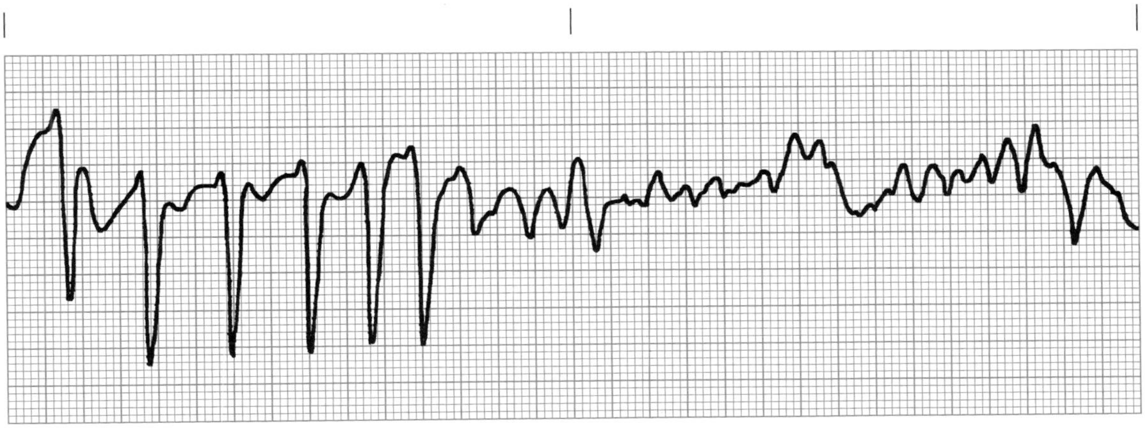

Regularity: _____   PRI: _____

Rate: _____   QRS: _____

P Waves: _____   Interp: _____

9.213

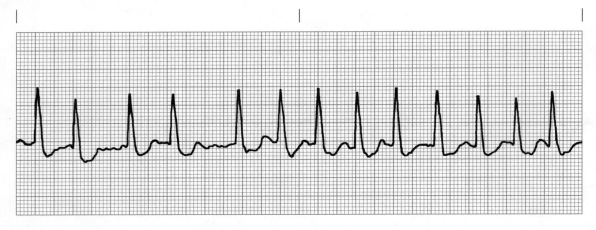

Regularity: _____	PRI: _____
Rate: _____	QRS: _____
P Waves: _____	Interp: _____

9.214

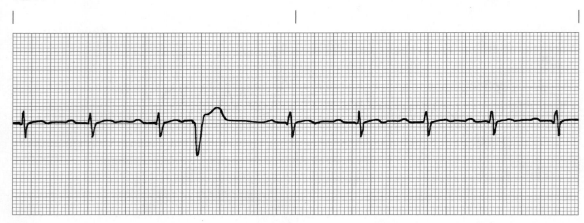

Regularity: _____	PRI: _____
Rate: _____	QRS: _____
P Waves: _____	Interp: _____

9.215

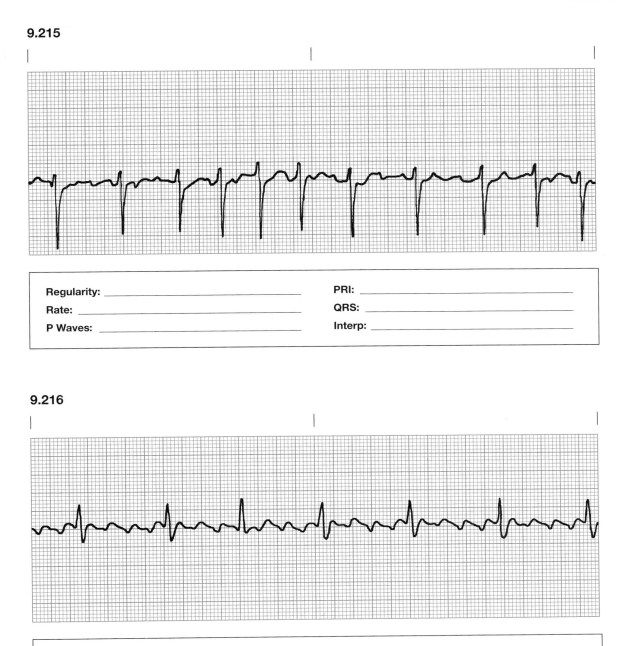

Regularity: _____   PRI: _____

Rate: _____   QRS: _____

P Waves: _____   Interp: _____

9.216

Regularity: _____   PRI: _____

Rate: _____   QRS: _____

P Waves: _____   Interp: _____

9.217

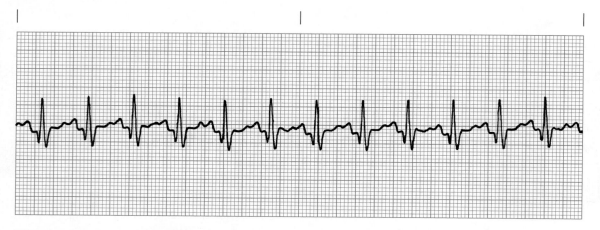

Regularity: _____	PRI: _____
Rate: _____	QRS: _____
P Waves: _____	Interp: _____

9.218

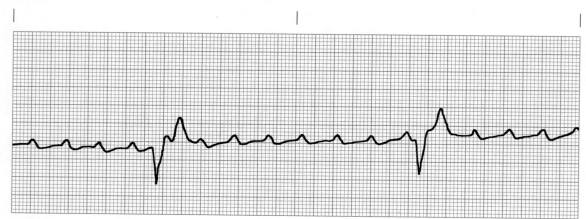

Regularity: _____	PRI: _____
Rate: _____	QRS: _____
P Waves: _____	Interp: _____

9.219

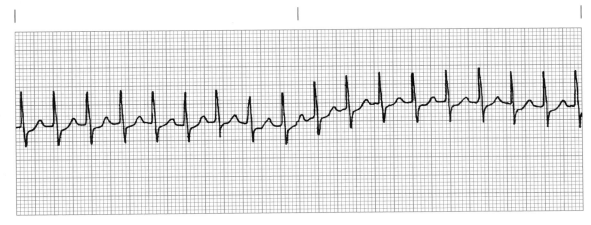

Regularity: _____		PRI: _____	
Rate: _____		QRS: _____	
P Waves: _____		Interp: _____	

9.220

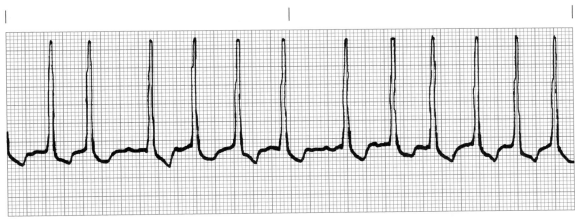

Regularity: _____		PRI: _____	
Rate: _____		QRS: _____	
P Waves: _____		Interp: _____	

9.221

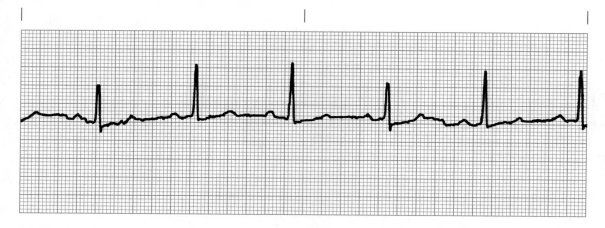

Regularity: _____	PRI: _____
Rate: _____	QRS: _____
P Waves: _____	Interp: _____

9.222

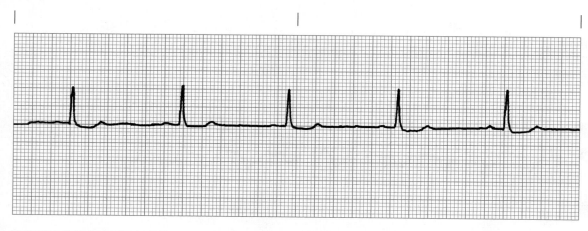

Regularity: _____	PRI: _____
Rate: _____	QRS: _____
P Waves: _____	Interp: _____

9.223

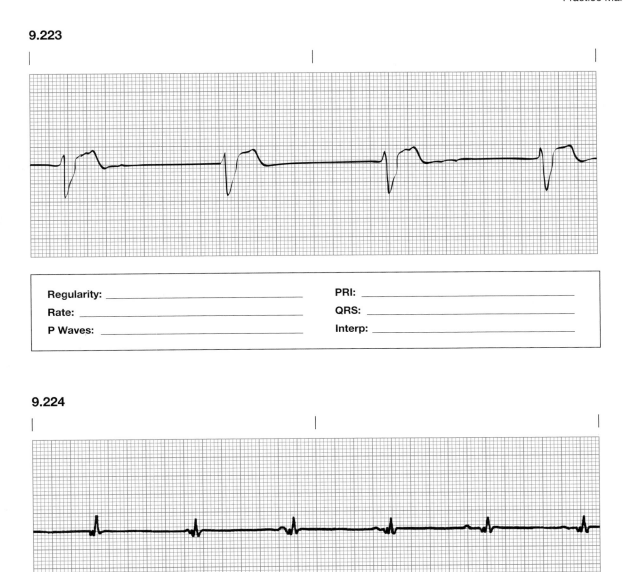

Regularity: _____		**PRI:** _____	
Rate: _____		**QRS:** _____	
P Waves: _____		**Interp:** _____	

9.224

Regularity: _____		**PRI:** _____	
Rate: _____		**QRS:** _____	
P Waves: _____		**Interp:** _____	

9.225

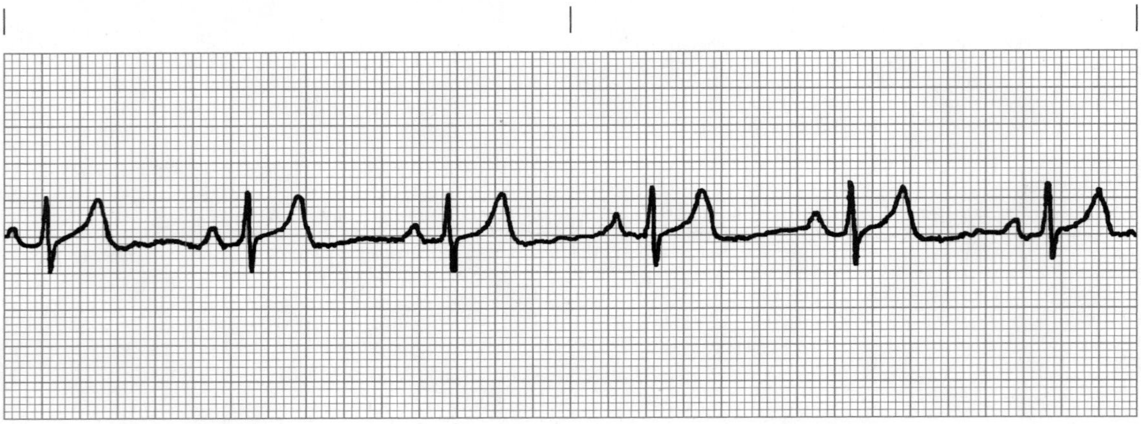

Regularity: _____	PRI: _____
Rate: _____	QRS: _____
P Waves: _____	Interp: _____

9.226

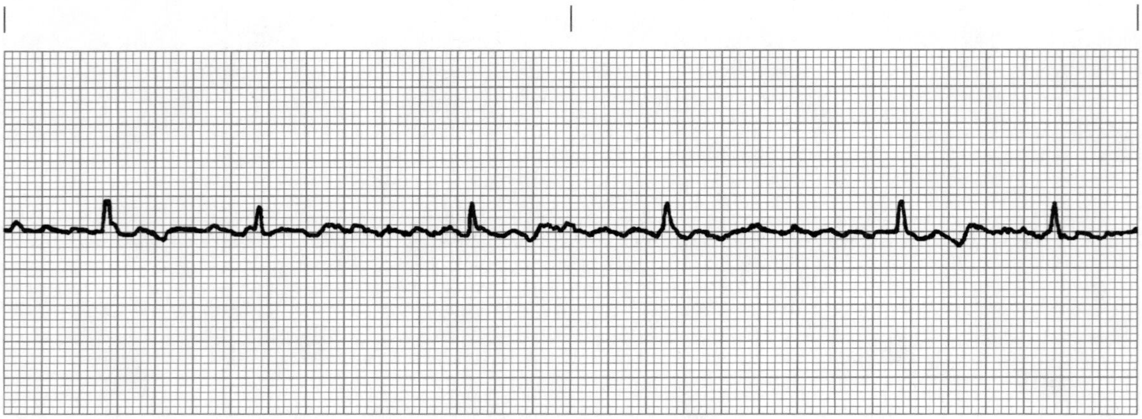

Regularity: _____	PRI: _____
Rate: _____	QRS: _____
P Waves: _____	Interp: _____

9.227

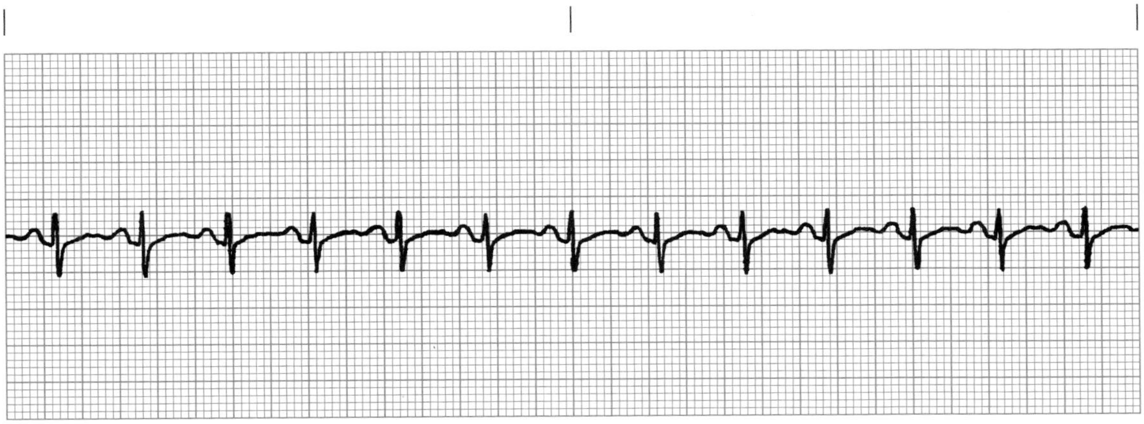

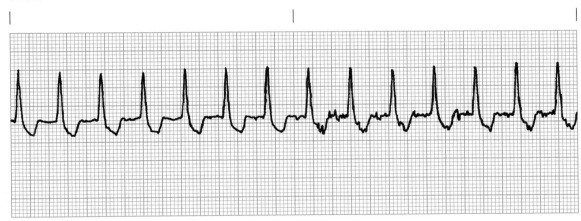

Regularity: _____	**PRI:** _____	
Rate: _____	**QRS:** _____	
P Waves: _____	**Interp:** _____	

9.228

Regularity: _____	**PRI:** _____	
Rate: _____	**QRS:** _____	
P Waves: _____	**Interp:** _____	

9.229

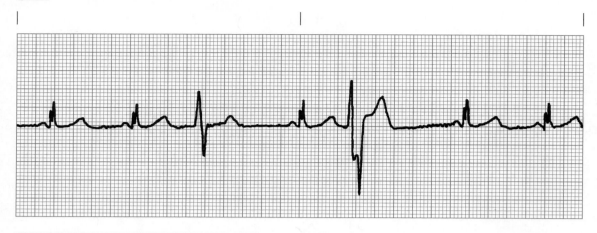

Regularity: _____   PRI: _____

Rate: _____   QRS: _____

P Waves: _____   Interp: _____

9.230

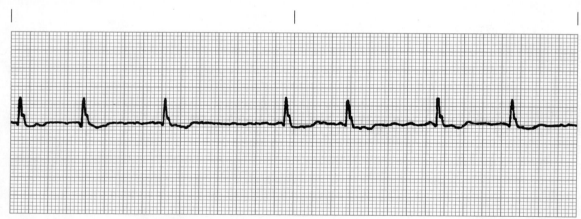

Regularity: _____   PRI: _____

Rate: _____   QRS: _____

P Waves: _____   Interp: _____

9.231

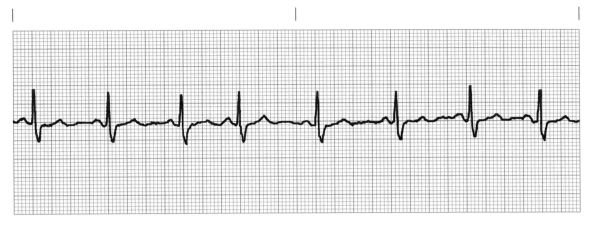

Regularity: _____	PRI: _____
Rate: _____	QRS: _____
P Waves: _____	Interp: _____

9.232

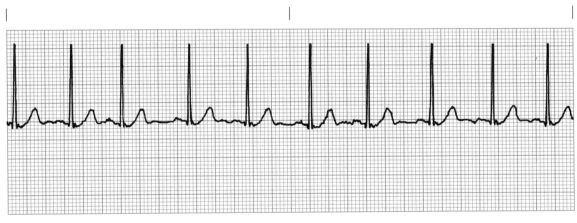

Regularity: _____	PRI: _____
Rate: _____	QRS: _____
P Waves: _____	Interp: _____

9.233

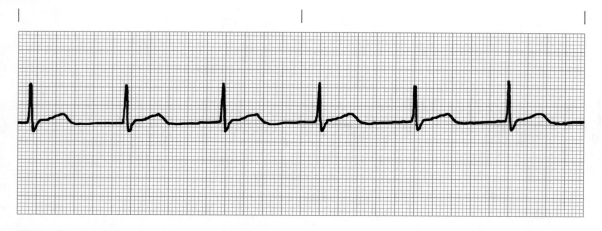

Regularity: _____	PRI: _____
Rate: _____	QRS: _____
P Waves: _____	Interp: _____

9.234

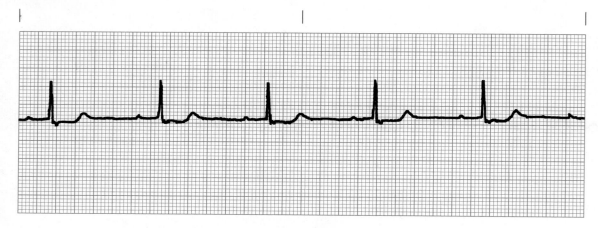

Regularity: _____	PRI: _____
Rate: _____	QRS: _____
P Waves: _____	Interp: _____

9.235

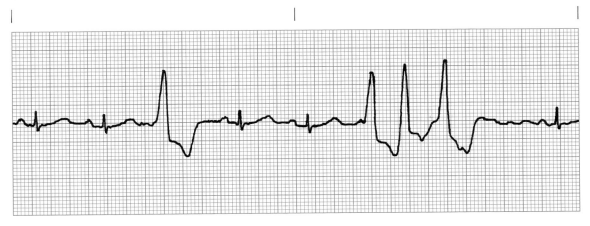

Regularity: _____	**PRI:** _____
Rate: _____	**QRS:** _____
P Waves: _____	**Interp:** _____

9.236

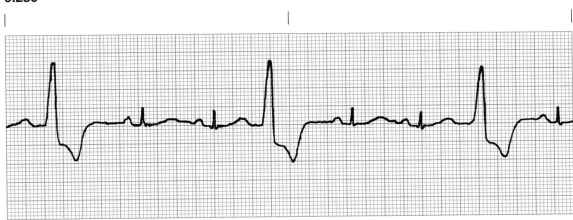

Regularity: _____	**PRI:** _____
Rate: _____	**QRS:** _____
P Waves: _____	**Interp:** _____

9.237

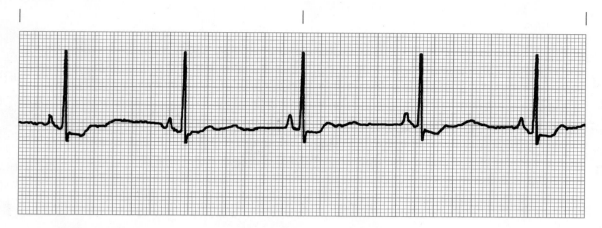

Regularity: _____	PRI: _____
Rate: _____	QRS: _____
P Waves: _____	Interp: _____

9.238

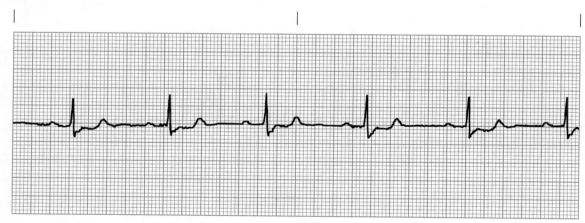

Regularity: _____	PRI: _____
Rate: _____	QRS: _____
P Waves: _____	Interp: _____

9.239

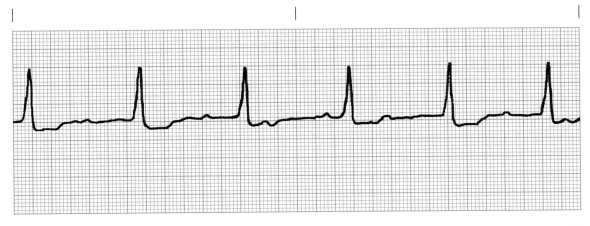

Regularity: _____	PRI: _____
Rate: _____	QRS: _____
P Waves: _____	Interp: _____

9.240

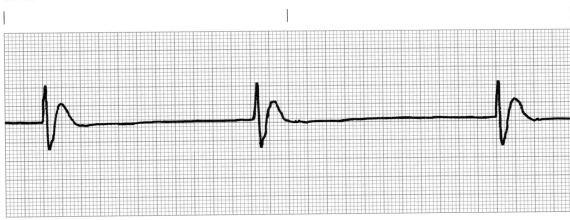

Regularity: _____	PRI: _____
Rate: _____	QRS: _____
P Waves: _____	Interp: _____

9.241

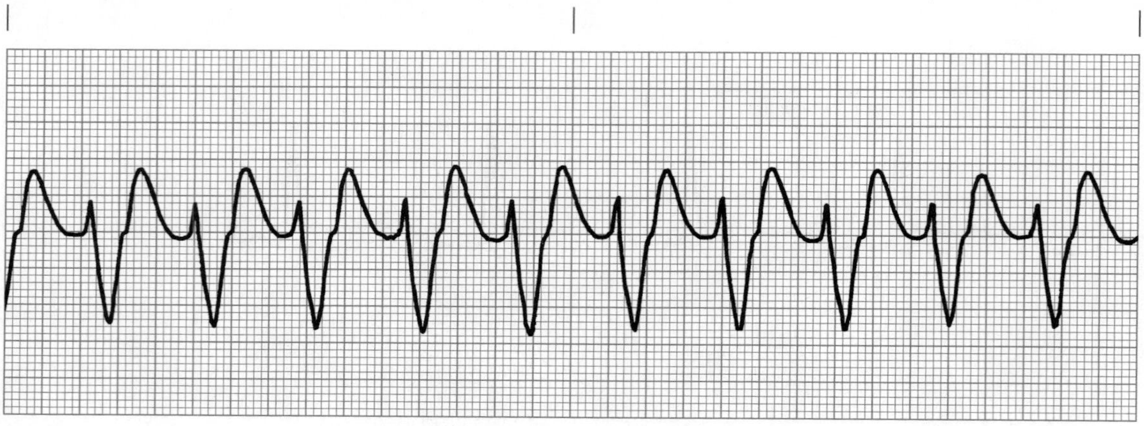

Regularity: _____   PRI: _____

Rate: _____   QRS: _____

P Waves: _____   Interp: _____

9.242

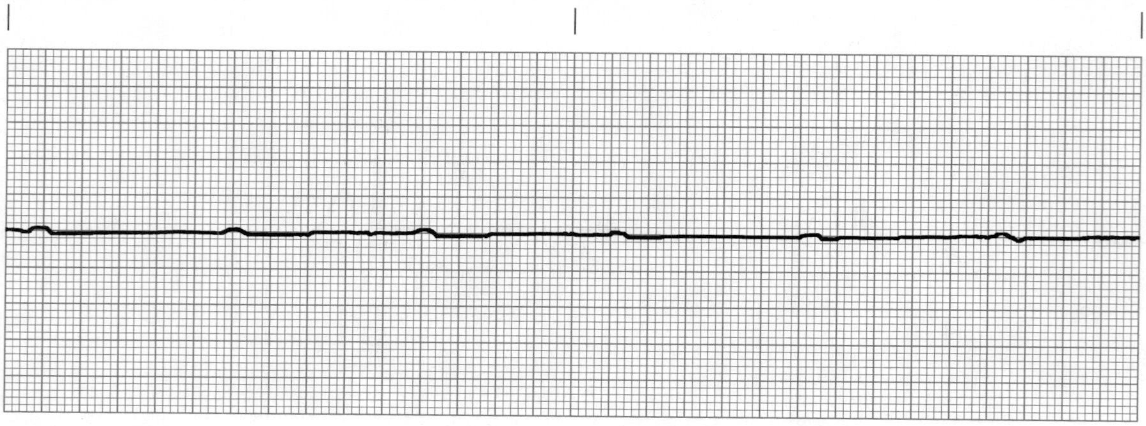

Regularity: _____   PRI: _____

Rate: _____   QRS: _____

P Waves: _____   Interp: _____

9.243

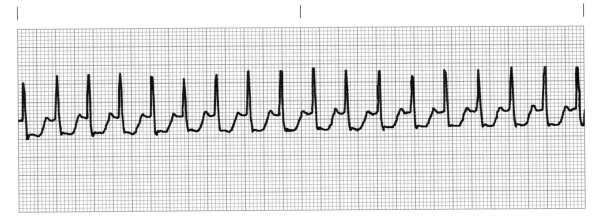

Regularity: _____	PRI: _____
Rate: _____	QRS: _____
P Waves: _____	Interp: _____

9.244

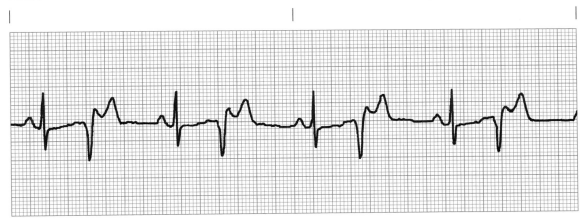

Regularity: _____	PRI: _____
Rate: _____	QRS: _____
P Waves: _____	Interp: _____

9.245

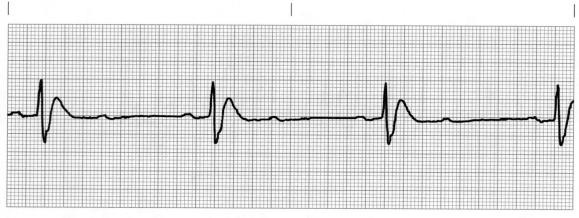

Regularity: _____		PRI: _____	
Rate: _____		QRS: _____	
P Waves: _____		Interp: _____	

9.246

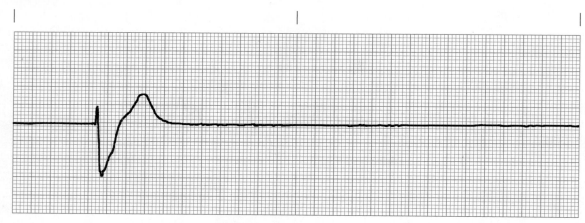

Regularity: _____		PRI: _____	
Rate: _____		QRS: _____	
P Waves: _____		Interp: _____	

9.247

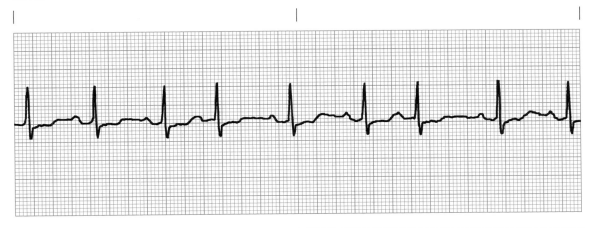

Regularity: _____   PRI: _____

Rate: _____   QRS: _____

P Waves: _____   Interp: _____

9.248

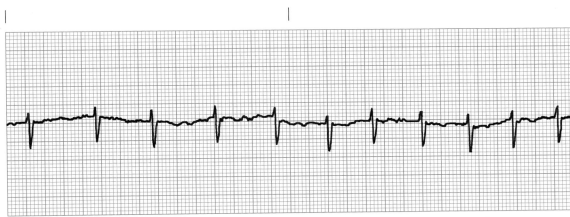

Regularity: _____   PRI: _____

Rate: _____   QRS: _____

P Waves: _____   Interp: _____

9.249

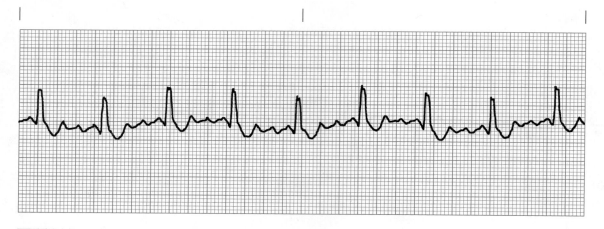

Regularity: _____	PRI: _____
Rate: _____	QRS: _____
P Waves: _____	Interp: _____

9.250

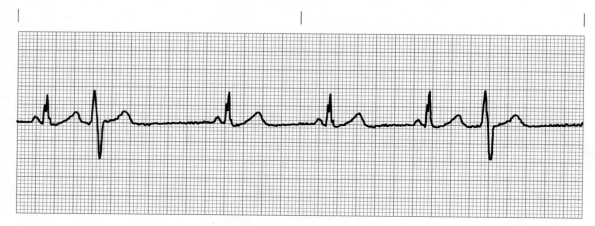

Regularity: _____	PRI: _____
Rate: _____	QRS: _____
P Waves: _____	Interp: _____

Chapter 10
Final Challenge

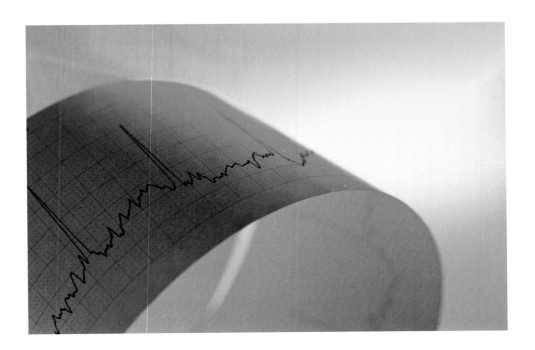

Introduction

Well, you've finished all the chapters, you've passed each of the chapter tests, and you've practiced, practiced, practiced. Do you think you're ready to take on the Final Challenge? Here's how to test yourself to see how good you really are.

First, set aside about an hour or two of uninterrupted time. This should be closed-book, so all you'll need is a pencil and your calipers. Tackle each strip in order; don't skip around. When you're done, turn to the answer key to correct yourself. If you want to score yourself, each strip is worth one percentage point (i.e., if you miss five, your score is 95%). On a standard scale, a score of 90% or above is an A, 80–89% is a B, 70–79% is a C, 60–69% is a D, and below 60% is failing.

Keep in mind that this isn't an algebra test, where all the questions have equal value. Some rhythms are more significant than others, so it's important for you to be able to interpret accurately across all the rhythm categories. After you've graded yourself, go back and tally any you missed. Look for clustering or any other pattern that might suggest a weak area; then use that information to target supplemental study.

Okay. Are you ready? Good luck, and enjoy it.

SELF-TEST (answers can be found in the Answer Key on page 579)

10.1

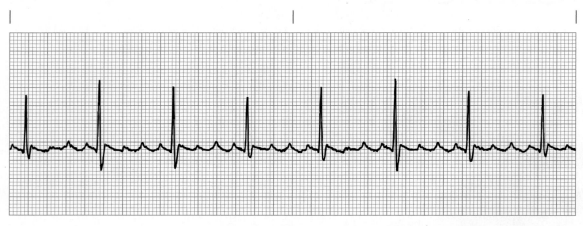

Regularity: _____   PRI: _____

Rate: _____   QRS: _____

P Waves: _____   Interp: _____

10.2

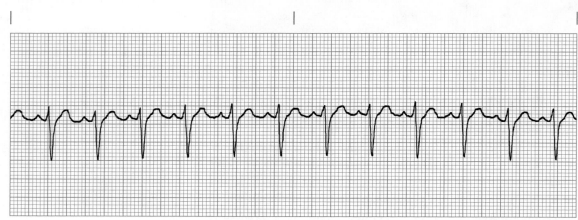

Regularity: _____   PRI: _____

Rate: _____   QRS: _____

P Waves: _____   Interp: _____

10.3

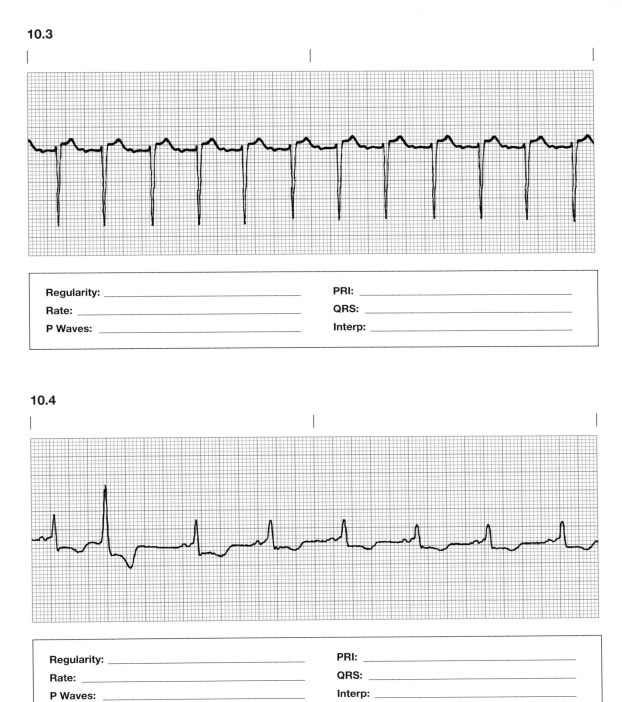

Regularity: _____	**PRI:** _____
Rate: _____	**QRS:** _____
P Waves: _____	**Interp:** _____

10.4

Regularity: _____	**PRI:** _____
Rate: _____	**QRS:** _____
P Waves: _____	**Interp:** _____

10.5

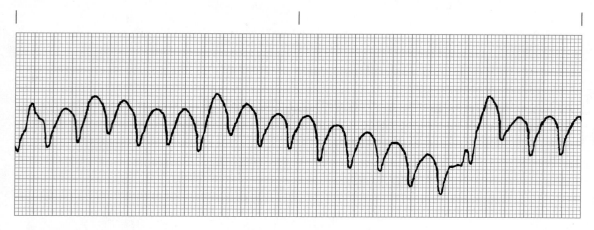

Regularity: _____	PRI: _____
Rate: _____	QRS: _____
P Waves: _____	Interp: _____

10.6

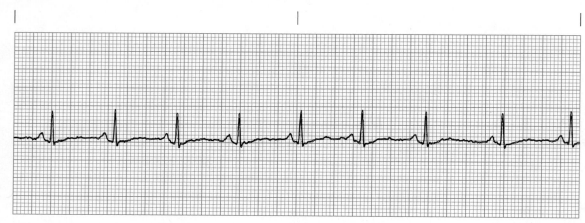

Regularity: _____	PRI: _____
Rate: _____	QRS: _____
P Waves: _____	Interp: _____

10.7

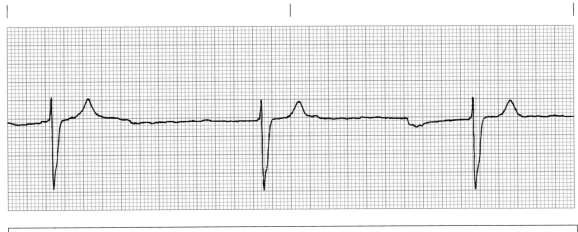

Regularity: _____	PRI: _____
Rate: _____	QRS: _____
P Waves: _____	Interp: _____

10.8

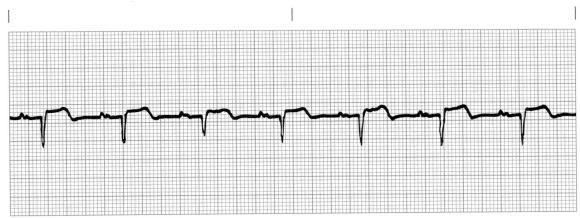

Regularity: _____	PRI: _____
Rate: _____	QRS: _____
P Waves: _____	Interp: _____

10.9

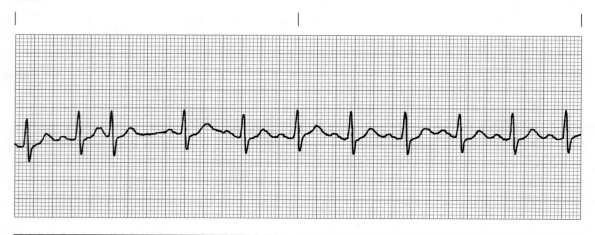

Regularity: _____	PRI: _____
Rate: _____	QRS: _____
P Waves: _____	Interp: _____

10.10

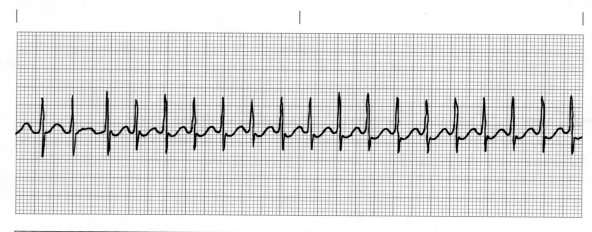

Regularity: _____	PRI: _____
Rate: _____	QRS: _____
P Waves: _____	Interp: _____

10.11

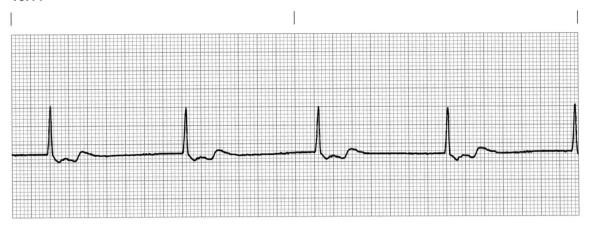

Regularity: _____	PRI: _____
Rate: _____	QRS: _____
P Waves: _____	Interp: _____

10.12

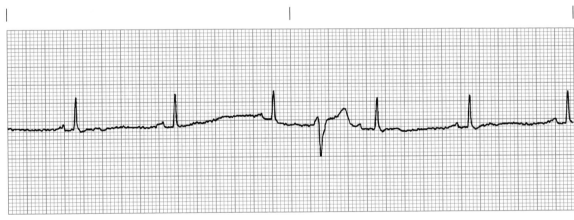

Regularity: _____	PRI: _____
Rate: _____	QRS: _____
P Waves: _____	Interp: _____

10.13

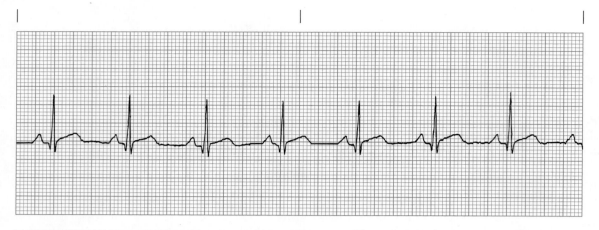

Regularity: _____	PRI: _____
Rate: _____	QRS: _____
P Waves: _____	Interp: _____

10.14

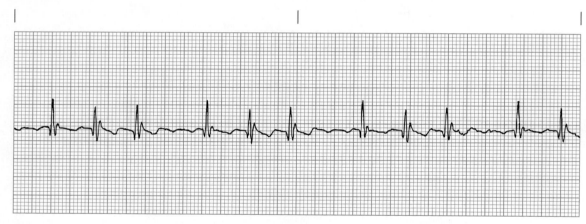

Regularity: _____	PRI: _____
Rate: _____	QRS: _____
P Waves: _____	Interp: _____

10.15

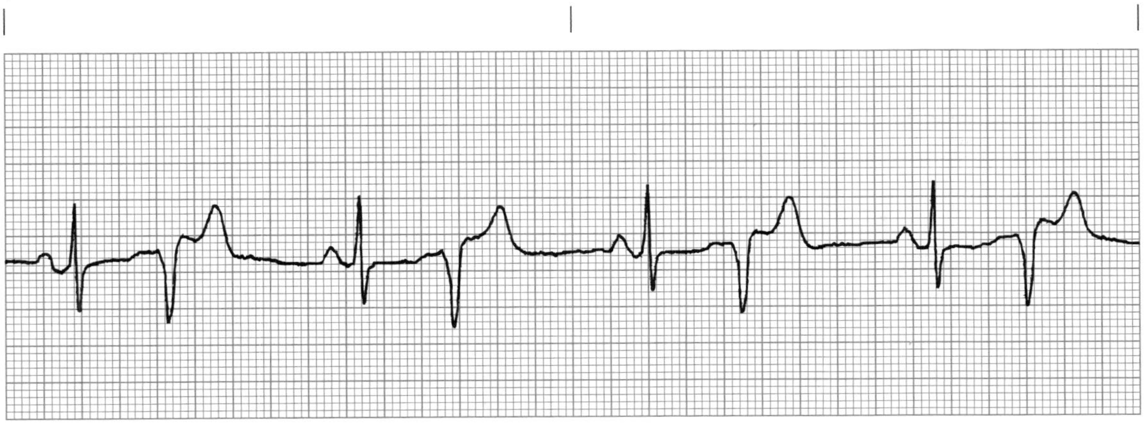

Regularity: _____	PRI: _____
Rate: _____	QRS: _____
P Waves: _____	Interp: _____

10.16

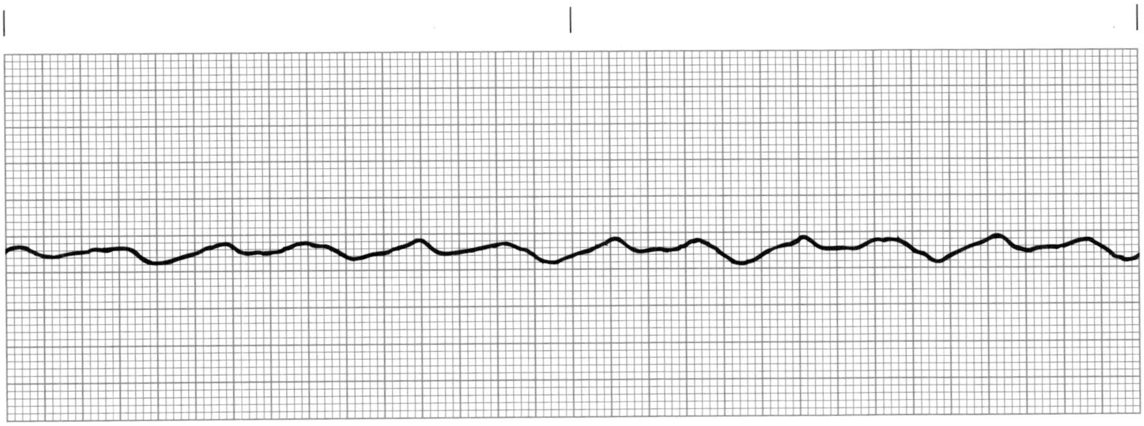

Regularity: _____	PRI: _____
Rate: _____	QRS: _____
P Waves: _____	Interp: _____

10.17

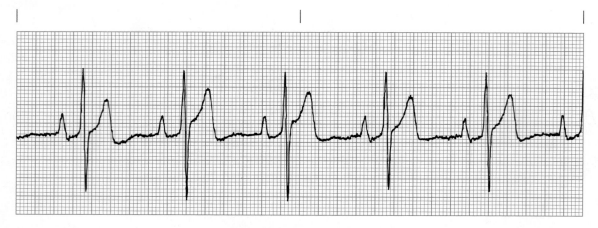

Regularity: _____	**PRI:** _____
Rate: _____	**QRS:** _____
P Waves: _____	**Interp:** _____

10.18

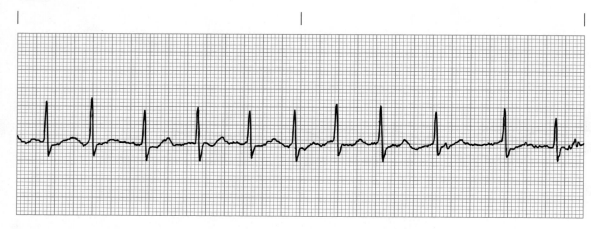

Regularity: _____	**PRI:** _____
Rate: _____	**QRS:** _____
P Waves: _____	**Interp:** _____

10.19

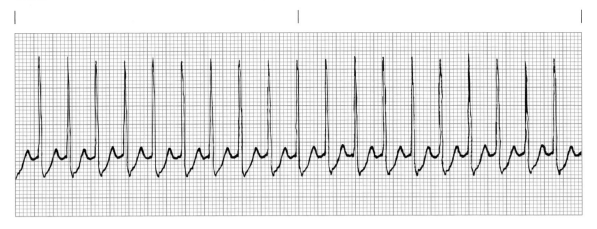

Regularity: _____	PRI: _____
Rate: _____	QRS: _____
P Waves: _____	Interp: _____

10.20

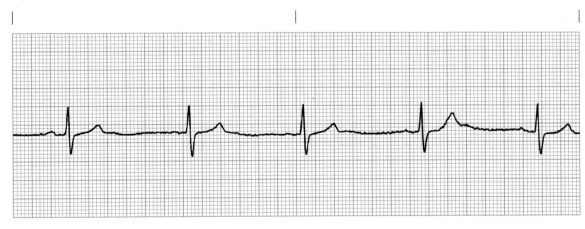

Regularity: _____	PRI: _____
Rate: _____	QRS: _____
P Waves: _____	Interp: _____

10.21

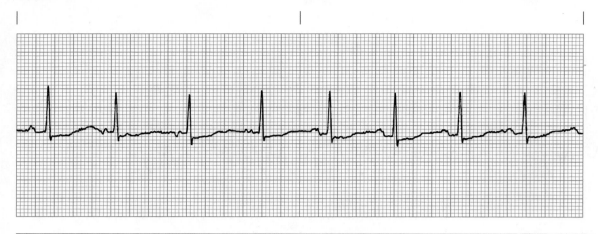

Regularity: _____	PRI: _____
Rate: _____	QRS: _____
P Waves: _____	Interp: _____

10.22

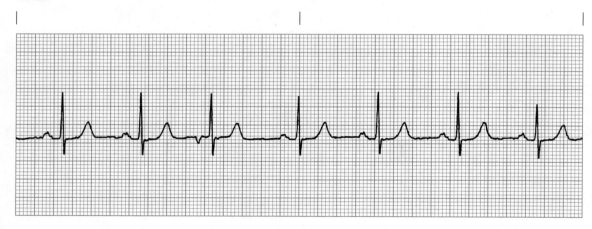

Regularity: _____	PRI: _____
Rate: _____	QRS: _____
P Waves: _____	Interp: _____

10.23

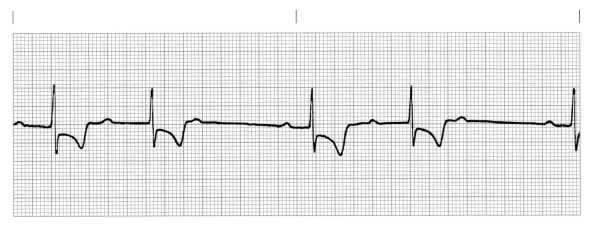

Regularity:	PRI:
Rate:	QRS:
P Waves:	Interp:

10.24

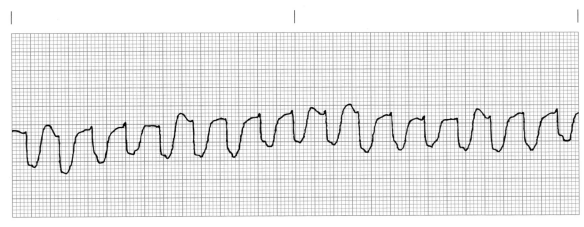

Regularity:	PRI:
Rate:	QRS:
P Waves:	Interp:

10.25

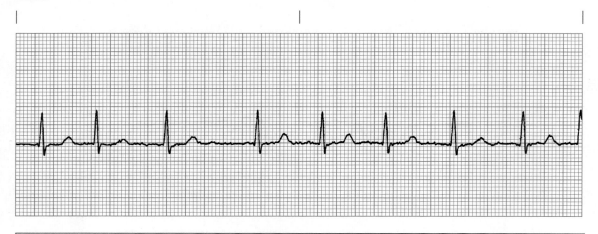

Regularity: _____ PRI: _____

Rate: _____ QRS: _____

P Waves: _____ Interp: _____

10.26

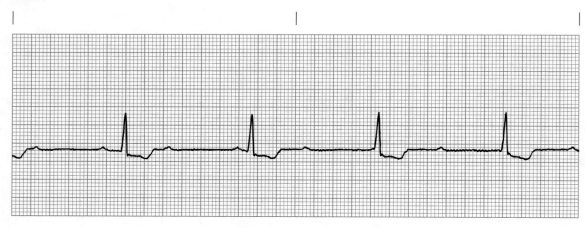

Regularity: _____ PRI: _____

Rate: _____ QRS: _____

P Waves: _____ Interp: _____

10.27

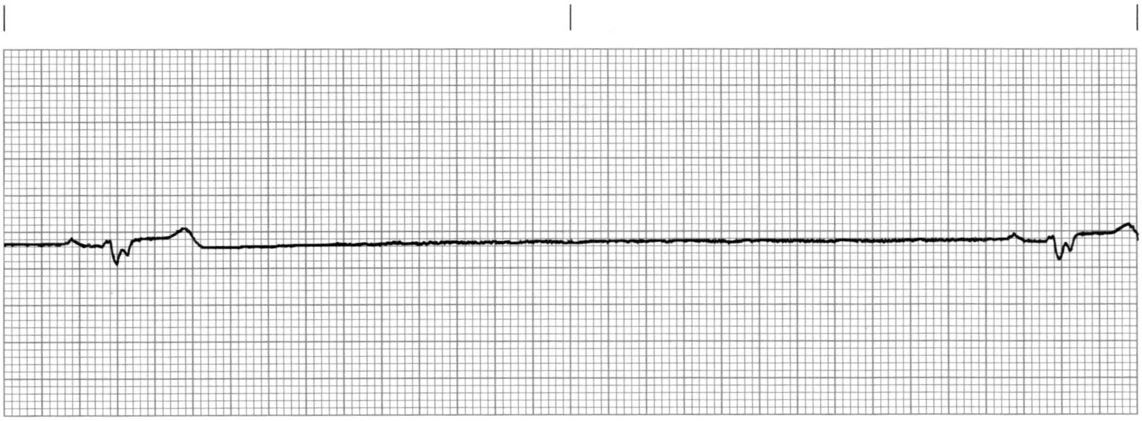

Regularity: _____	PRI: _____
Rate: _____	QRS: _____
P Waves: _____	Interp: _____

10.28

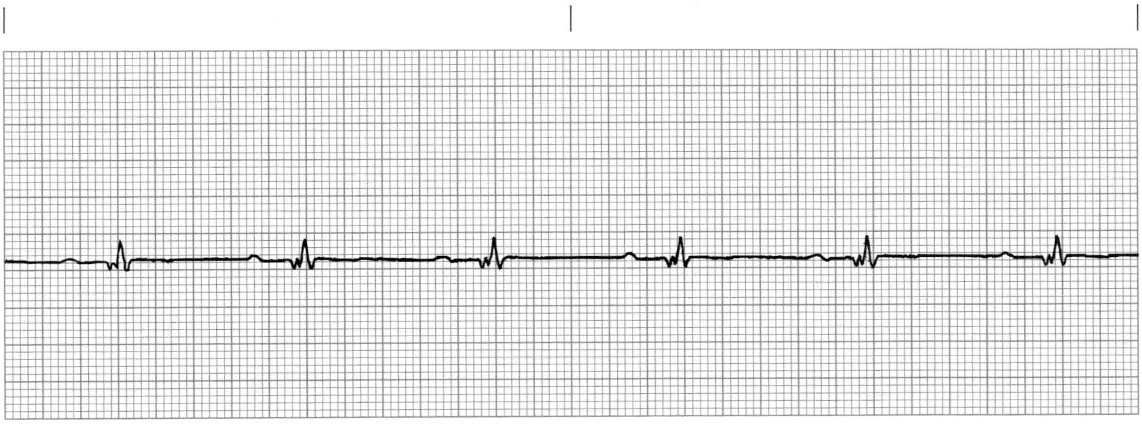

Regularity: _____	PRI: _____
Rate: _____	QRS: _____
P Waves: _____	Interp: _____

10.29

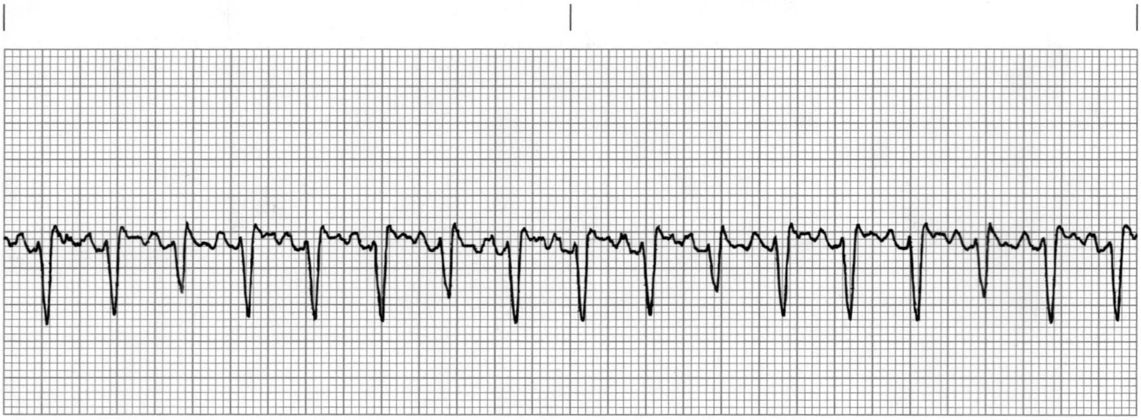

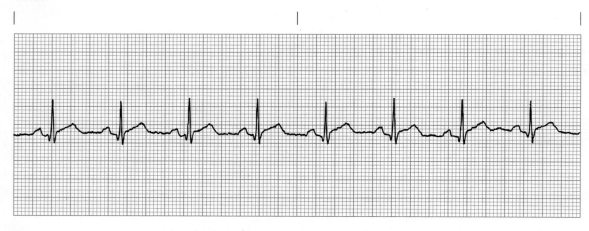

Regularity: _____   PRI: _____

Rate: _____   QRS: _____

P Waves: _____   Interp: _____

10.30

Regularity: _____   PRI: _____

Rate: _____   QRS: _____

P Waves: _____   Interp: _____

10.31

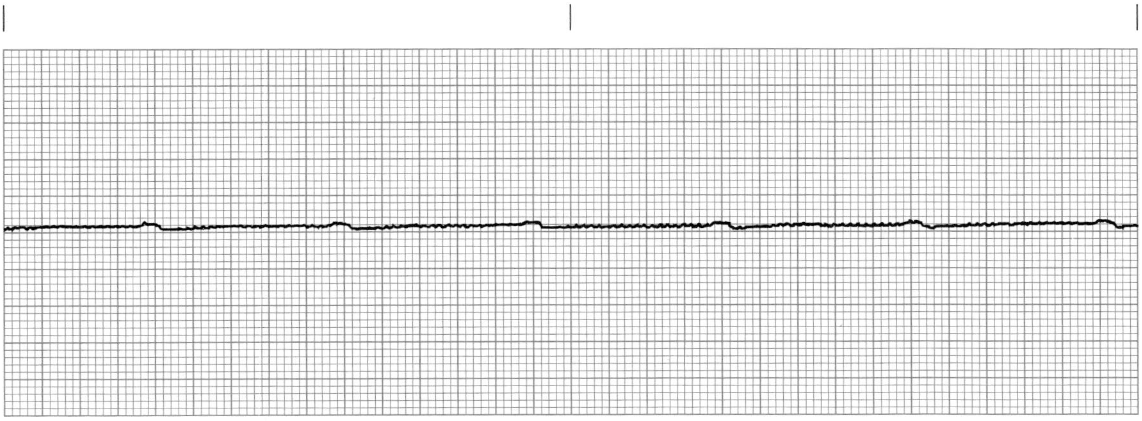

Regularity: _____	PRI: _____
Rate: _____	QRS: _____
P Waves: _____	Interp: _____

10.32

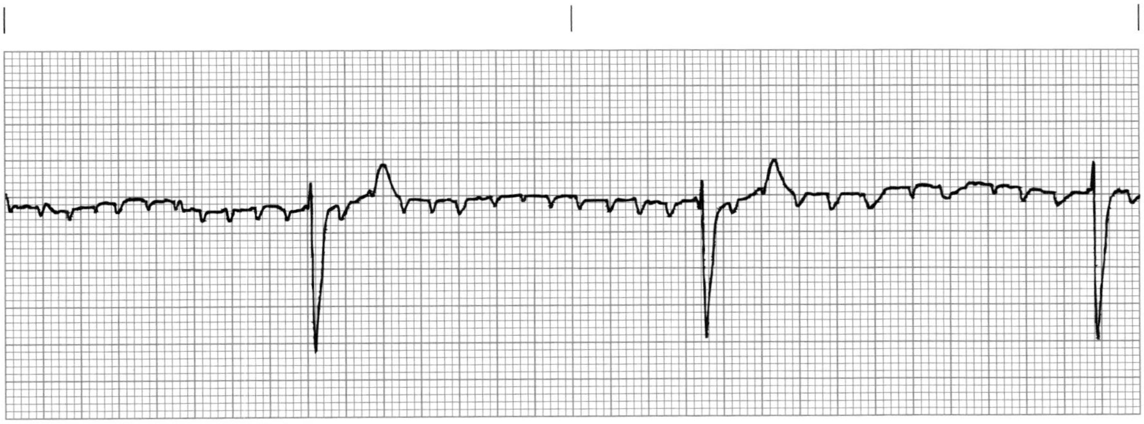

Regularity: _____	PRI: _____
Rate: _____	QRS: _____
P Waves: _____	Interp: _____

10.33

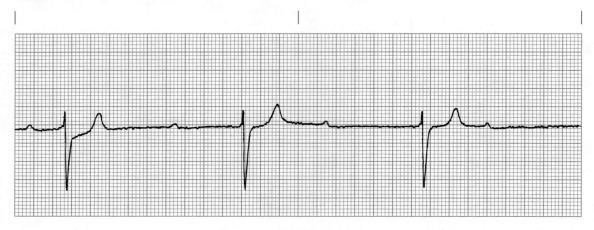

Regularity: _____   PRI: _____

Rate: _____   QRS: _____

P Waves: _____   Interp: _____

10.34

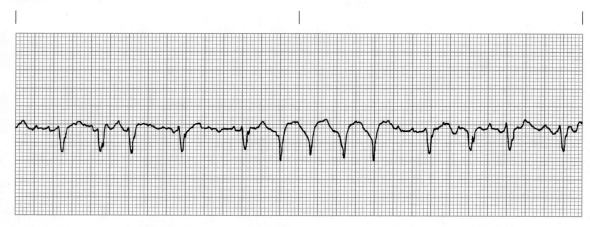

Regularity: _____   PRI: _____

Rate: _____   QRS: _____

P Waves: _____   Interp: _____

10.35

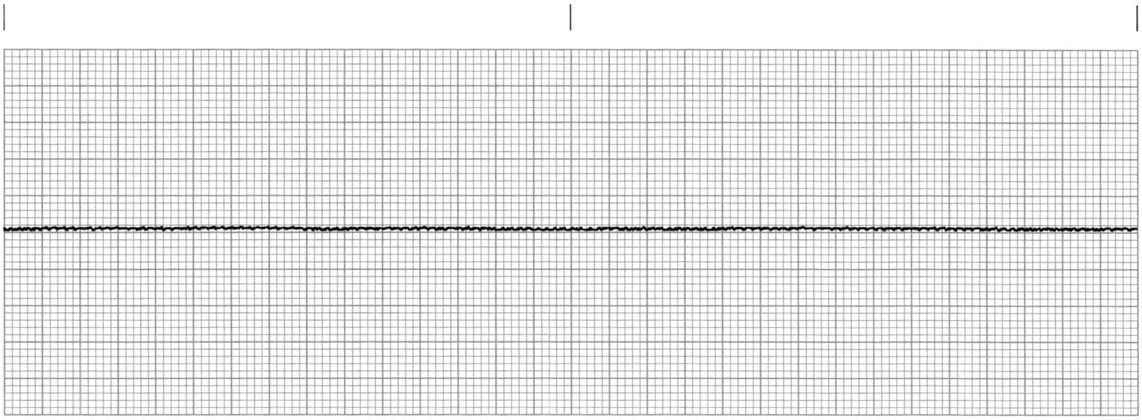

Regularity: _____	PRI: _____
Rate: _____	QRS: _____
P Waves: _____	Interp: _____

10.36

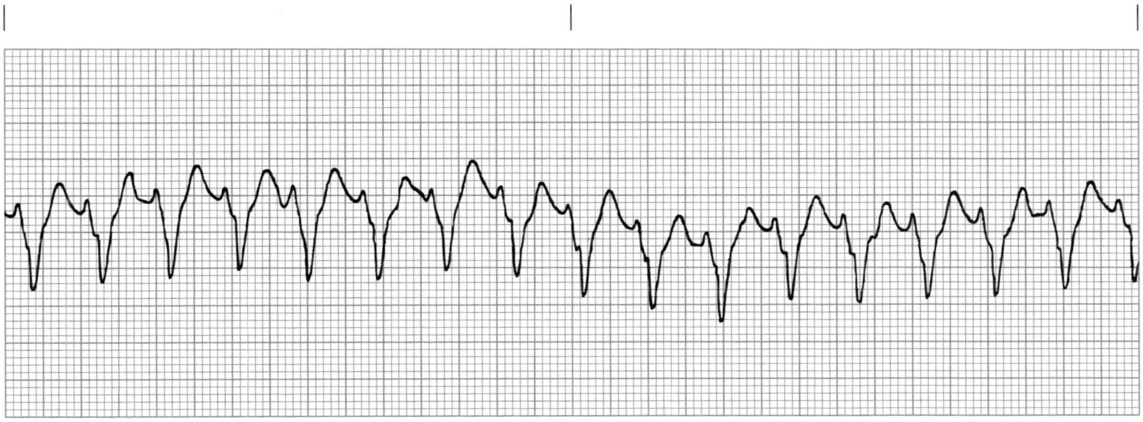

Regularity: _____	PRI: _____
Rate: _____	QRS: _____
P Waves: _____	Interp: _____

10.37

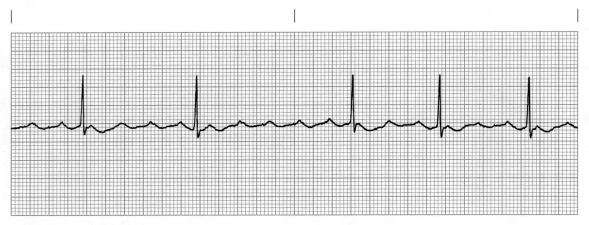

Regularity: _____	PRI: _____
Rate: _____	QRS: _____
P Waves: _____	Interp: _____

10.38

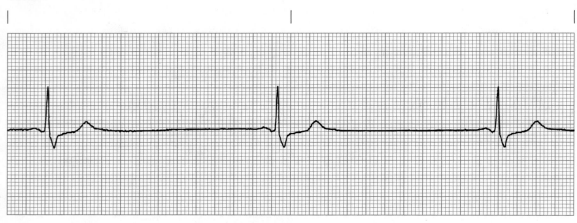

Regularity: _____	PRI: _____
Rate: _____	QRS: _____
P Waves: _____	Interp: _____

10.39

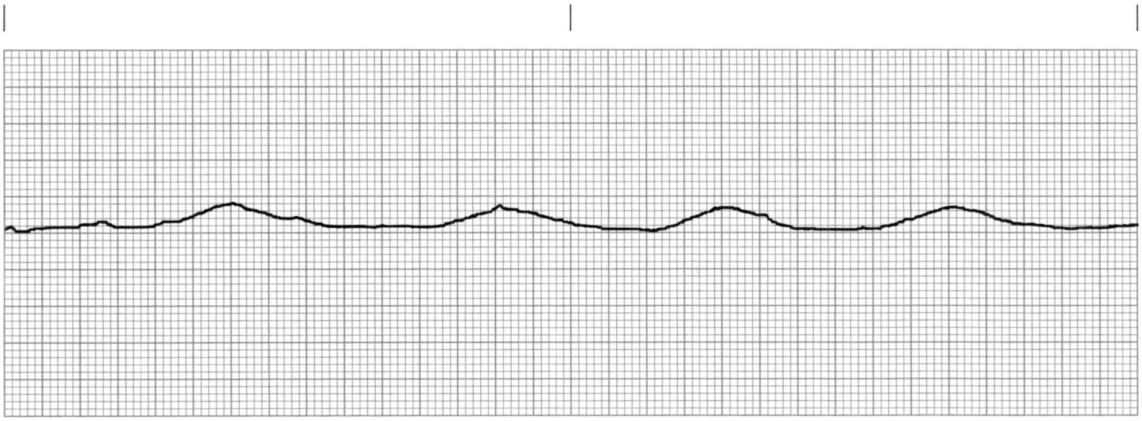

Regularity: _____	PRI: _____
Rate: _____	QRS: _____
P Waves: _____	Interp: _____

10.40

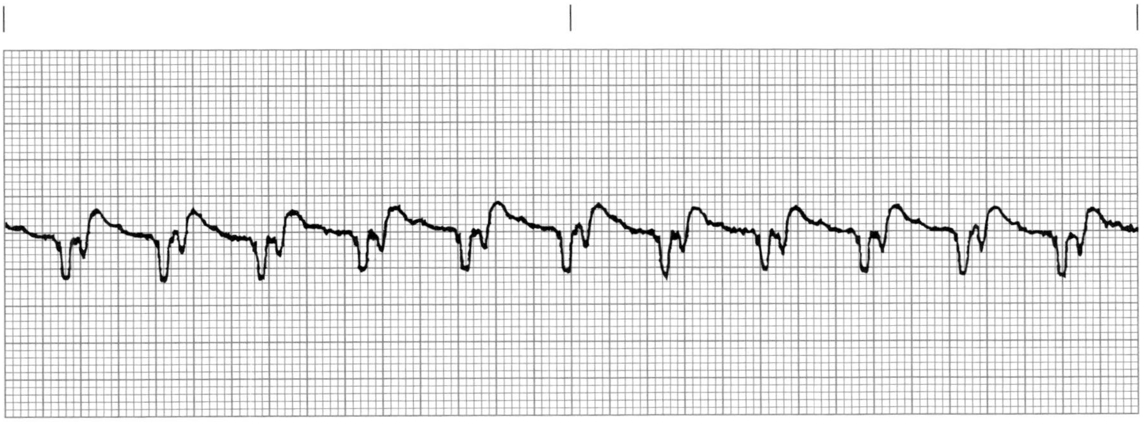

Regularity: _____	PRI: _____
Rate: _____	QRS: _____
P Waves: _____	Interp: _____

10.41

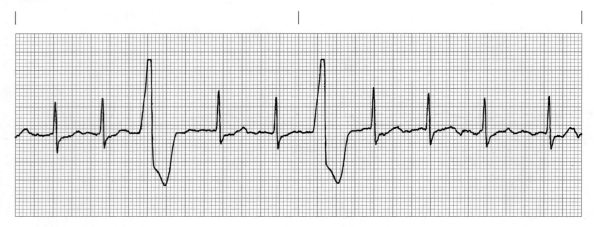

Regularity: _____	**PRI:** _____
Rate: _____	**QRS:** _____
P Waves: _____	**Interp:** _____

10.42

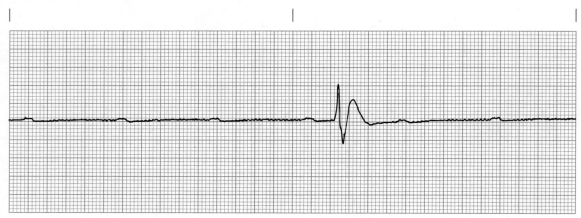

Regularity: _____	**PRI:** _____
Rate: _____	**QRS:** _____
P Waves: _____	**Interp:** _____

10.43

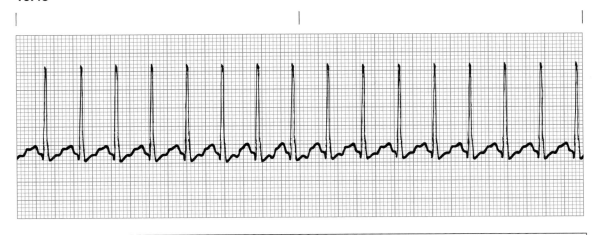

Regularity: _____	PRI: _____
Rate: _____	QRS: _____
P Waves: _____	Interp: _____

10.44

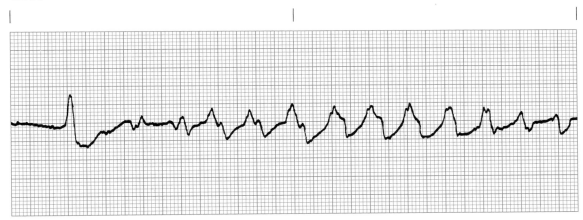

Regularity: _____	PRI: _____
Rate: _____	QRS: _____
P Waves: _____	Interp: _____

10.45

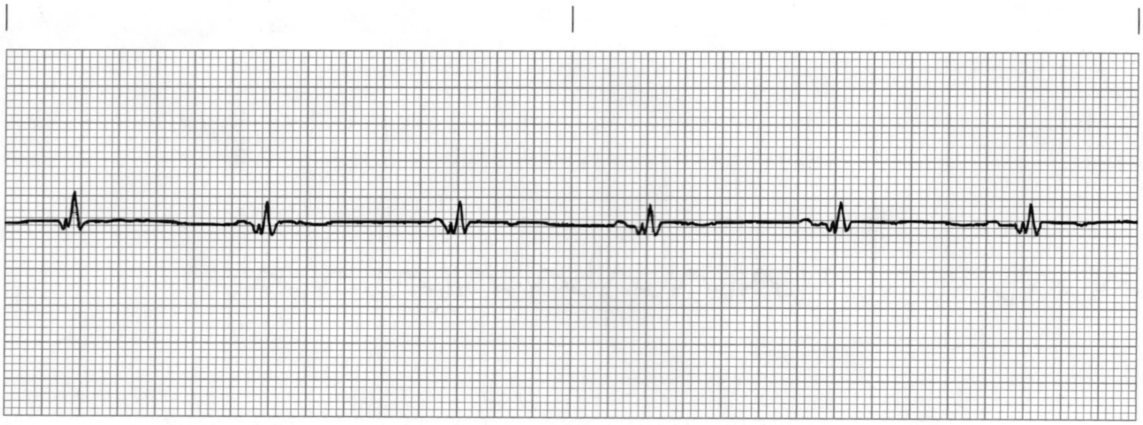

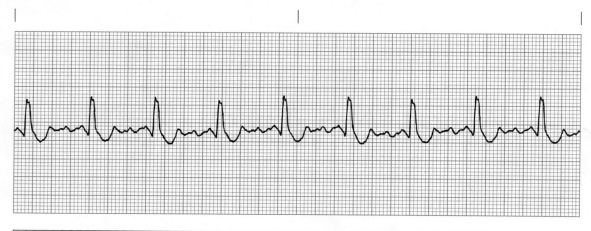

Regularity: _____	PRI: _____
Rate: _____	QRS: _____
P Waves: _____	Interp: _____

10.46

Regularity: _____	PRI: _____
Rate: _____	QRS: _____
P Waves: _____	Interp: _____

10.47

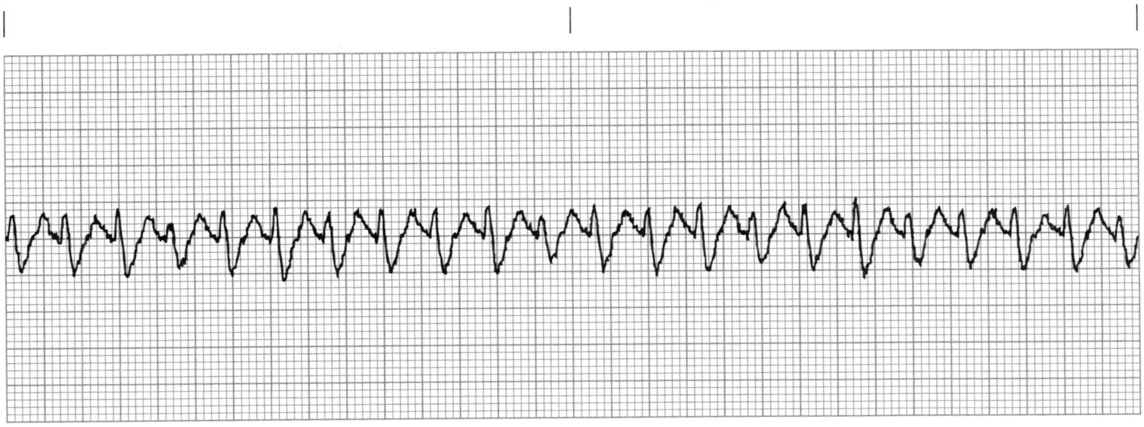

Regularity: _____	**PRI:** _____
Rate: _____	**QRS:** _____
P Waves: _____	**Interp:** _____

10.48

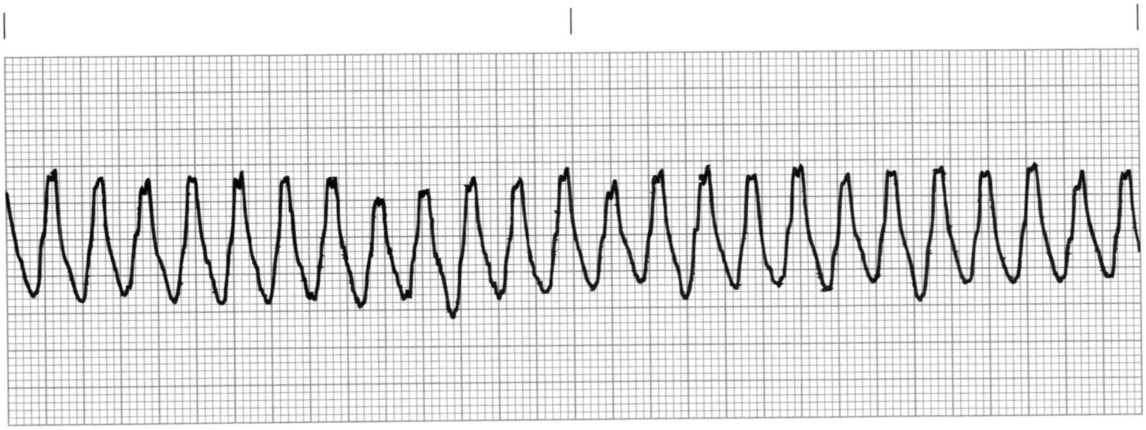

Regularity: _____	**PRI:** _____
Rate: _____	**QRS:** _____
P Waves: _____	**Interp:** _____

10.49

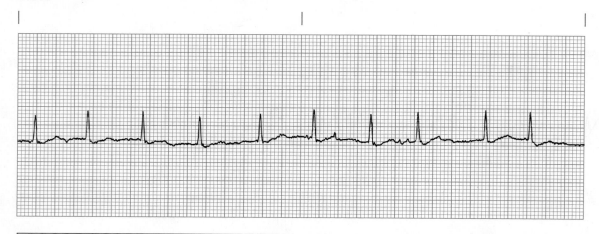

Regularity: _____	PRI: _____
Rate: _____	QRS: _____
P Waves: _____	Interp: _____

10.50

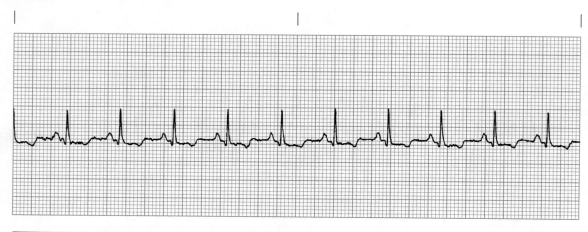

Regularity: _____	PRI: _____
Rate: _____	QRS: _____
P Waves: _____	Interp: _____

10.51

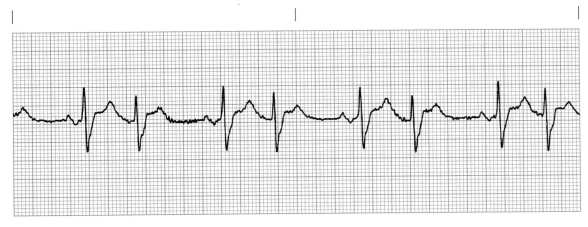

Regularity: _____	PRI: _____
Rate: _____	QRS: _____
P Waves: _____	Interp: _____

10.52

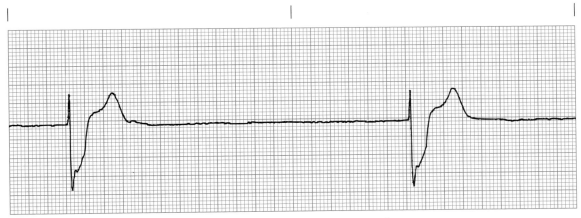

Regularity: _____	PRI: _____
Rate: _____	QRS: _____
P Waves: _____	Interp: _____

10.53

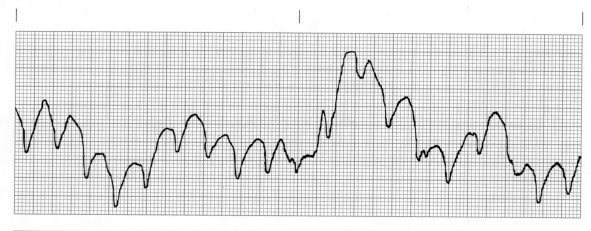

Regularity: _____	PRI: _____
Rate: _____	QRS: _____
P Waves: _____	Interp: _____

10.54

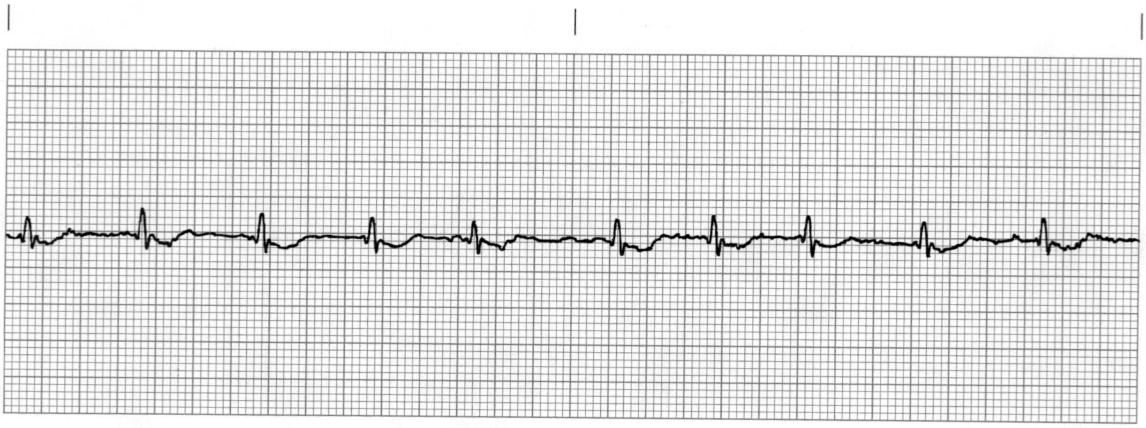

Regularity: _____	PRI: _____
Rate: _____	QRS: _____
P Waves: _____	Interp: _____

10.55

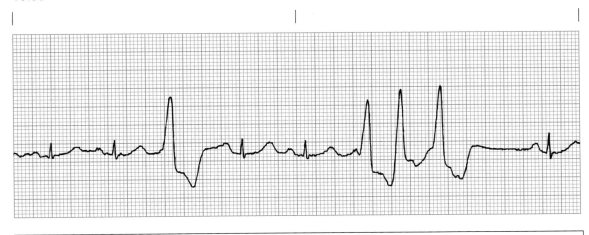

> Regularity: _____   PRI: _____
>
> Rate: _____   QRS: _____
>
> P Waves: _____   Interp: _____

10.56

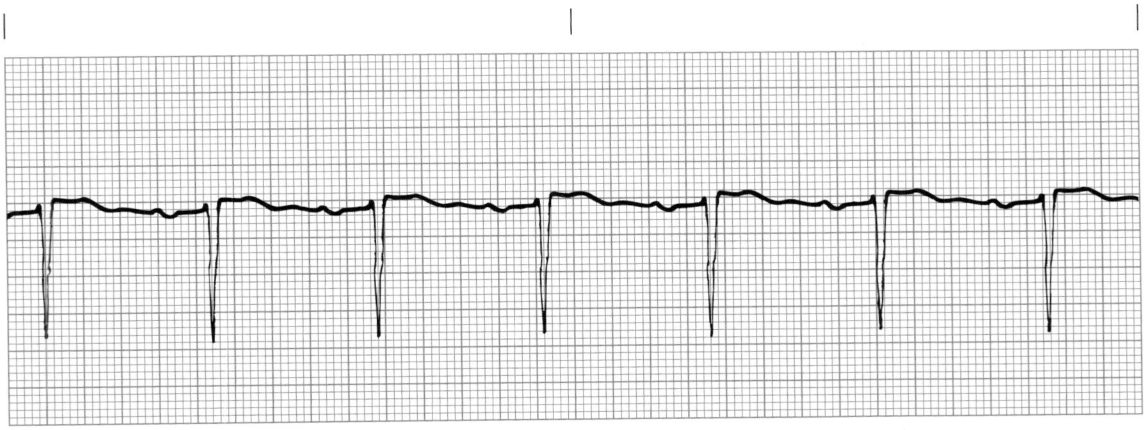

> Regularity: _____   PRI: _____
>
> Rate: _____   QRS: _____
>
> P Waves: _____   Interp: _____

10.57

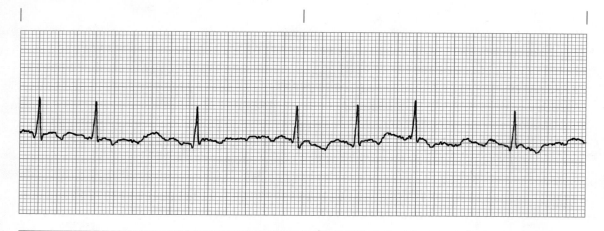

Regularity: _____   PRI: _____

Rate: _____   QRS: _____

P Waves: _____   Interp: _____

10.58

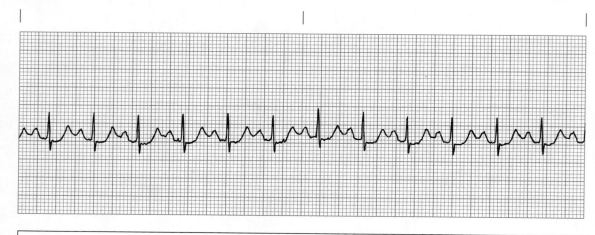

Regularity: _____   PRI: _____

Rate: _____   QRS: _____

P Waves: _____   Interp: _____

10.59

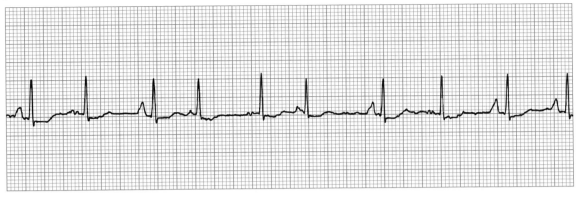

Regularity: _____	**PRI:** _____
Rate: _____	**QRS:** _____
P Waves: _____	**Interp:** _____

10.60

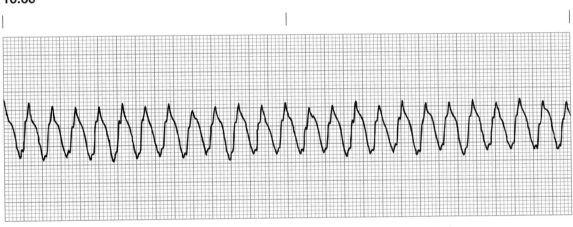

Regularity: _____	**PRI:** _____
Rate: _____	**QRS:** _____
P Waves: _____	**Interp:** _____

10.61

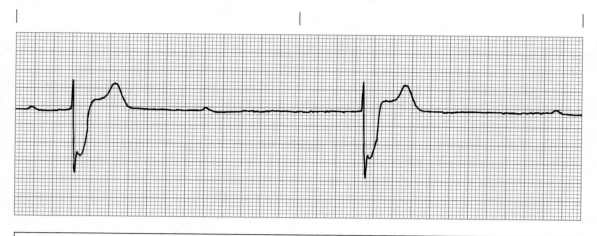

Regularity: _____ PRI: _____

Rate: _____ QRS: _____

P Waves: _____ Interp: _____

10.62

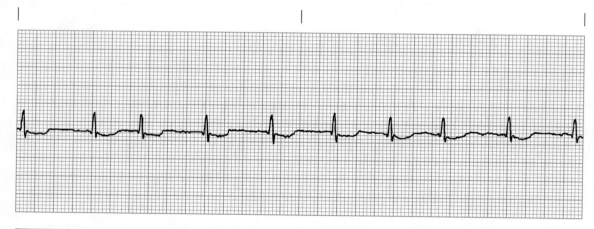

Regularity: _____ PRI: _____

Rate: _____ QRS: _____

P Waves: _____ Interp: _____

10.63

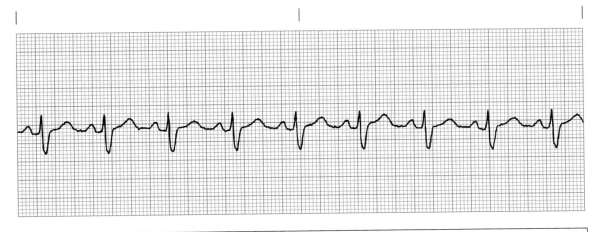

Regularity: _____	PRI: _____
Rate: _____	QRS: _____
P Waves: _____	Interp: _____

10.64

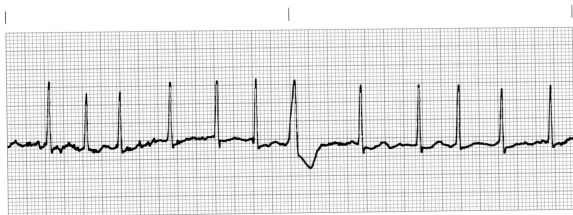

Regularity: _____	PRI: _____
Rate: _____	QRS: _____
P Waves: _____	Interp: _____

10.65

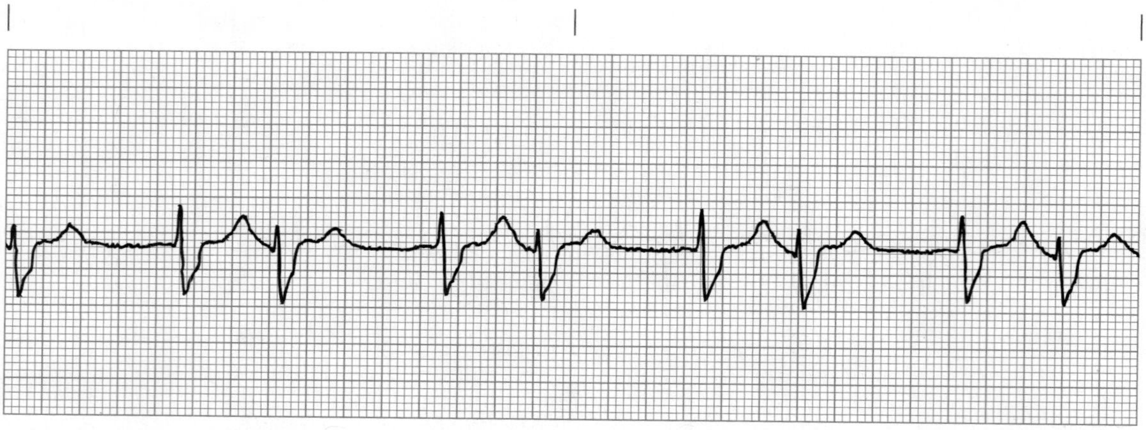

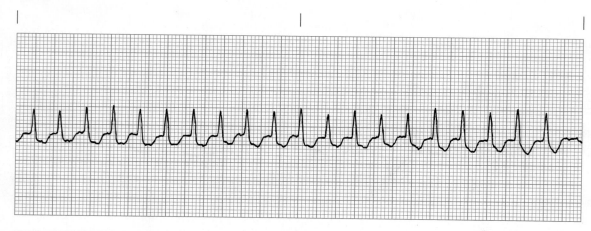

Regularity: _____	PRI: _____
Rate: _____	QRS: _____
P Waves: _____	Interp: _____

10.66

Regularity: _____	PRI: _____
Rate: _____	QRS: _____
P Waves: _____	Interp: _____

10.67

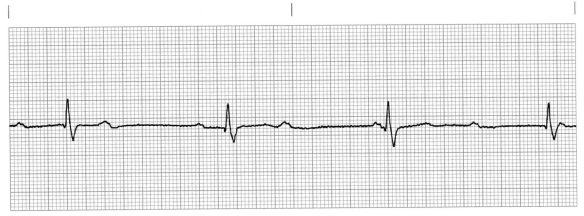

Regularity: _____	PRI: _____
Rate: _____	QRS: _____
P Waves: _____	Interp: _____

10.68

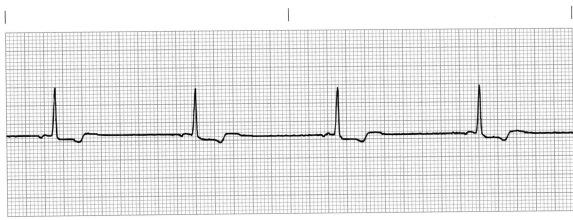

Regularity: _____	PRI: _____
Rate: _____	QRS: _____
P Waves: _____	Interp: _____

10.69

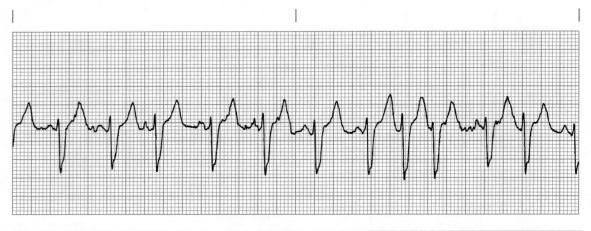

Regularity: _____	**PRI:** _____
Rate: _____	**QRS:** _____
P Waves: _____	**Interp:** _____

10.70

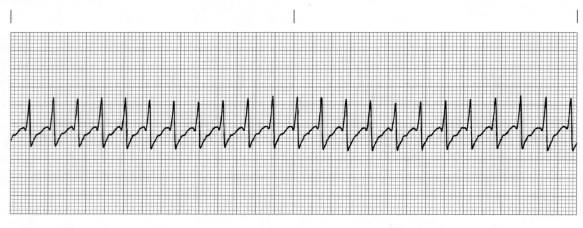

Regularity: _____	**PRI:** _____
Rate: _____	**QRS:** _____
P Waves: _____	**Interp:** _____

10.71

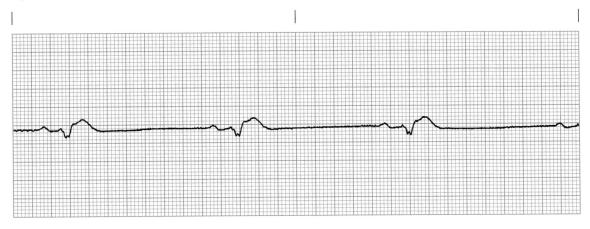

Regularity: _____	PRI: _____
Rate: _____	QRS: _____
P Waves: _____	Interp: _____

10.72

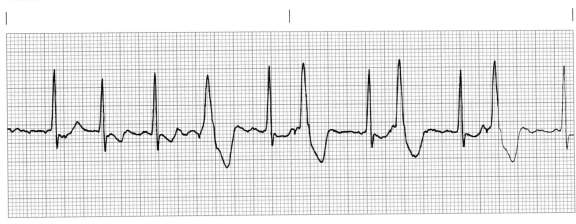

Regularity: _____	PRI: _____
Rate: _____	QRS: _____
P Waves: _____	Interp: _____

10.73

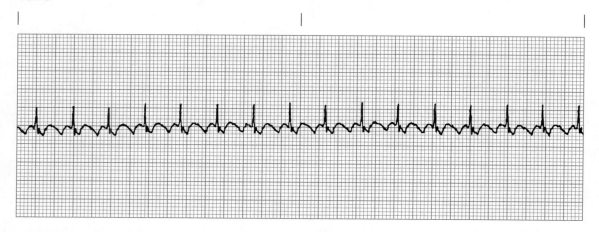

Regularity: _____		PRI: _____	
Rate: _____		QRS: _____	
P Waves: _____		Interp: _____	

10.74

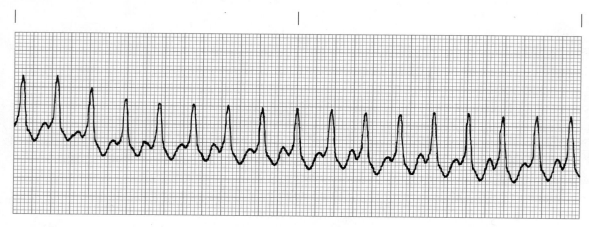

Regularity: _____		PRI: _____	
Rate: _____		QRS: _____	
P Waves: _____		Interp: _____	

10.75

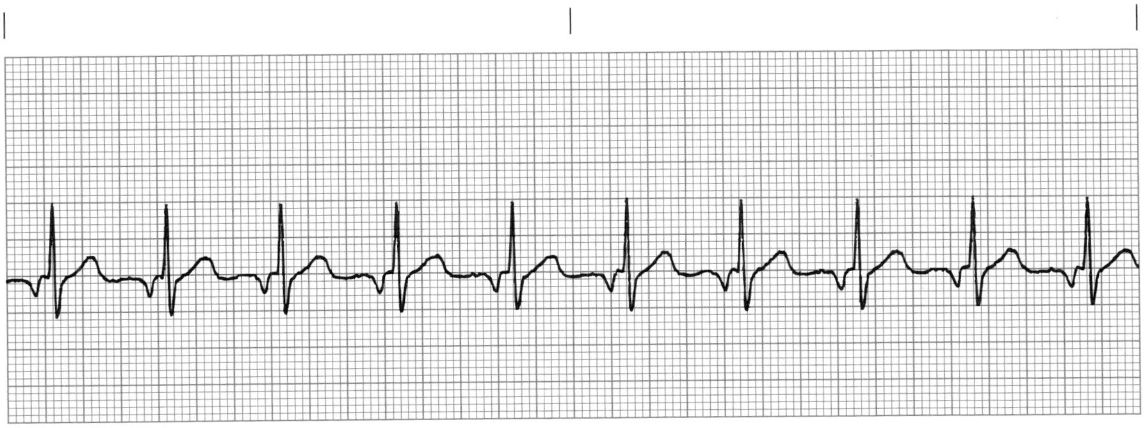

Regularity: _____	PRI: _____
Rate: _____	QRS: _____
P Waves: _____	Interp: _____

10.76

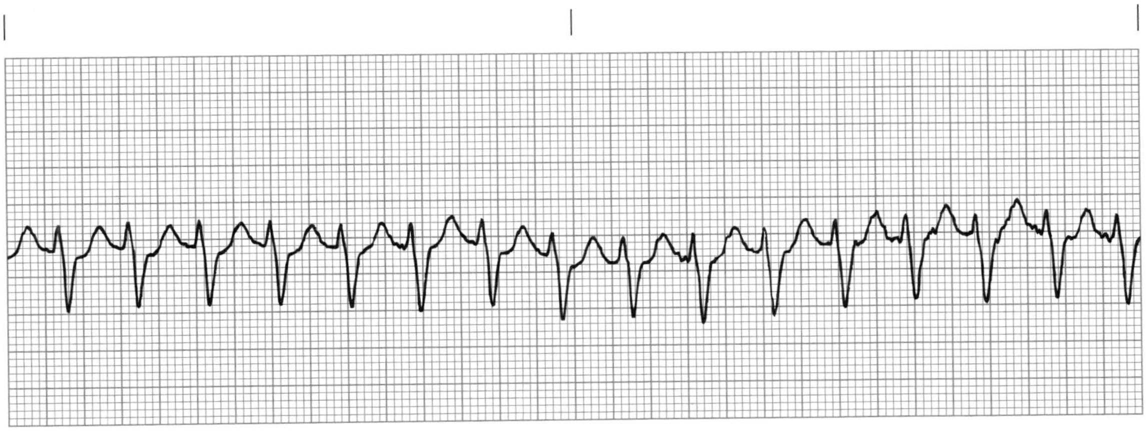

Regularity: _____	PRI: _____
Rate: _____	QRS: _____
P Waves: _____	Interp: _____

10.77

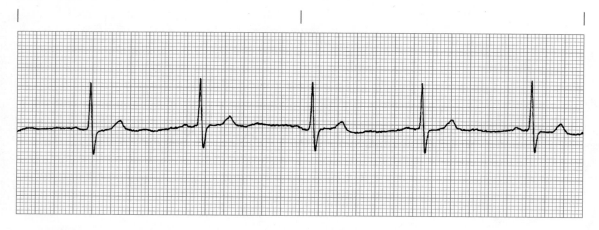

Regularity: _____	PRI: _____
Rate: _____	QRS: _____
P Waves: _____	Interp: _____

10.78

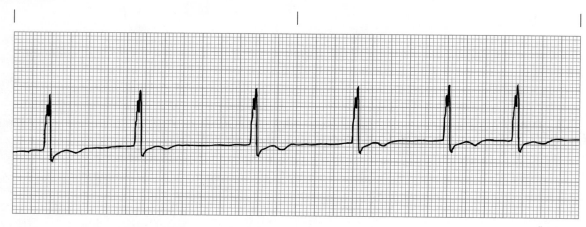

Regularity: _____	PRI: _____
Rate: _____	QRS: _____
P Waves: _____	Interp: _____

10.79

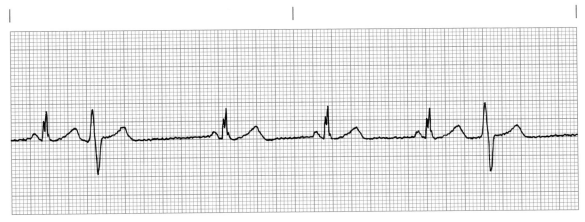

Regularity: _____	**PRI:** _____	
Rate: _____	**QRS:** _____	
P Waves: _____	**Interp:** _____	

10.80

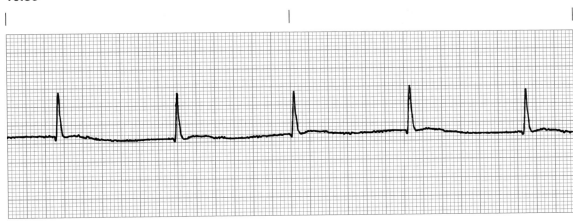

Regularity: _____	**PRI:** _____	
Rate: _____	**QRS:** _____	
P Waves: _____	**Interp:** _____	

10.81

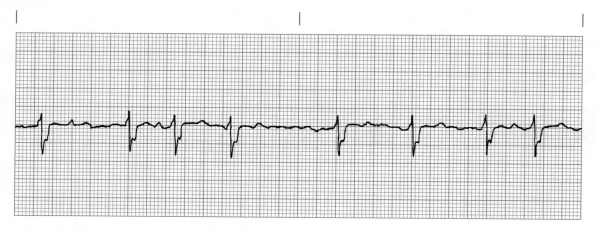

Regularity: _____	PRI: _____
Rate: _____	QRS: _____
P Waves: _____	Interp: _____

10.82

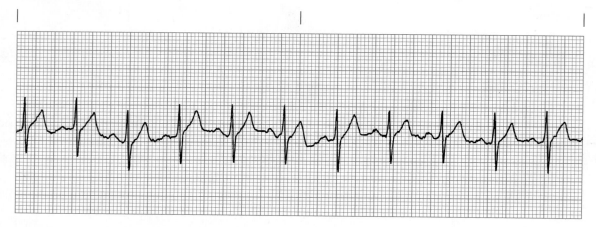

Regularity: _____	PRI: _____
Rate: _____	QRS: _____
P Waves: _____	Interp: _____

10.83

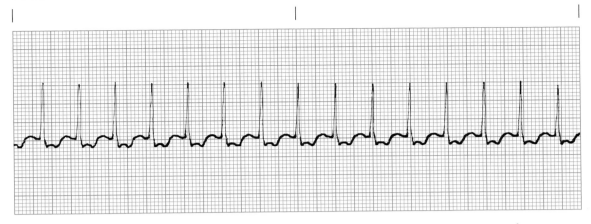

Regularity: _____	PRI: _____
Rate: _____	QRS: _____
P Waves: _____	Interp: _____

10.84

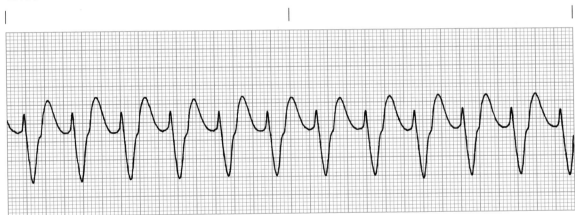

Regularity: _____	PRI: _____
Rate: _____	QRS: _____
P Waves: _____	Interp: _____

10.85

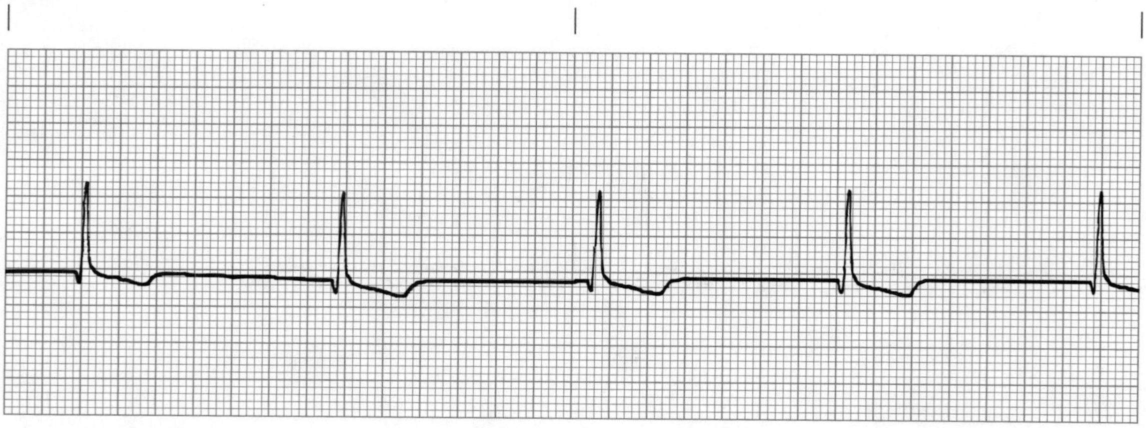

Regularity: _____   PRI: _____

Rate: _____   QRS: _____

P Waves: _____   Interp: _____

10.86

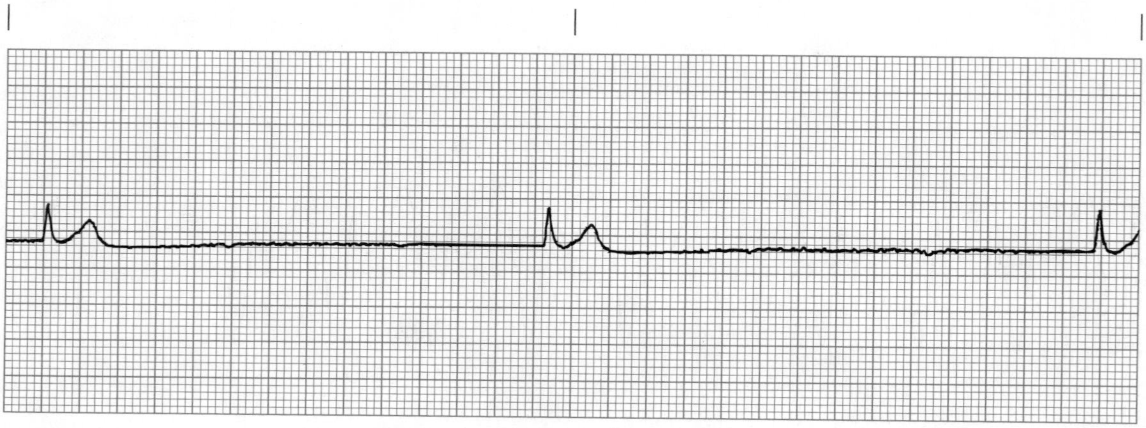

Regularity: _____   PRI: _____

Rate: _____   QRS: _____

P Waves: _____   Interp: _____

10.87

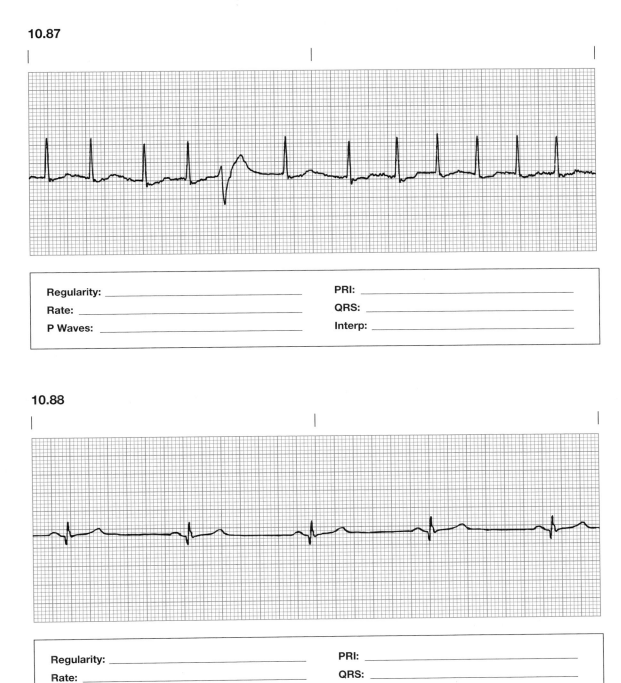

Regularity: _____	**PRI:** _____
Rate: _____	**QRS:** _____
P Waves: _____	**Interp:** _____

10.88

Regularity: _____	**PRI:** _____
Rate: _____	**QRS:** _____
P Waves: _____	**Interp:** _____

10.89

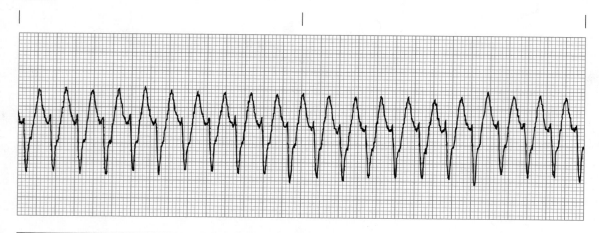

Regularity: _____   PRI: _____

Rate: _____   QRS: _____

P Waves: _____   Interp: _____

10.90

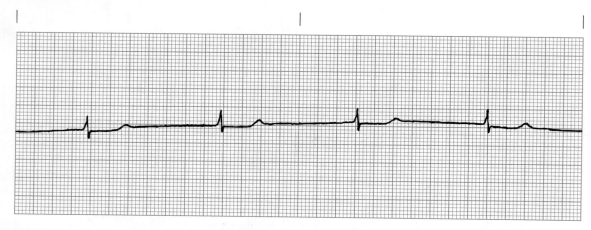

Regularity: _____   PRI: _____

Rate: _____   QRS: _____

P Waves: _____   Interp: _____

10.91

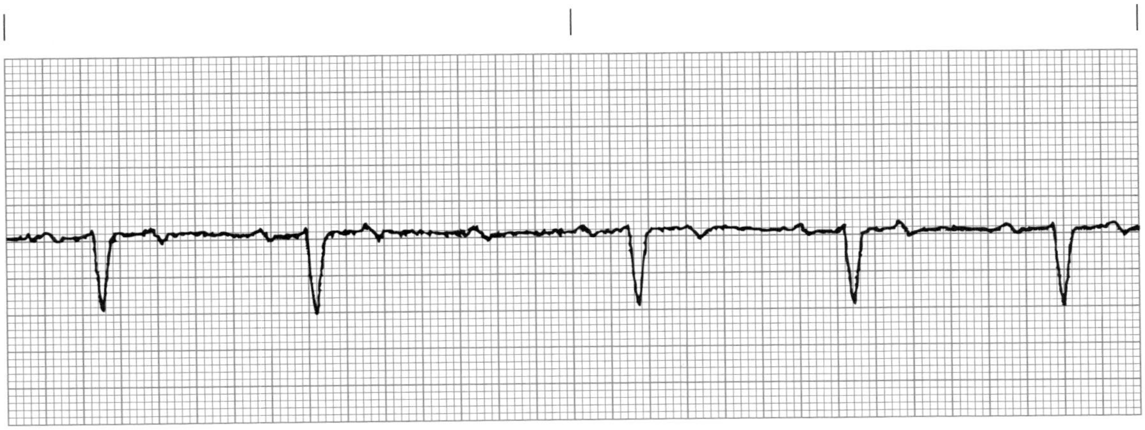

Regularity: _____   PRI: _____

Rate: _____   QRS: _____

P Waves: _____   Interp: _____

10.92

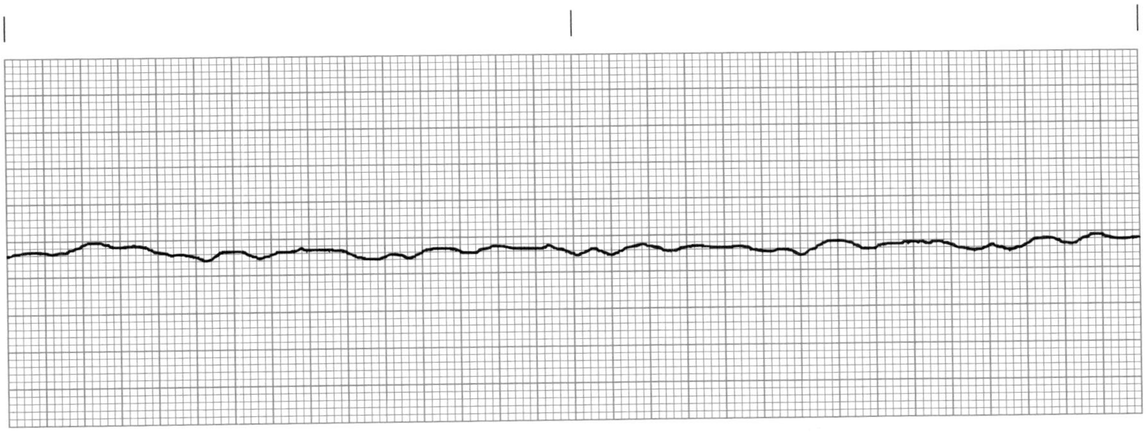

Regularity: _____   PRI: _____

Rate: _____   QRS: _____

P Waves: _____   Interp: _____

10.93

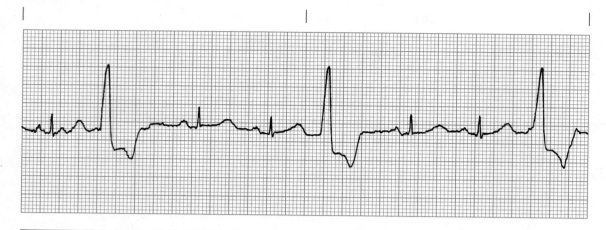

Regularity: _____	PRI: _____
Rate: _____	QRS: _____
P Waves: _____	Interp: _____

10.94

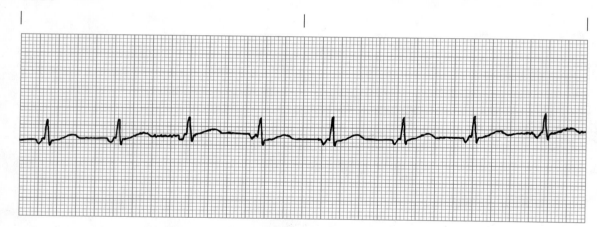

Regularity: _____	PRI: _____
Rate: _____	QRS: _____
P Waves: _____	Interp: _____

10.95

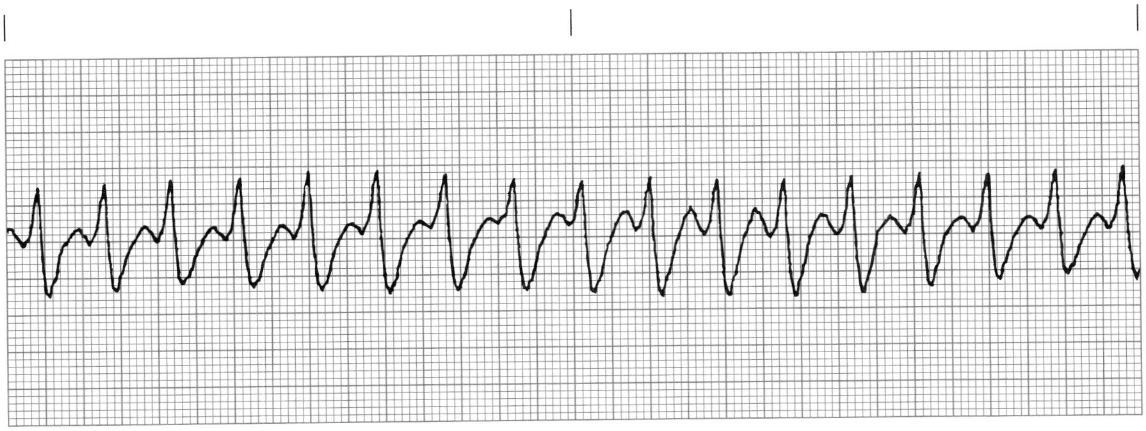

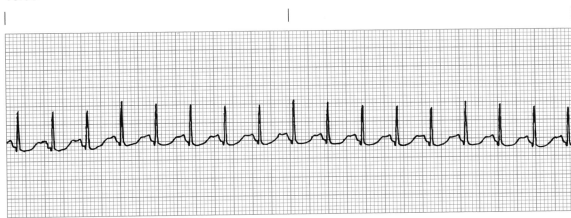

Regularity: _____	PRI: _____
Rate: _____	QRS: _____
P Waves: _____	Interp: _____

10.96

Regularity: _____	PRI: _____
Rate: _____	QRS: _____
P Waves: _____	Interp: _____

10.97

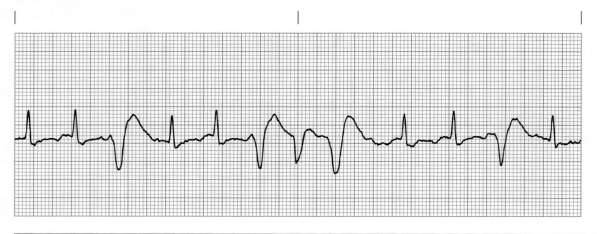

Regularity: _____	PRI: _____
Rate: _____	QRS: _____
P Waves: _____	Interp: _____

10.98

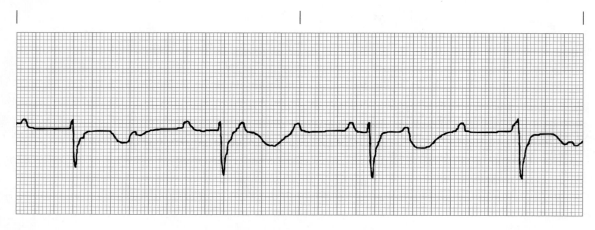

Regularity: _____	PRI: _____
Rate: _____	QRS: _____
P Waves: _____	Interp: _____

10.99

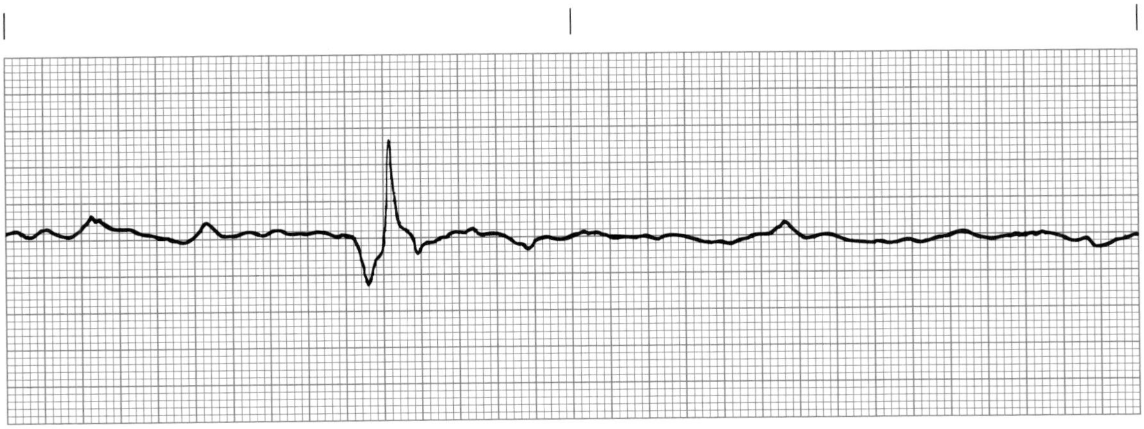

Regularity: _____   PRI: _____

Rate: _____   QRS: _____

P Waves: _____   Interp: _____

10.100

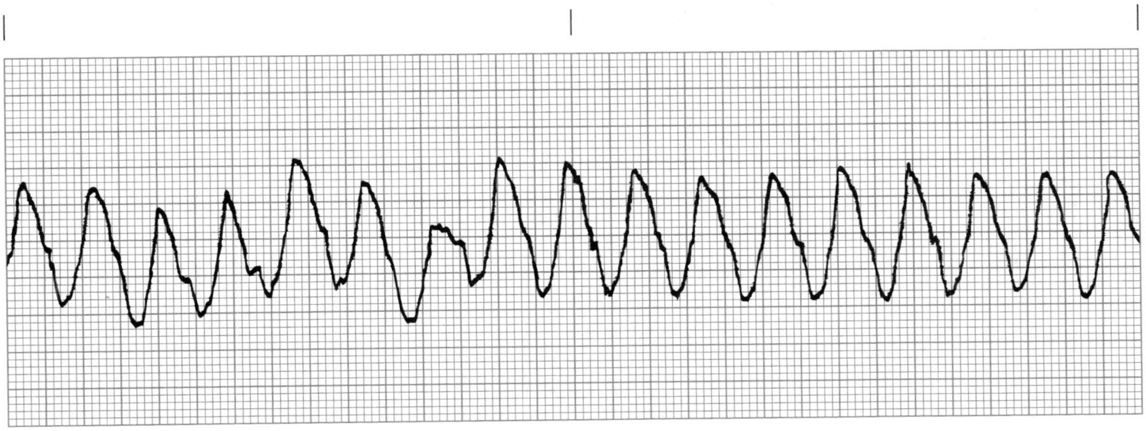

Regularity: _____   PRI: _____

Rate: _____   QRS: _____

P Waves: _____   Interp: _____

Appendix A
Cardiac Anatomy and Physiology

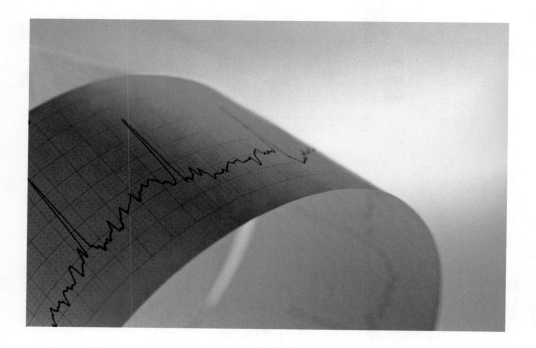

Overview

IN THIS APPENDIX, you will learn about the structure and function of the heart. You will learn about its chambers, valves, walls, surfaces, and surrounding pericardial sac. You will find out how the heart contracts in response to electrical stimulation, and you will learn about the stages of contraction: systole and diastole. You will also learn about the blood vessels that supply the heart itself: the coronary arteries, cardiac veins, and coronary sinus.

The cardiovascular system serves to carry oxygen from the lungs to tissues throughout the body. In a never-ending cycle, blood circles throughout the body, taking oxygen from the lungs to the tissues, then taking carbon dioxide from the tissues back to the lungs to exchange for new oxygen.

The heart's role in this process is to keep the blood circulating. To accomplish this task, it has two separate but interrelated systems: a mechanical mechanism that actually pumps the blood and an electrical system that tells the

mechanical system how and when to pump. This appendix outlines the heart's mechanical system, while the body of the book is devoted to cardiac electrical function.

Location and Structure

The heart is a hollow, muscular, cone-shaped organ, roughly the size of a fist. It is located in the chest, behind the sternum and between the lungs. Just above it are the great vessels

Figure A1 Location of the Heart

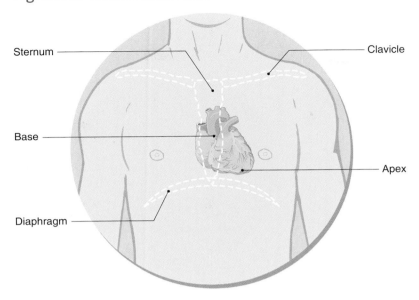

(aorta and superior vena cava), and below it is the diaphragm (Figure A1).

The heart sits slightly off center, with 2/3 of its mass lying to the left of the middle. It's also tilted slightly. The upper end (called the **base**) is pointed upward and to the right, while the lower point (called the **apex**) slants downward and to the left. The apex moves toward the anterior chest wall during contraction, allowing its beats to be felt just below the left nipple.

Internal Chambers

The heart consists of four hollow chambers: the two upper chambers are called **atria**, and the two lower chambers are the **ventricles**. The walls of the ventricles are much thicker than those of the atria, because the lower chambers have to pump blood much farther than do the atria.

Between the two upper chambers is a thin wall called the **interatrial septum**. A thicker, more muscular **interventricular septum** sits between the two lower chambers (Figure A2).

Heart Walls

All the walls of the heart consist of three layers (Figure A3):

Endocardium: contains the branches of the heart's electrical conduction system

Myocardium: made up of layers and bands of cardiac muscle fibers that are wound in complex spirals around the atria and ventricles

Figure A2 Internal Anatomy of the Heart

MyBRADYLab™

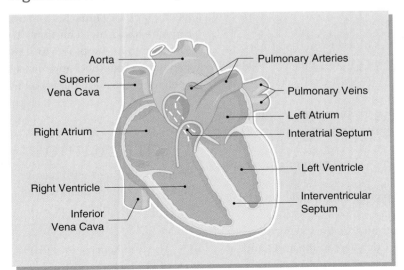

Figure A3 Walls of the Heart

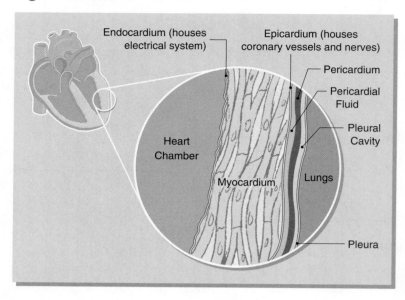

Epicardium: single layer of cells supported by connective tissues; contains nerves to the heart and coronary blood vessels

The entire cardiac structure (the heart and the beginnings of the great vessels) is housed in a fibroserous sac called the **pericardial sac**. Under normal conditions, the sac fits snugly around the heart, leaving space only for about 50 mL of lubricating fluid.

Blood Flow

The septum effectively divides the heart into right and left sides to form two separate pumps. The right side pumps blood through the lungs, and the left side maintains circulation through the body (Figure A4). The walls of the left ventricle are three times thicker than those of the right side because it takes more pressure to reach distal parts of the body.

The two pumps of the right and left heart function in close syncopation. This is a closed system, so the blood continues interminably in a cycle:

- The right atrium receives blood from distal parts of the body by way of the superior or inferior vena cava.
- Blood passes through the tricuspid valve to the right ventricle.
- The right ventricle pumps the blood out the pulmonic valve to the pulmonary artery and on to the lungs for a new supply of oxygen.
- Oxygenated blood returns via the pulmonary vein to the left atrium.
- From the left atrium, it passes through the mitral valve and into the left ventricle.
- When the left ventricle contracts, the oxygenated blood is ejected through the aortic valve to the aorta and distal body tissues.

MyBRADYLab™

Heart Valves

To keep all the blood flowing in the same direction, the heart has two sets of one-way valves. The first two, called the atrioventricular valves, are located at each of the two openings between the atria and the ventricles. The **tricuspid** valve lies between the right atrium and right ventricle, and the **mitral** (also called *bicuspid*) valve separates the left atria and left ventricle. The second pair is called the semilunar valves. One is located at each of the two exits leading from the ventricles into the great vessels. The **pulmonic** valve is at the exit from the right ventricle to the pulmonary artery, and the **aortic** valve is at the exit from the left ventricle to the aorta (Figure A5).

All of the valves consist of leaflets that open and close in response to changing pressures within the chambers. Structures called **chordate tendineae** connect the valve leaflets to **papillary muscles** that open and close the valves and prevent backflow. The two atrioventricular valves open together to allow blood to flow into the ventricles. Then they close together, and the aortic and pulmonic valves open together, allowing blood to pass out of the heart.

Heart Sounds

Sounds associated with blood flow through heart chambers and the closing of heart valves can be heard with the aid of a stethoscope placed against the chest wall. The normal heart has four distinct sound components.

1. The first heart sound (S_1) is associated with the closure of the mitral and tricuspid valves and corresponds to

Figure A4 Flow of Blood through the Body

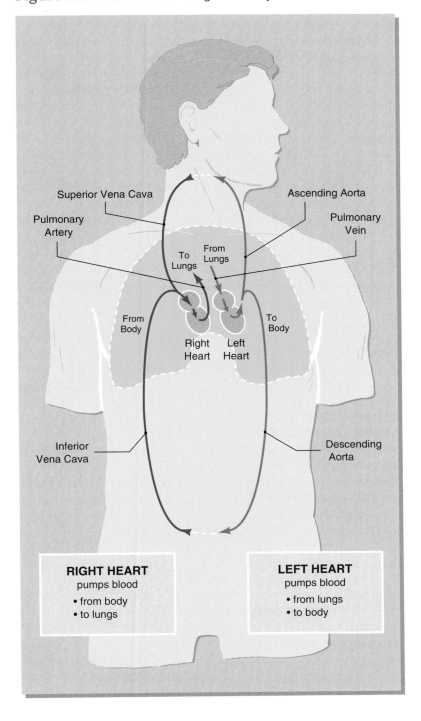

the onset of ventricular systole. Since mitral closure precedes tricuspid closure by a split second, S_1 has two separate components, but these are generally not audible.

2. The second heart sound (S_2) is associated with the closure of the aortic and pulmonic valves. S_2 also has two components: the first is closure of the aortic valve, and

the second is the pulmonic. The first and second heart sounds are normal findings.

3. The third heart sound (S_3) is a sign of pathology in an adult. It occurs early in ventricular diastole, during the phase of rapid ventricular filling.

4. The fourth heart sound (S_4) is related to atrial contraction that is more forceful than normal.

Figure A5 Heart Valves

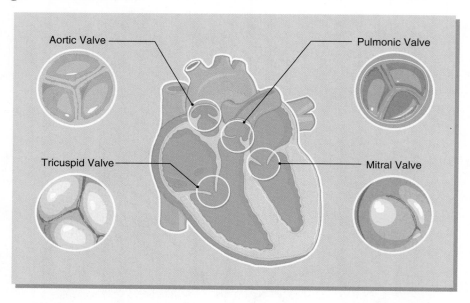

Gallop Rhythms

Gallop rhythms are so called because the heart sounds are grouped together so they sound like galloping horses. There are three distinct types of gallop rhythms: *ventricular gallop rhythm*, due to an exaggerated third heart sound; *atrial gallop rhythm*, which occurs late in diastole or just before systole; and *summation gallop rhythm*, heard when a tachycardia is so rapid that the third and fourth heart sounds are blended into one.

Murmurs

Murmurs reflect turbulence that can be caused by high flow rates, damaged valves, dilated chambers or vessels, or backward flow through a regurgitant valve. Murmurs are described by timing, intensity, quality, pitch, location, and radiation.

Systole and Diastole

In the first phase of a cardiac cycle the atria are at rest, allowing blood to pour in from the body and lungs. This phase is called **atrial diastole**. As the pressure rises, the tricuspid and mitral valves open to allow blood to pass into the relaxed ventricles. Next, the atria contract (**atrial systole**) to fill the ventricles. The period during which the ventricles are relaxed and filling is called **ventricular diastole**. As the pressures equalize, the tricuspid and mitral valves close and the aortic and pulmonic valves open. The ventricles contract (**ventricular systole**) and eject blood from the heart, into either the pulmonary system or the distal circulation (Figure A6).

Coronary Circulation

The heart is never without blood *inside* its chambers, but it can't use this blood for its own nourishment. The tissues of the heart itself have a separate blood supply that flows on the *outside* of the heart to provide oxygen to heart tissues.

As blood leaves the left ventricle and enters the aorta for general circulation, it comes immediately to the coronary arteries, which siphon off a share of oxygenated blood to supply the heart muscle itself. There are two main vessels, the left and right coronary arteries, each supplying the major portion of their respective ventricles. The left coronary artery quickly branches into the anterior descending artery, which supplies the anterior surface of the heart, and the circumflex artery, which passes around to the left and back between the left atrium and left ventricle (Figure A7).

Occasionally, the circumflex branch continues around to supply the back side of the heart, including the septum. In such a case, the coronary circulation would be considered **dominant left**. However, in 80 percent of people, the right coronary artery supplies the posterior side of the heart and interventricular septum. This is called a **dominant right** heart.

Figure A6 Systole and Diastole

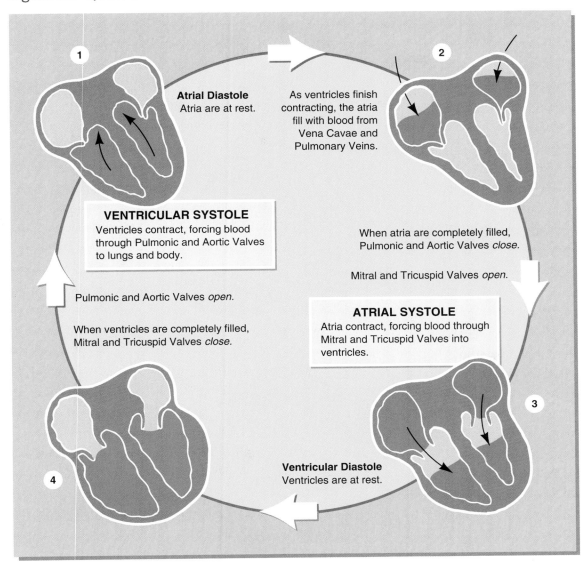

Atrial Diastole
Atria are at rest.

As ventricles finish contracting, the atria fill with blood from Vena Cavae and Pulmonary Veins.

VENTRICULAR SYSTOLE
Ventricles contract, forcing blood through Pulmonic and Aortic Valves to lungs and body.

When atria are completely filled, Pulmonic and Aortic Valves *close.*

Mitral and Tricuspid Valves *open.*

Pulmonic and Aortic Valves *open.*

ATRIAL SYSTOLE
Atria contract, forcing blood through Mitral and Tricuspid Valves into ventricles.

When ventricles are completely filled, Mitral and Tricuspid Valves *close.*

Ventricular Diastole
Ventricles are at rest.

Deoxygenated blood is returned to general circulation by way of cardiac veins, which empty into the **coronary sinus**, located within the right atrium.

Surfaces of the Heart

The heart has four surfaces, or planes. The **anterior surface** faces forward, abutting the chest wall. On the opposite plane, facing the spine, is the **posterior surface**. The **diaphragmatic surface** refers to the under portion of the heart that rests against the diaphragm. The **lateral surface** is the side wall, on the side above the diaphragmatic surface (Figure A8).

Figure A7 Coronary Circulation

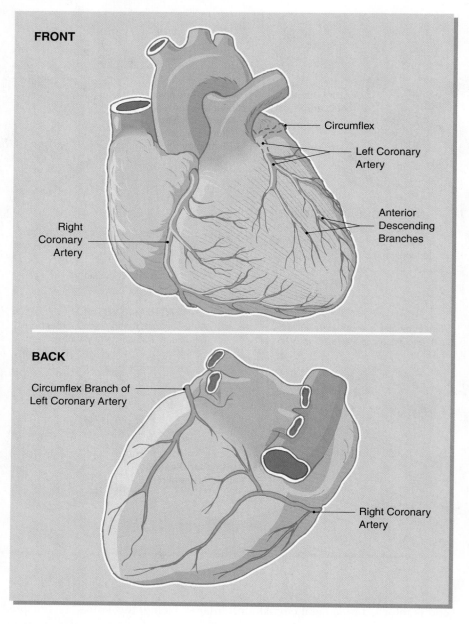

FRONT

Circumflex

Left Coronary
Artery

Anterior
Descending
Branches

Right
Coronary
Artery

BACK

Circumflex Branch of
Left Coronary Artery

Right Coronary
Artery

Figure A8 Surfaces of the Heart

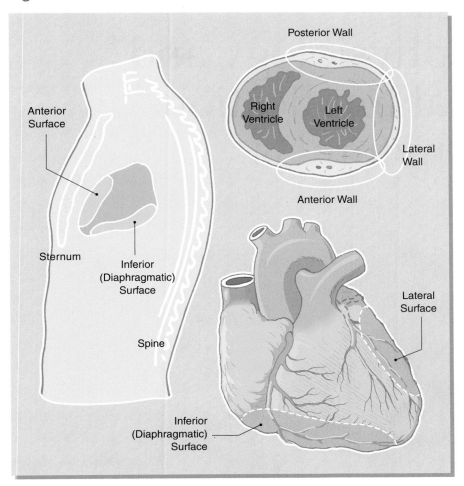

Anterior Surface

Sternum

Inferior (Diaphragmatic) Surface

Spine

Posterior Wall

Right Ventricle

Left Ventricle

Lateral Wall

Anterior Wall

Lateral Surface

Inferior (Diaphragmatic) Surface

Appendix B
Pathophysiology and Clinical Implications of Arrhythmias

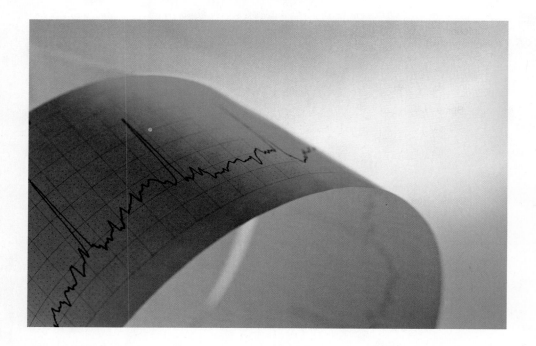

Overview

IN THIS APPENDIX, you will be exposed to the clinical importance of each of the basic cardiac arrhythmias you learned in earlier chapters. You will learn about cardiac output, and how it is affected by arrhythmias, and about the symptoms produced when it is impaired. You will also learn general treatment principles that apply when arrhythmias cause clinical problems. Then, for each arrhythmia, you will find out its significance and clinical presentation.

Pathophysiology

Arrhythmias are manifestations of *electrical* activity in the heart. Ideally, each electrical impulse results in a *mechanical* contraction of the heart to pump blood and produce a pulse. Arrhythmias cause problems when this process breaks down. When a rhythm fails to produce adequate pulses, the patient begins to have symptoms. Symptoms arise when arrhythmias reduce *cardiac output*, the volume of blood pumped by the heart.

Cardiac Output

Cardiac output is defined as the total volume of blood pumped by the heart in one minute. If you measured the volume pumped during each ventricular contraction (called *stroke volume*) and multiplied that by the number of contractions (heartbeats) per minute, you would have a *measured cardiac output*. The formula for measured cardiac output is:

Heart Rate × Stroke Volume = Cardiac Output

Anything that alters either heart rate or stroke volume will also affect cardiac output. Arrhythmias have the ability to lower cardiac output (and thus cause symptoms) in two ways:

Heart Rate: Any rhythm with an extreme rate (either bradycardia or tachycardia) can reduce cardiac output.

Stroke Volume: Normal stroke volume relies on synchronous electrical stimulation to produce an efficient pumping action. Rhythms originating from ventricular foci cause the heart to contract erratically, which reduces stroke volume and ultimately lowers cardiac output.

You can use this basic understanding to organize all the arrhythmias according to each one's likelihood of causing symptoms and therefore needing treatment. One such organization scheme is called the **Matrix of Clinical Impact**, which uses the two variables of *Rate* and *Pacemaker Site* (Figure B1).

Each of the basic arrhythmias is placed in its appropriate place on the matrix. They then can be clustered according to their threat to cardiac output. The three areas known to produce symptoms are *Bradycardias, Tachycardias,* and *Ventricular Irritability.*

Symptoms of Impaired Cardiac Output

When cardiac output is diminished, it produces symptoms in the patient. Regardless of which arrhythmia is causing the problem, the symptoms of reduced cardiac output are the same. These symptoms can include:

- Anxiety
- Chest pain
- Shortness of breath
- Diaphoresis
- Hypotension
- Cool, clammy skin
- Cyanosis
- Decreased
- Consciousness

These symptoms are indications that cardiac output is inadequate to perfuse body tissues. When you see these symptoms, you know that perfusion is impaired and the arrhythmia should be treated.

Treating Arrhythmias

ACLS Recommendations
The American Heart Association's Advanced Cardiac Life Support (ACLS) recommendations are the recognized standard for treatment of arrhythmias associated with cardiac events such as acute myocardial infarction and cardiac arrest. The ACLS guidelines are prepared by leading researchers and clinicians to provide detailed considerations for management of all aspects surrounding treatment of arrhythmias. The ACLS standards are published and updated regularly and should be used as the guide for clinical management of arrhythmias. The material presented here is an introductory overview of management principles and should not be used to direct clinical treatment.

General Treatment Principles

Arrhythmias are treated when they cause (or are likely to cause) clinical symptoms. All patients with arrhythmias or the potential for them should be monitored and receive oxygen and a keep-open IV as a precaution. If arrhythmias do occur, the patient's various perfusion parameters (blood pressure, pulses, skin, etc.) should be assessed to determine impact on cardiac output. When arrhythmias cause symptoms, treatment should be initiated immediately.

Support Perfusion

In addition to treating the specific presenting arrhythmia, it may be necessary to provide general supportive measures such as ventilation to improve oxygenation, chest compression to maintain circulation, and drugs to stabilize blood pressure.

Look for Correctable Underlying Conditions

To enhance conversion of an arrhythmia, any contributing conditions should be identified and corrected: bicarbonate if the patient is acidotic, fluids if hypovolemic, oxygen if hypoxic, and so on.

Figure B1 Matrix of Clinical Impact

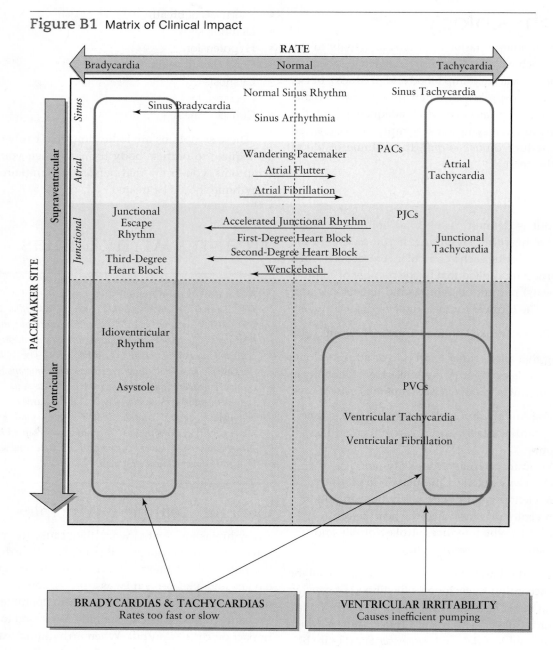

Treatment Concepts

The old adage in electrocardiography is that you do not treat rhythms, you treat patients. As you can see in Figure B1, many arrhythmias produce no symptoms in the patient. These rhythms do not require treatment, though they may bear watching.

Treat the three groups that are likely to cause symptoms by removing the threat to cardiac output, as shown in Figure B2.

The likelihood of any given arrhythmia producing symptoms or causing clinical concerns depends on both rate and pacemaker site. The expected significance and clinical picture of each of the arrhythmias is shown in Figure B3.

Figure B2 Treatment Concepts

Rhythm	Concept	Treatment Goals
Tachycardias	Heart rate is too fast to allow the ventricles to fill completely before contraction.	• Slow the heart rate.
Bradycardias	Heart rate is too slow to maintain cardiac output.	• Speed up heart rate. • When bradycardia is caused by block at the AV node, the goal is to increase conduction through the junction.
Ventricular Irritability	Erratic ventricular contraction is not effective enough to maintain stroke volume.	• Suppress irritable focus.

Figure B3 Arrhythmia Significance and Clinical Picture

Arrhythmia	Significance	Clinical Picture
NSR	• Normal cardiac pattern	• Does not produce symptoms
Sinus Bradycardia	• Can precede blocks or Asystole • Can precipitate escape rhythms or ventricular irritability • Can be caused by AMI, vagal stimulation, increased intracranial pressure • Can reflect normal, athletic heart	• Slow, regular pulse • Can cause signs/symptoms of decreased cardiac output
Sinus Tachycardia	• Usually a compensatory response to fever, activity, pain, anxiety, hypovolemia, heart failure, etc. • Dangerous in AMI (can extend infarct)	• Rapid, regular pulse • Probably asymptomatic • Possibly palpitations, dyspnea
Sinus Arrhythmia	• Common in children and young adults	• Irregular pulse • Rarely causes symptoms
Premature Atrial Complex	• Usually benign • Can be early sign of CHF • Can lead to atrial tachyarrhythmias • Causes include fatigue, hypoxia, dig-toxicity, caffeine, ischemia, CHF, alcohol	• Irregular pulse • Rarely causes symptoms
Wandering Pacemaker	• Normal; often seen in very old, very young, or in athletes • Persistence of junctional rhythm can indicate heart disease	• Rarely causes symptoms
Atrial Tachycardia	• Very dangerous in AMI or heart disease • Commonly caused by dig-toxicity	• Rapid, regular pulse • May show signs/symptoms of drop in cardiac output • Can cause pulmonary edema, CHF, shock
Atrial Flutter	• Rapid ventricular rate and loss of atrial kick can drop cardiac output • Risk of pulmonary and cerebral emboli • Can cause CHF or myocardial ischemia • Seen in CAD, rheumatic heart disease	• Pulse can be regular or irregular, fast or slow • Rapid ventricular rate can cause signs/symptoms of low cardiac output
Atrial Fibrillation	• Very rapid rate can lead to CHF or myocardial ischemia • Threat of pulmonary or cerebral emboli • Commonly caused by dig-toxicity	• Irregular pulse, can be fast or slow • Can have pulse deficit • Can cause signs/symptoms of low cardiac output
Premature Junctional Complex	• May precede AV block	• Rarely causes signs/symptoms
Junctional Escape Rhythm	• Failsafe mechanism • Can be normal, as with athletes	• Slow pulse • If rate is slow enough, can cause signs/symptoms of low cardiac output
Accelerated Junctional Rhythm	• Indicates irritable junction overriding normal pacemaker • Often caused by AMI, open-heart surgery, myocarditis, dig-toxicity	• Usually asymptomatic
Junctional Tachycardia	• Indicates irritable junction overriding normal pacemaker • Often caused by AMI, open-heart surgery, myocarditis, dig-toxicity	• Rapid, regular pulse • Can cause signs/symptoms of low cardiac output
First-Degree Heart Block	• Can be caused by anoxia, ischemia, AV node malfunction, edema following open-heart surgery, dig-toxicity • Can lead to more serious AV block	• Usually asymptomatic
Second-Degree Heart Block Type I Wenckebach	• Common following inferior MI • Can progress to more serious AV block	• Irregular pulse • Usually asymptomatic
Second-Degree Heart Block Type II	• Can be caused by anoxia, edema after open-heart surgery, dig-toxicity, hyper-kalemia, anterior MI	• Slow rate can cause signs/symptoms of low cardiac output

Figure B3 Continued

Arrhythmia	Significance	Clinical Picture
Third-Degree Heart Block	• Can progress to ventricular standstill	• Very slow rate and abnormal pacemaker site severely impair cardiac output • Patients will frequently be unconscious from poor perfusion • Cardiac failure can follow quickly
Premature Ventricular Complex	• Indicates ventricular irritability; increasing frequency indicates increasing irritability • Causes include ischemia/infarction, hypoxia, acidosis, hypovolemia, electrolyte imbalance, caffeine, smoking, alcohol • PVCs considered to be extremely dangerous include: —frequent, or increasing in frequency —patterns (bigeminy, trigeminy, etc.) —couplets —runs —R on T phenomenon —multifocal	• Patients can feel PVCs and be distressed by them • Pulse is irregular • Perfusion is generally not impaired unless PVCs become frequent • Many adults have chronic PVCs from underlying respiratory disease, smoking, caffeine, etc.
Ventricular Tachycardia	• Can quickly progress to Ventricular Fibrillation	• Patient will begin to lose consciousness as perfusion drops
Ventricular Fibrillation	• Lethal arrhythmia • Indicative of extreme myocardial irritability	• Patient is clinically dead
Idioventricular Rhythm	• Carries poor prognosis • Often associated with large MI and damage to large amount of ventricular muscle mass	• Patient is clinically dead
Asystole	• Carries very poor prognosis • Often seen after patient has been in arrest for some time	• Patient is clinically dead

Appendix C
12-Lead Electrocardiography

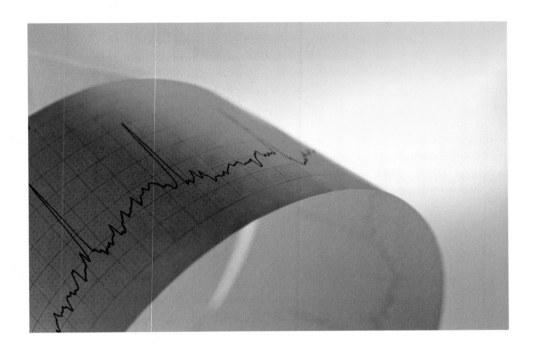

Overview

IN THIS APPENDIX, you will learn how 12-lead EKGs are different from the basic arrhythmias you learned in the first part of the book, and you will learn the uses and limitations of a 12-lead EKG. You will learn the fundamental rules of electrocardiography, leads, and electrode placement. Then you will explore vectors, vector relationships, and axis. Finally, you will learn the standardized format for a printed 12-lead EKG. In general, you will learn everything you need to know to understand what you are looking at when you first approach a 12-lead EKG.

The rhythm strips that you studied in the first part of this book were single-lead strips. They all showed cardiac activity from one angle (Lead II). A single-lead strip provides enough information to analyze rate, determine pacemaker control, identify conduction problems, and, ultimately, to identify threats to perfusion.

A 12-lead EKG gives you twelve short strips, allowing you to view the heart from twelve different directions, both top to bottom and front to back. The added angles provide a more complete picture of cardiac function. In addition to information from the rhythm strip, the 12-lead EKG enables you to locate tissue damage caused by myocardial hypoxia and to determine whether the chambers are abnormally enlarged as a result of valve problems or pulmonary disease. It also provides more detailed information about conduction, such as which branches of the conduction system are blocked or whether the entire electrical flow is slightly off kilter, and it can reveal certain metabolic and chemical abnormalities.

That much information packed into a single-page report can be intimidating at first glance. But so was this book when you first opened it, and by now you're probably quite comfortable with rhythm strips. The same will happen with 12-lead EKGs. Just take one step at a time. Don't try to go from A to Z in the first sitting. This appendix will take you from A to B, or maybe C. From there, you can add information from a variety of sources until you have all the knowledge you want.

Fundamental Rules of Electrocardiography

As you learn about 12-lead EKGs, remember the fundamental rules that apply to all tracings produced by EKG machines:

- Current flowing *toward* a *positive* electrode creates an **upright** deflection; current flowing *away from* a *positive* electrode creates a **downward** deflection.
- Current flowing *toward* a *negative* electrode creates a **downward** deflection; current flowing *away from* a *negative* electrode creates an **upright** deflection.
- When the lead that detects the current is at *right angles* (perpendicular) to the current, the line will be **isoelectric**—that is, neither upright nor downward.

Leads and Electrode Placement

Single-Lead Rhythm Strips

A **lead** is a combination of electrodes that reflects the flow of electricity between two points on opposing sides of the heart. Some leads have one positive and one negative electrode, making them **bipolar** leads. Other leads have a single positive electrode, but the opposing electrode is created by combining other electrodes into a **central terminal**, an electrically neutral point situated to reference the center of the heart. Since only the positive electrode is polarized, these leads are considered **unipolar** leads.

Regardless of whether a lead is unipolar or bipolar, it provides information only in one dimension: it shows only the view of the heart as seen between two points. Many times, a single perspective is sufficient. It can tell you whether the heart is beating, and, if so, you can identify the underlying rate and rhythm. A single lead used for this purpose is called a **monitoring lead**.

When monitoring is all that's needed, it is usually done in Lead II. Lead II is also the most common lead used as the rhythm strip on a 12-lead EKG.

Another popular monitoring lead is called Modified Chest Left, or MCL_1. MCL_1 is a bipolar lead that can be useful in differentiating rhythms with broad QRS complexes. MCL_1 requires different electrode positioning than Lead II: the negative electrode goes on the left upper chest, with the positive electrode at the right side of the sternum in the fourth intercostal space (Figure C1). MCL_1 is not included on standard 12-lead EKGs.

Multiple Lead Recordings

You can learn more about the heart's electrical function by using multiple leads, each one providing a view that is slightly different from other leads. By carefully positioning electrodes to cover the various areas of the heart, you can see a more thorough picture of cardiac electrical activity.

Practically speaking, there are two dimensions in which electrodes can be placed: up and down across the **frontal plane** of the body and around the chest on the **horizontal plane** (Figure C2). A standardized format has been developed that places six leads on each of these two planes,

Figure C1 Electrode Placement for MCL_1

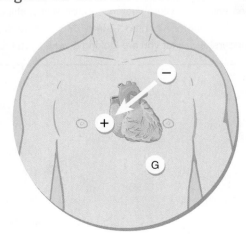

Figure C2 Frontal and Horizontal Planes

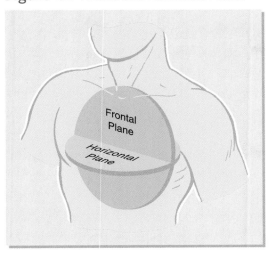

thereby providing information from a total of twelve different angles. This record is called a **conventional 12-lead EKG**. Once electrodes are placed in the standard locations, the machine automatically measures flow between the electrodes needed to produce the desired lead.

Frontal Plane Leads

Four limb electrodes are used to view the frontal plane: right arm (RA), left arm (LA), left leg (LL), and right leg (RL). These electrodes are often placed in corresponding positions on the anterior chest wall, both for convenience and in hopes of reducing movement artifact (Figure C3).

These electrodes are used to produce the **Standard Limb Leads:** I, II, and III (Figure C4). All of these are bipolar leads, meaning they use both a positive and a negative electrode. They view electrical flow as follows:

Lead I: right arm to left arm
Lead II: right arm to left leg
Lead III: left arm to left leg

Figure C3 Electrode Placement, Frontal Plane
MyBRADYLab™

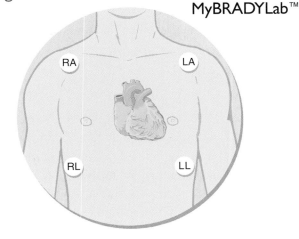

Figure C4 The Standard Limb Leads

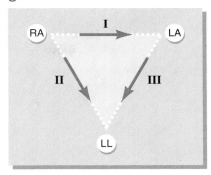

The equilateral triangle formed by the standard limb leads is called Einthoven's Triangle.

By using a central terminal, it is possible to create three more frontal leads, called **Augmented Leads:** augmented voltage right arm (aVR), augmented voltage left arm (aVL), and augmented voltage left leg (aVF) (Figure C5). (*Note:* The abbreviation is for "foot" to avoid confusion with aVL.)

The augmented leads are unipolar; they measure information from the central terminal to a positive electrode. They view electrical flow as follows:

aVR: central terminal to right arm
aVL: central terminal to left arm
aVF: central terminal to left leg

These leads can also be illustrated graphically on the triangle:

The three standard limb leads and the three augmented leads all view the heart from the frontal plane (Figure C6).

Horizontal Plane Leads

To visualize electrical flow on a horizontal plane (that is, around the circumference of the chest) we use additional electrodes to create six more leads. These leads are called chest leads, or **Precordial** leads (Figure C7).

Six different positive electrodes are used to produce the six precordial leads. The leads are obtained by pairing each positive electrode with the electrically neutral central terminal composed of the combined limb electrodes. Thus,

Figure C5 The Augmented Leads

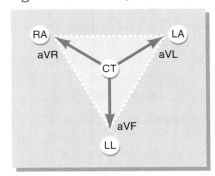

Figure C6 Frontal Plane Leads

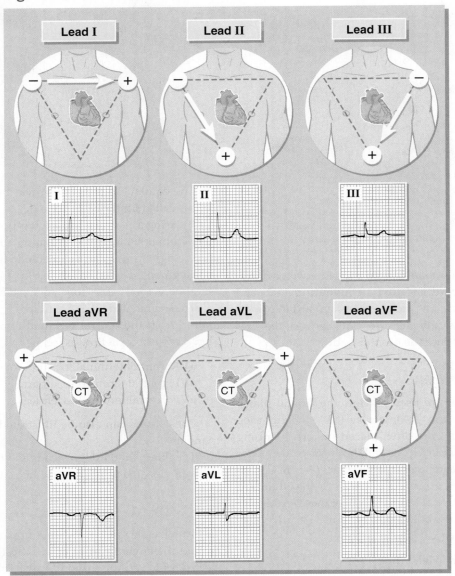

the precordial leads are unipolar, and they view current flowing from the heart toward the chest wall.

To ensure accurate readings of chest leads, the precordial electrodes must be placed with care. The standardized locations for the precordial electrodes are as follows:

V_1: Right sternal border, fourth intercostal space
V_2: Left sternal border, fourth intercostal space
V_3: Midway between V_2 and V_4
V_4: Midclavicular line, fifth intercostal space
V_5: Anterior axillary line, fifth intercostal space
V_6: Midaxillary line, fifth intercostal space

The six chest leads can be localized to provide information about specific areas of the heart: V_1 and V_2 view the septum, V_3 and V_4 view the anterior myocardial wall, and the lateral myocardial wall is reflected in V_5 and V_6.

The precordial leads provide information on the horizontal plane. When combined with the leads of the frontal plane, we see a more detailed view of the heart's electrical activity.

Vectors and Axis

Electrical Flow through the Heart

We think of the heart as having a single electrical flow that goes roughly from the sinus node down toward the apex. We've used large arrows to show how the direction of flow changes slightly with rhythm changes. For example, with junctional rhythms, the retrograde flow is shown by one arrow from the AV junction up toward the sinus

Figure C7 Horizontal Plane Leads

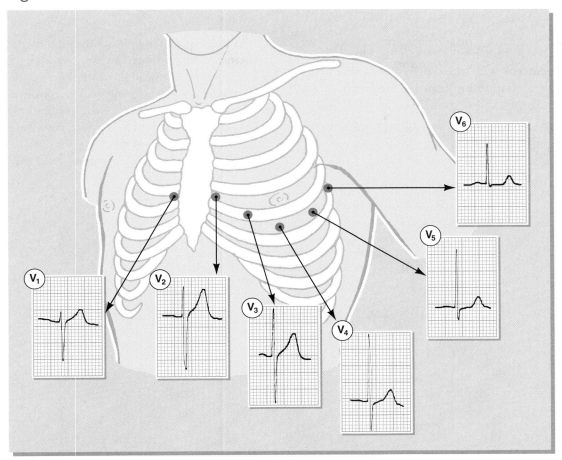

node, while a second arrow goes from the AV junction down through the ventricles. These arrows are called vectors. They are used to depict the direction of flow, with the point of the arrow indicating the positive electrode. Vectors also indicate magnitude; the larger the arrow, the greater the amplitude of the flow.

There is one slight problem with our thinking at this point. The heart doesn't depolarize as a single event. During each cardiac cycle, every depolarizing myocardial cell generates its own current moving in all directions at once and continuously changing direction. Each of these countless electrical currents has its own small vector showing its magnitude and direction of flow. The much larger vector we're used to seeing is actually a combined vector of all these various currents.

This larger, aggregate vector is called the **axis**, or the sum direction of electrical flow. The axis of the heart as a whole is called the **mean QRS axis**. The mean QRS axis shows the overall direction of flow within the heart. In a normal heart, the depolarization wave of the right ventricle proceeds down and to the right. The much larger left ventricle produces a stronger vector that goes down and to the left. Thus, the combined vector of both ventricles, the mean

QRS axis, flows down and to the left, reflecting the left ventricle's larger muscle mass.

Lead Axis

Each lead also has its own axis. All the leads detect current between two points on opposing sides of the heart. An imaginary line between these two points is called the axis of the lead. The axis of each lead is shown by an arrow, or vector, drawn from its negative electrode (or central terminal) to its positive electrode.

The lead vectors are the physiologic basis for interpreting 12-lead EKGs. In a rhythm strip, you look at the wave patterns and work backward to determine what went on in the heart. The rules you use to draw your conclusions are based on a single lead, Lead II, in which the vector goes from the right atrium to the left ventricle. When the P wave is inverted, you conclude that the vector was going the wrong direction; thus, the impulse originated in the AV junction.

The same principle applies when interpreting 12-lead EKGs, except that now you will compare direction of flow for electrodes placed in twelve different places, reflecting twelve different lead vectors. Begin by learning how the vectors of each lead relate to the others and to the vector of the heart as a whole.

Interpretation of EKG Deflections

The heart's current will cause deflections on the EKG according to the relationship between the lead's axis and the heart's mean QRS axis (Figure C8).

- Complexes are most positive when lead axis and QRS axis are *parallel* (or most negative if the current flows toward the negative electrode).

- When lead axis and QRS axis are *perpendicular*, each complex will be both upright and inverted (biphasic, or equiphasic).

As depolarization spreads through the ventricles, the changing vectors produce a QRS wave form reflecting the axis of the particular lead in which it is viewed. The 12-lead EKG displays the heart's mean axis from twelve different angles. Thus, the individual wave configurations will normally vary from one lead to the next. Before exploring these differences, we must first review terms used to define some of the specific waves and measurements (Figure C9).

Figure C8 EKG Deflections

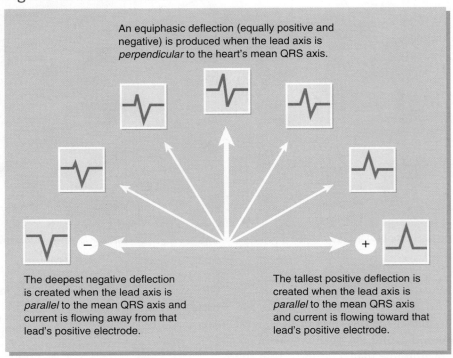

An equiphasic deflection (equally positive and negative) is produced when the lead axis is *perpendicular* to the heart's mean QRS axis.

The deepest negative deflection is created when the lead axis is *parallel* to the mean QRS axis and current is flowing away from that lead's positive electrode.

The tallest positive deflection is created when the lead axis is *parallel* to the mean QRS axis and current is flowing toward that lead's positive electrode.

Figure C9 Wave Definitions

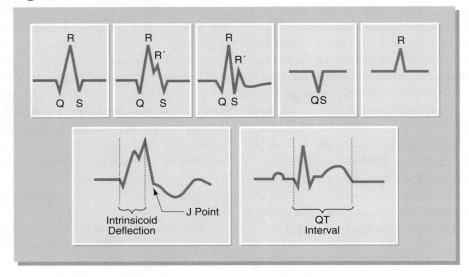

R Waves: All positive deflections within the QRS complex are R waves.

If there are two R waves in the same complex, the second is named *prime* ('). Two R waves in the same complex without an intervening S wave produce a pattern that is technically an RR', though it is most commonly called a notched R wave, or "rabbit ears."

NOTE: It is common to use upper and lowercase letters to indicate the relative size of waves: uppercase denotes large waves, while small waves are indicated by lowercase. Thus, qRSr' would indicate a small Q wave, large initial R wave, large S wave, and small second R wave. Many combinations are possible: qR, Rs, rSR', etc. For our purposes, we will use only uppercase letters.

Q Waves: A negative deflection before the R wave is a Q.

S Waves: A negative deflection following an R wave is an S.

QS Waves: If there is no R wave, the combined negative deflection is a QS.

Intrinsicoid Deflection: This reflects the time it takes for peak voltage to develop within the ventricles. It is measured from the onset of the QRS to the peak of the R wave. A prolonged intrinsicoid deflection (> 0.06 second) is considered a "late R wave."

J Point: This is the demarcation between the end of the QRS complex and the beginning of the ST segment.

QT Interval: This reflects the total duration of ventricular depolarization and repolarization. It is measured from the beginning of the QRS complex to the end of the T wave. The QT interval varies with heart rate.

The presence or absence of individual wave forms is determined by the vectors produced within the heart, relative to the axis of the lead being viewed.

Vector Relationships

Since the goal is to compare each lead's axis to that of the heart's mean axis, we need to give them all a common reference point. We can do this by drawing a circle, with the center being the AV node. For each lead, draw an arrow from the center of the circle to that lead's positive electrode. You will find that the vectors cross the perimeter of the circle in increments of 30 degrees. Each arrow shows the *angle* the vector has in its lead; thus, the vectors are shown in relation to the heart and can be quantified in terms of degrees. The first six leads show the vectors of the frontal plane (Figure C10). The vectors of the six V leads, showing the horizontal plane, can be similarly illustrated (Figure C11).

Axis Deviation

This same format can be used to quantify the mean QRS axis, the aggregate flow of electrical current through the heart (Figure C12). By dividing the circle into four quadrants, we see that the QRS axis normally falls in the lower right quadrant, between 0° and +90°. When the heart is damaged, displaced, or enlarged, the electrical flow changes, shifting the mean QRS axis. When the vector shifts beyond the boundaries of normal, it is called **axis deviation**. Axis deviation can be found in normal EKGs, or it can be associated with myocardial infarction, ventricular hypertrophy, or ventricular conduction defect.

Figure C10 Frontal Plane Vectors

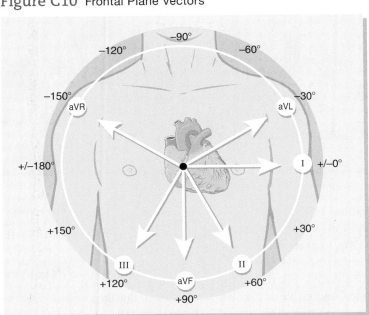

Figure C11 Horizontal Plane Vectors

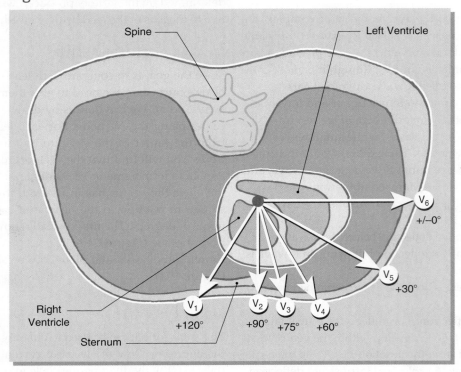

Figure C12 Mean QRS Axis

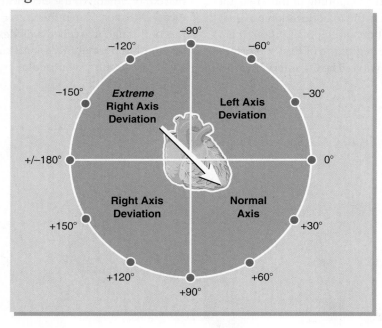

A shift in vector to the patient's left (0° to −90° on the circle) is called left axis deviation and can be associated with left ventricular hypertrophy, hypertension, aortic stenosis, and other disorders affecting the left ventricle. When the vector shifts to the patient's right (+90° to +180°), it is called right axis deviation and is suggestive of problems in the right heart and pulmonary system. The upper left quadrant, between +/−180° and −90°, is considered extreme right axis deviation, or indeterminate axis.

Estimating QRS Axis

Understanding normal QRS axis, and recognizing abnormal deviations, is essential to accurate interpretation of lead vectors. However, the information gleaned from axis analysis can be quite esoteric and can sidetrack you from some of the more practical elements of basic 12-lead EKG interpretation. For this reason, axis calculation has been greatly simplified here.

A quick method for estimating axis relies on evaluating leads I and aVF. In both these leads, the QRS complex is normally upright. Axis deviation is indicated when the QRS complex in either or both of these leads is negative—that is, where the sum of the individual Q, R, and S waves is *not* positive (Figure C13).

Standardized Format

Most 12-lead EKGs are printed in a standard format that prints patient information across the top, followed by about 3 seconds of each lead. Any effort to analyze a 12-lead EKG must necessarily begin with locating lead layout. The transition between leads is often obscure, so you won't know what you're looking at unless you know the standard layout (Figure C14).

The standard layout places the twelve leads in four columns of three rows each. Starting at the upper left, you'll read top to bottom, left to right. Column one holds leads I, II, and III, and column two holds aVR, aVL, and aVF. The V leads are in the last two columns; column three holds V$_1$, V$_2$, and V$_3$, and you'll find V$_4$, V$_5$, and V$_6$ in the last column.

The last thing you see is a rhythm strip, usually lead II, running across the bottom of the page. However, it is increasingly common to find the rhythm strip run in leads I, II, and III simultaneously, occupying an entire second page of the report.

Normal 12-Lead EKG

Before you can recognize abnormalities, you must first learn to recognize normal. Because each lead has its own axis, which may or may not align with the mean QRS axis, you should expect to see a wide range of complexes from lead to lead. A wave form that is normal for one lead could be abnormal in another. The better you understand the electrical forces that produced the waves, the better you will be able to remember what each lead normally looks like (Figure C15).

Use the tracing in Figure C15, along with its definition of features, to analyze the two normal tracings in Figures C16 and C17. You may want to refer to these "normal" EKGs as you explore the abnormalities discussed in Appendix D.

Figure C13 Estimating QRS Axis

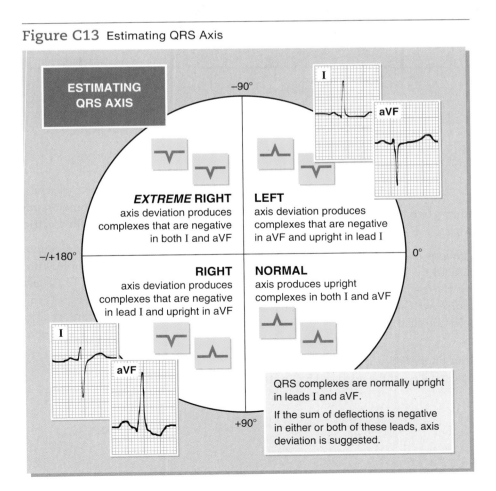

ESTIMATING QRS AXIS

−90°

I
aVF

EXTREME RIGHT axis deviation produces complexes that are negative in both I and aVF

LEFT axis deviation produces complexes that are negative in aVF and upright in lead I

−/+180°

0°

RIGHT axis deviation produces complexes that are negative in lead I and upright in aVF

NORMAL axis produces upright complexes in both I and aVF

I
aVF

+90°

QRS complexes are normally upright in leads I and aVF.

If the sum of deflections is negative in either or both of these leads, axis deviation is suggested.

Figure C14 Standard Layout of 12-Lead EKG

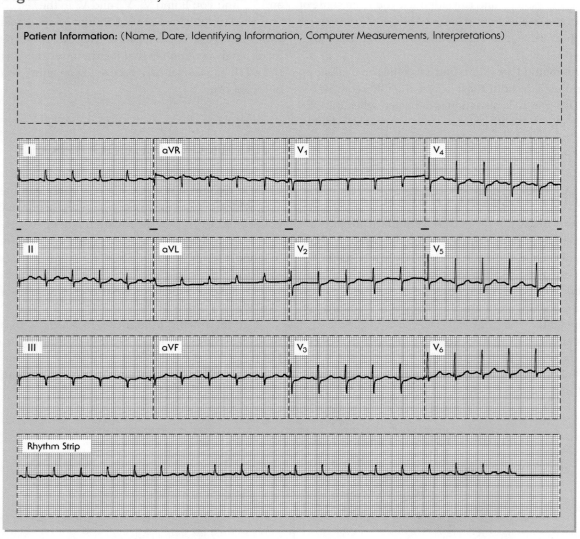

Patient Information: (Name, Date, Identifying Information, Computer Measurements, Interpretations)

I   aVR   V₁   V₄

II   aVL   V₂   V₅

III   aVF   V₃   V₆

Rhythm Strip

Limitations of 12-Lead EKGs

Twelve-lead EKGs share two distinct limitations with single-lead rhythm strips:

1. They are representations of *electrical* activity. They provide information about the heart's electrical status but can't tell us how the heart's mechanical pump is functioning. Of course, we can draw conclusions when the electrical patterns are clearly inadequate to produce mechanical response.

2. They show us what happened *when the recording was made*, but they don't show what the heart did 5 minutes later, and they can't predict what it will do tomorrow. Again, we can make some assumptions based on the physiology underlying the electrical patterns.

The 12-lead EKG can provide more information about cardiac activity than is possible with a single monitoring strip. However, with 12-lead EKGs as well as rhythm strips and all other diagnostic tools, it is important to assess the patient and consider the context of current and previous clinical circumstances. It is always the patient who receives the treatment, not the EKG.

Figure C15 Features of a Normal 12-Lead EKG

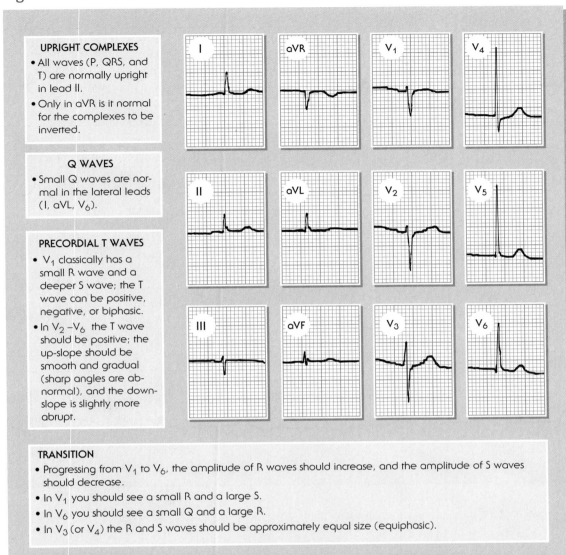

UPRIGHT COMPLEXES
- All waves (P, QRS, and T) are normally upright in lead II.
- Only in aVR is it normal for the complexes to be inverted.

Q WAVES
- Small Q waves are normal in the lateral leads (I, aVL, V_6).

PRECORDIAL T WAVES
- V_1 classically has a small R wave and a deeper S wave; the T wave can be positive, negative, or biphasic.
- In V_2–V_6 the T wave should be positive; the up-slope should be smooth and gradual (sharp angles are abnormal), and the down-slope is slightly more abrupt.

TRANSITION
- Progressing from V_1 to V_6, the amplitude of R waves should increase, and the amplitude of S waves should decrease.
- In V_1 you should see a small R and a large S.
- In V_6 you should see a small Q and a large R.
- In V_3 (or V_4) the R and S waves should be approximately equal size (equiphasic).

Figure C16 Normal 12-Lead Wave Forms—Example #1

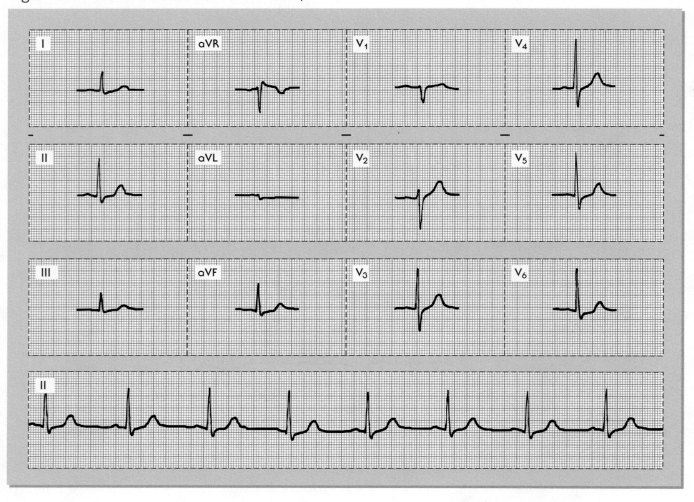

Figure C17 Normal 12-Lead Wave Forms—Example #2

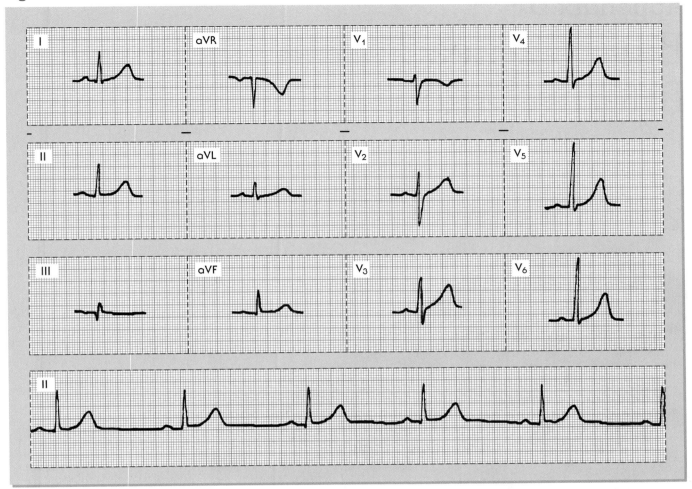

Appendix D
Basic 12-Lead Interpretation

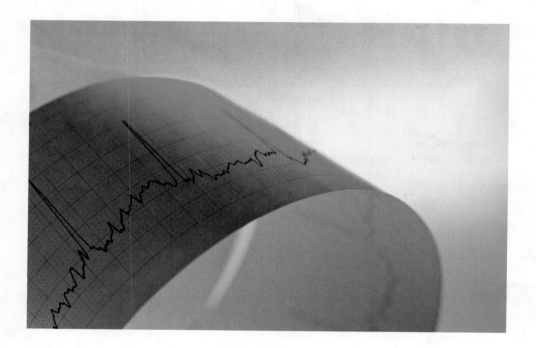

Overview

IN THIS APPENDIX, you will begin to analyze and interpret what you are seeing on a 12-lead EKG. You will learn to recognize EKG changes caused by myocardial damage, chamber enlargement, bundle branch block, and miscellaneous conditions such as pericarditis, digitalis toxicity, and abnormal calcium and potassium levels. You will learn a methodical format for analyzing 12-lead EKGs.

From Appendix C you know that the 12-lead EKG provides information about cardiac rhythm and mean QRS axis. The 12-lead EKG is also used routinely for a range of other information. In this appendix you will learn to interpret a 12-lead EKG to determine all of the following:

- *Myocardial Damage:* age, extent, and location of damage

- *Bundle Branch Block:* which branches of the ventricular conduction system are blocked
- *Chamber Enlargement:* caused by dilation or hypertrophy
- *Miscellaneous Effects:* drugs, electrolytes, pericarditis

Myocardial Damage

Extent of Injury

When blood flow is obstructed within a coronary artery, the portion of myocardial wall that was fed by the obstructed vessel is deprived of oxygen and begins to die. The initial lack of oxygen is called **ischemia**, and if allowed to continue, it causes **injury** to the myocardium. If untreated, the tissues eventually die completely—a condition called **myocardial infarction** (Figure D1).

When the area of infarction extends completely through the wall of the ventricle, the infarction is called **transmural**. The term **subendocardial** has been used to describe infarctions that extend only partially through the wall (Figure D2).

Ischemic Changes on the EKG

The effects of ischemia appear on the EKG as changes in Q waves, ST segments, and T waves as outlined below:

ST Segment:	• depression
	• elevation
T Wave:	• peaking
	• flattening
	• inversion
Q Wave:	• deepening and widening of Q waves
	• loss of R wave resulting in deep QS wave

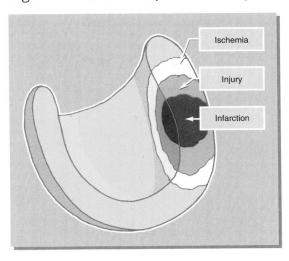

Figure D1 Grades of Myocardial Damage

These changes are considered **ischemic changes** and are indicative of myocardial damage. They can be found alone or, more commonly, in combination with one another to produce a variety of patterns (Figure D3).

In infarctions limited to partial wall thickness (subendocardial infarctions), the damage may be insufficient to produce classically abnormal Q waves. For this reason, you may see subendocardial infarctions referred to as **"non-Q" infarctions**. In such situations the Q wave is not a diagnostic feature.

Evolution of Ischemic Changes

Ischemic changes are the result of abnormal depolarization around the area of damage. As the damage evolves, the

Figure D2 Extent of Infarction

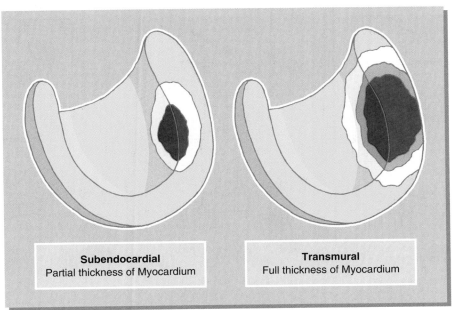

Subendocardial
Partial thickness of Myocardium

Transmural
Full thickness of Myocardium

Figure D3 Ischemic Changes

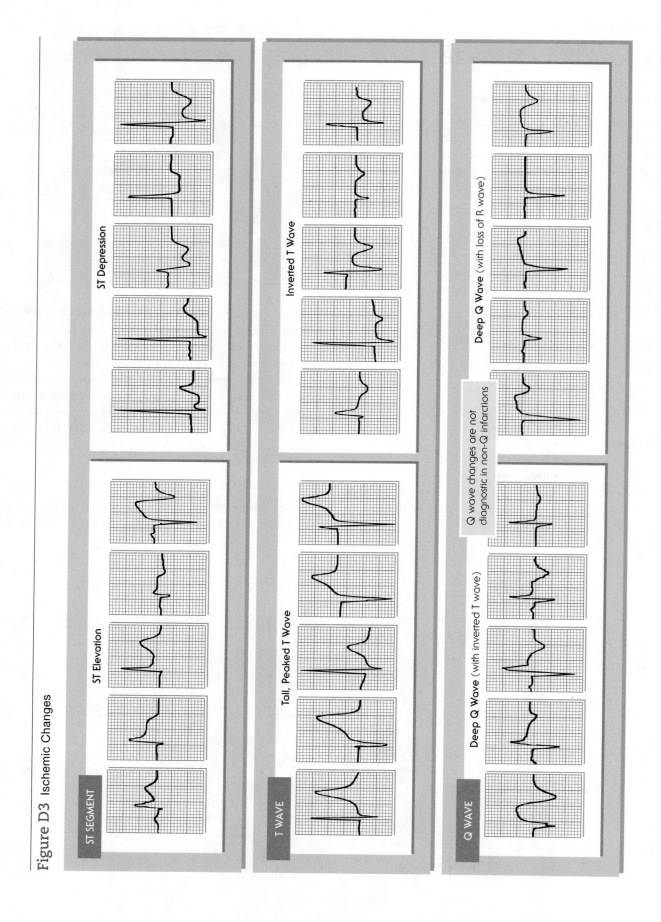

EKG continues to change (Figure D4). Thus, the EKG picture will change over time and may show any combination of these changes depending on when the tracing was made. Generally speaking, the changes evolve as follows:

First Hours: Almost immediately, the ST segment rises, and the T wave becomes more prominent; it may be tall, peaked, or possibly inverted. You may also see an increase in R wave amplitude.

First Day: Over the course of the first day or two, the R wave begins to diminish, while the Q wave becomes deeper and wider. The ST segment elevation may increase. The T wave can be upright, flattened, or inverted, but it usually becomes less prominent.

First Week: Within a week or so, the ST segment begins returning to normal, though the T wave can remain inverted, upright, or flat. The most prominent feature at this point is loss of the R wave, resulting in a deep QS wave.

Months Later: Weeks or months later, the ST segment returns to normal, though T wave abnormalities can persist. The R wave may return partially, but the Q wave often remains a permanent feature of the EKG.

MyBRADYLab™
Infarction Location

Most infarctions cause damage to one or more walls of the left ventricle. Abnormal depolarization in the damaged area will cause ischemic changes in the leads directly over

---

Figure D4 Age of Infarction (Transmural MI)

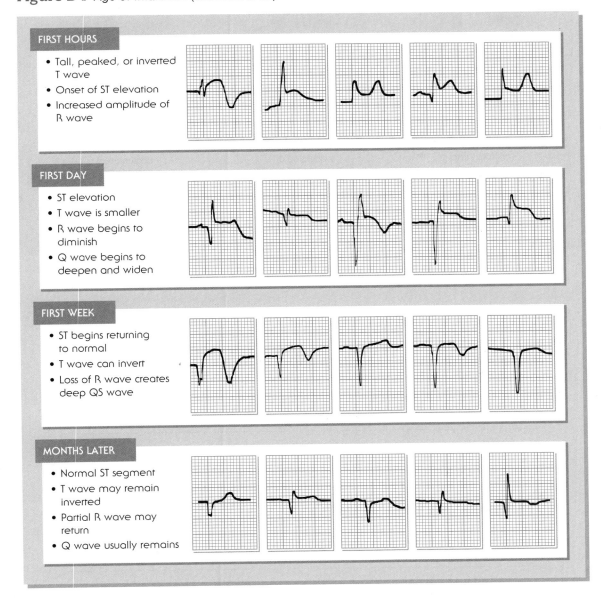

FIRST HOURS
- Tall, peaked, or inverted T wave
- Onset of ST elevation
- Increased amplitude of R wave

FIRST DAY
- ST elevation
- T wave is smaller
- R wave begins to diminish
- Q wave begins to deepen and widen

FIRST WEEK
- ST begins returning to normal
- T wave can invert
- Loss of R wave creates deep QS wave

MONTHS LATER
- Normal ST segment
- T wave may remain inverted
- Partial R wave may return
- Q wave usually remains

that heart surface. Leads that correlate with myocardial surfaces are called **facing** leads. By isolating ischemic changes in facing leads, we can localize the area of damage.

The three heart surfaces most commonly damaged by infarction are the anterior, lateral, and inferior walls (Figure D5). See the facing lead clusters that correlate with these surfaces in Figure D6.

Begin by looking across all the leads for ischemic changes. Note the leads in which these changes are visible. The ischemic changes should correlate with the facing lead clusters.

Anterior wall damage is reflected by ischemic changes in leads V_1–V_4 (Figure D7). When the changes are seen only in V_2 and/or V_3, it indicates **anteroseptal** damage. When both anterior (V_1–V_4) and lateral (V_5–V_6) leads show ischemic changes, it indicates **anterolateral** damage (Figure D8).

Lateral wall damage shows up as ischemic changes in the lateral precordial leads (V_5 and V_6) and in left lateral limb leads (I and aVL) (Figure D9).

Inferior wall damage creates ischemic changes in the lower limb leads (II, III, and aVF) (Figure D10).

Figure D5 Infarction Location

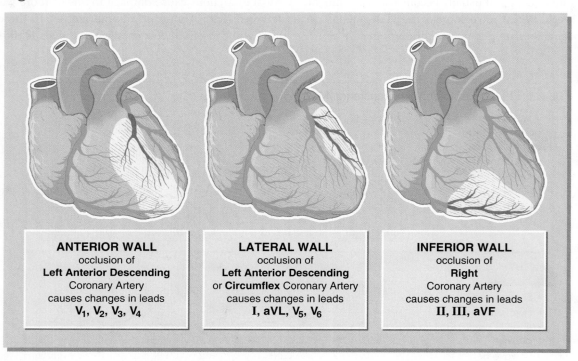

| **ANTERIOR WALL** occlusion of **Left Anterior Descending** Coronary Artery causes changes in leads **V_1, V_2, V_3, V_4** | **LATERAL WALL** occlusion of **Left Anterior Descending** or **Circumflex** Coronary Artery causes changes in leads **I, aVL, V_5, V_6** | **INFERIOR WALL** occlusion of **Right** Coronary Artery causes changes in leads **II, III, aVF** |

Figure D6 Localizing Myocardial Damage Using Facing Leads

Damage to These Surfaces ...	Will be Reflected in These Changing Lead Clusters ...
Anterior	V_1, V_2, V_3, V_4
Lateral	I, aVL, V_5, V_6
Inferior	II, III, aVF

Figure D7 Anterior Wall Facing Leads

These Leads ...	Are Directly Over These Surfaces ...
V_1	anterior wall of the *right* ventricle
V_2, V_3	anterior wall over the septum
V_3, V_4	anterior wall of the *left* ventricle

Figure D8 Anterior Wall Infarctions

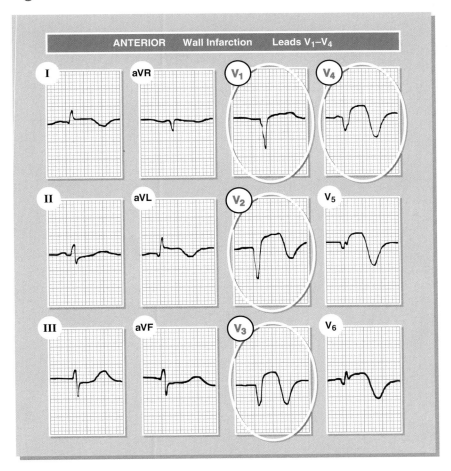

ANTERIOR Wall Infarction Leads V₁–V₄

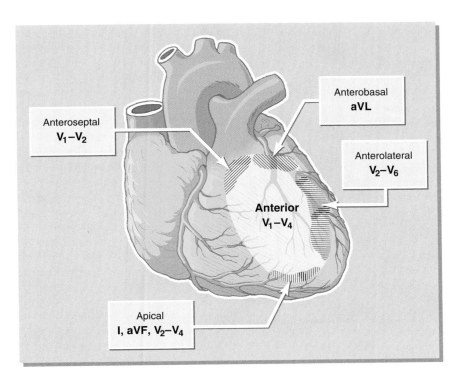

Figure D9 Lateral Wall Infarctions

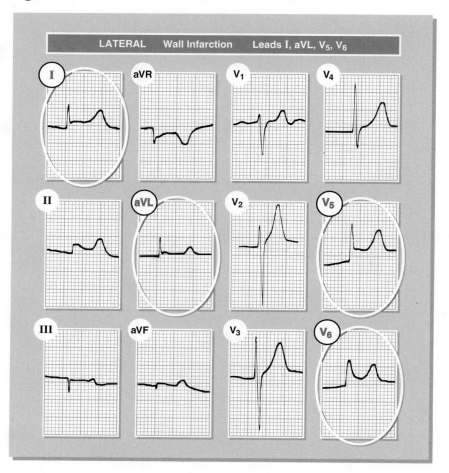

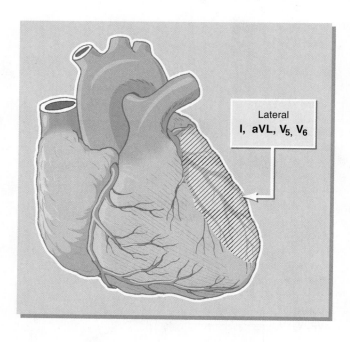

Figure D10 Inferior Wall Infarctions

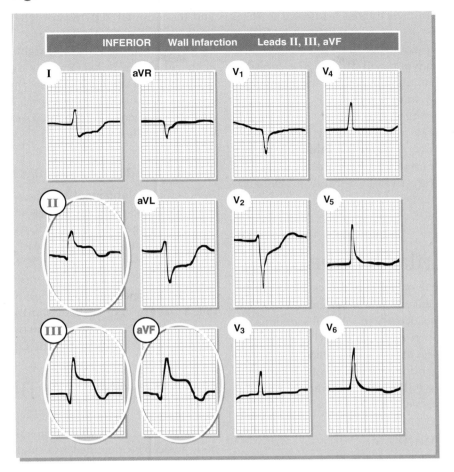

INFERIOR   Wall Infarction   Leads II, III, aVF

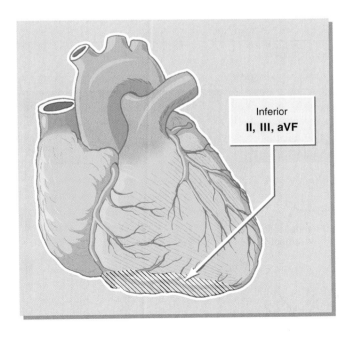

Inferior
II, III, aVF

Less commonly, the **posterior** surface is damaged. The ischemic changes of posterior infarctions are seen in the anterior leads (V_1–V_4), but since those leads face the back side of the damaged area, the changes will be **reciprocal**, or the reverse of what you would see in an anterior MI. Specifically, a posterior infarction will present ST depression (rather than elevation), an upright T wave, and a tall, broad R wave (the Q wave seen in reverse).

When ischemic changes are random across the 12 leads—that is, they fail to correlate readily with coronary artery distribution—it may indicate something other than myocardial ischemia or infarction. **Pericarditis** is the most common cause of widespread or random ischemic changes.

Chamber Enlargement

Excesses of either volume or pressure can cause any of the four heart chambers to enlarge. Chamber enlargement can be due either to *dilation* (increase in internal size of chamber) or to *hypertrophy* (increase in mass of chamber walls). When either happens, the abnormal depolarization waves produce vectors of longer duration and greater magnitude. Atrial enlargement affects P waves, whereas ventricular enlargement affects QRS complexes.

Atrial Enlargement

Atrial enlargement will produce a biphasic P wave in V_1. Right atrial enlargement produces a sharply biphasic P,

with an initial upright deflection that is larger than the terminal deflection. With left atrial enlargement, the P is broad and the terminal, downward deflection is larger than the initial deflection (Figure D11).

In Lead II, the P wave of right atrial enlargement will characteristically be tall (amplitude > 7.25 mm) and peaked, with a normal duration (0.10 second or less). This distinctive P wave is called *P pulmonale*. Left atrial enlargement produces a broad, notched P (0.11 second or more) in Lead II, commonly called *P mitrale*.

Ventricular Enlargement

Ventricular enlargement will be seen as unusually high amplitude QRS complexes across all the V leads. Right ventricular enlargement has tall R waves in V_1 and deep S waves in V_6. Left ventricular enlargement produces deep S waves in V_1 and tall R waves in V_6 (Figure D12).

Rule of 35: To verify the presence of left ventricular enlargement, measure the deepest wave in V_1 or V_2 and the tallest wave in V_5 or V_6. If the sum of the two measurements is greater than 35 mm in a patient over 35 years old, the criteria for LVE are satisfied (Figure D13).

Bundle Branch Block

In Chapter 7 of this book you learned about AV Heart Blocks, a type of heart block that originates in the area of the AV node and can be identified on a single-lead monitoring strip.

There is another kind of block, called **bundle branch block** (BBB), that originates below the AV node within the

Figure D11 Atrial Enlargement

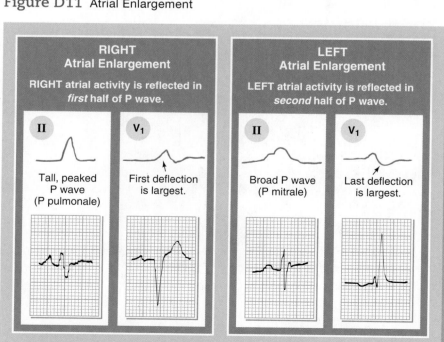

Figure D12 Ventricular Enlargement

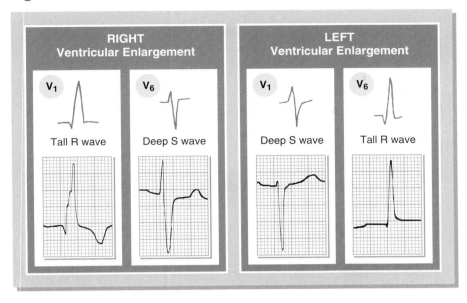

Figure D13 Rule of 35

RULE OF 35	
Criteria for Left Ventricular Enlargement	
1	Measure depth of deepest wave in V_1 or V_2.
2	Add height of tallest wave in V_5 or V_6.
3	If sum is > 35mm and patient is > 35 years old, criteria for LVE are met.

bundle branches. Since conduction above the ventricles is normal, the only abnormal feature of BBB is an unexpectedly wide QRS complex. You'll recall that many of the strips in this book had unexpectedly wide QRS complexes, and you were directed to identify the underlying rhythm and note that it had a "wide QRS." That's because you need more than one lead to determine which of the bundle branches is causing the problem.

A prolonged QRS measurement (> 0.12 second) suggests defective conduction within the bundle branches. This feature will be apparent across all leads, but you look at V_1 and V_6 to determine whether the blockage is in the right or left bundle branch. The normal QRS complex in V_1 has a small R wave and a deep S wave. The normal QRS complex in V_6 has a very small Q wave and a large R wave.

> **Right Bundle Branch Block (RBBB):** In V_1, RBBB produces a notched QRS complex, commonly referred to as "rabbit ears." With RBBB, the QRS complex in V_6 is characterized by a very broad S wave (Figure D14a).
> **Left Bundle Branch Block (LBBB):** In V_1, LBBB produces a small initial R wave, followed by a wide, deep S wave; the QRS complex is predominantly negative

in V_1. In V_6, the R wave is large, very broad, and often notched. There is no Q wave or S wave, so the QRS complex is totally positive in V_6 (Figure D14b).

The QRS changes associated with LBBB obscure the ST changes associated with myocardial injury. Thus, the presence of LBBB greatly reduces the value of the EKG in diagnosing acute MI.

Miscellaneous EKG Abnormalities

A number of drug and electrolyte imbalances cause EKG changes that are detectable on a 12-lead EKG (Figure D15). Some common anomalies are outlined below:

> **Pericarditis:** The injury caused by an inflamed pericardium produces ST changes similar to those of ischemia/infarction. However, they will not correlate with coronary artery distribution.
> **Digitalis:** Digitalis toxicity produces ST changes characterized by a "scooped" appearance. The QT interval is also shortened.
> **Potassium:** Hyperkalemia produces characteristic peaked T waves and merging of the QRS and T waves. Hypokalemia is reflected in flat T waves, widening of QRS complexes, and appearance of U waves.
> **Calcium:** Hypercalcemia produces QT intervals that are unexpectedly short for the rate, whereas in hypocalcemia, the QT intervals are longer than expected.

The types of EKG changes suggestive of these various effects are outlined in Figure D16.

Figure D14 (a) Right Bundle Branch Block; (b) Left Bundle Branch Block

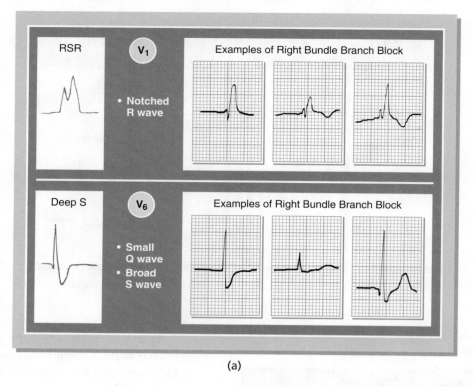

(a)

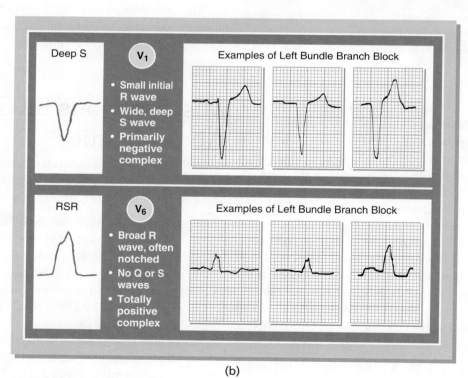

(b)

Analysis Format

As with arrhythmia interpretation, the key to easy and effective analysis of 12-lead EKGs is use of a methodical process (Figure D17). There are many acceptable formats, and you will adjust your approach in response to the context. However, it is advisable to develop a routine approach and use it regularly until it becomes second nature to you. One such approach is outlined below.

Context: Before beginning analysis, consider the context in which you find yourself looking at the EKG.

Figure D15 Miscellaneous Changes

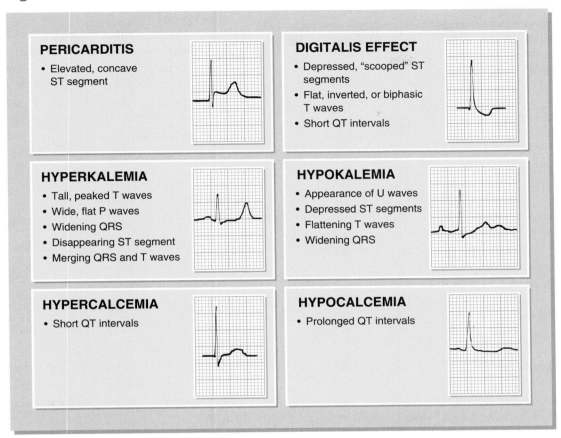

PERICARDITIS
- Elevated, concave ST segment

DIGITALIS EFFECT
- Depressed, "scooped" ST segments
- Flat, inverted, or biphasic T waves
- Short QT intervals

HYPERKALEMIA
- Tall, peaked T waves
- Wide, flat P waves
- Widening QRS
- Disappearing ST segment
- Merging QRS and T waves

HYPOKALEMIA
- Appearance of U waves
- Depressed ST segments
- Flattening T waves
- Widening QRS

HYPERCALCEMIA
- Short QT intervals

HYPOCALCEMIA
- Prolonged QT intervals

Figure D16 Miscellaneous Abnormalities

	Abnormality …	Suggestive of …
P Waves	• wide, flat P waves • no P waves	Hyperkalemia
QRS Complexes	• widening of QRS • merging QRS and T • widening of QRS • prolonged QT interval • short QT interval • short QT interval	Hyperkalemia Hypokalemia Hypocalcemia Hypercalcemia Digitalis Toxicity
ST Segments	• disappearing ST segments • ST depression • sloping ST segments • depressed, "scooped" ST segments • elevated, concave ST segments	Hyperkalemia Hypokalemia Digitalis Toxicity Pericarditis
T Waves	• tall, peaked T waves • flattening of T wave • diphasic or inverted T waves	Hyperkalemia Hypokalemia Digitalis Toxicity
U Waves	• development of U waves	Hypokalemia

Why was it ordered? Is this a middle-aged patient with sudden onset of chest pain, diaphoresis, and shortness of breath? Is this a repeat EKG on a post-operative orthopedic patient whose pre-op EKG had non-specific changes? Is it a pre-admission EKG for an elective admission? Is the patient stable or coding? Are you looking for something specific, or just "fishing"? The context often guides the order in which you approach the tracing and may dictate the depth of your analysis.

Figure D17 Analysis Format for 12-Lead EKG Interpretation

STEP	LOOK FOR	LOOK AT
1	Rhythm	Rhythm strip
2	Axis deviation	I, aVF
3	Bundle branch block	V_1, V_6
4	Ischemia/infarction	V_1, V_4 II, III, aVF I, aVL, V_5, V_6
5	Chamber enlargement	V_1, II
6	Miscellaneous changes	All leads

Rhythm: Look first at the rhythm strip at the bottom of the page to identify the underlying rhythm and rate. Name the arrhythmia and note its potential to impact perfusion.

Axis Deviation: Check Lead I and aVF to determine axis. An underlying axis abnormality affects vectors of all leads, so it should be ruled out before drawing conclusions from the remainder of the tracing.

Bundle Branch Block: Look at V_1 and V_6 to detect bundle branch block. It's useful to identify conduction defects before looking for ischemic changes because the ST pattern of left bundle branch block can obscure the ST changes associated with myocardial ischemia and infarction.

Ischemia and Infarction: This step has many components and involves virtually all leads. The major clusters are the anterior leads (V_1–V_4), the inferior leads (II, III, and aVF), and the lateral leads (I, aVL, and V_5–V_6).

Chamber Enlargement: A thorough 12-lead analysis will include inspection for both atrial and ventricular enlargement. The best leads for analyzing atrial enlargement are V_1 and Lead II, while ventricular enlargement is best viewed in V_1 and V_6.

Miscellaneous Changes: The final inspection goes back over all leads to look for fine points indicative of chemical, metabolic, or mechanical disorders.

Summary of Findings

Your summary analysis should answer these questions:

1. What's the rhythm? Is it a threat to perfusion?
2. Are there any ischemic changes? If so, which leads? Which wall is involved?
3. Is the axis normal? If not, what is the deviation?
4. Is there a ventricular conduction defect? If so, which branch?
5. Are there signs of hypertrophy? If so, which chambers?
6. Are there any other unusual findings that might indicate drug toxicity, electrolyte imbalance, pericarditis, etc.?

Never forget that it's the patient you treat, not the EKG. All findings should be considered in context of the patient's overall status. See Figure D18.

Figure D18 Summary of EKG Features

ASSESSMENT	LOOK AT	LOOK FOR
Context	Patient, chart	• Clinical condition • Changes over time
Rhythm and Rate	Rhythm strip (Lead II)	• Arrhythmias • Threats to perfusion
Ischemia/Infarction	All leads • V_1–V_4 (anterior) • V_5, V_6, aVL, I (lateral) • II, III, aVF (inferior)	• ST changes • T wave changes • Q waves • Loss of R waves
Axis	Leads I and aVF	• QRS upright in I and aVF (normal axis) • QRS up in I, down in aVF (LAD) • QRS down in I, up in aVF (RAD) • QRS down in I and aVF (ERAD)
Chamber Enlargement	Atrial enlargement V_1 II Ventricular enlargement V_1	*Diphasic P:* • Initial deflection is larger (RAE) • Terminal deflection is larger (LAE) *Unusual P morphology:* • Tall, peaked P wave (RAE) • Notched P wave (LAE) *High-amplitude QRS complexes:* • R wave longer than S (RVE) • Extremely deep S (LVE)
	V_6	• S wave larger than R (RVE) • Extremely tall R (LVE)
Intraventricular Conduction Defects	V_1 V_6	*Wide QRS:* • Notched R wave (RBBB) • Deep, slurred S wave (LBBB) • Broad S wave (RBBB) • Broad notched R wave (LBBB)
Miscellaneous Abnormalities		
• Hyperkalemia	All leads	• Tall, peaked T waves • Wide, flat P waves • Widening of QRS • Disappearing ST segment • Merging QRS and T
• Hypokalemia	All leads	• Flat T waves • Increasingly prominent U waves
• Hypocalcemia	All leads	• Prolonged QT interval (for rate)
• Hypercalcemia	All leads	• Short QT interval (for rate)
• Digitalis Toxicity	All leads	• Sloping ST segment • ST depression • Diphasic or inverted T wave • Short QT interval
• Pericarditis	All leads	• Elevated, concave ST segment • Diffuse ST changes not correlated to coronary vessels

SECTION 1 Introduction
Practice 12-Lead EKGs

In this section, you will find 18 12-lead EKGs for you to practice applying the things you've learned up to this point. These 18 tracings are intentionally "simplified" to get you used to looking at 12-leads. That means that each of the 12 leads has been reduced to a single complex, rather than the usual 2-4 complexes. This helps you get the feel of a 12-lead without becoming overwhelmed.

Following these 18 "simplified" tracings, you'll find another 20 tracings in Section 2. The tracings in Section 2 have not been simplified. They are just the way they come out of the EKG machine. By the time you get to Section 2, you should be comfortable enough to find your way around the format.

Approach each tracing in the methodical format you learned in Figure D17. Look at Rhythm, Axis, Bundle Branch Block, Ischemia/Infarction, Chamber Enlargement, and finally Miscellaneous Changes.

Figure D19 12-Lead EKG—Practice Tracing #1

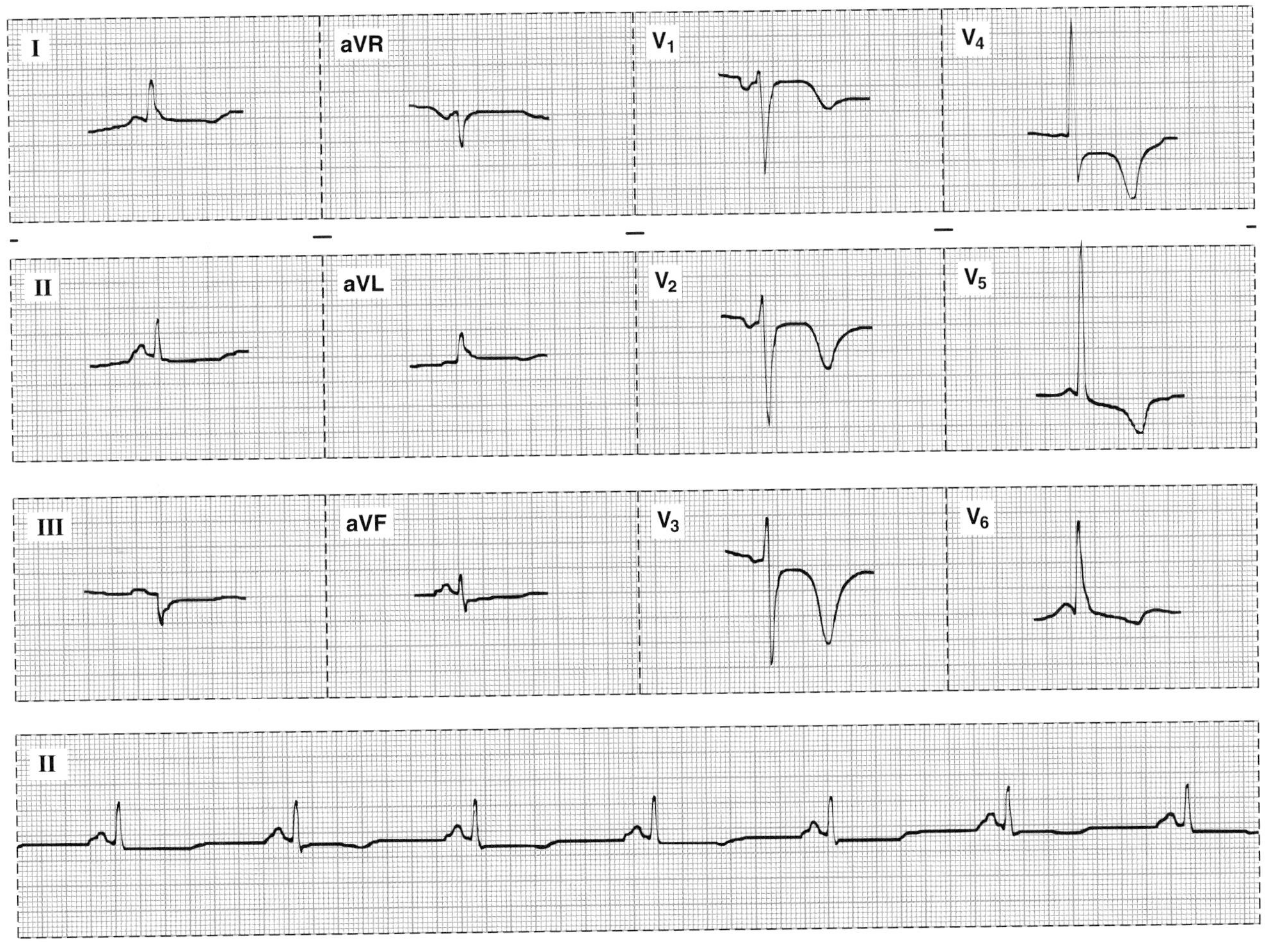

SIGNIFICANT FINDINGS

- Sinus Rhythm, rate 72 bpm

- Left Atrial Enlargement

- Left Ventricular Enlargement

- Acute anterior ischemia

Figure D20 12-Lead EKG—Practice Tracing #2

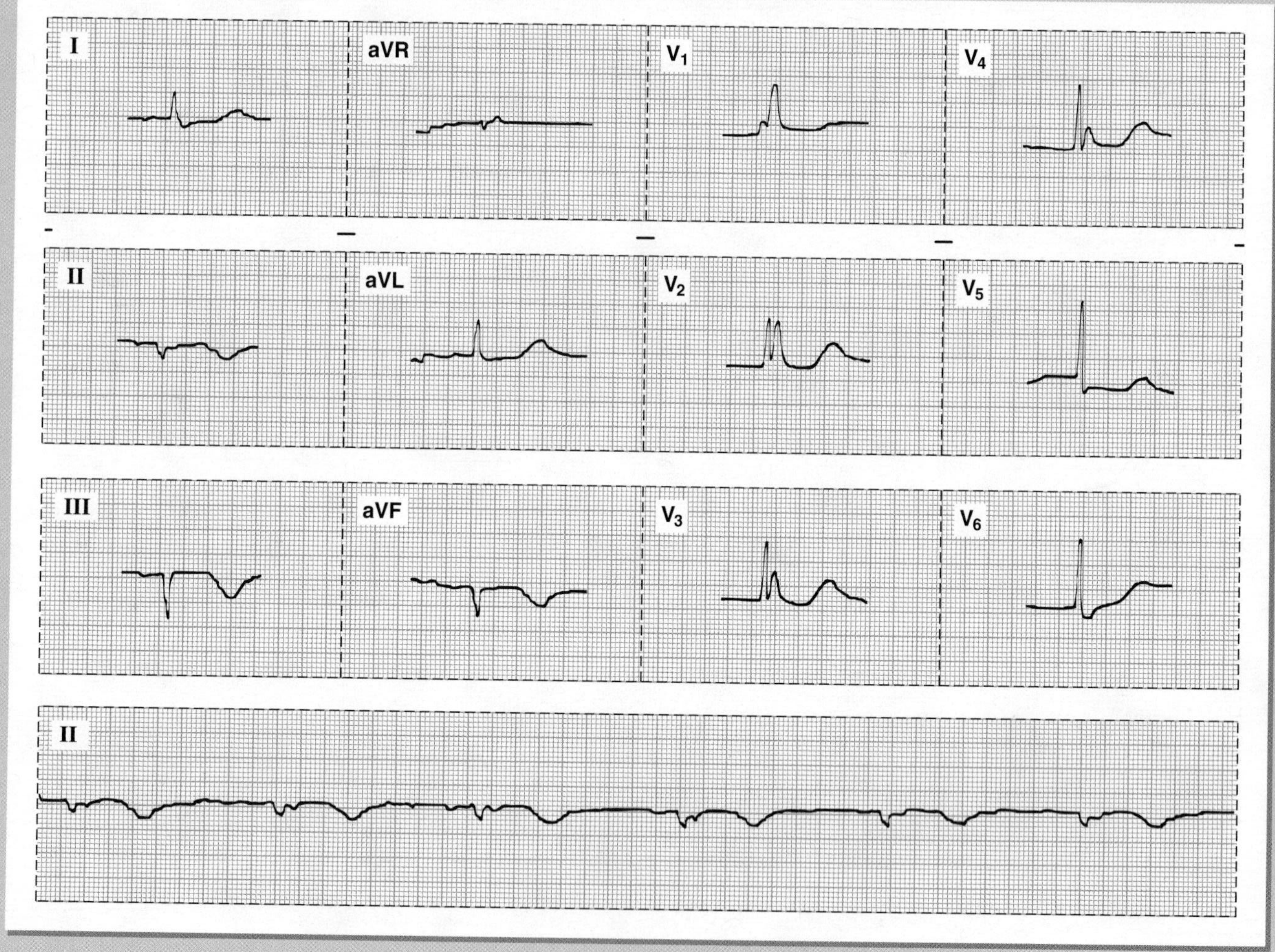

SIGNIFICANT FINDINGS

- Sinus rhythm, rate 60 bpm
- Left axis deviation
- Inferior wall ischemia (acute evolving inferior wall MI)
- Right bundle branch block

Figure D21 12-Lead EKG—Practice Tracing #3

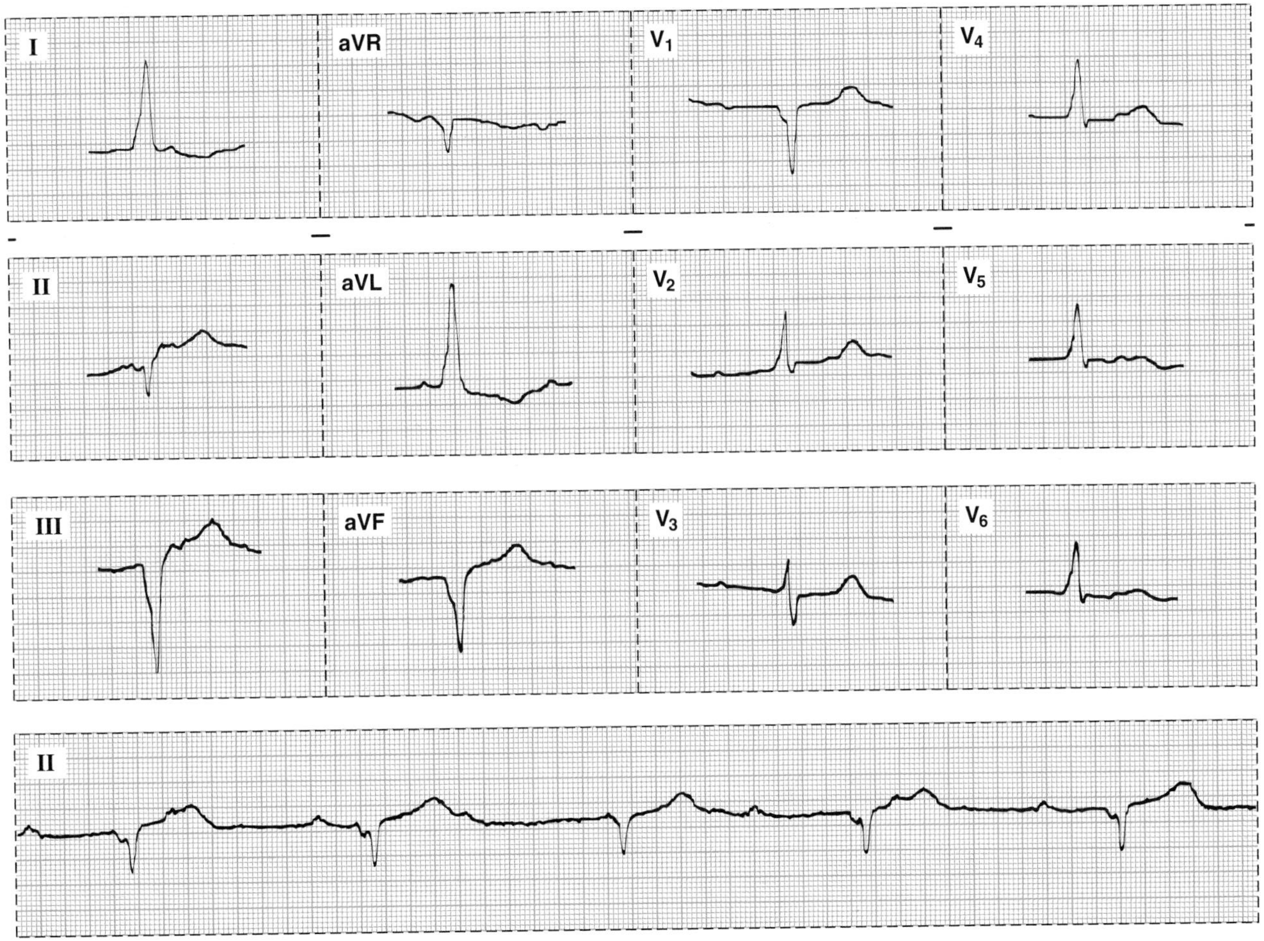

SIGNIFICANT FINDINGS

- Third-degree AV block (CHB) with junctional escape pacemaker
  —atrial rate: 84 bpm
  —ventricular rate: 50 bpm (irregular rhythm)

- Left bundle branch block

- Left axis deviation

NOTE: The underlying rhythm is potentially lethal, making it the most important feature of this EKG.

Figure D22 12-Lead EKG—Practice Tracing #4

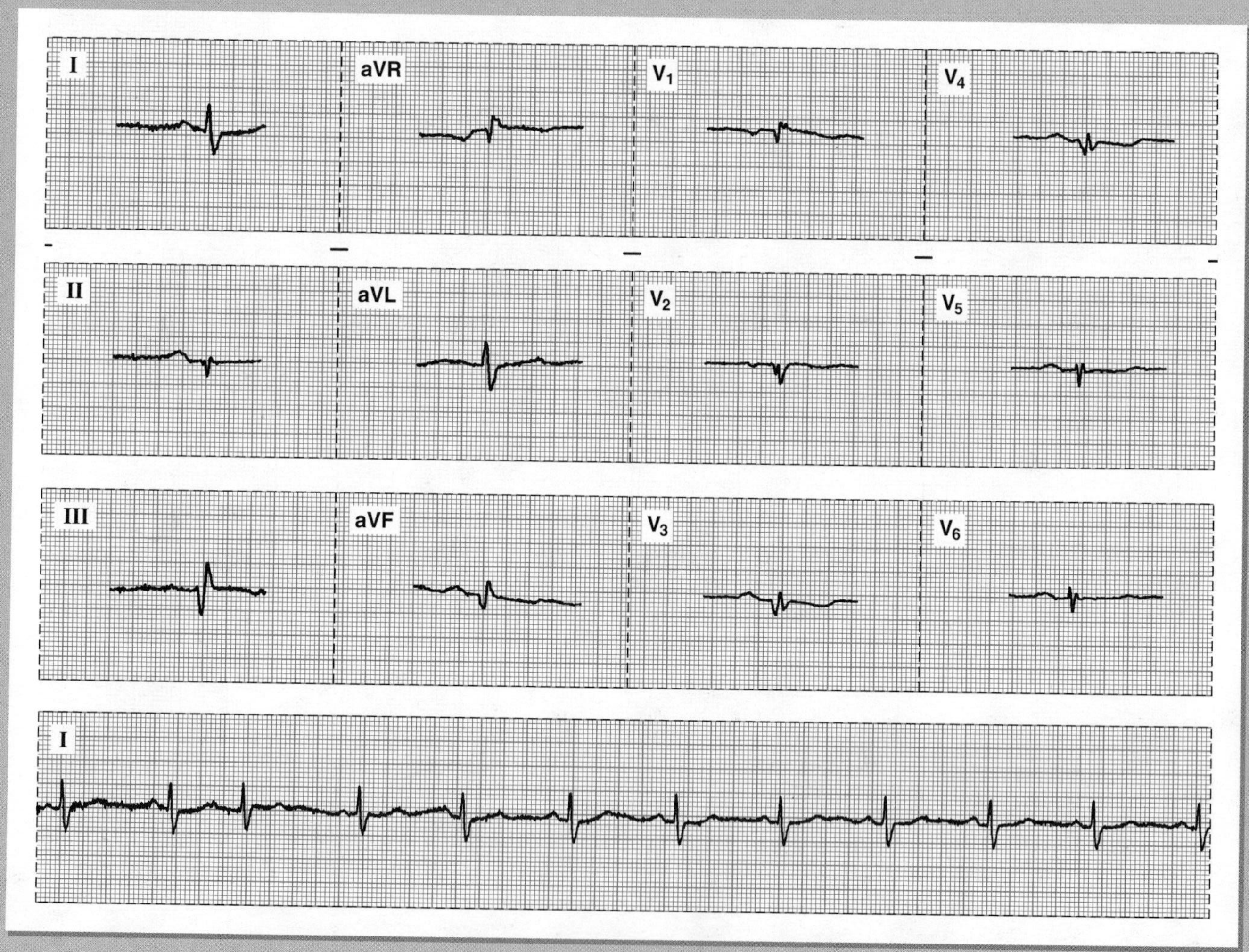

SIGNIFICANT FINDINGS

- Sinus rhythm, rate 67 bpm
- Premature atrial complex
- Inferior infarct, age indeterminate
- Anterolateral infarct, age indeterminate

Figure D23 12-Lead EKG—Practice Tracing #5

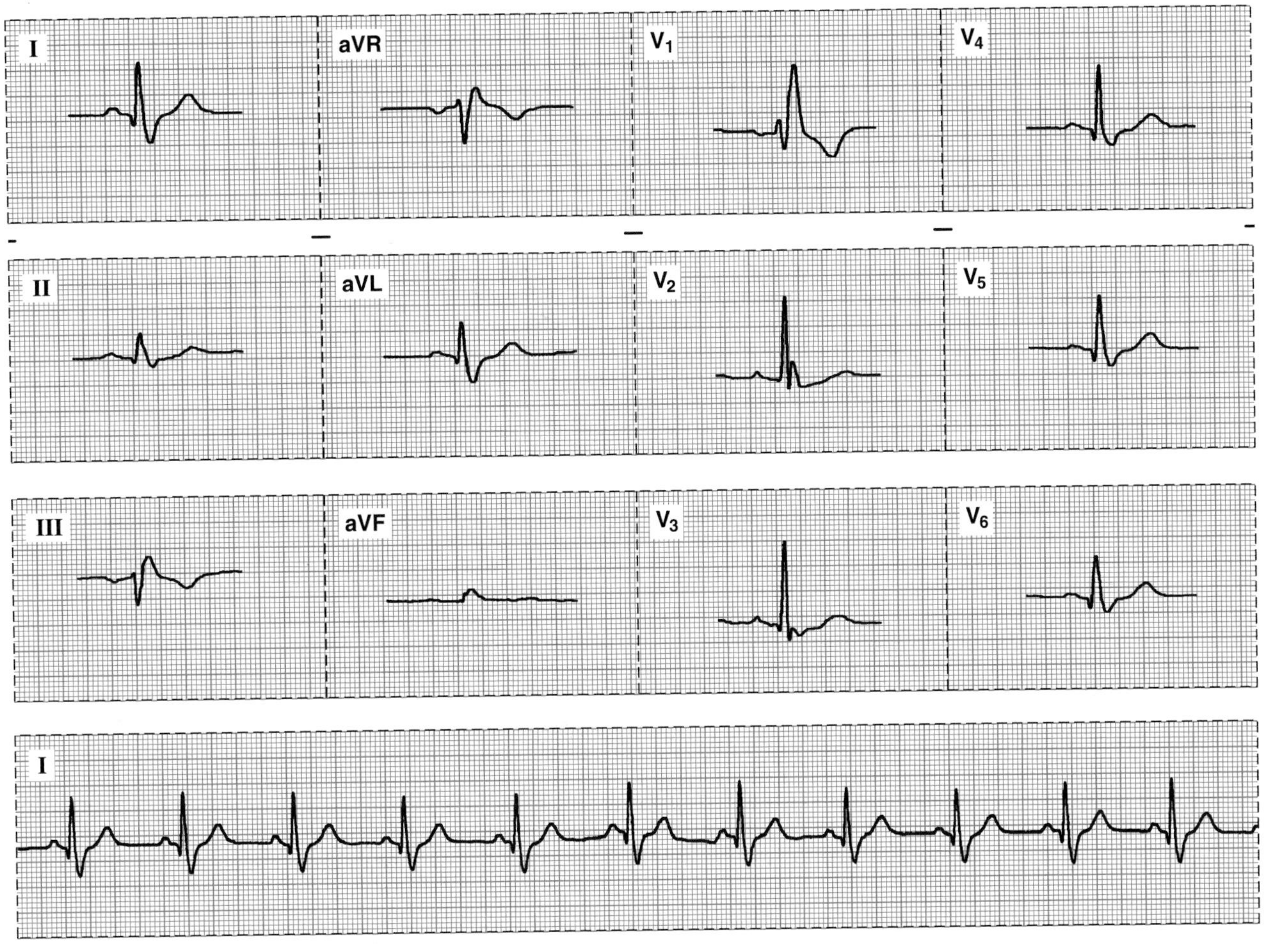

SIGNIFICANT FINDINGS

- Sinus rhythm, rate 69 bpm
- Right bundle branch block
- Possible lateral infarct

Figure D24 12-Lead EKG—Practice Tracing #6

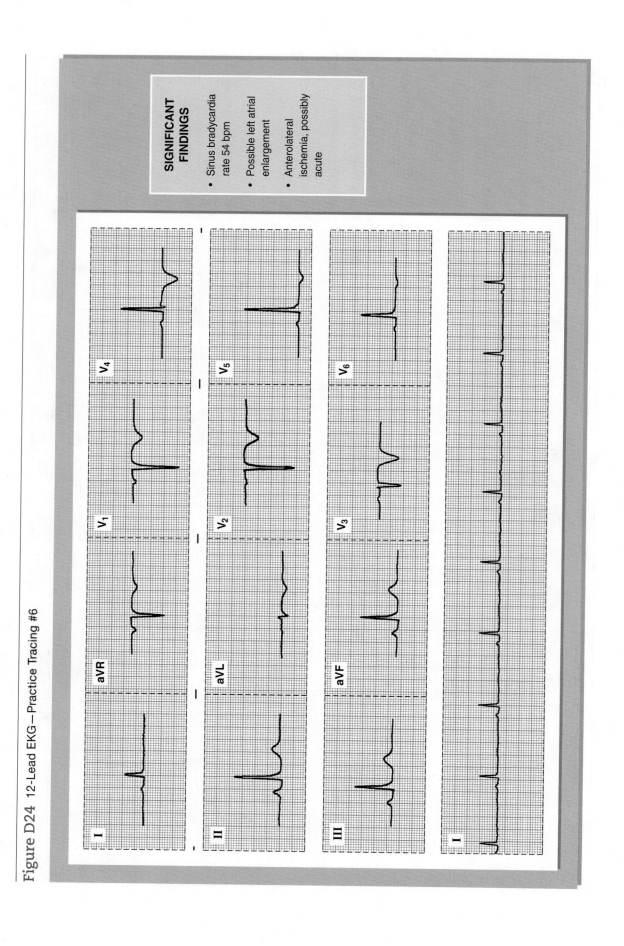

SIGNIFICANT FINDINGS

- Sinus bradycardia rate 54 bpm
- Possible left atrial enlargement
- Anterolateral ischemia, possibly acute

Figure D25 12-Lead EKG—Practice Tracing #7

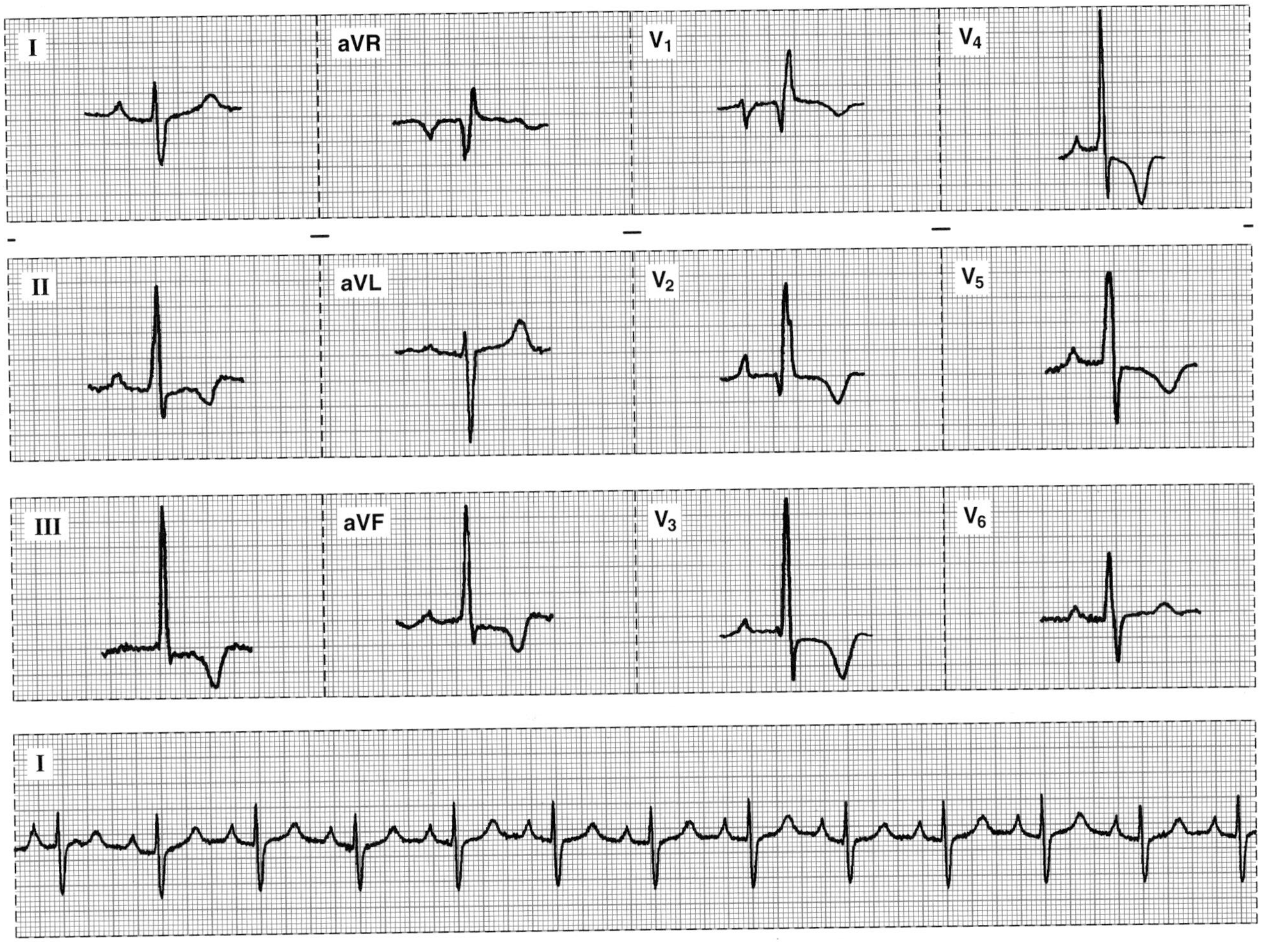

SIGNIFICANT
FINDINGS

- Sinus rhythm, rate 77 bpm
- First-degree heart block
- Incomplete right bundle branch block
- Biatrial enlargement
- Probable anteroseptal MI, age indeterminate

491

Figure D26 12-Lead EKG—Practice Tracing #8

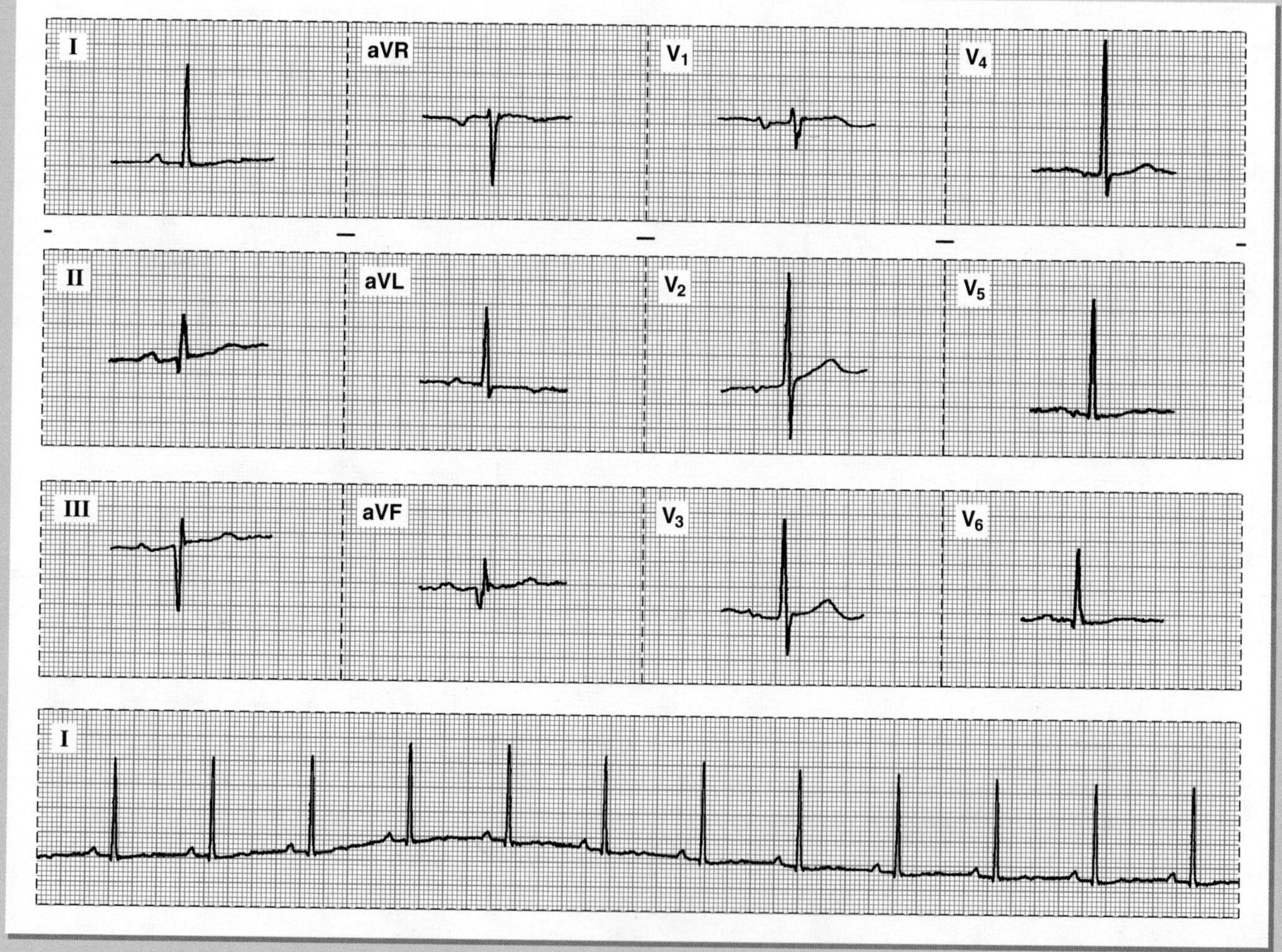

SIGNIFICANT FINDINGS

- Sinus rhythm, rate 76 bpm
- Left atrial enlargement
- Inferior infarct

Figure D27 12-Lead EKG—Practice Tracing #9

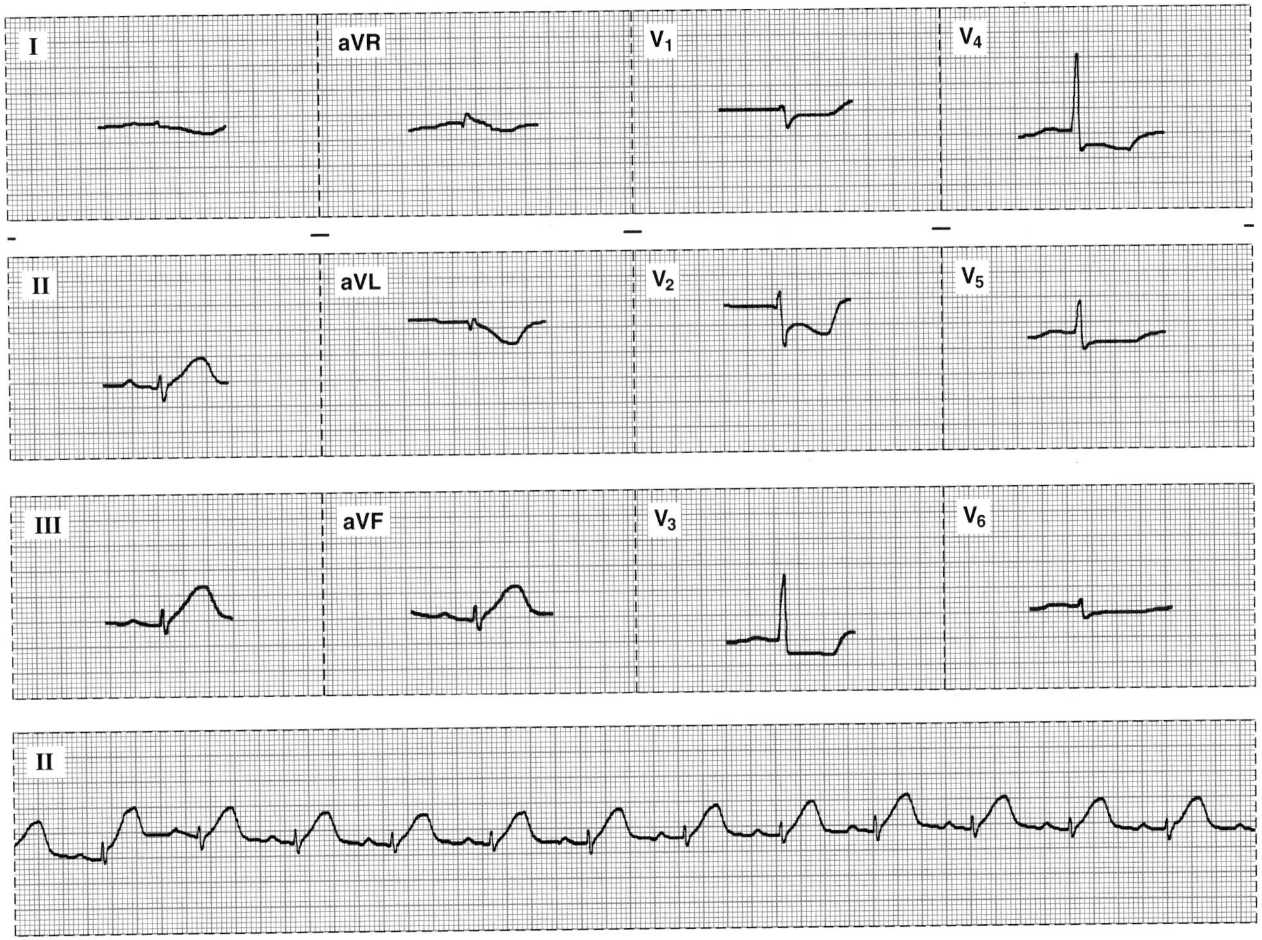

SIGNIFICANT FINDINGS

- Sinus rhythm, rate is 86 bpm

- Acute inferior subepicardial injury

Figure D28 12-Lead EKG—Practice Tracing #10

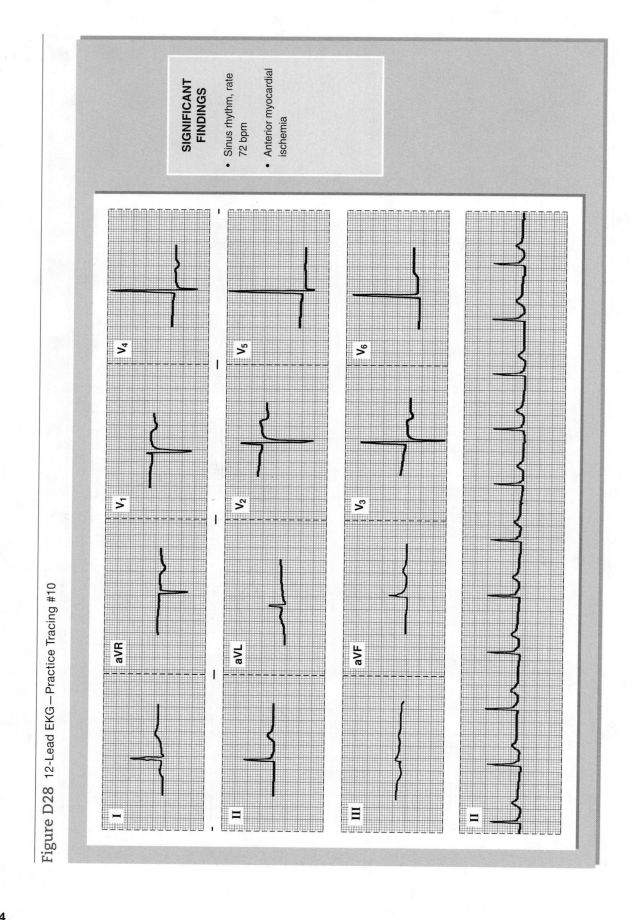

SIGNIFICANT FINDINGS

- Sinus rhythm, rate 72 bpm
- Anterior myocardial ischemia

Figure D29 12-Lead EKG—Practice Tracing #11

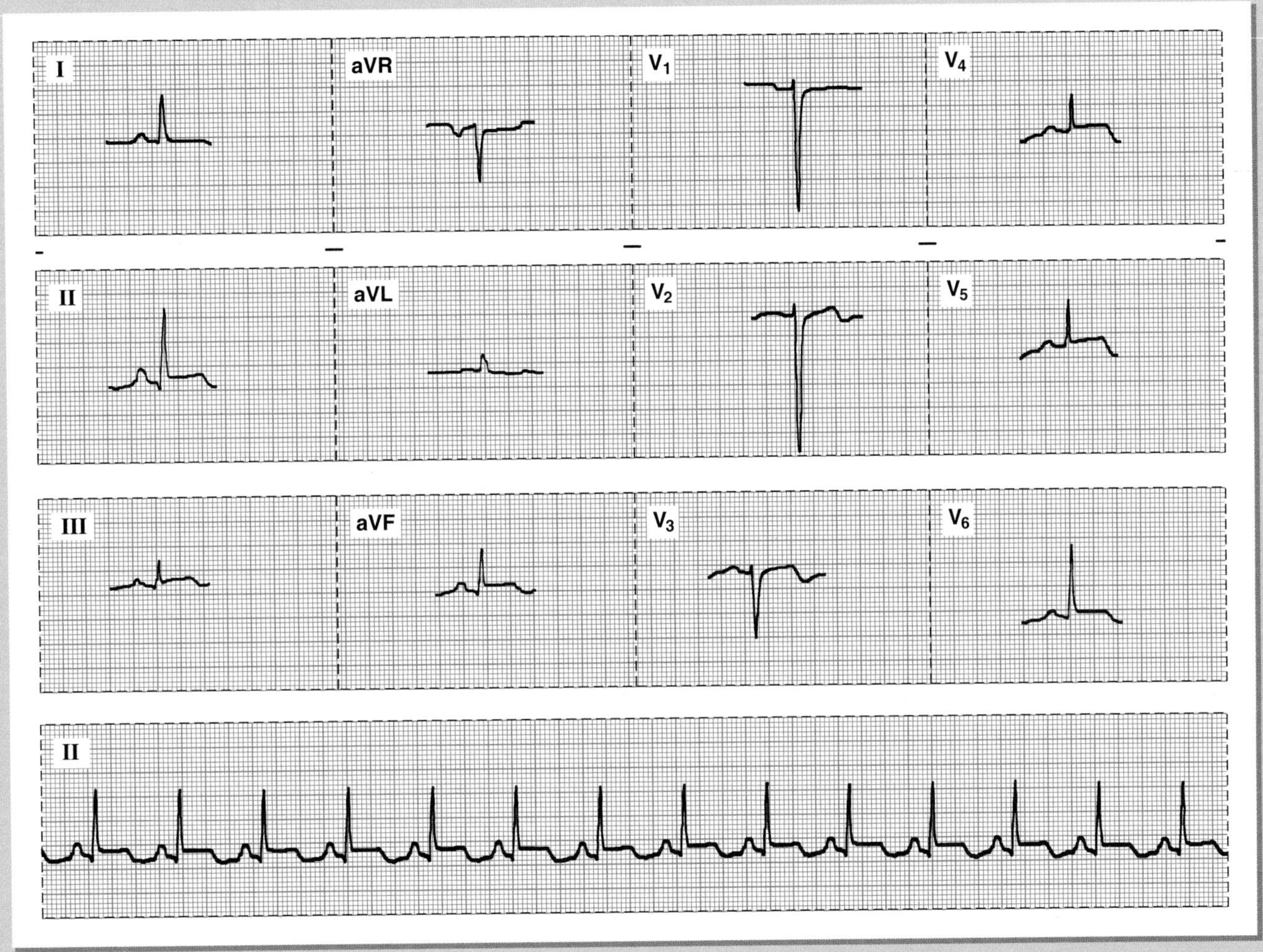

SIGNIFICANT FINDINGS

- Sinus rhythm, rate 100 bpm
- Recent inferior wall MI
- Possible previous anterior MI

Figure D30 12-Lead EKG—Practice Tracing #12

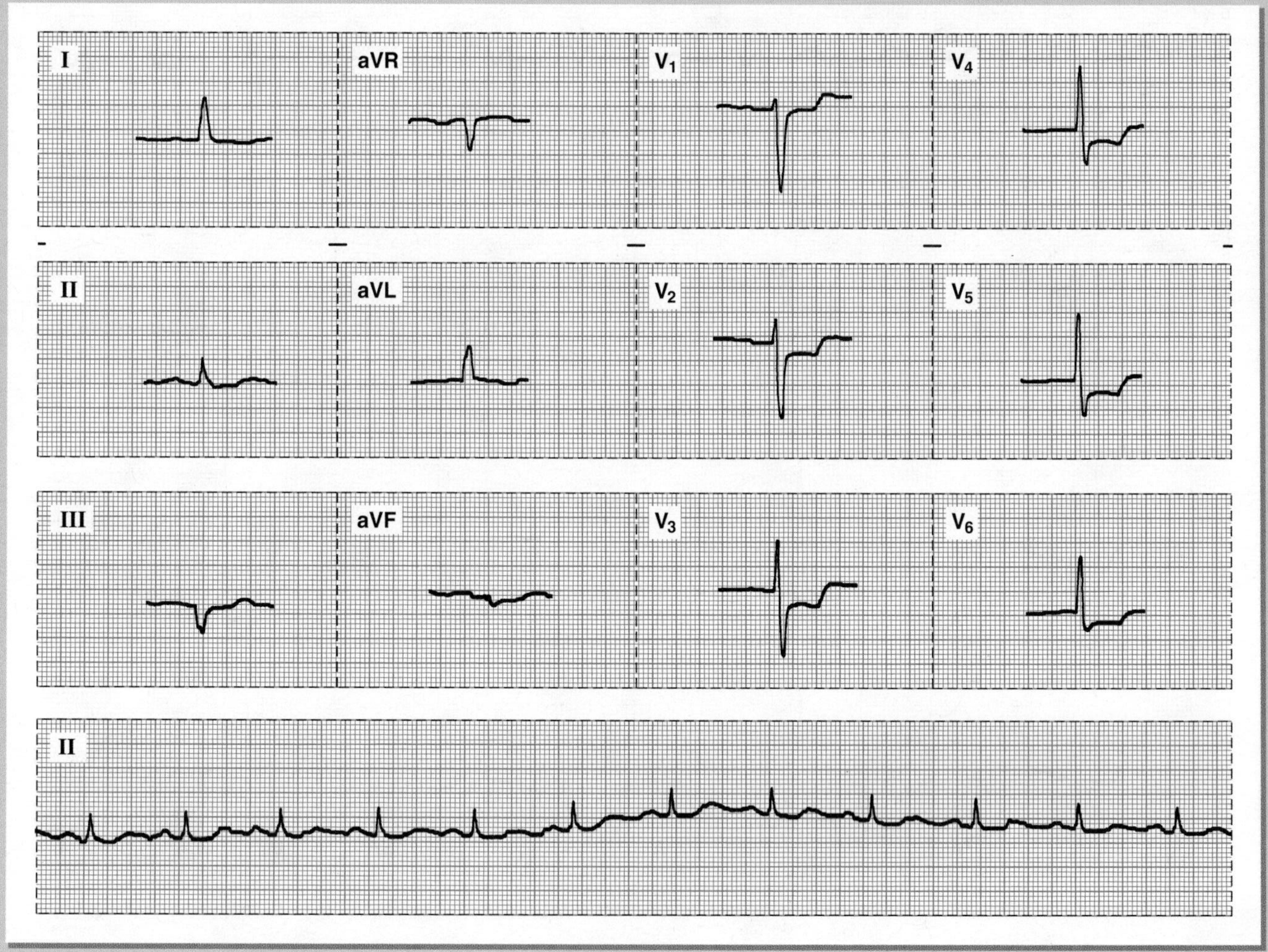

SIGNIFICANT FINDINGS

- Sinus rhythm, rate 82 bpm
- Anterolateral ischemia

I aVR V1 V4

II aVL V2 V5

III aVF V3 V6

II

Figure D31 12-Lead EKG—Practice Tracing #13

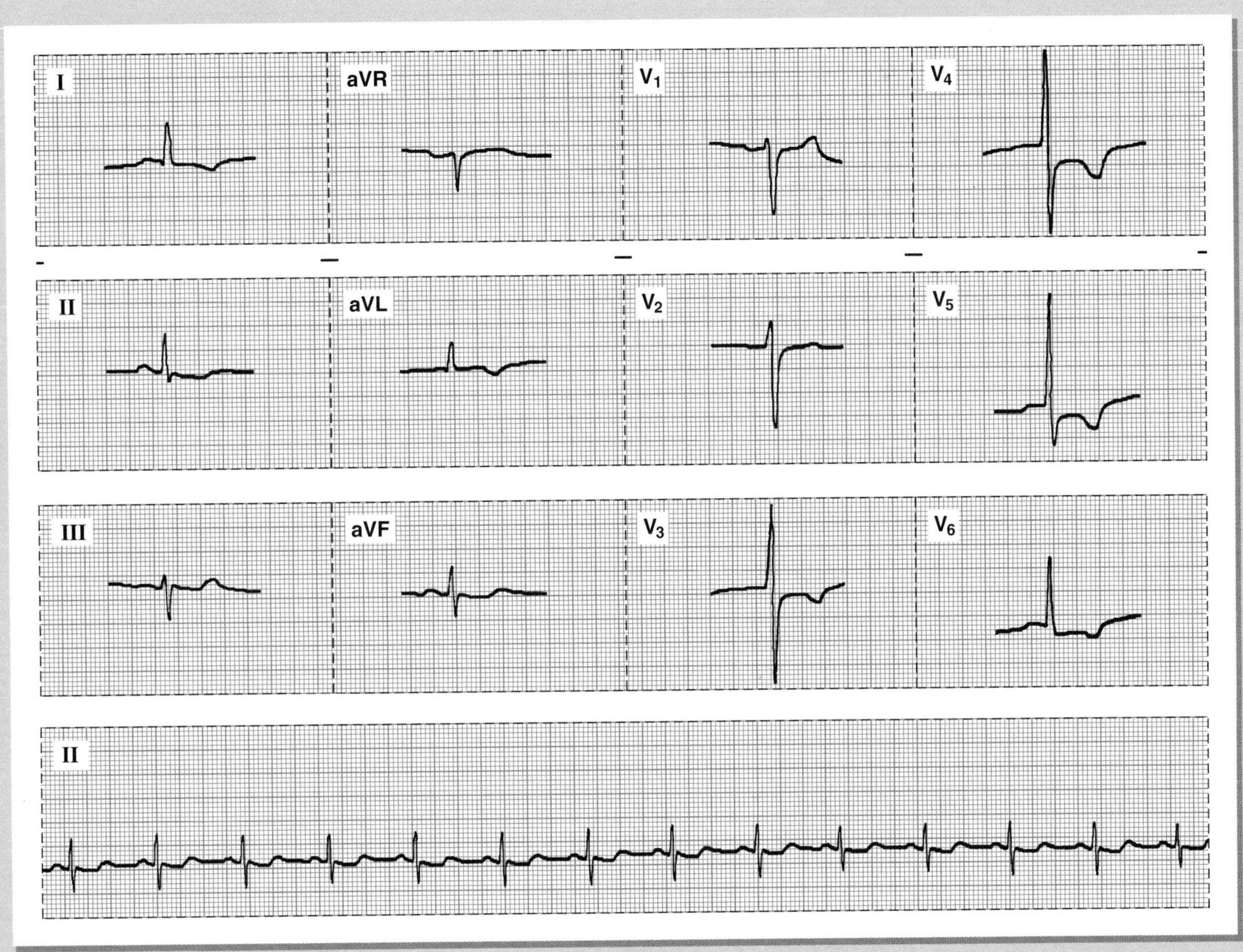

SIGNIFICANT FINDINGS

- Sinus rhythm, rate 79 bpm
- Less-than-transmural MI is possible
- Actual anterolateral ischemia

497

Figure D32 12-Lead EKG—Practice Tracing #14

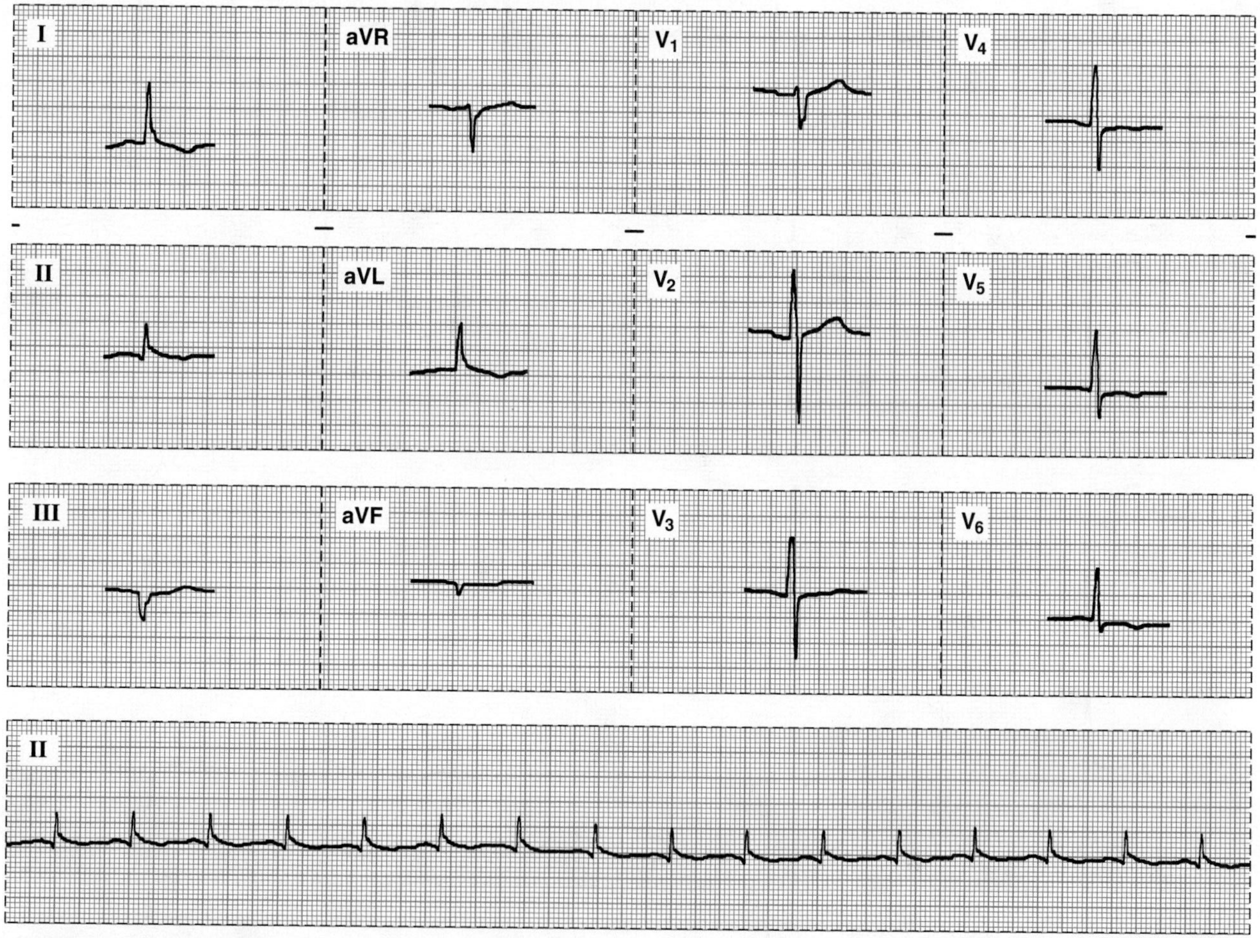

SIGNIFICANT FINDINGS

- Sinus tachycardia, rate 107 bpm
- Old inferior infarct
- Repolarization abnormality consisent with pericarditis following recent surgery

I   aVR   V₁   V₄

II   aVL   V₂   V₅

III   aVF   V₃   V₆

II

Figure D33 12-Lead EKG—Practice Tracing #15

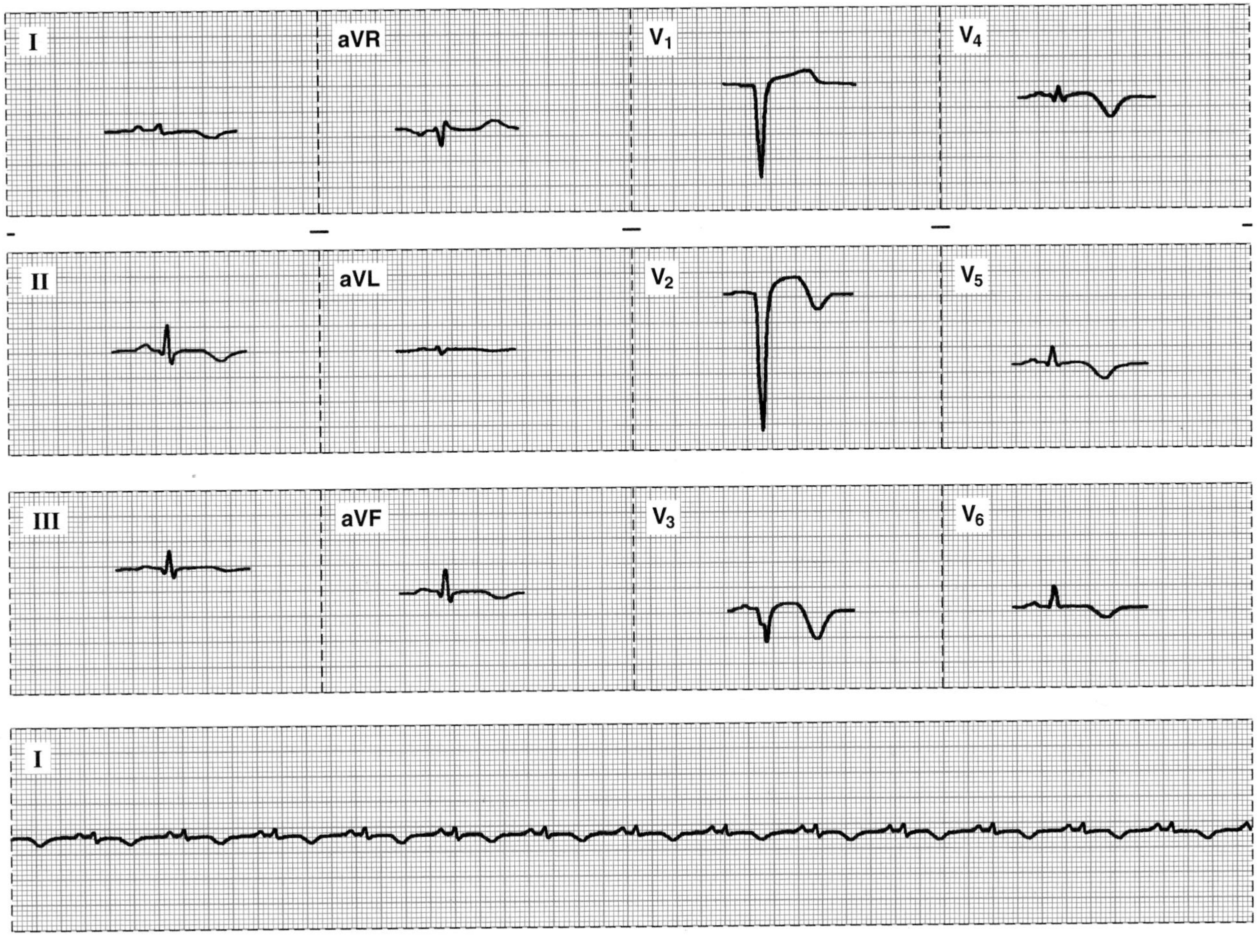

SIGNIFICANT FINDINGS

- Sinus rhythm, rate 85 bpm
- Anterior infarct, age indeterminate
- Diffuse nondiagnostic T wave changes

I   aVR   V₁   V₄

II   aVL   V₂   V₅

III   aVF   V₃   V₆

I

Figure D34 12-Lead EKG—Practice Tracing #16

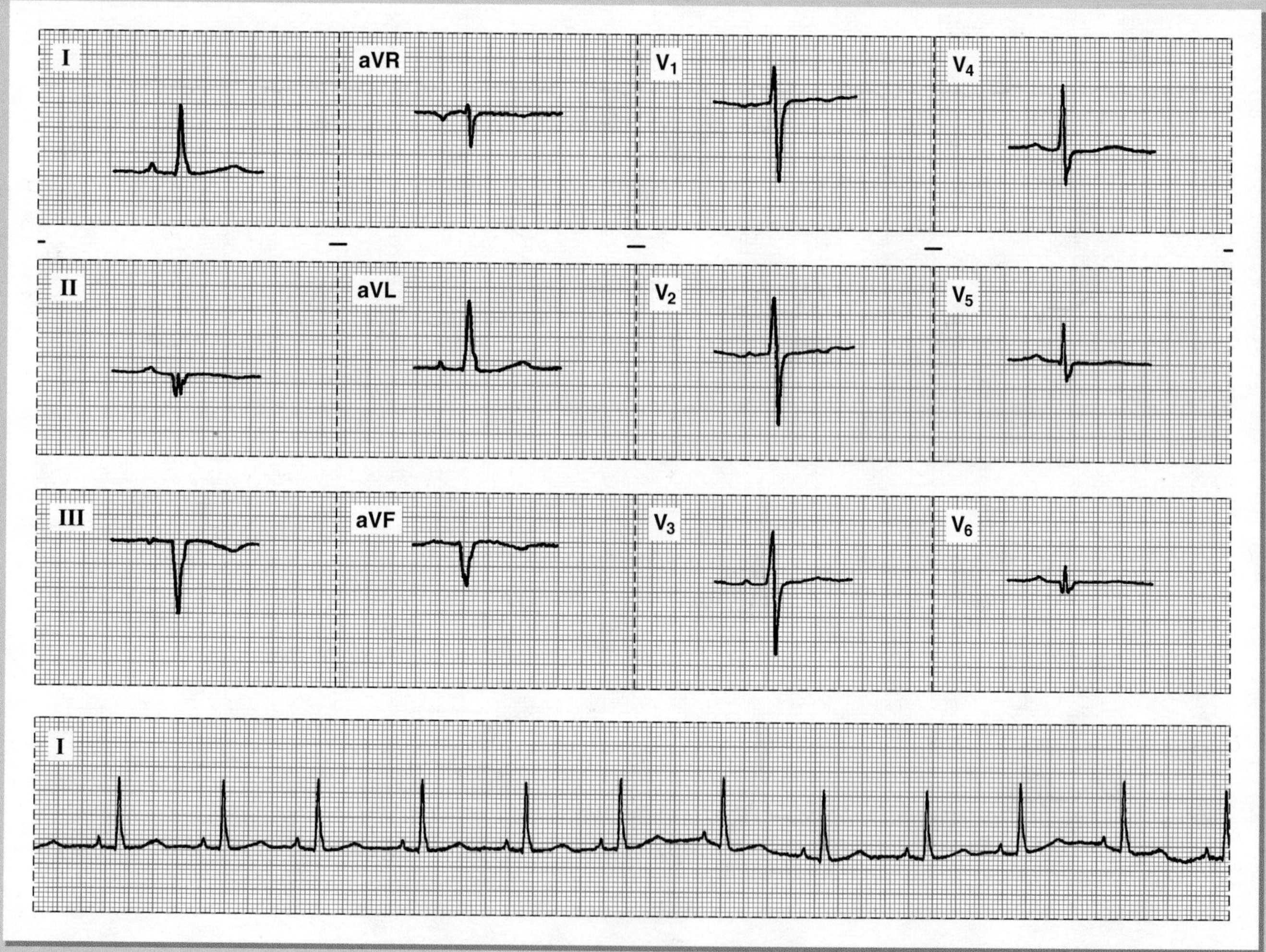

SIGNIFICANT FINDINGS

- Sinus rhythm, rate 73 bpm
- Left axis deviation
- Inferior infarct, age indeterminate
- Nondiagnostic anterolateral T wave changes

Figure D35 12-Lead EKG—Practice Tracing #17

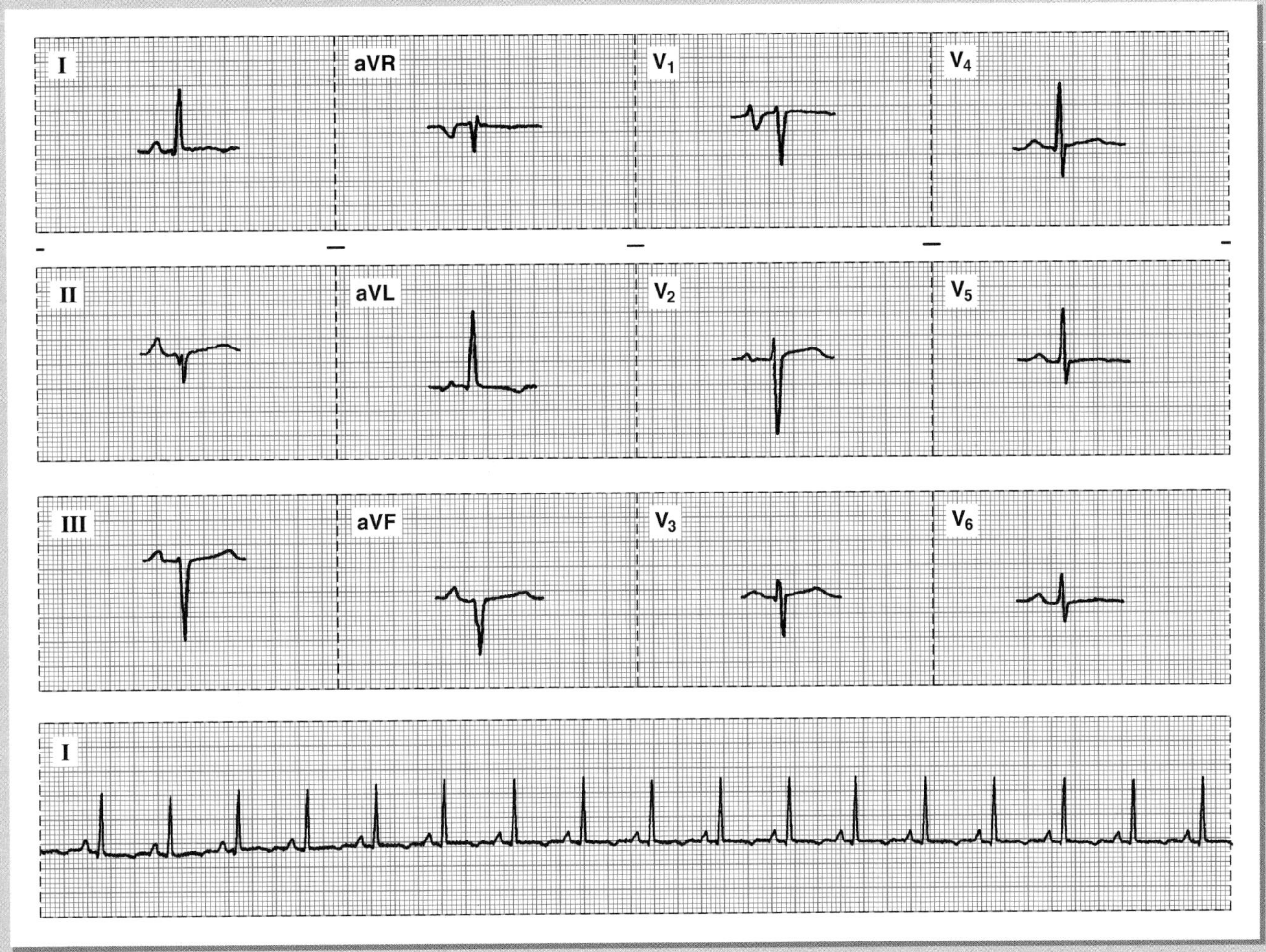

SIGNIFICANT FINDINGS

- Sinus tachycardia, rate 107 bpm
- Left axis deviation
- Left atrial enlargement
- Inferior infarct
- Nondiagnostic lateral T wave changes

Figure D36 12-Lead EKG—Practice Tracing #18

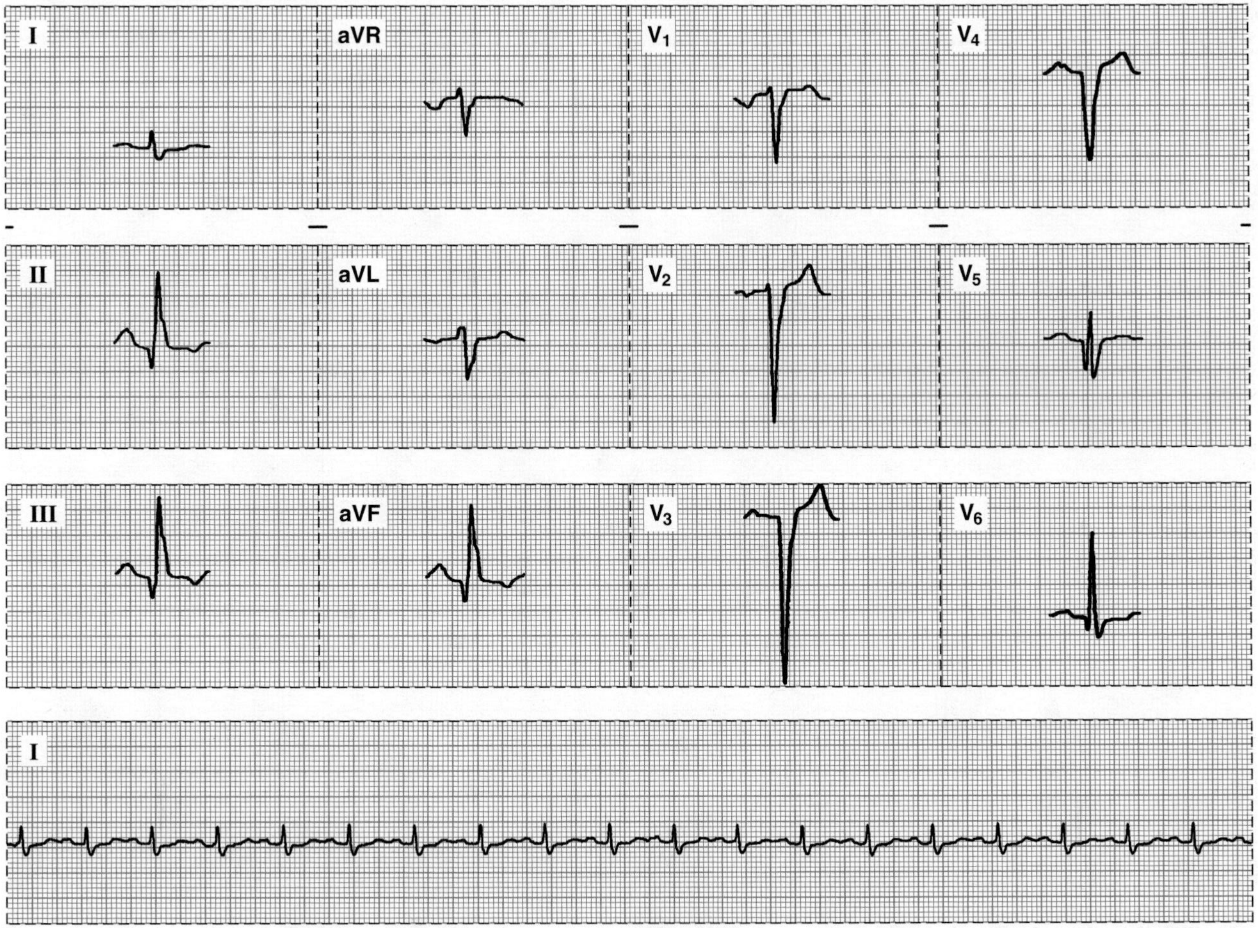

SIGNIFICANT FINDINGS

- Sinus tachycardia, rate 115 bpm
- Right axis deviation
- Inferior infarct, age indeterminate
- Recent anterolateral infarct

SECTION 2 Introduction

Practice 12-Lead EKGs

In this section you'll have an opportunity to practice reading 12-Lead EKGs as they are typically found. Unlike SECTION 1, the EKGs in this section are not simplified as single complexes, but are left in their original state of a running EKG. This will help you transition from a textbook to the "real" EKGs you will find in your work. The purpose of this section is to get you used to "real life" EKGs.

Some of the EKGs are normal while others have various abnormalities. Approach each strip according to the format shown in Figure D17. Consider the Context – why are you taking the EKG? Then analyze Rhythm, Axis Deviation, Bundle Branch Block, Ischemia/Infarction, Chamber Enlargement, and Miscellaneous Changes.

Figure D37 12-Lead EKG—Practice Tracing #19

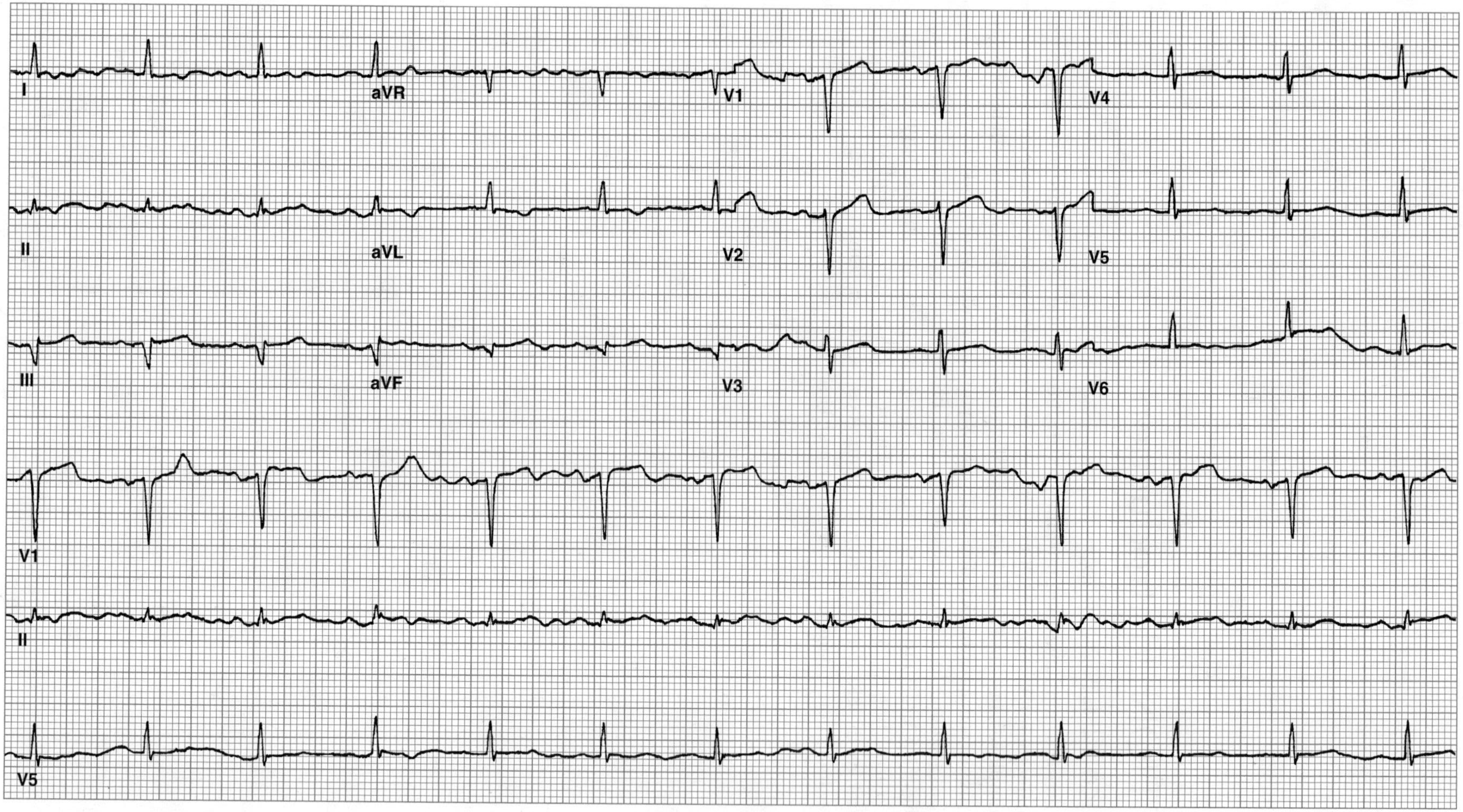

Ventricular Rate	76 bpm	Normal Sinus Rhythm
PR Interval	0.20 sec	Inferior infarct, age undetermined
QRS Duration	0.08 sec	Abnormal EKG

Figure D38 12-Lead EKG—Practice Tracing #20

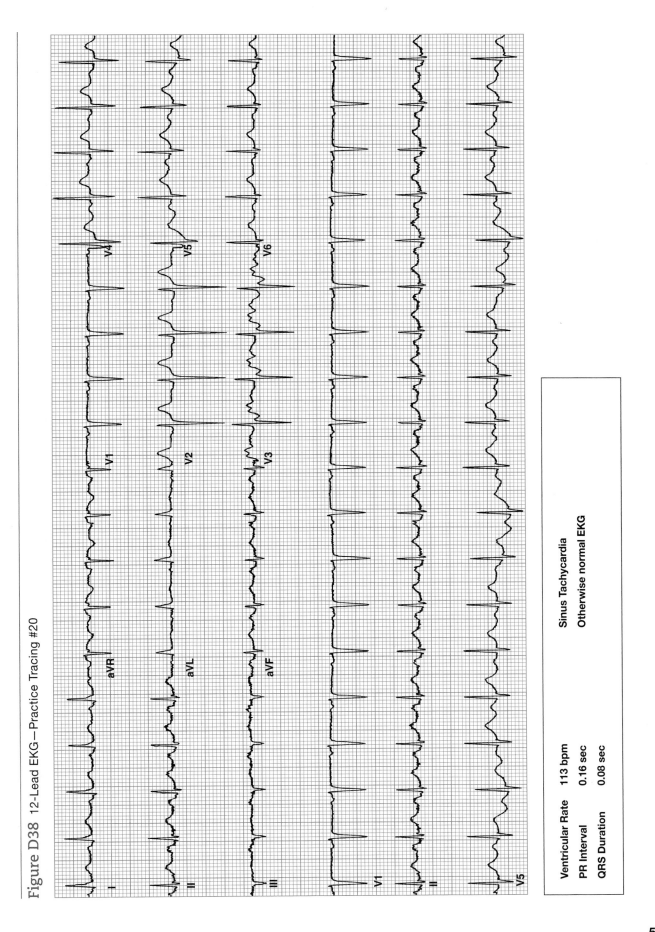

Ventricular Rate	113 bpm	Sinus Tachycardia
PR Interval	0.16 sec	Otherwise normal EKG
QRS Duration	0.08 sec	

Figure D39 12-Lead EKG—Practice Tracing #21

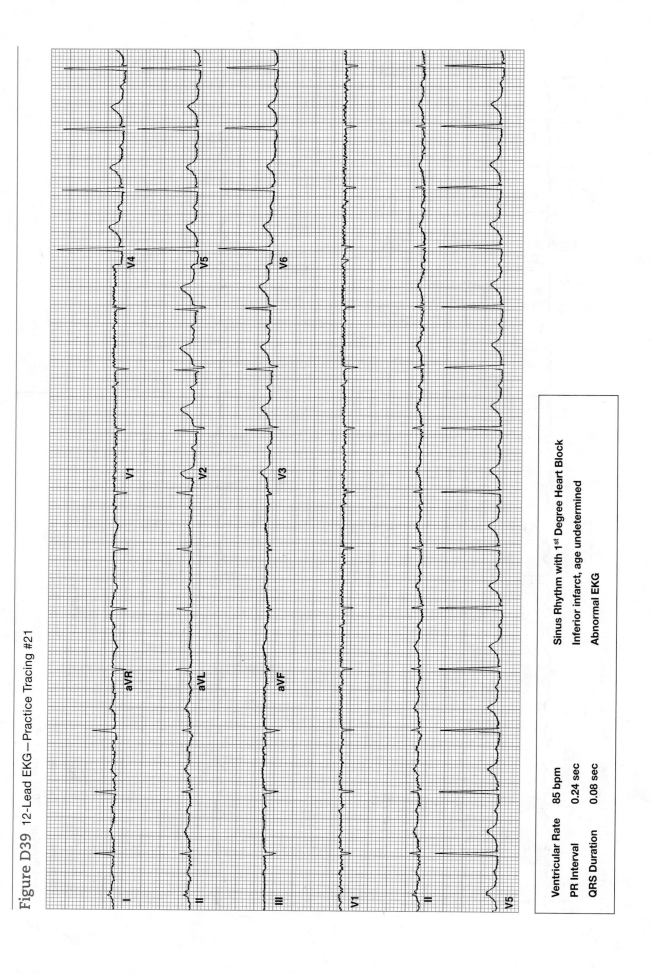

Ventricular Rate	85 bpm	Sinus Rhythm with 1st Degree Heart Block
PR Interval	0.24 sec	Inferior infarct, age undetermined
QRS Duration	0.08 sec	Abnormal EKG

Figure D40 12-Lead EKG—Practice Tracing #22

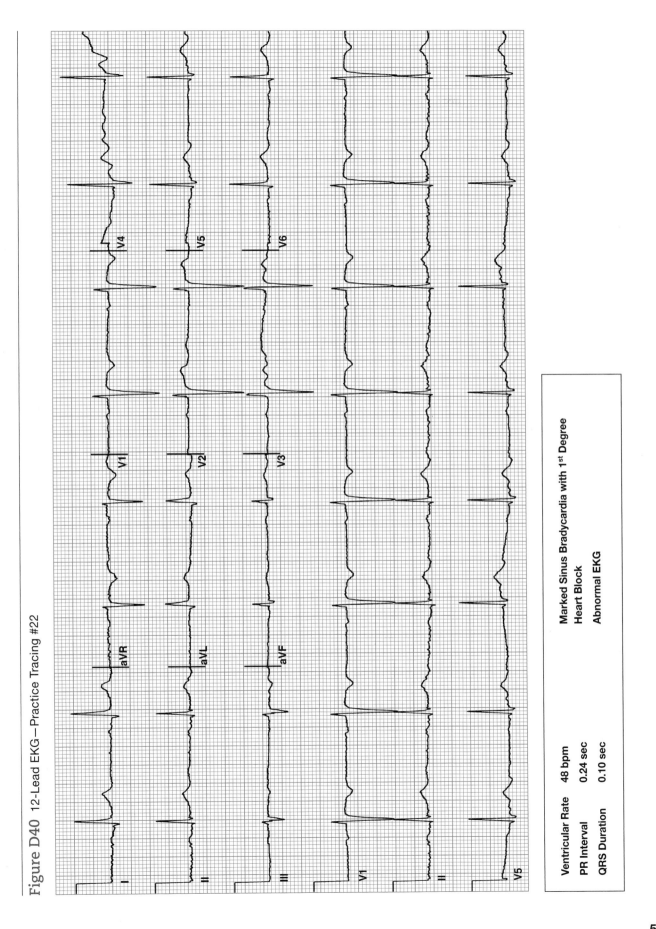

Ventricular Rate	48 bpm
PR Interval	0.24 sec
QRS Duration	0.10 sec

Marked Sinus Bradycardia with 1st Degree
Heart Block
Abnormal EKG

Figure D41 12-Lead EKG—Practice Tracing #23

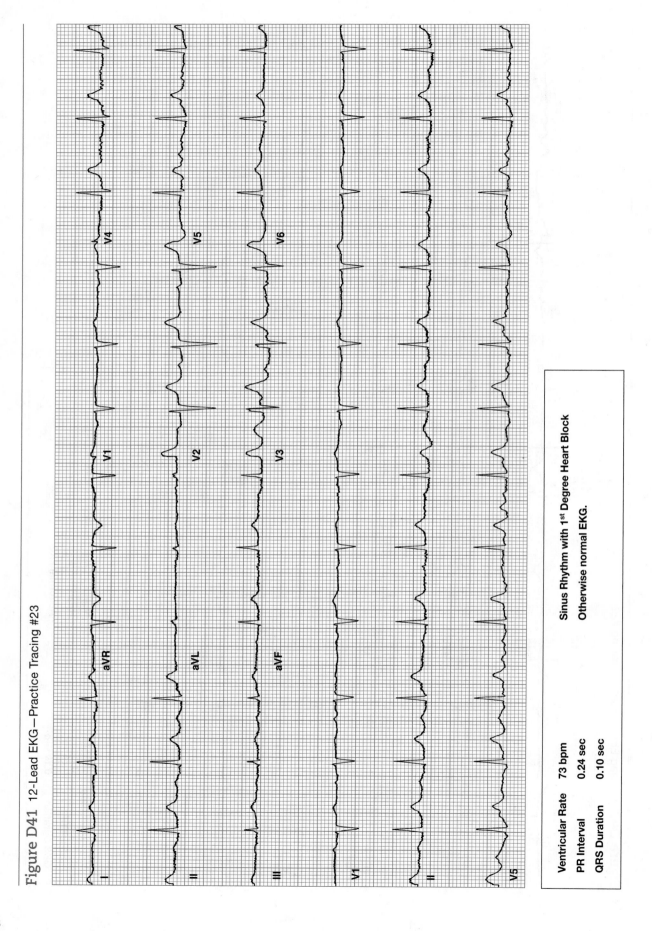

Ventricular Rate	73 bpm	Sinus Rhythm with 1st Degree Heart Block
PR Interval	0.24 sec	Otherwise normal EKG.
QRS Duration	0.10 sec	

Figure D42 12-Lead EKG – Practice Tracing #24

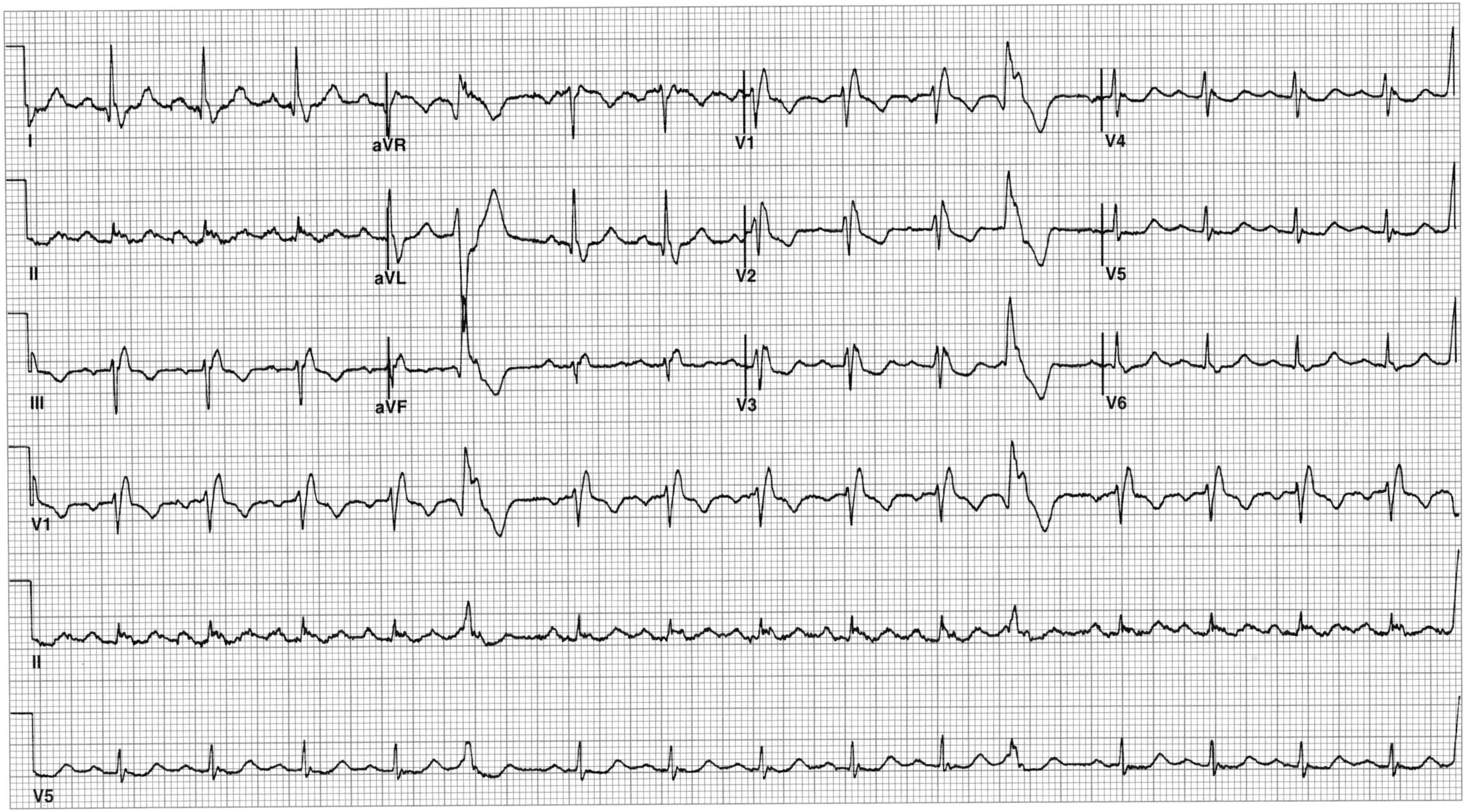

Ventricular Rate	94 bpm	Sinus Rhythm with occasional PVCs
PR Interval	0.20 sec	Possible left atrial enlargement
QRS Duration	0.10 sec	Right Bundle Branch Block
		Abnormal EKG

Figure D43 12-Lead EKG—Practice Tracing #25

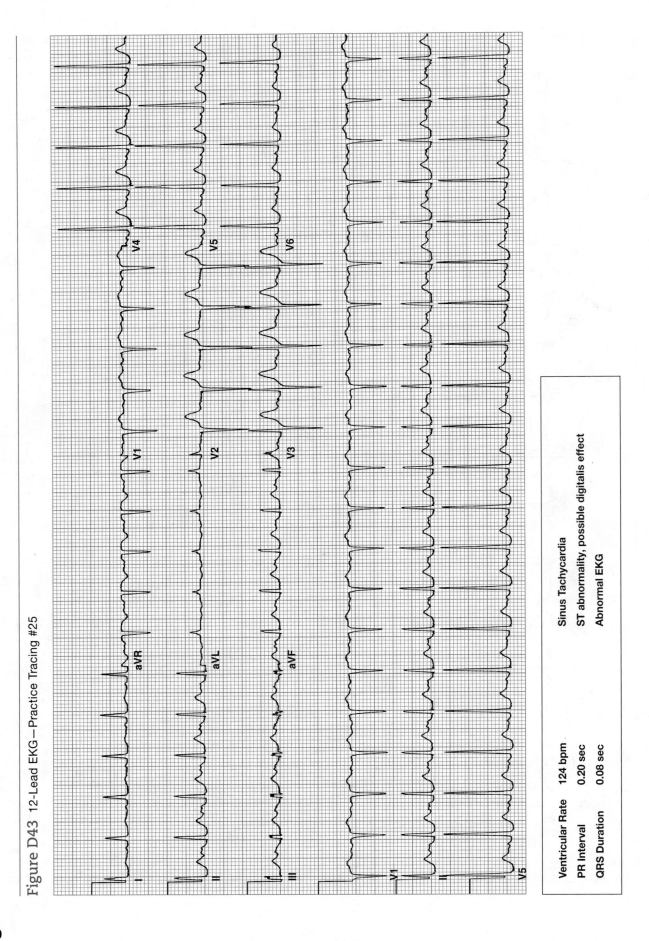

Ventricular Rate	124 bpm	Sinus Tachycardia
PR Interval	0.20 sec	ST abnormality, possible digitalis effect
QRS Duration	0.08 sec	Abnormal EKG

Figure D44 12-Lead EKG—Practice Tracing #26

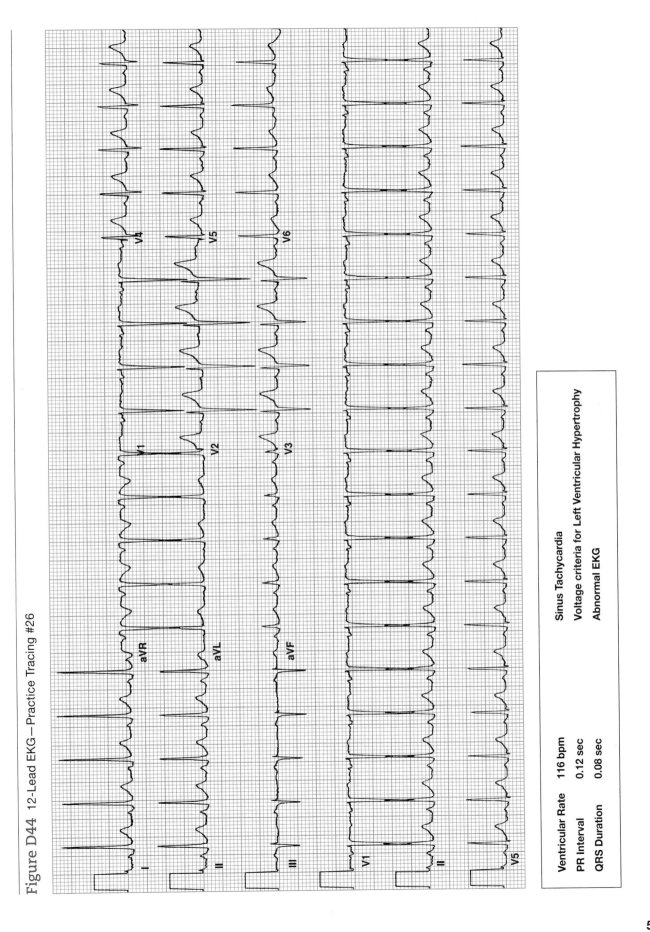

Ventricular Rate	116 bpm	Sinus Tachycardia
PR Interval	0.12 sec	Voltage criteria for Left Ventricular Hypertrophy
QRS Duration	0.08 sec	Abnormal EKG

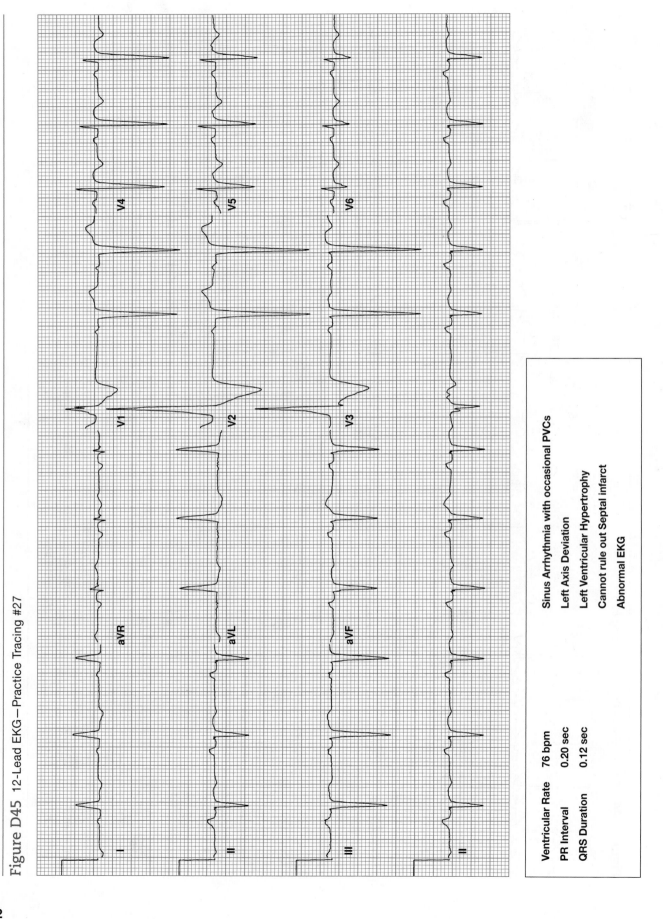

Figure D45 12-Lead EKG—Practice Tracing #27

Ventricular Rate	76 bpm	Sinus Arrhythmia with occasional PVCs
PR Interval	0.20 sec	Left Axis Deviation
QRS Duration	0.12 sec	Left Ventricular Hypertrophy
		Cannot rule out Septal infarct
		Abnormal EKG

Figure D46 12-Lead EKG—Practice Tracing #28

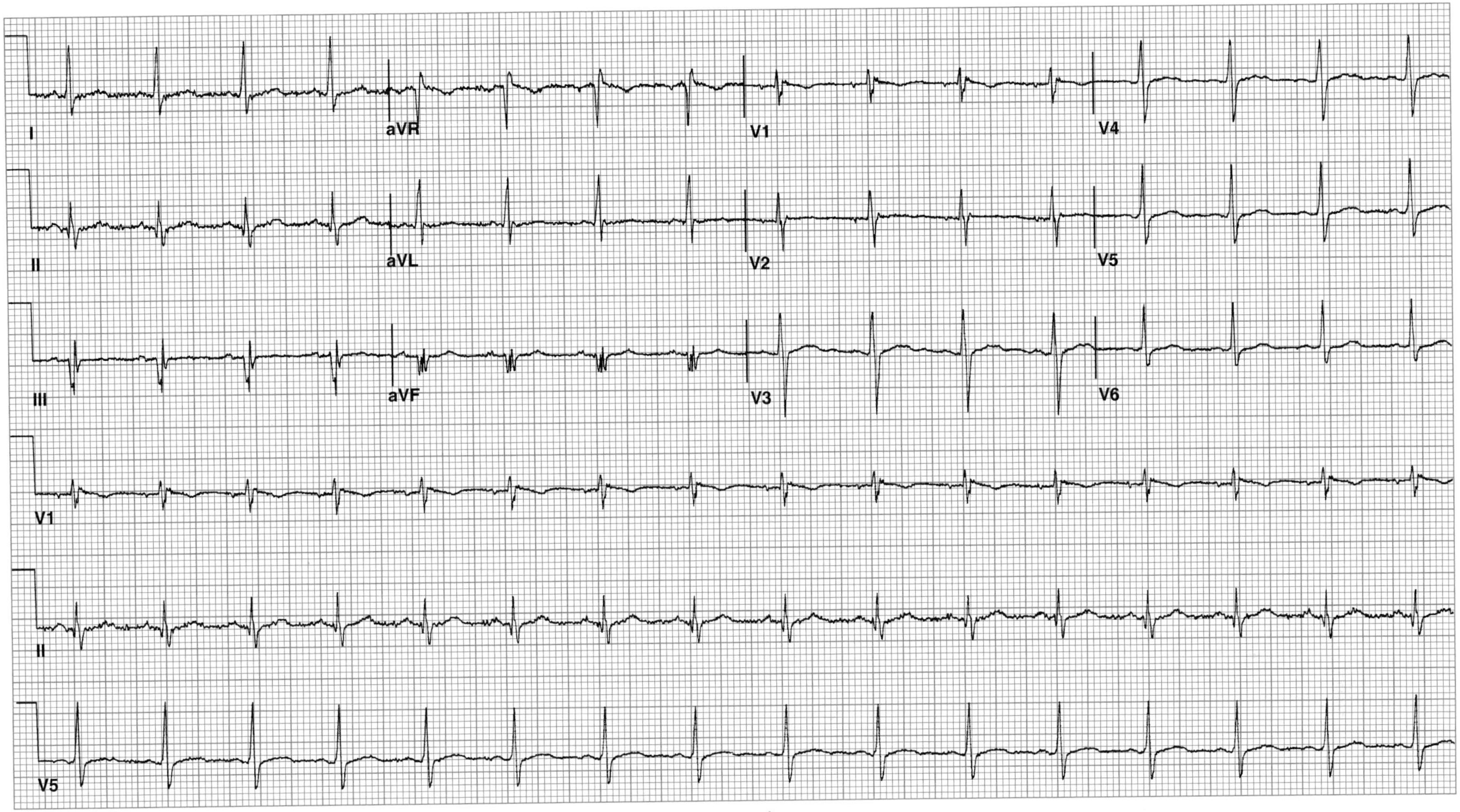

I

II

III

aVR

aVL

aVF

V1

V2

V3

V4

V5

V6

V1

II

V5

Ventricular Rate	95 bpm
PR Interval	0.12 sec
QRS Duration	0.08 sec

Normal Sinus Rhythm

Incomplete Right Bundle Branch Block

Inferior infarct, age undetermined

Abnormal EKG

Figure D47 12-Lead EKG—Practice Tracing #29

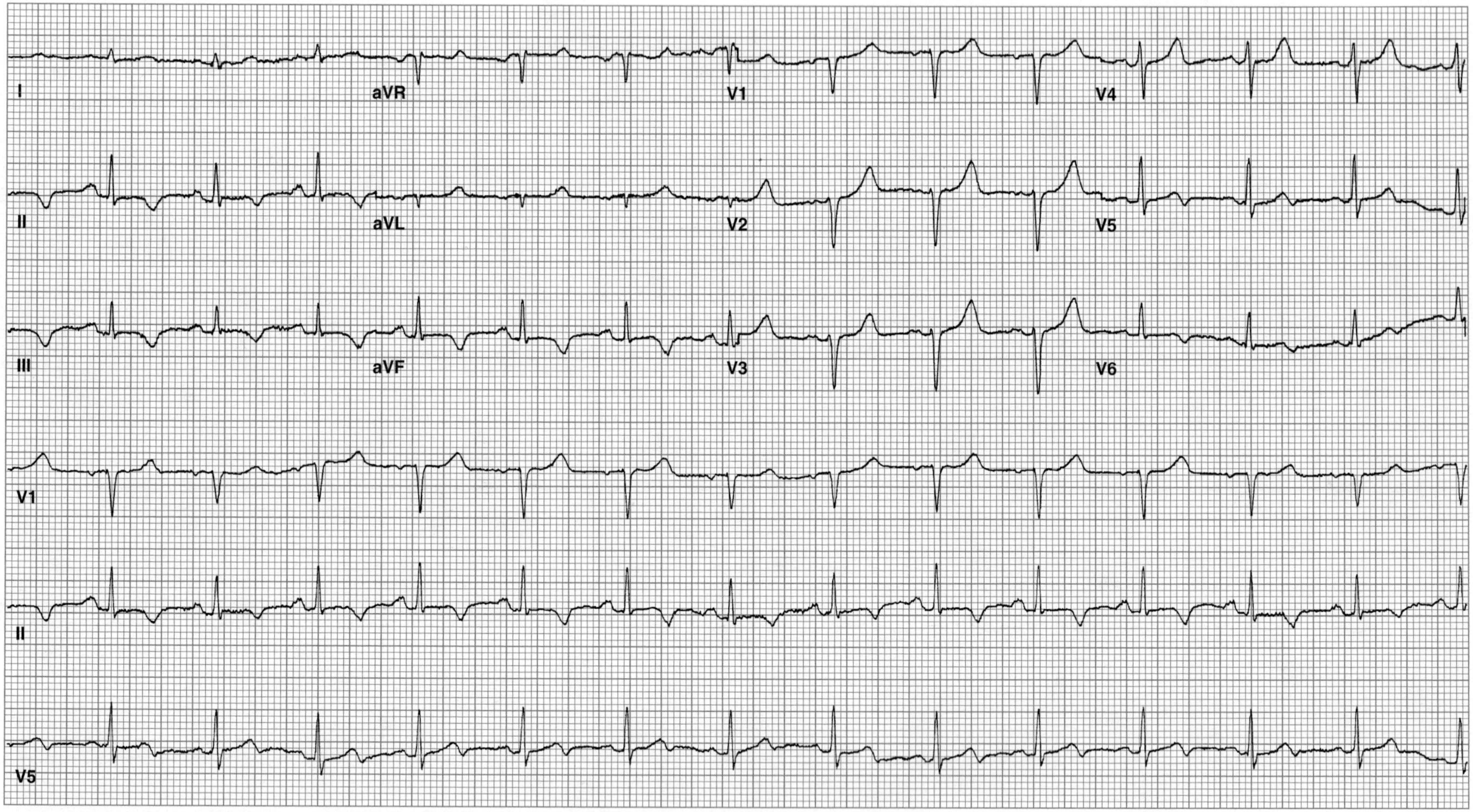

Ventricular Rate	84 bpm	Normal Sinus Rhythm
PR Interval	0.16 sec	Cannot rule out Anterior infarct, age undetermined
QRS Duration	0.08 sec	T wave abnormality, consider inferior ischemia
		Abnormal EKG

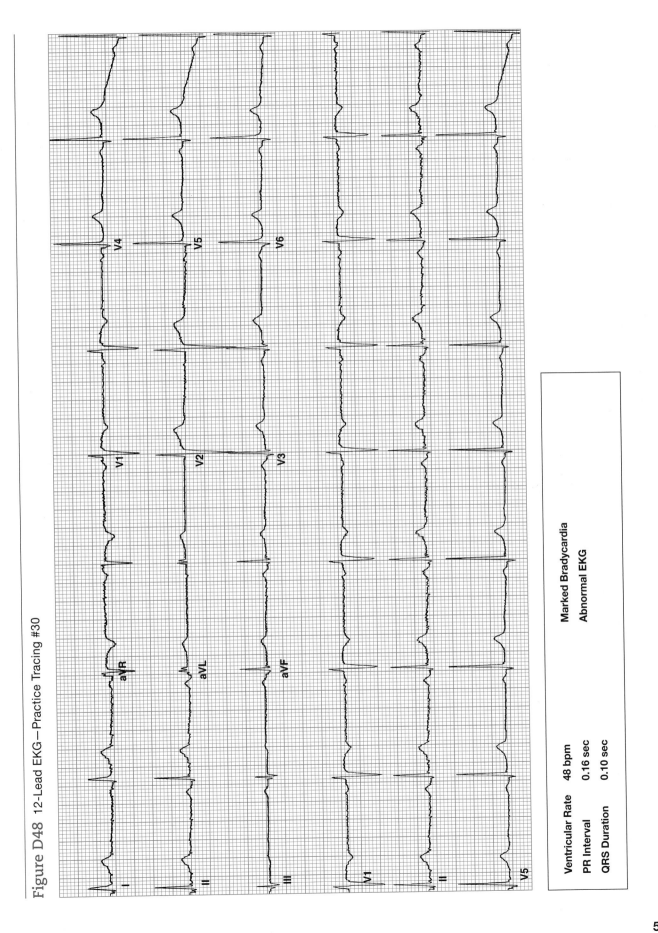

Figure D48 12-Lead EKG—Practice Tracing #30

Ventricular Rate	48 bpm	Marked Bradycardia
PR Interval	0.16 sec	Abnormal EKG
QRS Duration	0.10 sec	

Figure D49 12-Lead EKG—Practice Tracing #31

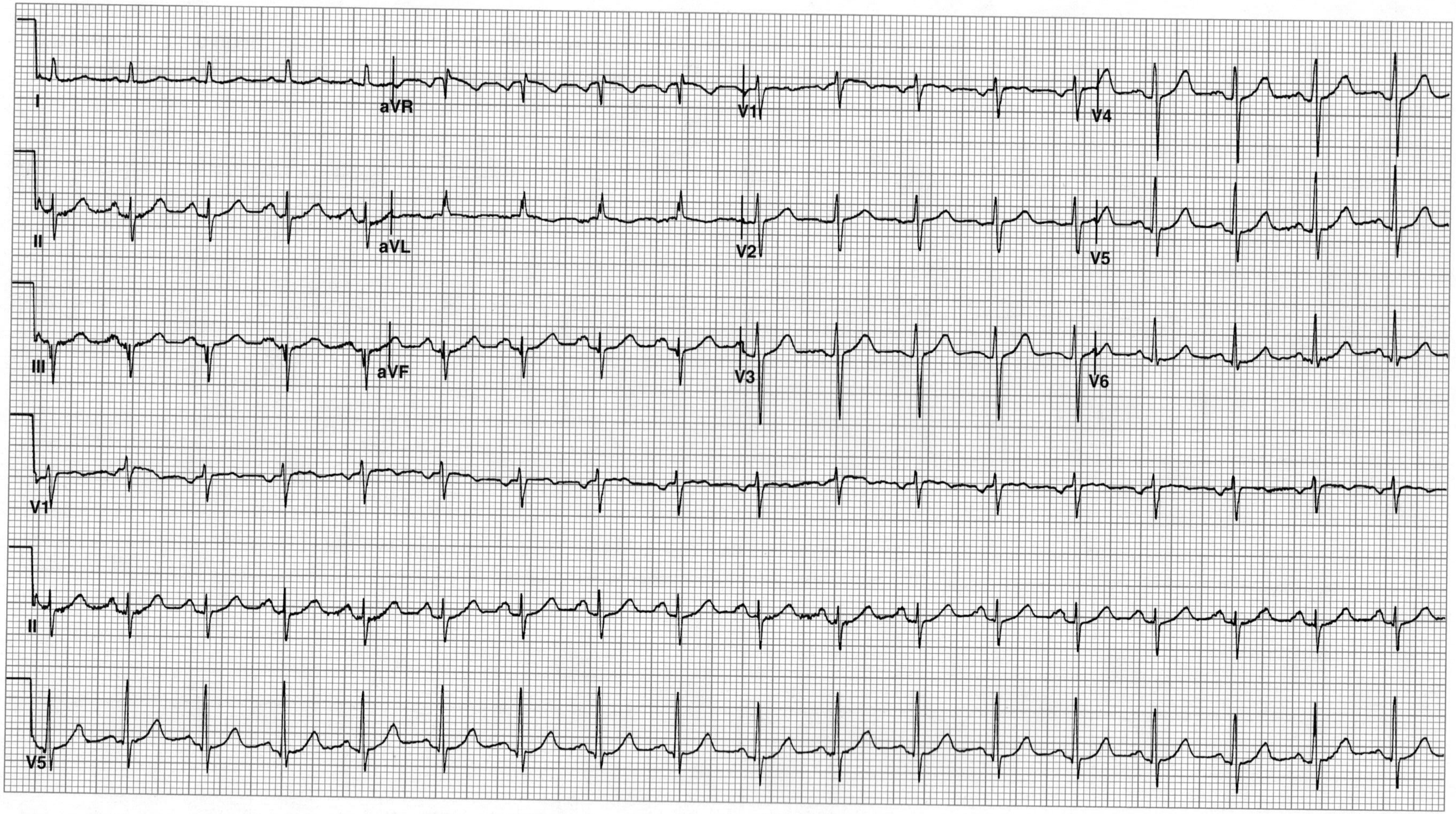

Ventricular Rate	107 bpm		Sinus Tachycardia
PR Interval	0.16 sec		Left Axis Deviation
QRS Duration	0.08 sec		Possible Inferior infarct, age undetermined
			Abnormal EKG

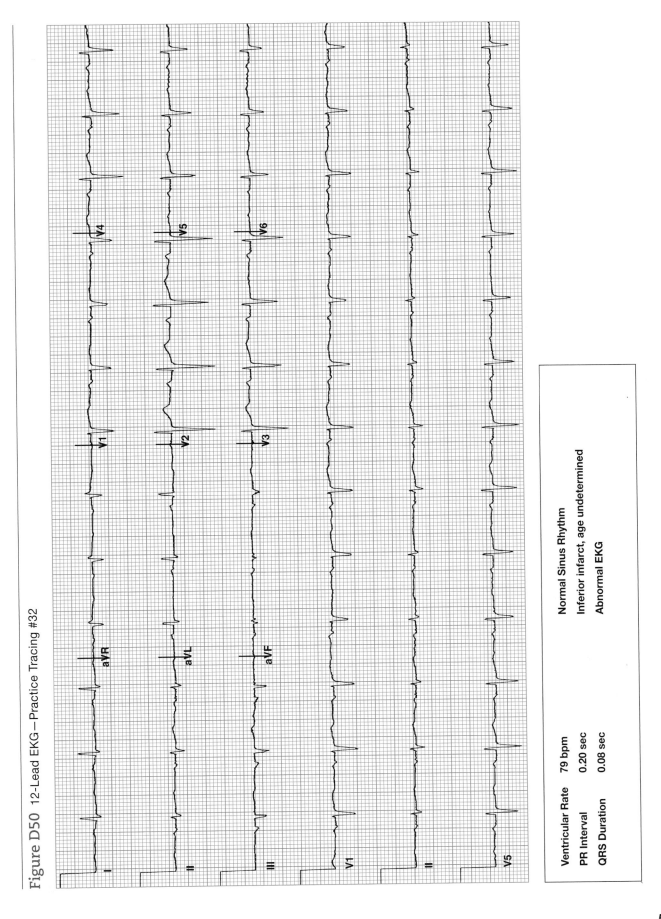

Figure D50 12-Lead EKG – Practice Tracing #32

Ventricular Rate	79 bpm	Normal Sinus Rhythm
PR Interval	0.20 sec	Inferior infarct, age undetermined
QRS Duration	0.08 sec	Abnormal EKG

Figure D51 12-Lead EKG – Practice Tracing #33

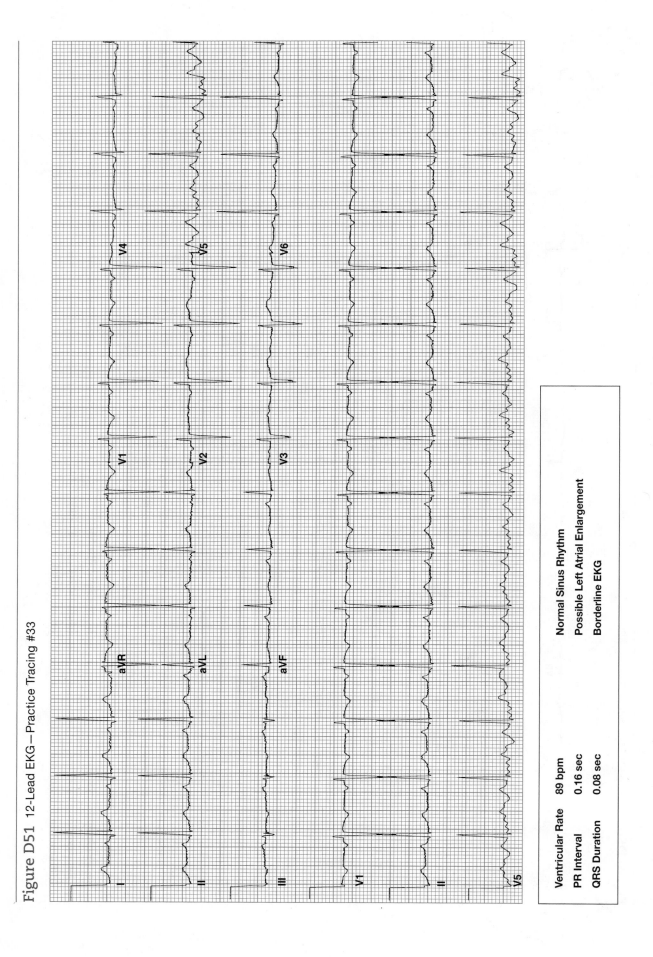

Ventricular Rate	89 bpm	**Normal Sinus Rhythm**
PR Interval	0.16 sec	**Possible Left Atrial Enlargement**
QRS Duration	0.08 sec	**Borderline EKG**

Figure D52 12-Lead EKG—Practice Tracing #34

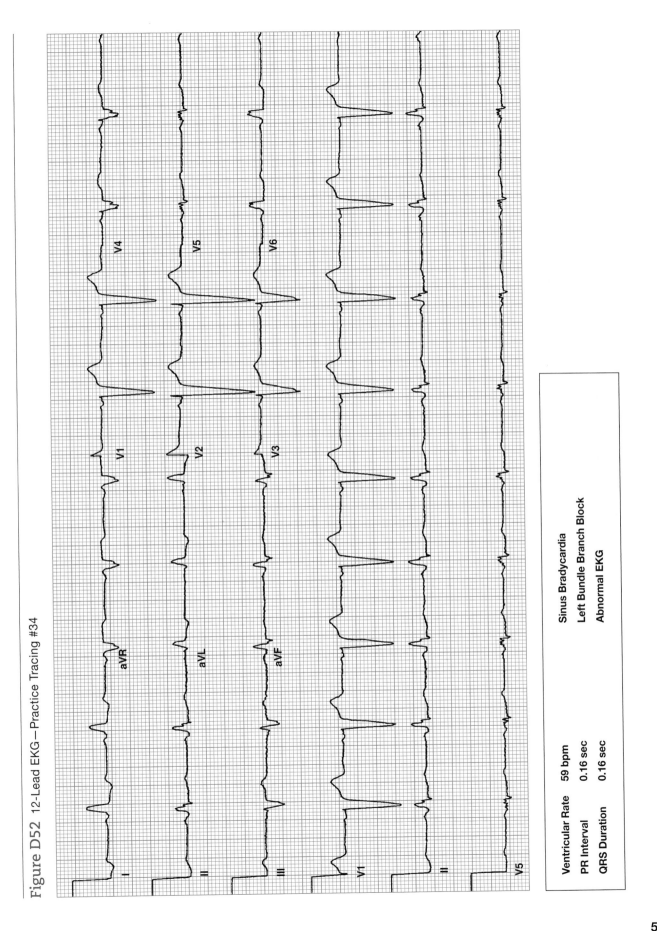

Ventricular Rate	59 bpm	Sinus Bradycardia
PR Interval	0.16 sec	Left Bundle Branch Block
QRS Duration	0.16 sec	Abnormal EKG

Figure D53 12-Lead EKG—Practice Tracing #35

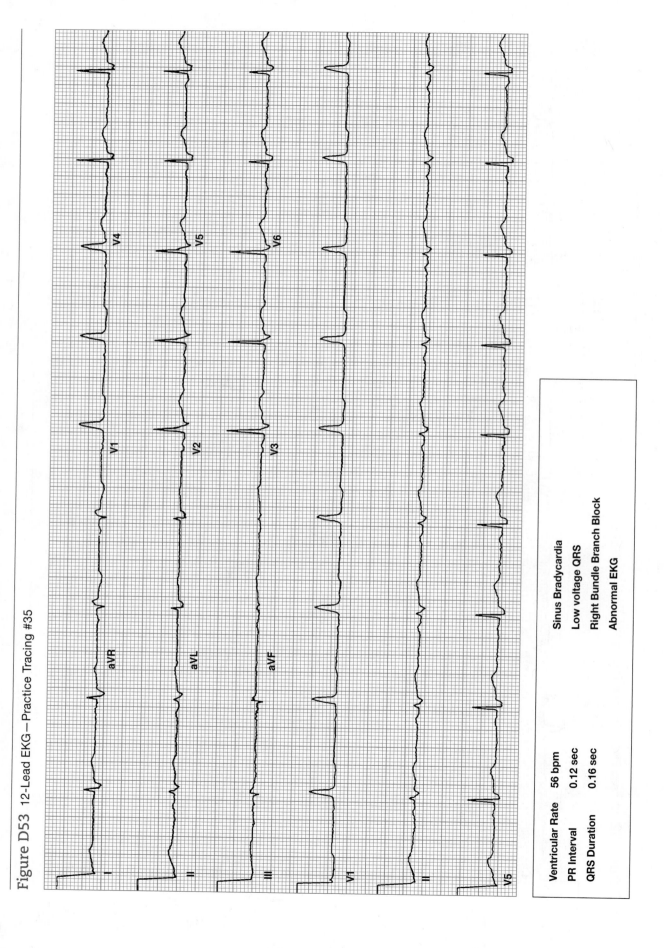

Ventricular Rate	56 bpm	Sinus Bradycardia
PR Interval	0.12 sec	Low voltage QRS
QRS Duration	0.16 sec	Right Bundle Branch Block
		Abnormal EKG

Figure D54 12-Lead EKG – Practice Tracing #36

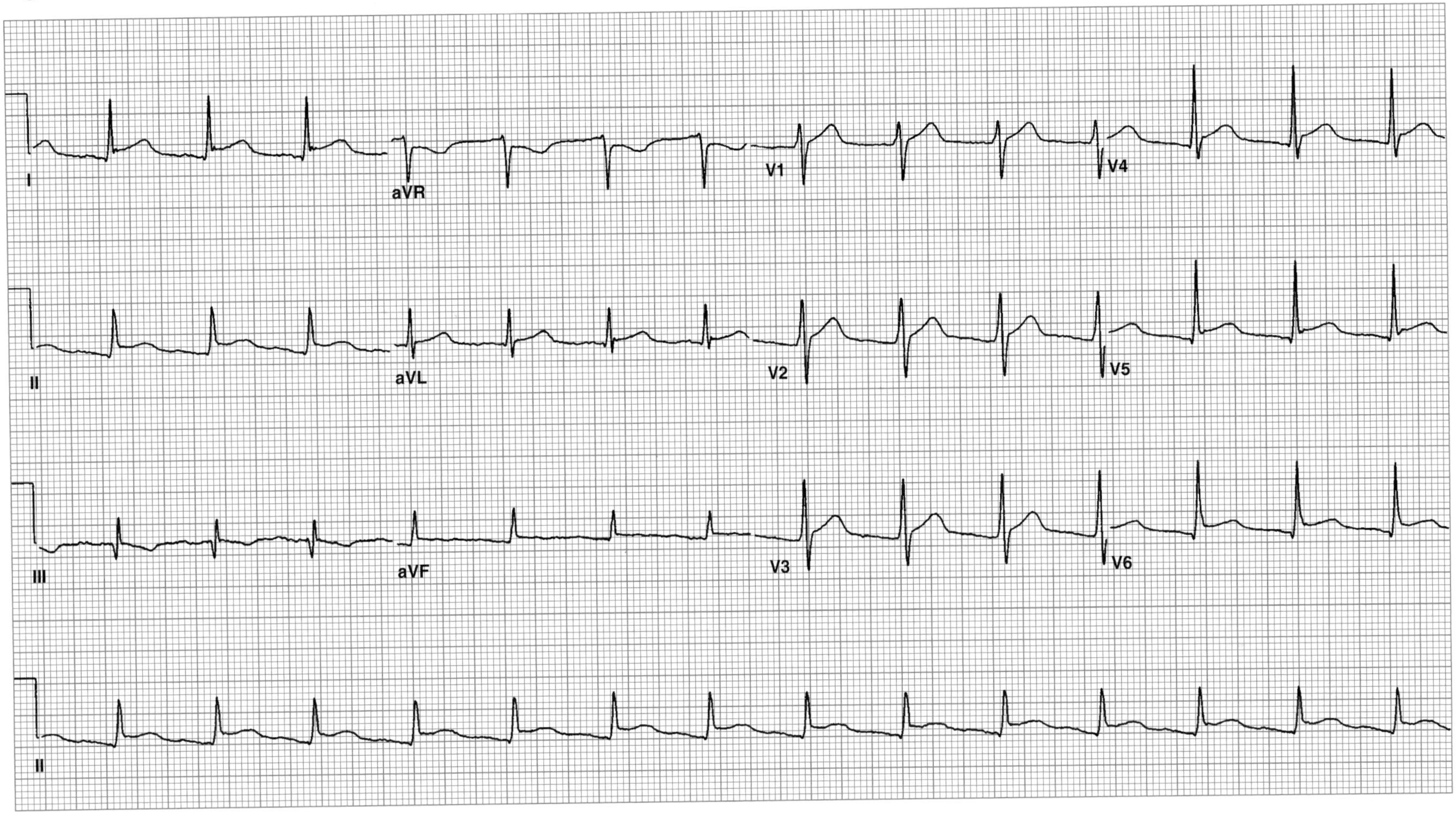

Ventricular Rate	87 bpm	**Normal Sinus Rhythm**
PR Interval	0.08 sec	**ST elevation, consider inferolateral injury or**
QRS Duration	0.10 sec	acute infarct
		Abnormal EKG

Figure D55 12-Lead EKG—Practice Tracing #37

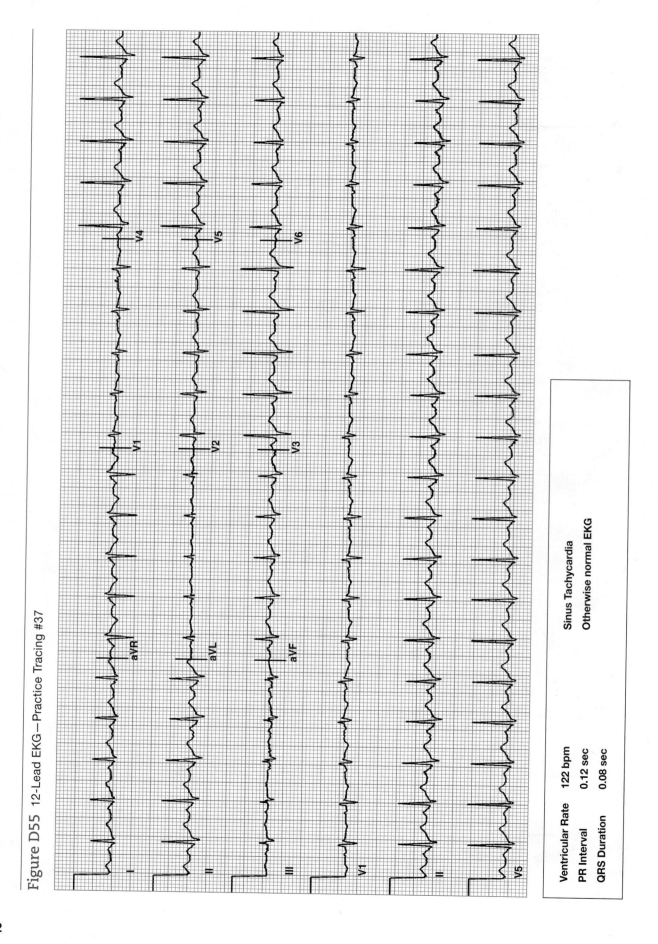

Ventricular Rate	122 bpm	Sinus Tachycardia
PR Interval	0.12 sec	Otherwise normal EKG
QRS Duration	0.08 sec	

Figure D56 12-Lead EKG—Practice Tracing #38

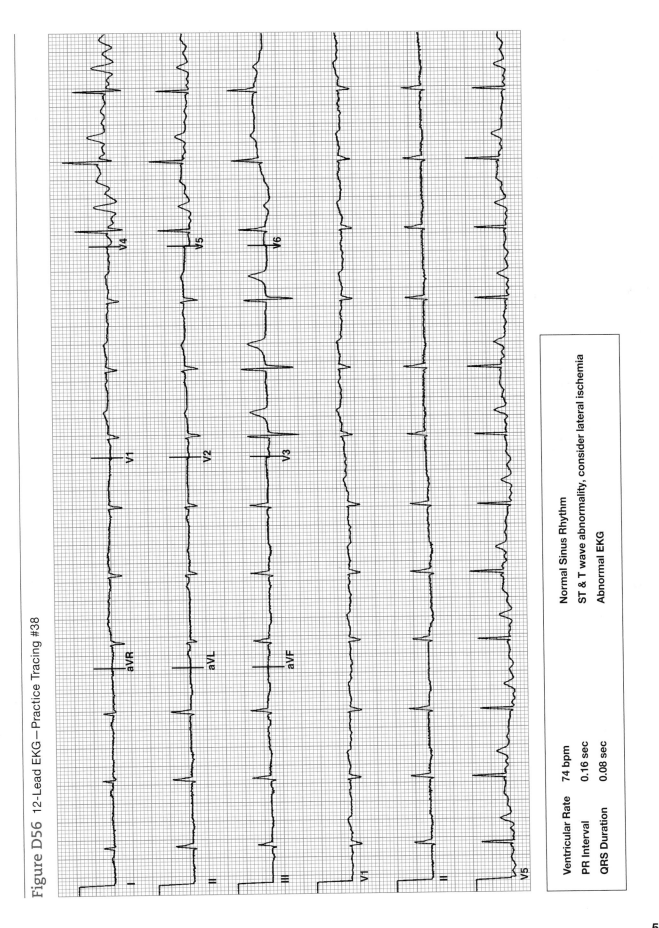

Ventricular Rate	74 bpm	Normal Sinus Rhythm
PR Interval	0.16 sec	ST & T wave abnormality, consider lateral ischemia
QRS Duration	0.08 sec	Abnormal EKG

Appendix E
Pacemakers

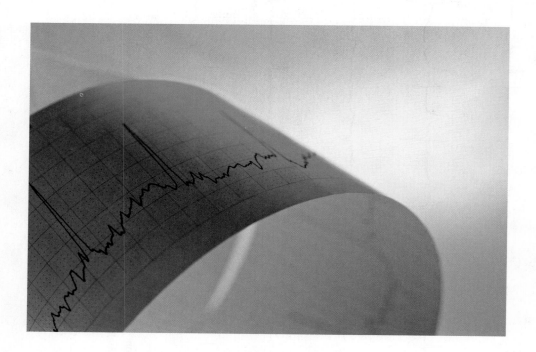

Overview

IN THIS APPENDIX, you will learn about artificial pacemakers, why and how they are used, and the various ways they work. You will find out how different types of pacemakers produce different wave forms on an EKG. You will learn to recognize pacemaker spikes and to differentiate between functioning and malfunctioning pacemakers. You will learn how to interpret what is happening in the heart based on what is seen on the rhythm strip.

When the heart's normal pacemaker is unreliable and causes bradyarrhythmias, it becomes essential to restore ventricular function. This can be done by applying an artificial stimulus to heart muscle, resulting in depolarization. Pacemaker-induced depolarization is called **capture**. Pacemakers use three components to produce a repetitive electrical stimulus and convey it directly to the myocardium:

Power Source: Battery unit called a *pulse generator*
Conducting Wire: *Electrode* that goes to the heart to provide the stimulus
Return Wire: Wire that returns to the battery unit to complete the electrical circuit

Pacemakers can be used temporarily or permanently. **Temporary** pacemakers are usually employed in acute settings to stabilize and maintain the patient for short periods. The wires of a temporary pacemaker are usually inserted transvenously, or occasionally transcutaneously, and the pacing unit is positioned outside the body. Temporary pacemakers are just that—they rarely stay in place longer than a few days (Figure E1).

When extended pacing support is needed, a **permanent** pacemaker is used. The wires are inserted surgically and the pacing unit is implanted in the fatty layer under the skin of the chest or abdomen.

Figure E1 Pacemaker Placement

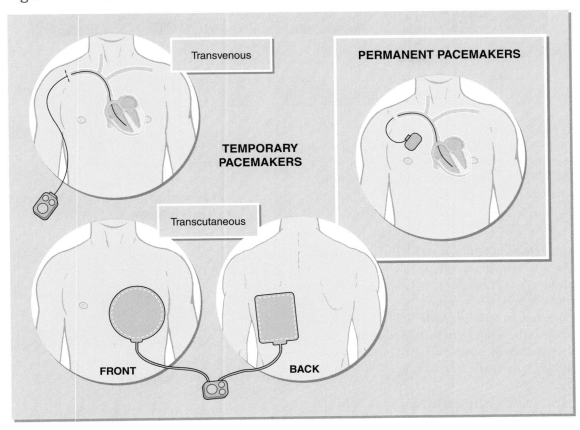

Chambers Paced

Pacemakers that stimulate only the ventricles are called **ventricular pacemakers**. Since ventricular function is essential, virtually all pacemakers have this capability. In occasional patients, the pathology is within the atrial conduction system while ventricular conduction is known to be reliable. In such cases, an **atrial pacemaker** is used to depolarize the atria, and the heart's own conduction system is relied upon to depolarize the ventricles.

Some pacemakers stimulate both atria and ventricles in sequence. Called **AV synchronous** pacemakers, these advanced sequential pacemakers are physiologically superior because they restore atrial kick.

Pacemakers that stimulate either the atria or the ventricles, but not both, are considered **single-chamber** pacemakers. Pacemakers that can stimulate both atrial and ventricular chambers are considered **dual-chamber** pacemakers.

Sensing Ability

Semiconductors enable tiny pacemakers to sense intrinsic electrical activity and respond appropriately, either by pacing or withholding stimulation in synchrony with the patient's rhythm. This microelectronic technology enables them to manage complex information, making them "smart" devices that are more responsive to changing patient needs.

Pacing Response

There are two basic ways in which pacemakers can initiate impulses:

Triggered: These are fixed-rate pacemakers that fire according to a predetermined plan, regardless of the patient's underlying cardiac activity.

Inhibited: These pacemakers fire only when needed—they are demand pacemakers capable of inhibiting their stimulus when they sense a patient's complex.

It is possible for pacemakers to be both triggered and inhibited. That is, they ignore atrial complexes but hold back if they sense a ventricular beat.

Classification of Pacemakers

Pacemakers can be described according to the chamber *paced*, the chamber *sensed*, and the *response* of the pacemaker to the sensed impulse (Figure E2). A three-letter code correlating to these categories is used to describe

Figure E2 Pacemaker Classification

Chamber PACED	Chamber SENSED	Pacemaker RESPONSE
V Ventricle	V Ventricle	T Triggered (fires even when it senses a beat)
A Atrium	A Atrium	I Inhibited (holds back when it senses a beat; fires only on demand)
D Dual (both)	D Dual (both)	D Dual (atrial triggered and ventricular inhibited)
	O Neither (no sensing)	

pacemaker types. For example, a VVI pacemaker paces the *ventricles*, senses the *ventricles*, and is *inhibited* when it senses a beat. Some of the more common types of pacemakers are listed below.

Single-Chamber Pacemakers

Ventricular Demand Pacemaker (VVI): This is by far the most common type of pacemaker. It senses spontaneous ventricular impulses and paces the ventricles only when needed.

Atrial Demand Pacemaker (AAI): This is a pacemaker similar to the VVI except that it senses and paces the atria, thereby maintaining the sequence of atrial and ventricular contraction.

Dual-Chamber Pacemakers

AV Synchronous Pacemaker (VDD): This unit senses atrial and ventricular activity but paces only in the ventricle.

AV Sequential Pacemaker (DVI): This unit paces both chambers sequentially, though it senses only in the ventricle.

Optimal Pacemaker (DDD): This pacemaker is also referred to as *fully automatic, universal,* and *physiologic.* It senses both atrial and ventricular activity and as needed, paces the atria, the ventricles, or both in synchrony.

EKG Analysis

The electrical impulse produced by the pacemaker appears on the EKG tracing as an unnaturally sharp spike superimposed on the patient's underlying rhythm (shown in figures as ⓟ). Pacemaker spikes can be small and difficult to detect, so EKG machines often augment pacemaker signals to make spikes more visible. See Figures E3–E5.

When the pacemaker captures, it produces an EKG wave consistent with the chamber being paced. That is, if it's an atrial pacemaker, the spike will be followed immediately by a P wave, but if the pacemaker is stimulating the ventricles, the spike will be followed immediately by a wide QRS configured like a PVC. If both chambers are paced, there will be two spikes for each cardiac cycle.

Figure E3 Paced Complexes

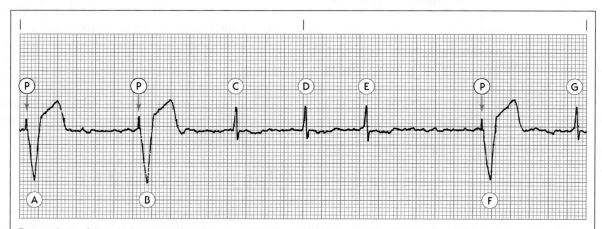

Pacemakers often supplement, rather than supplant, the patient's own rhythm. This rhythm strip shows a ventricular demand pacemaker that fires occasionally to supplement the patient's underlying atrial fibrillation. Complexes C, D, E, and G are the patient's normally conducted beats (note narrow QRS complexes). Complexes A, B, and F are initiated by the artificial ventricular pacemaker (note spikes preceding each wide QRS).

Figure E4 Pacemaker Rhythms

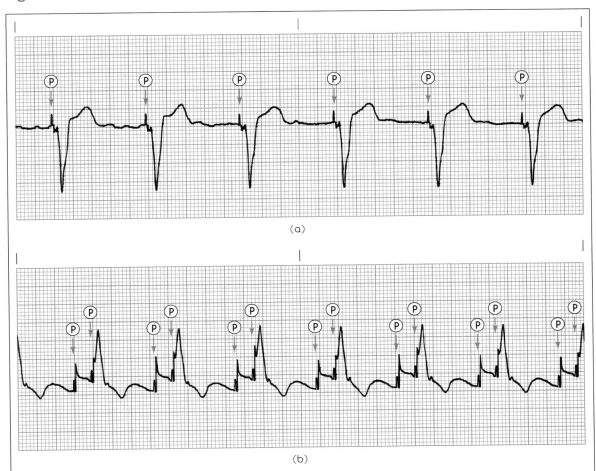

(a)

(b)

A properly functioning pacemaker will show a sharp spike, followed immediately by depolarization of the chamber it is intended to pace. (a) *Ventricular Pacemaker:* This rhythm strip shows ventricular pacemaker capturing every beat. Note absence of mappable P waves and sharp spikes followed immediately by wide QRS complexes. (b) *AV Synchronous Pacemaker:* This rhythm strip shows an AV synchronous pacemaker capturing every beat. Note pacemaker spikes preceding both atrial and ventricular depolarization.

Figure E5 Properly Functioning Ventricular Demand Pacemaker

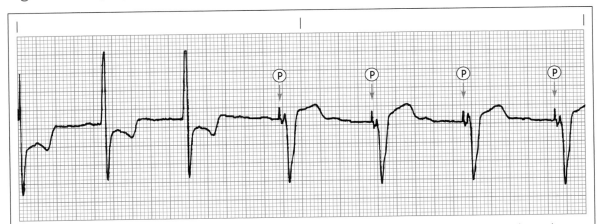

This pacemaker is set to fire whenever the patient's intrinsic rate falls below 60 bpm. The first three complexes show the patient's heart depolarizing at about 68 bpm, so the pacemaker inhibited itself. It kicked in at the fourth complex when the rate dropped and continued to pace at a rate of 60 bpm.

Assessment

Assessment must begin with the patient. Check pulses and other perfusion parameters. Remember that the EKG can't tell you whether or not the heart is actually beating in response to the pacemaker's stimuli.

Next, determine whether the pacemaker is doing what it was intended to do. By establishing the relationship between pacemaker spikes and the patient's complexes, you should be able to answer the following questions:

1. Does each spike capture?
2. Is the rate reasonable?
3. Are spikes competing with the patient's rhythm (are they falling near T waves)?
4. Is the pacemaker functioning consistently and reliably?

Pacemaker Malfunction

Today's pacemakers are far more reliable than earlier models, but they still experience occasional problems. Some of the more common malfunctions are listed below.

Failure to Capture (Figure E6): Occasionally, a pacemaker fires normally but no capture occurs; this is called a non-capturing pacemaker. This is seen on the EKG as pacemaker spikes that are not followed by depolarization complexes.

Competition (Figure E7): If a demand pacemaker fails to sense an underlying rhythm, it can fire in complete disregard to the patient's own rhythm, thereby competing for control of the heart. Competition can also occur if the heart's intrinsic pacemaker fires in a patient with a fixed-rate pacemaker, thus allowing competition between the two pacemakers. In either case, there is danger that the pacemaker spike can fall during the heart's relative refractory period (downslope of the T wave) and instigate a rapid, repetitive rhythm such as VT or VF.

Runaway Pacemaker: This occurs when the pacemaker fires too rapidly but still captures, causing the heart to respond in a tachycardia. The problem is caused by a malfunctioning impulse generator and is usually associated with older pacemaker units. Runaway pacemaker is not common with today's sophisticated units.

Battery Failure: As with all battery-operated products, the pacemaker is useless when the battery fails. This would appear on the EKG as the complete absence of pacemaker spikes in a rhythm that would normally be paced. Since pacemakers are most often used to support non-viable rhythms, a simple problem like battery failure can throw the patient into a life-threatening situation. Fortunately, this problem is not common with today's close patient monitoring and longer battery life.

Additional sample pacemaker rhythms are shown in Figures E8–E19.

Patient Management

Pacemakers are themselves a treatment; hence, it is a mistake to try to "treat" a malfunctioning pacemaker. When pacemakers malfunction, treatment is directed at the patient and the underlying rhythm. See Figures E8–E19.

Pacemaker Malfunctions

Figure E6 Failure to Capture / Failure to Sense

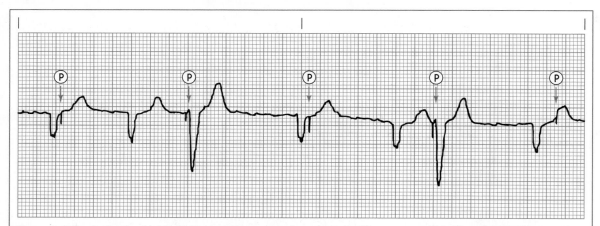

The underlying rhythm is atrial fibrillation, and the ventricular pacemaker is set at an unusually slow rate of 44 bpm. It fails to sense the patient's own complexes and continues to fire regularly, regardless of underlying ventricular activity. When the pacemaker stimulus finds the ventricles refractory, it fails to capture.

Figure E7 Competition

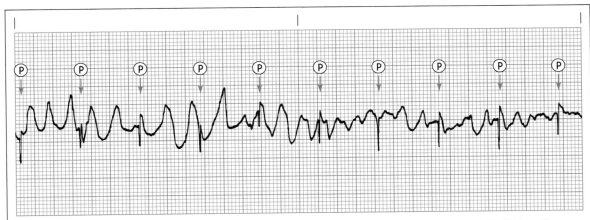

This strip shows pacemaker spikes at a rate of 100 bpm, with an underlying ventricular tachycardia/fibrillation. The pacemaker is competing for control of the heart, but the irritable ventricular foci are winning.

Sample Pacemaker Rhythm Strips

Figure E8 Fully Functional Atrial Pacemaker Showing 100% Capture

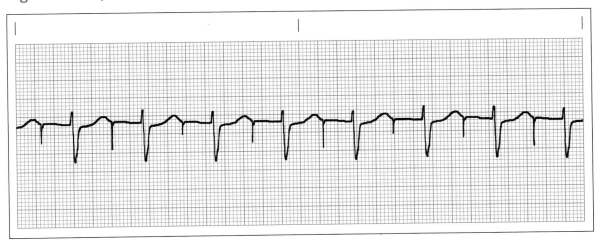

Figure E9 Ventricular Pacemaker Showing 100% Capture (with Underlying Complete Heart Block)

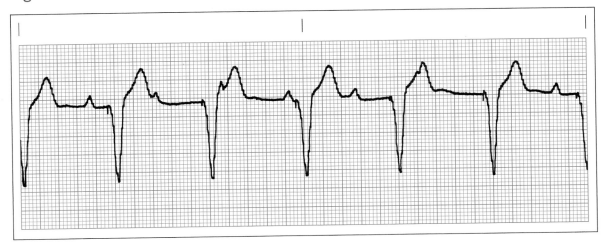

Figure E10 AV Sequential (DVI) Pacemaker

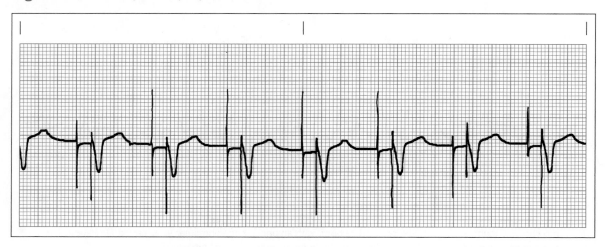

Figure E11 Properly Functioning Demand Pacemaker

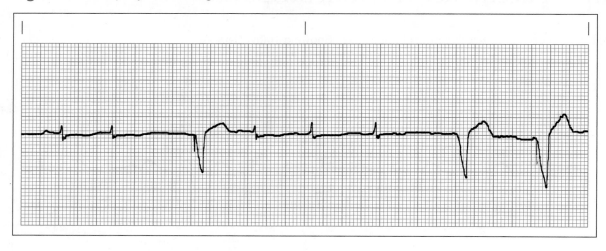

Figure E12 DDD Pacemaker in AV Sequential Mode

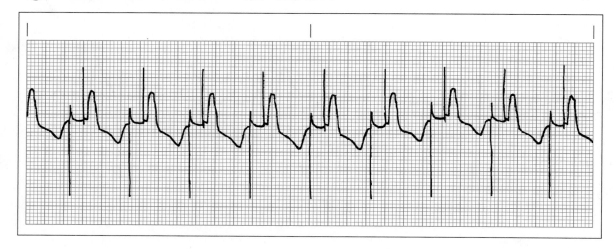

Figure E13 Sinus Rate Accelerates and Regains Control from Ventricular Demand Pacemaker

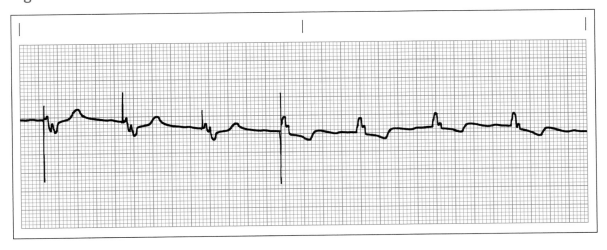

Figure E14 Pacemaker Fails to Depolarize Consistently, Indicating Lead Fracture or Displacement

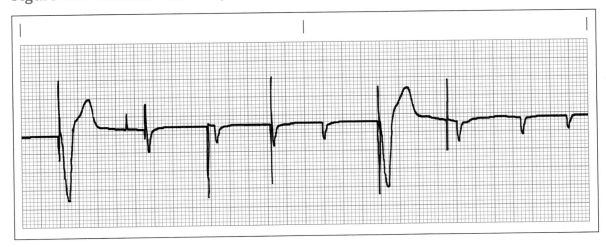

Figure E15 Ventricular Pacemaker (with Underlying Complete Heart Block) with 100% Capture

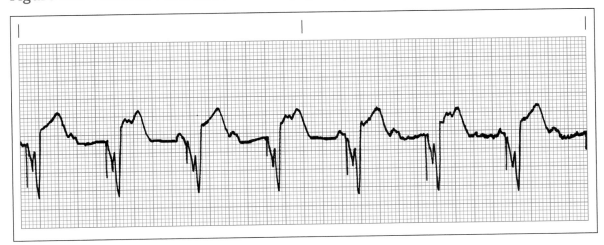

Figure E16 Atrial Pacemaker with 100% Capture

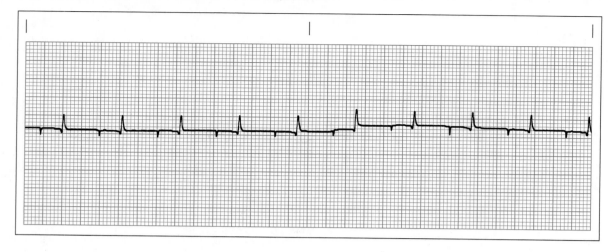

Figure E17 Non-Capturing Pacemaker Competing with Supraventricular Rhythm in First Part of Strip, Converting to Ventricular Tachycardia Competing with Pacemaker at End of Strip

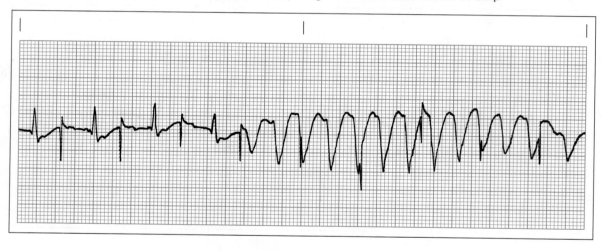

Figure E18 Ventricular Demand Pacemaker (with Underlying Atrial Fibrillation)

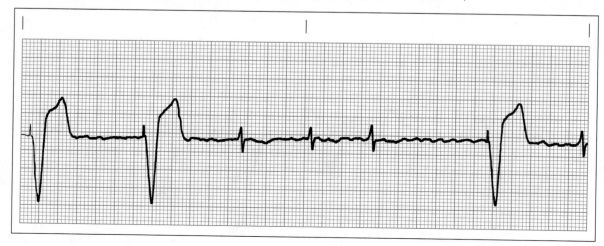

Figure E19 Ventricular Pacemaker Showing 100% Capture

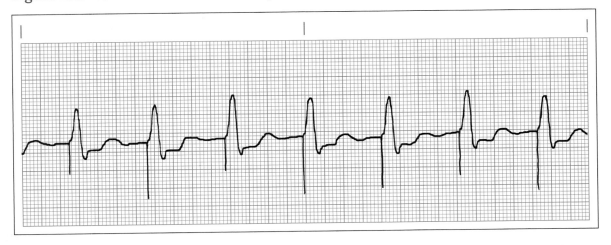

Glossary

ACLS: Advanced cardiac life support.

AF: Atrial Flutter.

Af: Atrial Fibrillation.

AMI: Acute myocardial infarction.

ANS: Autonomic nervous system.

Anterior MI: Infarction of the anterior wall of the heart, most often caused by occlusion of the Left Anterior Descending coronary artery.

Anterior Surface: The plane of the heart that faces forward, abutting the chest wall.

Anterobasal MI: Anterior wall infarction localized to the base (top) of the heart.

Anterolateral MI: Anterior wall infarction localized to the area of the lateral wall.

Anteroseptal MI: Anterior wall infarction localized to the area of the septum.

Aorta: Artery that carries oxygenated blood from the left ventricle to distal parts of the body.

Aortic Valve: The valve that controls passage of blood from the left ventricle to the aorta.

Apex: The lower point of the heart.

Apical MI: Infarction localized to the apex (bottom) of the heart.

Arrhythmia: The graphic representation of the heart's electrical activity; the term is loosely used to mean an abnormality of the heart's electrical function, but it is also used to categorize patterns of electrical activity, not all of which are necessarily abnormal or bad; also called *dysrhythmia*; it can also be used to mean that a rhythm is not regular.

Artifact: Electrical activity displayed on graph paper that is superimposed on cardiac tracings, interfering with interpretation of the rhythm; can be caused by outside electrical sources, muscle tremors, patient movement; also called *interference.*

Asystole: The absence of any cardiac electrical activity; appears as a straight line on graph paper.

AT: Atrial Tachycardia.

Atria: The upper two chambers of the heart.

Atrial Arrhythmia: A cardiac arrhythmia originating from the conduction system within the atria.

Atrial Fibrillation (Af): The cardiac arrhythmia in which the atria are controlled by numerous irritable foci, thereby causing ineffectual, chaotic atrial activity and irregular ventricular response.

Atrial Flutter (AF): The cardiac arrhythmia in which an irritable focus in the atria produces a rapid, repetitive discharge, resulting in rhythmic atrial depolarizations at a rate of 250–350 bpm, some of which are usually blocked by the AV node to keep the ventricular rate in a more normal range.

Atrial Hypertrophy: Enlargement of myocardial wall in one or more of the atria.

Atrial Kick: The increased pressure of atrial contraction immediately before ventricular contraction; this "priming" force increases ventricular efficiency, and can account for up to 30% of cardiac output.

Atrial Pacemaker: An electrical stimulus originating in the atria that paces the heart; an artificial pacemaker that stimulates only the atria.

Atrial Tachycardia (AT): The cardiac arrhythmia in which a single irritable focus in the atria takes over control of the heart to produce a rate of 150–250 bpm; this arrhythmia is often paroxysmal in nature—that is, it starts and stops suddenly; in that instance it is called *Paroxysmal Atrial Tachycardia* (PAT).

Atrioventricular Dissociation: A conduction defect that causes the atria and ventricles to depolarize and function independently; AV Dissociation.

Augmented Leads: Unipolar leads that measure electrical flow on the frontal plane from the center of the heart to each of three limb electrodes: Leads aVR, aVL, and aVF.

Automaticity: The unique ability of cardiac pacemaker cells to initiate spontaneous excitation impulses.

Autonomic Nervous System: The system responsible for control of involuntary bodily functions, including cardiac and vascular activity; branches are sympathetic nervous system and parasympathetic nervous system.

AV: Atrioventricular.

aVF: Augmented voltage, foot (left leg).

AV Heart Block: Arrhythmias caused by disturbances in conduction through the AV node.

AV Junction: That part of the cardiac conduction system that connects the atria and the ventricles; contains the AV node and the non-branching part of the Bundle of His.

aVL: Augmented voltage, left.

AV Node: A part of the cardiac conduction system located within the AV junction; does not contain pacemaking cells; its purpose is to slow conduction of impulses through the AV junction.

aVR: Augmented voltage, right.

AV Sequential Pacemaker: A type of artificial pacemaker that senses ventricular activity and, in its absence, paces atria and ventricles in a normal sequence.

AV Synchronous Pacemaker: A type of artificial pacemaker that senses both atria and ventricles and paces the ventricles when a spontaneous P wave is not followed by a QRS. The ventricles are depolarized in synchrony with P waves so that atrial and ventricular contractions are coordinated.

Axis: Sum direction of electrical flow through the heart. The axis of a given lead is the *lead axis*. The sum direction of electrical flow through the heart as a whole is the *mean QRS axis.*

Axis Deviation: Shift in mean QRS axis reflecting myocardial damage, enlargement, or conduction defect.

Base: The upper end of the heart.

Baseline: The isoelectric line; the line on EKG graph paper that indicates lack of electrical activity and from which all other cardiac wave impulses deviate.

BBB: Bundle branch block.

Bigeminy: A pattern of cardiac electrical activity in which every other beat is an ectopic, usually a PVC.

Biological Death: The second phase of death, following clinical death; defined by brain death, usually following 4–6 minutes of cardiac arrest if no resuscitation is instituted.

Biphasic: A single EKG wave that has two deflections, one upright and the other inverted.

Bipolar Lead: A lead composed of one positive and one negative electrode.

Block: A defect in conduction within the heart's electrical system.

Bolus: A single loading dose of a drug; used to achieve a rapid high therapeutic blood level prior to instituting IV drip therapy.

bpm: Beats per minute.

Bradyarrhythmia: Any cardiac arrhythmia with a rate below 60 bpm.

Bradycardia: A heart rate less than 60 bpm.

Bundle Branches: The portion of the cardiac conduction system within the ventricles that conducts impulses from the Bundle of His to the Purkinje fibers; consists of right and left bundle branches.

Bundle Branch Block (BBB): A conduction disturbance that prevents or delays passage of impulses from the Bundle of His through to the Purkinje network; can involve the right or left bundle branch or, less frequently, both.

Bundle of His: That part of the cardiac conduction system that conducts impulses from the AV Junction through to the bundle branches.

Ca: Calcium.

CAD: Coronary artery disease.

Calibration: The act of standardizing the graphic display of electrical activity; the calibration mark should measure 1 millivolt on the graph paper.

Capture: The act of responding to an electrical stimulus with depolarization; generally refers to an arrhythmia's response to an artificial pacemaker.

Cardiac Arrest: The cessation of cardiac function, resulting in sudden drop in perfusion and resultant clinical death.

Cardiac Cycle: The interval from the beginning of one heartbeat to the beginning of the next; on the EKG it encompasses the PQRST complex.

Cardiac Output (CO): The amount of blood pumped by the left ventricle in one minute; it is calculated by multiplying the stroke volume by the heart rate and is measured in liters per minute.

Cardioversion: A maneuver used to convert various tachyarrhythmias to more viable rhythms; consists of application of electrical countershock (DC current) to the chest wall; the electrical discharge is usually synchronized to fall on the R wave, thus avoiding the relative refractory period.

Carotid Sinus Massage: A maneuver used to convert various supraventricular tachycardias to a more viable rhythm; consists of gentle massage with fingertips over the carotid sinus in the neck.

Central Terminal: An electrically neutral reference point created by combining two or more electrodes. It is used to oppose the positive electrode in unipolar leads.

CHB: Complete Heart Block.

CHF: Congestive Heart Failure.

Chordae Tendineae: Specialized fibers that connect heart valve leaflets to papillary muscles to prevent backflow during contractions.

Classical Second-Degree Heart Block: The term formerly used to describe the type of AV heart block that is now called Type II Second-Degree Heart Block, in which the AV node intermittently blocks sinus impulses, preventing them from being conducted through to the ventricles.

Clinical Death: The absence of pulse and blood pressure; occurs immediately following cardiac arrest.

CO: Cardiac output.

Compensatory Pause: The time lag following an ectopic beat before the next normal beat occurs; is identified by measuring the interval from the R wave immediately preceding the ectopic to the R wave immediately following it; a fully compensatory pause (such as occurs following most PVCs) will be exactly two times the normal R–R interval.

Competition: Condition in which an artificial pacemaker competes with the patient's intrinsic pacemaker for control of the heart.

Complete Heart Block (CHB): Third-Degree AV Block; a form of AV dissociation.

Conduction Ratio: The number of P waves to QRS complexes. One P wave for every QRS complex is a 1:1 conduction ratio. Three P waves for every QRS complex would be a 3:1 conduction ratio.

Conduction System: The pathways of conductive tissues within the heart that facilitate passage of electrical impulses throughout the myocardium.

Conductivity: The property of some cardiac cells that enables them to transmit electrical impulses.

Contractility: The ability of heart muscle to contract in response to electrical stimulation.

Conventional 12-Lead EKG: Electrocardiogram that provides images of cardiac electrical activity from 12 perspectives simultaneously.

Coronary Arteries: Those blood vessels that supply the heart muscle itself. The major branches are the Left Coronary Artery (with the Left Anterior Descending branches and the Circumflex branch) and the Right Coronary Artery.

Coronary Sinus: The reentry point within the right atrium where deoxygenated blood returns after having supplied the heart muscle itself.

CPR: Cardiopulmonary resuscitation.

CT: Central terminal.

DDD: Double paced, double sensed, double response (optimal pacemaker).

Defibrillation: Application of electrical countershock (DC current) to the chest wall to terminate ventricular tachyarrhythmias.

Demand Pacemaker: Pacemaker that senses patient's intrinsic complexes and fires only when needed.

Depolarization: The electrical process of discharging polarized cells, usually resulting in muscle contraction.

Diaphragmatic Surface: The plane of the heart that faces downward, resting against the diaphragm.

Diastole: The phase of the cardiac cycle in which chambers are relaxing.

Digitalis Toxicity: Excessive blood levels of the heart drug digitalis; also called dig-toxicity.

Dissociation: Independent function of two parts, generally the atria and ventricles.

Dual-Chamber Pacemaker: Paces both atria and ventricles.

DVI: Double paced, ventricle sensed, inhibited response (AV sequential pacemaker).

Dysrhythmia: Arrhythmia.

ECG: Electrocardiogram; see EKG.

Ectopic: Originating from a focus other than the primary pacemaker.

Einthoven's Triangle: The triangle created by an imaginary line connecting the three chest electrodes used to create the standard limb leads.

EKG: Electrocardiogram; electrocardiograph.

Electrocardiogram (EKG; ECG): Graphic representation of the electrical activity in the heart.

Electrode: Metal wire attached to the patient's body for the purpose of conveying electrical impulses to a machine for recording or displaying.

EMD: Electromechanical dissociation.

Endocardium: The inner layer of the heart wall, which contains the branches of the heart's electrical system.

Epicardium: The outside layer of the heart wall, which contains the coronary blood vessels and nerves.

Equiphasic: A single EKG wave that has two deflections of equal magnitude, one upright and the other inverted.

ERAD: Extreme right axis deviation.

Escape: The mechanism that allows a lower pacemaker site to assume pacemaking responsibilities when a higher site fails.

Evolving Infarction: The changing EKG picture associated with the passage of time following myocardial infarction.

Failure to Capture: Situation in which the pacemaker fires but the patient's heart does not respond with depolarization.

Fibrillation: Chaotic, ineffective movement of the heart muscle.

First-Degree Heart Block: A type of AV heart block characterized by prolonged but consistent conduction of atrial impulses through to the ventricles.

Fixed-Rate Pacemaker: Pacemaker that is set at a predetermined rate and fires regardless of the patient's underlying rhythm.

Flutter: Rhythmic, rapid beating of the heart muscle.

F waves: Flutter waves.

f waves: Fibrillatory waves.

Gallop Rhythms: Heart sounds that are grouped together so they sound like galloping horses.

Heart Block: AV heart block.

Heart Rate (HR): The number of heart beats per minute.

Heart Sounds: Sounds associated with flow of blood through heart chambers and closing of heart valves. The four components are S_1: closure of mitral and tricuspid valves; S_2: closure of aortic and pulmonic valves; S_3: abnormally rapid ventricular filling; S_4: abnormally forceful atrial contraction.

His–Purkinje System: The lower part of the cardiac conduction system that transmits impulses throughout the ventricles; located in the interventricular septum and ventricular walls.

HR: Heart rate.

Hyperkalemia: High blood potassium level.

Hypertrophy: Enlargement of myocardial wall in one or more of the chambers of the heart.

Hypokalemia: Low blood potassium level.

IAS: Interatrial septum.

Idioventricular Rhythm: A ventricular escape rhythm; characterized by a rate less than 40 bpm.

Impulse Formation: The process by which cardiac electrical cells create an electrical impulse without stimulation from another source. See Automaticity.

Inferior MI: Infarction of the inferior wall of the heart, most often caused by occlusion of the right coronary artery.

Inferior Vena Cava (IVC): Vein that carries deoxygenated blood from the lower body back to the right atrium.

Interference: *See* Artifact.

Interpolation: The placement of an ectopic (especially PVCs) between two normal beats without disturbing the regularity of the underlying rhythm.

Interval: Distance between two points on an EKG tracing.

Interventricular Septum (IVS): The muscular wall dividing the right and left ventricles.

Intraatrial Pathways: Branches of the cardiac conduction system that service the atria.

Intraventricular Conduction Defect (IVCD): Disturbance in conduction involving one or more of the bundle branches. Also called Bundle Branch Block.

Intrinsicoid Deflection: Reflection of the time it takes for peak voltage to develop within the ventricles; measured from the onset of the QRS to the peak of the R wave; a prolonged intrinsicoid deflection (> 0.06 sec) is considered a "late R wave."

Ischemic Changes: Changes on the EKG that reflect myocardial ischemia: ST elevation, ST depression, Q wave deepening, and T wave inversion.

Isoelectric Line: The line created on EKG graph paper when no electrical current is flowing; *see also* Baseline.

IV: Intravenous.

IVC: Inferior vena cava.

IVCD: Intraventricular conduction defect.

IVS: Interventricular septum.

J Point: The demarcation between the end of the QRS complex and the beginning of the ST segment.

JT: Junctional Tachycardia.

Junction: *See* AV Junction.

Junctional Escape Rhythm: An arrhythmia resulting from failure of a higher pacemaker site, allowing the AV junction to pace the heart at a bradycardia rate.

Junctional Tachycardia (JT): A rapid arrhythmia originating in the AV junction.

K: Potassium.

LA: Left atrium; left arm.

LAD: Left axis deviation; left anterior descending branch of the left coronary artery.

LAE: Left atrial enlargement.

Lateral MI: Infarction of the lateral wall of the heart, most often caused by occlusion of the Left Anterior Descending coronary artery.

Lateral Surface: The plane of the heart that faces the side, just above the diaphragmatic surface.

LBB: Left bundle branch.

LBBB: Left bundle branch block.

LCA: Left coronary artery.

Lead: An electrocardiographic view of the heart, gained by recording the electrical activity between two or more electrodes.

LV: Left ventricle.

LVE: Left ventricular enlargement.

MCL$_1$: Modified Chest Left; a monitoring lead that mimics V$_1$ and is useful in differentiating tachycardias.

MI: Myocardial Infarction.

Millivolts (mV): A measure of electricity; 1 volt equals 1,000 millivolts.

Mitral Valve: The valve that controls passage of blood from the left atrium to the left ventricle.

mm: Millimeter.

Monitor: The machine on which electrocardiographic impulses are displayed; oscilloscope.

Monitoring Lead: A lead that clearly shows individual wave forms and is useful for monitoring cardiac rhythm, most often Lead II or MCL$_1$.

Multifocal: Term used to describe ectopic beats that originate from more than one irritable focus. Also called Multiformed.

Murmurs: Heart sounds caused by abnormal turbulence associated with high flow rates, damaged valves, dilated chambers, or backward flow.

mV: Millivolt.

Myocardial Infarction (MI): Tissue death caused by lack of oxygen to the myocardium.

Myocardial Injury: Heart tissue damage caused by sustained lack of oxygen.

Myocardial Ischemia: Initial heart tissue response to lack of oxygen.

Myocardium: The center layer of the heart wall, consisting of cardiac muscle fibers.

Na: Sodium.

Noise: Electrical interference displayed on graph paper that interferes with interpretation of the underlying arrhythmia; *see* Artifact.

Non-Q Infarction: Myocardial infarction that fails to produce classic Q wave changes, most often because the infarcted area is limited to partial thickness of the myocardium; subendocardial infarction.

Normal Sinus Rhythm (NSR): The usual cardiac electrical pattern of healthy people.

NSR: Normal Sinus Rhythm.

Oscilloscope: Display device with a screen for viewing EKG and other physiological information; monitor.

PAC: Premature Atrial Complex.

Pacemaker: The source of electrical stimulation for cardiac rhythm.

Pacemaker, Artificial: A device used to provide artificial electrical stimuli to myocardial tissue to cause myocardial depolarization.

Pacemaker Electrode: The conducting wire that connects to the myocardium to deliver the pacemaker stimulus.

Pacemaker Site: The site of origin of the electrical stimulation that is causing the cardiac rhythm.

Palpitations: The feeling the patient senses when the heart is beating abnormally.

Papillary Muscles: Specialized muscles in the ventricles that attach to heart valves by way of chordae tendineae, enabling the valves to open and close.

Parasympathetic Nervous System: A branch of the autonomic nervous system involved in control of involuntary bodily functions; depresses cardiac activity in opposition to the sympathetic branch of the ANS; effects include slowing of heart rate and conduction and diminished myocardial irritability.

Paroxysmal: Sudden onset and cessation; often used to describe Atrial Tachycardia if it is characterized by abrupt onset and termination.

Paroxysmal Atrial Tachycardia (PAT): The term used to describe an Atrial Tachycardia characterized by abrupt onset and cessation.

PAT: Paroxysmal Atrial Tachycardia.

PEA: Pulseless Electrical Activity. A condition in which the EKG shows a viable rhythm, but no pulse is detectible in the patient. The electrical activity in the heart is not producing a mechanical response (pulse.)

Pericarditis: Inflammation of the pericardial sac surrounding the heart. Causes ischemic changes on EKG and can thus be misinterpreted to be MI.

Pericardium: A thin layer of tissue that forms the pericardial sac to encase the heart in lubricating fluid.

Permanent Pacemaker: Pacemaker that is surgically implanted within the patient's body for an extended time.

PJC: Premature Junctional Complex.

Posterior Surface: The plane of the heart that faces backward, abutting the spine.

PQRST: A single cardiac cycle on the EKG graph paper; includes the P wave, QRS complex, and T wave and any segments and intervals between.

Precordial Leads: Leads that measure electrical flow on the horizontal plane, from the center of the heart to locations around the anterior and lateral chest walls. The V leads: V_1, V_2, V_3, V_4, V_5, and V_6.

Premature Atrial Complex (PAC): An ectopic beat originating from an irritable focus in the atria.

Premature Junctional Complex (PJC): An ectopic beat originating from an irritable focus in the AV Junction.

Premature Ventricular Complex (PVC): An ectopic beat originating from an irritable focus in the ventricles.

PR Interval (PRI): The time interval on EKG graph paper measured from the beginning of the P wave to the beginning of the R wave; includes both the P wave and the PR segment; indicates time of atrial depolarization.

PRI: P–R interval.

PR Segment: The time interval on EKG graph paper measured from the end of the P wave to the beginning of the R wave; indicates delay in the AV node.

Pulmonary Artery: Artery that carries deoxygenated blood from the right ventricle to the lungs.

Pulmonary Vein: Vein that carries oxygenated blood from the lungs back to the left atrium.

Pulmonic Valve: The valve that controls passage of blood from the right ventricle to the pulmonary artery.

Pulse Deficit: The situation in which the heart is contracting, but not all of the pulsations are reaching the periphery; the difference between heart beats heard with a stethoscope and the pulse rate measured at the periphery.

Pulseless Electrical Activity: A condition in which the EKG shows a viable rhythm, but no pulse is detectible in the patient. The electrical activity in the heart is not producing a mechanical response (pulse.)

Pulse Generator: The power source (battery unit) that drives an artificial pacemaker.

Pump (Sodium): *See* Sodium Pump.

Purkinje System: The part of the cardiac conduction system that transmits impulses from the bundle branches to the myocardial cells in the ventricles; consists of Purkinje fibers and terminal branches.

PVC: Premature Ventricular Complex.

P Wave: The first wave form in the normal cardiac cycle; indicates atrial depolarization.

QRS Complex: The wave form on an EKG that represents ventricular depolarization; includes the Q, R, and S waves.

QT Interval: The time interval from the beginning of the QRS complex to the end of the T wave; varies with heart rate.

Quadrigeminy: A cardiac rhythm in which ectopics replace every fourth normal beat, resulting in a cycle of three normal beats and one ectopic, repeated continuously.

Q Wave: The first negative deflection following the P wave, but before the R wave.

RA: Right atrium; right arm.

RAD: Right axis deviation.

RAE: Right atrial enlargement.

RBB: Right bundle branch.

RBBB: Right bundle branch block.

RCA: Right coronary artery.

Reciprocal Changes: EKG deflections seen in leads that are opposite of each other and thus are mirror images. For example, ST elevation in a facing lead would be ST depression in an opposite lead. Reciprocal changes in anterior leads are used to locate posterior infarctions.

Refractory: The state wherein the electrical cells are unable to respond to electrical stimulation because they have not yet recovered from the previous discharge.

Refractory Period: That portion of the cardiac cycle in which the heart is unable to respond to electrical stimulation because it has not yet recovered from the preceding depolarization; consists of the Absolute Refractory Period (QRS complex and upslope of the T wave) and the Relative Refractory Period (downslope of the T wave).

Relative Refractory Period: The terminal portion of the cardiac refractory period, during which a strong enough electrical stimulus could discharge the heart, resulting in inefficient and potentially dangerous arrhythmias; located on the downslope of the T wave.

Repolarization: The process of recharging depolarized cells back to their "ready" (polarized) state.

Retrograde Conduction: Electrical current that arises from the area of the AV junction and travels backward up toward the SA node to depolarize the atria in the opposite direction of normal.

Rhythm: The regularity of a cardiac pattern; generally used to refer to the arrhythmia itself, rather than its rhythmicity (i.e., "The patient's rhythm is Atrial Fibrillation"), even though Atrial Fibrillation is an irregular arrhythmia; synonymous with arrhythmia.

"R on T" Phenomenon: The situation in which the R wave of a PVC occurs on or near the downslope of the preceding T wave, thereby falling in the vulnerable phase of the cardiac cycle, the Relative Refractory Period, and threatening to cause premature discharge and result in an ineffective pattern, such as Ventricular Tachycardia or Ventricular Fibrillation.

Runaway Pacemaker: A malfunction of an artificial pacemaker that causes it to fire at an excessive rate.

RV: Right ventricle.

RVE: Right ventricular enlargement.

R Wave: The first upright deflection following the P wave, or the first positive wave of the QRS complex.

S/S: Signs/symptoms.

SA: Sino-atrial.

SA: Sinus Arrhythmia.

SB: Sinus Bradycardia.

sec: Second.

Second-Degree Heart Block, Type I: A type of Second-Degree Heart Block in which sinus impulses are delayed at the AV node for increasingly long periods, until conduction is blocked completely, then the cycle repeats itself; Wenckebach. (Formerly called Mobitz Type I.)

Second-Degree Heart Block, Type II: A type of Second-Degree Heart Block in which the AV node selectively blocks some beats while allowing others to pass through to the ventricles. The EKG shows more P waves than QRS complexes; some P waves are not followed by QRS complexes. (Formerly called Classical Second-Degree Heart Block, or Mobitz Type II.)

Septum: The wall that divides the heart into right and left sides. The thin wall between the atria is called the interatrial septum. The thicker wall between the ventricles is the interventricular septum.

Single-Chamber Pacemaker: Paces only the atria or the ventricles, but not both.

Sinus Arrhythmia (SA): The arrhythmia in which the pacemaker is located in the SA node but discharges irregularly; usually correlated with respirations; rate increases on inspiration, and decreases on expiration.

Sinus Bradycardia (SB): The arrhythmia in which the pacemaker is located in the SA node but discharges at a rate less than 60 bpm.

Sinus Node: The normal pacemaker of the heart; located at the junction of the superior vena cava and the right atrium; SA node; sinoatrial node.

Sinus Rhythm: Any rhythm that originates in the sinus (SA) node; used loosely to refer to Normal Sinus Rhythm.

Sinus Tachycardia (ST): The arrhythmia in which the pacemaker is located in the SA node but discharges at a rate greater than 100 bpm.

Sodium Pump: The chemical phenomenon that takes place at a cellular level within the cardiac electrical conduction system, in which sodium and potassium trade places across the cell wall, thereby initiating the flow of electrical current within the heart.

Standardization: The act of calibrating the EKG machine or oscilloscope to a standard (1 millivolt).

Standard Limb Leads: The bipolar leads showing the frontal plane: Leads I, II, and III.

Stroke Volume: The amount of blood ejected with each contraction of the left ventricle.

ST: Sinus Tachycardia.

ST Segment: The portion of the cardiac cycle between the S wave and the T wave.

Subendocardial Infarction: Infarcted area too small to extend all the way through the ventricular wall; also called a *less-than-transmural* infarction, or *non-Q* infarction, since the damage is often insufficient to create the classic Q wave changes seen with larger infarctions.

Superior Vena Cava (SVC): Vein that carries deoxygenated blood from the upper body back to the right atrium.

Supraventricular (SV): Originating above the ventricles.

Supraventricular Tachycardia (SVT): Term used to describe a rapid arrhythmia that is regular, has no visible P waves, and has a rate range common to other arrhythmias, thereby making more accurate identification impossible; commonly applied to Atrial Tachycardia, Junctional Tachycardia, Sinus Tachycardia, and Atrial Flutter with 1:1 response; loosely used to refer to any tachycardia that originated above the ventricles.

SV: Supraventricular.

SVC: Superior vena cava.

SVT: Supraventricular tachycardia.

S Wave: The second negative deflection following the P wave, or the first negative deflection following the R wave.

Sympathetic Nervous System: One of the two main branches of the autonomic nervous system, which controls involuntary bodily functions; stimulates cardiac activity in opposition to the parasympathetic branch; effects include increased heart rate and conduction and increased myocardial irritability.

Systole: The phase of the cardiac cycle in which the chambers are contracting.

Tachyarrhythmia: Any cardiac arrhythmia with a ventricular rate greater than 100 bpm.

Tachycardia: Heart rate greater than 100 bpm.

Temporary Pacemaker: An artificial pacemaker used in acute setting to stabilize and maintain patient for short periods.

Third-Degree Heart Block: The arrhythmia in which all atrial impulses are prevented from reaching the ventricles because of a complete block at the AV node; constitutes a form of AV dissociation because atria and ventricles function totally independent of each other; Complete Heart Block (CHB).

Transcutaneous Pacemaker: Pacemaker stimulus delivered across the skin via external pads.

Transmural Infarction: Infarcted area large enough to extend completely through the wall of the ventricle.

Transvenous Pacemaker: Pacemaker wire inserted through a vein.

Tricuspid Valve: The valve that controls passage of blood from the right atrium to the right ventricle.

Trigeminy: A pattern in which ectopics occur every third beat, producing a repetitive cycle of two normal beats and one ectopic.

Unifocal: Refers to ectopic beats that originate from a single irritable focus. Also called Uniformed.

Uniphasic: A single EKG wave that has only one phase, either upright or inverted.

Unipolar Lead: A lead that has only one charged electrode (positive electrode). The opposing pole is created by combining other electrodes into an electrically neutral reference point (the *central terminal*).

U Wave: Low-voltage wave following the T wave, having the same polarity as the T wave. Usually not apparent but becomes more pronounced in hypokalemia.

Variable Conduction: A changing conduction ratio within a given strip. For example, rather than having a consistent ratio of 2 Ps for every QRS complex (a 2:1 ratio) across an entire strip, a variable conduction would show 2:1, then 3:2, then back to 2:1, or maybe 4:3, all within the same strip.

VDD: Ventricle paced, double sensed, double response (AV synchronous pacemaker).

Vector: Direction of flow of cardiac electrical activity; represented by an arrow with the point indicating the positive pole and the size of arrow indicating magnitude of current.

Ventricles: The lower two chambers of the heart.

Ventricular Depolarization: Discharge of electrical activity throughout the ventricles to stimulate ventricular contraction; produces the QRS complex on an EKG.

Ventricular Fibrillation (VF):   The arrhythmia in which the ventricles are controlled by numerous irritable foci, producing chaotic, ineffective muscle activity rather than the normal contraction.

Ventricular Flutter (VF):   The arrhythmia in which a single irritable focus in the ventricles depolarizes the heart at a rate greater than 250 bpm; usually considered to be a rapid form of Ventricular Tachycardia.

Ventricular Hypertrophy: Enlargement of myocardial wall in one or more of the ventricles.

Ventricular Pacemaker: An electrical stimulus from the ventricles that controls heart rhythm; an artificial pacemaker that stimulates only the ventricles.

Ventricular Standstill: The arrhythmia in which the ventricles are not depolarized by any electrical stimulation and therefore do not contract; if atrial activity is present, it is not conducted through the AV node; if no atrial activity is present, it is called Asystole.

Ventricular Tachycardia (VT):   The arrhythmia in which a single irritable focus in the ventricles depolarizes the heart at a rate of 150–250 bpm.

VF: Ventricular Fibrillation, Ventricular Flutter.

VT: Ventricular Tachycardia.

Vulnerable Period: The period in the cardiac cycle when the heart is most susceptible to premature discharge, with a resultant ineffective pattern if it receives a strong enough electrical stimulus; the Relative Refractory Period; corresponds with the downslope of the T wave.

VVI: Ventricle paced, ventricle sensed, inhibited response (ventricular demand pacemaker).

Wandering Pacemaker (WP):   The arrhythmia in which the pacemaker site shifts from the SA node to the atrium and back again, sometimes dropping as low as the AV junction.

Waves: Deflections on the electrocardiograph caused by changes in electrical activity in the heart.

Wenckebach: The form of Second-Degree AV Block in which the node progressively holds each impulse longer until one is eventually not conducted, then the cycle starts over; Type I Second-Degree Heart Block.

WP: Wandering Pacemaker.

Answers Key

Chapter 2,

Practice Strips Answers

PART I: LABELING WAVES

2.1

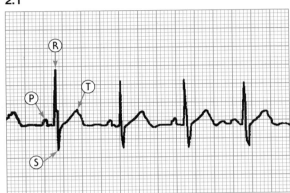

2.2

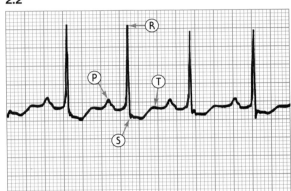

2.3

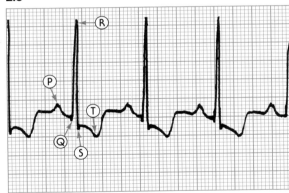

2.4

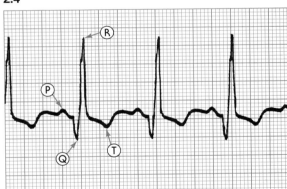

2.5

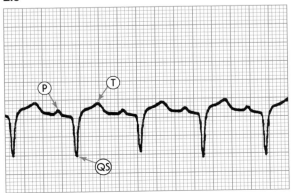

2.6

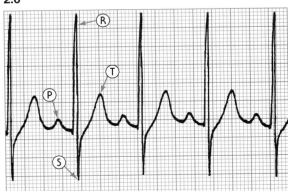

2.7

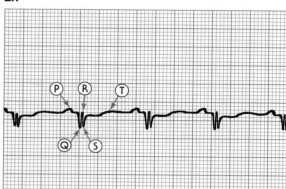

2.8

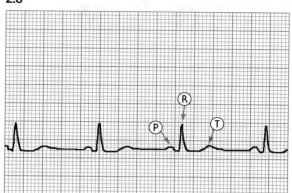

2.9

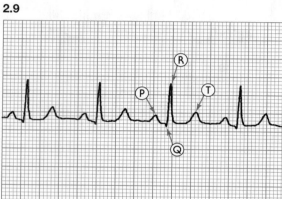

2.10

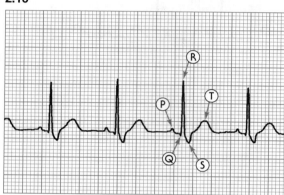

2.11

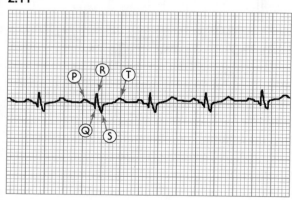

2.12

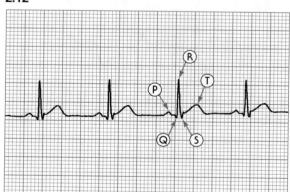

PART II: MEASURING INTERVALS

2.13

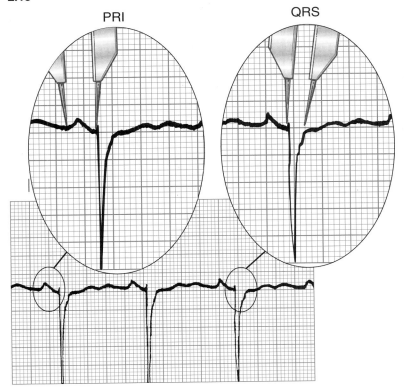

PRI: 0.20 second

QRS: 0.12 second

2.14

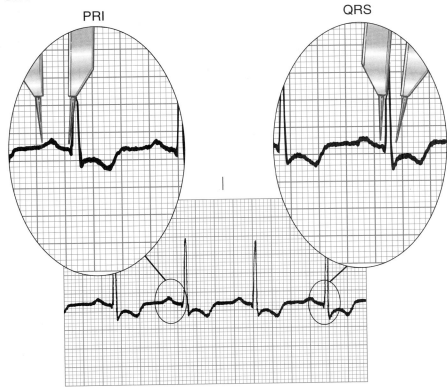

PRI: 0.20 second

QRS: 0.10 second

2.15

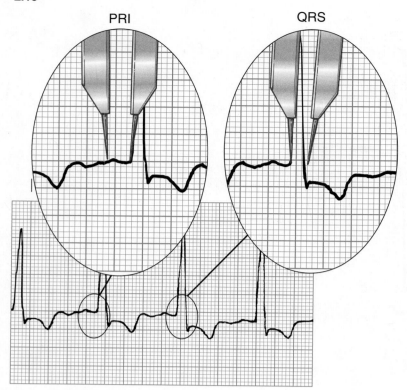

PRI: 0.16 second

QRS: 0.12 second

2.16

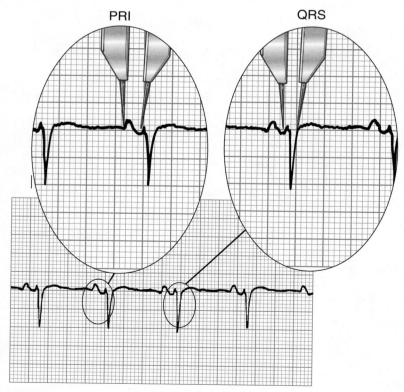

PRI: 0.12 second

QRS: 0.10 second

2.17

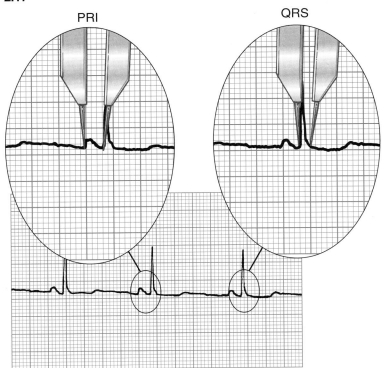

PRI: 0.14 second

QRS: 0.08 second

2.18

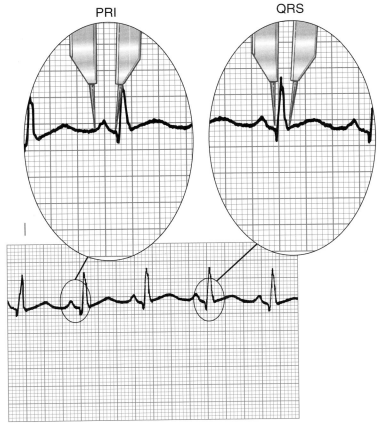

PRI: 0.14 second

QRS: 0.10 second

2.19

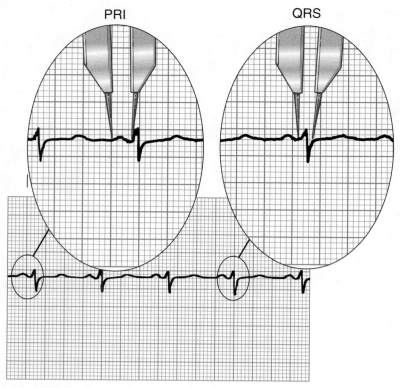

PRI: 0.14 second

QRS: 0.10 second

2.20

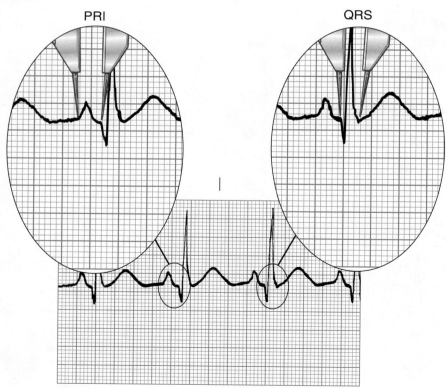

PRI: 0.16 second

QRS: 0.14 second

2.21

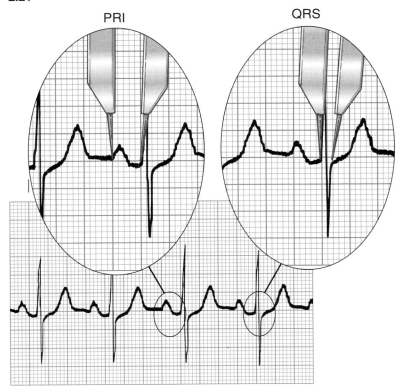

PRI: 0.20 second
QRS: 0.08 second

2.22

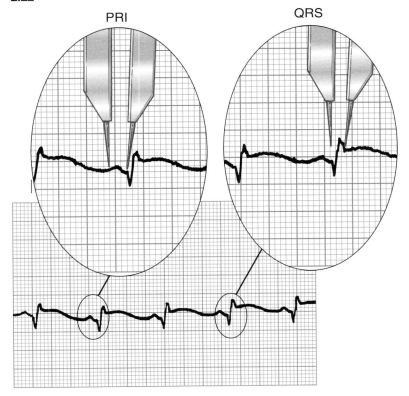

PRI: 0.12 second
QRS: 0.10 second

2.23

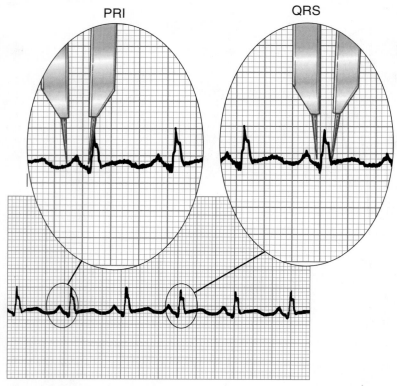

PRI: 0.16 second

QRS: 0.11 second

2.24

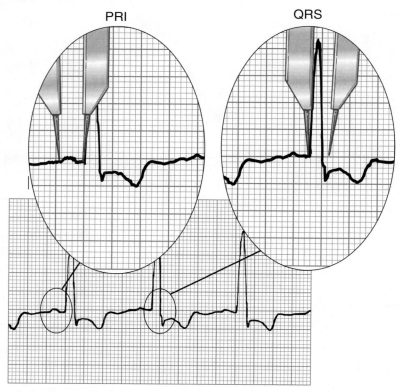

PRI: 0.16 second

QRS: 0.14 second

2.25

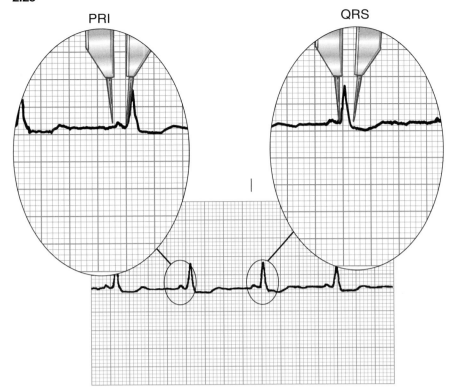

PRI: 0.10 second

QRS: 0.10 second

2.26

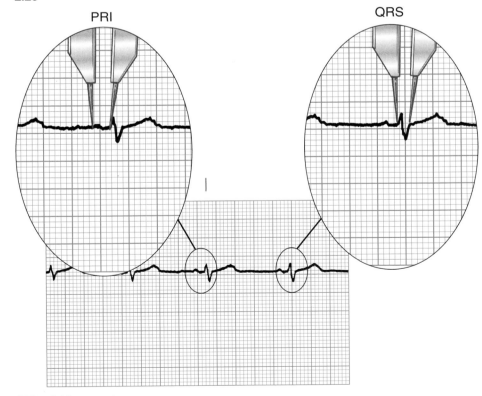

PRI: 0.12 second

QRS: 0.08 second

2.27

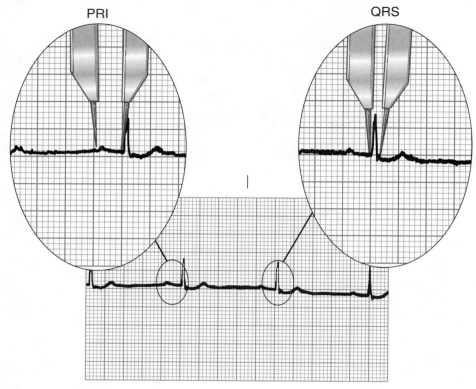

PRI: 0.18 second
QRS: 0.06 second

2.28

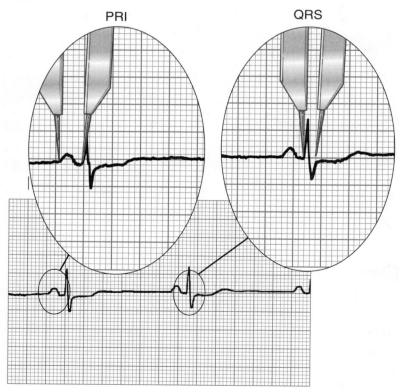

PRI: 0.16 second
QRS: 0.08 second

2.29

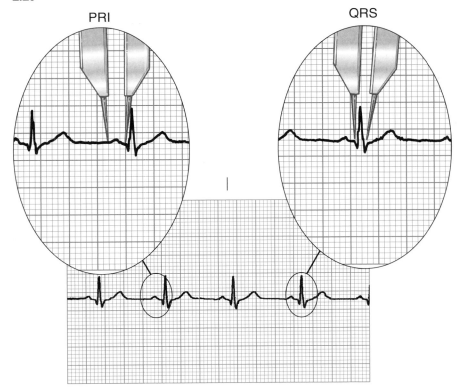

PRI: 0.12 second
QRS: 0.08 second

2.30

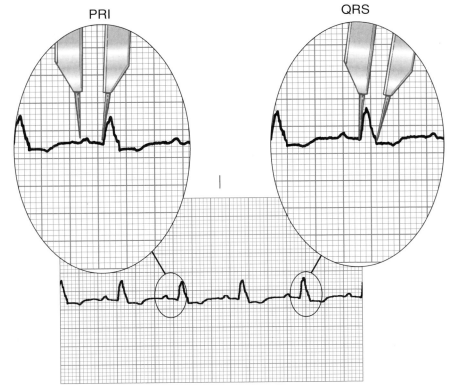

PRI: 0.16 second
QRS: 0.12 second

Chapter 3

3.1 Regularity: regular
Rate: 79 bpm
P Waves: regular
P–P interval; uniform
waves

PRI: 0.16 second and
constant
QRS: 0.08 second

3.2 Regularity: regular (very
slightly irregular)
Rate: approximately 90 bpm
P Waves: uniform; regular
P–P interval

PRI: 0.12 second and
constant
QRS: 0.08 second

3.3 Regularity: regular
Rate: 63 bpm
P Waves: uniform; regular
P–P interval

PRI: 0.16 second and
constant
QRS: 0.10 second

3.4 Regularity: regular
Rate: 125 bpm
P Waves: uniform, regular
P–P interval

PRI: 0.16 second and
constant
QRS: 0.08 second

3.5 Regularity: regular
Rate: 83 bpm
P Waves: uniform; regular
P–P interval

PRI: 0.16 second and
constant
QRS: 0.12 second

3.6 Regularity: regular
Rate: 107 bpm
P Waves: uniform; regular
P–P interval

PRI: 0.20 second and
constant
QRS: 0.10 second

3.7 Regularity: regular
Rate: 79 bpm
P Waves: uniform; regular
P–P intervals

PRI: 0.10 second and
constant
QRS: 0.06 second

3.8 Regularity: regular
Rate: 79 bpm
P Waves: uniform; regular
P–P interval

PRI: 0.16 second and
constant
QRS: 0.10 second

3.9 Regularity: regular
Rate: 83 bpm
P Waves: uniform; regular
P–P interval

PRI: 0.20 second and
constant
QRS: 0.08 second

3.10 Regularity: irregular
Rate: approximately
80 bpm
P Waves: uniform; irregular
P–P interval

PRI: 0.16 second and
constant
QRS: 0.10 second

3.11 Regularity: regular (very
slightly irregular)
Rate: 83 bpm
P Waves: upright and
uniform

PRI: 0.14 second
QRS: 0.10 second

3.12 Regularity: regular
Rate: 50 bpm
P Waves: upright and
uniform

PRI: 0.12 second
QRS: 0.08 second

3.13 Regularity: regular
Rate: 79 bpm
P Waves: upright and
uniform

PRI: 0.12 second
QRS: 0.08 second

3.14 Regularity: irregular
Rate: 70 bpm
P Waves: upright and
uniform

PRI: 0.16 second
QRS: 0.08 second

3.15 Regularity: regular (very
slightly irregular)
Rate: 79 bpm
P Waves: upright and
uniform

PRI: 0.16 second
QRS: 0.08 second

Chapter 4

4.1 Regularity: regular (slightly
irregular)
Rate: 48 bpm
P Waves: uniform and up-
right; regular P–P interval

PRI: 0.18 second and
constant
QRS: 0.12 second
Interp: Sinus Bradycardia
(with wide QRS)

4.2 Regularity: irregular
Rate: approximately 80 bpm
P Waves: uniform and up-
right; regular P–P interval

PRI: 0.14 second and
constant
QRS: 0.06 second
Interp: Sinus Arrhythmia

4.3 Regularity: regular
Rate: 75 bpm
P Waves: uniform and
upright; regular
P–P interval

PRI: 0.16 second and
constant
QRS: 0.08 second
Interp: Normal Sinus
Rhythm

4.4 Regularity: regular
Rate: 136 bpm
P Waves: uniform and up-
right; regular P–P interval

PRI: 0.16 second and
constant
QRS: 0.06 second
Interp: Sinus Tachycardia

4.5 Regularity: irregular
Rate: approximately 80 bpm
P Waves: uniform P waves
with an irregular P–P
interval

PRI: 0.16 second and
constant
QRS: 0.08 second
Interp: Sinus Arrhythmia

4.6 Regularity: regular
Rate: 107 bpm
P Waves: uniform and
upright; regular
P–P interval

PRI: 0.16 second and
constant
QRS: 0.12 second
Interp: Sinus Tachycardia
(with a wide QRS)

4.7 Regularity: regular
Rate: 50 bpm
P Waves: uniform and up-
right; regular P–P interval

PRI: 0.12 second and
constant
QRS: 0.08 second
Interp: Sinus Bradycardia

4.8 Regularity: regular
Rate: 83 bpm
P Waves: uniform and up-
right; regular P–P interval

PRI: 0.16 second and
constant
QRS: 0.08 second
Interp: Normal Sinus
Rhythm

4.9 Regularity: regular
Rate: 94 bpm
P Waves: uniform and upright; regular P–P interval

PRI: 0.16 second and constant
QRS: 0.12 second
Interp: Normal Sinus Rhythm (with a wide QRS)

4.10 Regularity: slightly irregular
Rate: approximately 30 bpm
P Waves: uniform and upright; irregular P–P interval

PRI: 0.18 second and constant
QRS: 0.08 second
Interp: Sinus Bradyarrhythmia

4.11 Regularity: regular
Rate: 75 bpm
P Waves: uniform and upright; regular P–P interval

PRI: 0.18 second and constant
QRS: 0.06 second
Interp: Normal Sinus Rhythm

4.12 Regularity: irregular
Rate: 90 bpm
P Waves: uniform and upright; irregular P–P interval

PRI: 0.20 second and constant
QRS: 0.06 second
Interp: Sinus Arrhythmia

4.13 Regularity: regular
Rate: 48 bpm
P Waves: uniform and upright; regular P–P interval

PRI: 0.20 second and constant
QRS: 0.08 second
Interp: Sinus Bradycardia

4.14 Regularity: irregular
Rate: approximately 70 bpm
P Waves: uniform and upright; regular P–P interval

PRI: 0.14 second and constant
QRS: 0.06 second
Interp: Sinus Arrhythmia

4.15 Regularity: regular
Rate: 65 bpm
P Waves: uniform and upright; regular P–P interval

PRI: 0.16 second and constant
QRS: 0.08 second
Interp: Normal Sinus Rhythm

4.16 Regularity: regular
Rate: 115 bpm
P Waves: uniform and upright; regular P–P interval

PRI: 0.14 second and constant
QRS: 0.16 second
Interp: Sinus Tachycardia (with wide QRS)

4.17 Regularity: regular
Rate: 65 bpm
P Waves: uniform and upright; regular P–P interval

PRI: 0.12 second and constant
QRS: 0.08 second
Interp: Normal Sinus Rhythm

4.18 Regularity: irregular
Rate: approximately 80 bpm
P Waves: uniform and upright; regular P–P interval

PRI: 0.12 second and constant
QRS: 0.08 second
Interp: Sinus Arrhythmia

4.19 Regularity: regular
Rate: 88 bpm
P Waves: uniform and upright; regular P–P interval

PRI: 0.16 second and constant
QRS: 0.08 second
Interp: Normal Sinus Rhythm

4.20 Regularity: regular
Rate: 150 bpm
P Waves: upright and uniform

PRI: 0.12 second
QRS: 0.08 second
Interp: Sinus Tachycardia

4.21 Regularity: regular
Rate: 83 bpm
P Waves: upright and uniform

PRI: 0.20 second
QRS: 0.12 second
Interp: Normal Sinus Rhythm (with wide QRS)

4.22 Regularity: regular
Rate: 54 bpm
P Waves: upright and uniform

PRI: 0.16 second
QRS: 0.08 second
Interp: Sinus Bradycardia

4.23 Regularity: regular
Rate: 107 bpm
P Waves: upright and uniform

PRI: 0.12 second
QRS: 0.08 second
Interp: Sinus Tachycardia

4.24 Regularity: irregular
Rate: 70 bpm
P Waves: upright and uniform

PRI: 0.20 second
QRS: 0.10 second
Interp: Sinus Arrhythmia

4.25 Regularity: irregular
Rate: 50 bpm
P Waves: upright and uniform

PRI: 0.16 second
QRS: 0.08 second
Interp: Sinus Bradyarrhythmia

4.26 Regularity: regular
Rate: 88 bpm
P Waves: upright and uniform

PRI: 0.14 second
QRS: 0.08 second
Interp: Normal Sinus Rhythm

4.27 Regularity: irregular
Rate: 50 bpm
P Waves: upright and uniform

PRI: 0.14 second
QRS: 0.08 second
Interp: Sinus Bradyarrhythmia

4.28 Regularity: regular
Rate: 107 bpm
P Waves: upright and uniform

PRI: 0.16 second
QRS: 0.08 second
Interp: Sinus Tachycardia

4.29 Regularity: regular (very slightly irregular)
Rate: 43 bpm
P Waves: upright and uniform

PRI: 0.18 second
QRS: 0.11 second
Interp: Sinus Bradycardia

4.30 Regularity: irregular
Rate: 70 bpm
P Waves: upright and uniform

PRI: 0.12 second
QRS: 0.08 second
Interp: Sinus Arrhythmia

Interpretation of Chapter 3 Rhythm Strips

3.1 Normal Sinus Rythm

3.2 Normal Sinus Rhythm (only very slightly irregular)

3.3 Normal Sinus Rhythm

3.4 Sinus Tachycardia

3.5 Normal Sinus Rhythm

3.6 Sinus Tachycardia

3.7 Normal Sinus Rhythm

3.8 Normal Sinus Rhythm

3.9 Normal Sinus Rhythm

3.10 Sinus Arrhythmia

3.11 Normal Sinus Rhythm

3.12 Sinus Bradycardia

3.13 Normal Sinus Rhythm

3.14 Sinus Arrhythmia

3.15 Normal Sinus Rhythm

Chapter 5

5.1   Regularity: irregular
Rate: approximately 100 bpm
P Waves: not discernible; only undulations are present
PRI: none
QRS: 0.08 second
Interp: Atrial Fibrillation, controlled

5.2   Regularity: regular
Rate: atrial rate is 300 bpm; ventricular rate is 150 bpm
P Waves: uniform; sawtooth appearance
PRI: none
QRS: 0.10 second (QRS is difficult to measure due to obscuring by Flutter waves)
Interp: Atrial Flutter with 2:1 response

5.3   Regularity: regular underlying rhythm interrupted by an ectopic
Rate: 71 bpm
P Waves: uniform in underlying rhythm; one differently shaped P wave before ectopic
PRI: 0.16 second and constant
QRS: 0.10 second
Interp: Sinus Rhythm with one PAC

5.4   Regularity: irregular
Rate: approximately 90 bpm
P Waves: not discernible; undulations present
PRI: none
QRS: 0.12 second
Interp: Atrial Fibrillation, controlled (with wide QRS)

5.5   Regularity: regular
Rate: atrial rate is 328 bpm; ventricular rate is 82 bpm
P Waves: uniform; sawtooth appearance
PRI: none
QRS: 0.08 second
Interp: Atrial Flutter with 4:1 response

5.6   Regularity: irregular
Rate: approximately 50 bpm
P Waves: not discernible; undulations present
PRI: none
QRS: 0.08 second (QRS complexes are sometimes obscured by fibrillatory waves)
Interp: Atrial Fibrillation, controlled

5.7   Regularity: regular underlying rhythm interrupted by ectopics
Rate: 115 bpm
P Waves: uniform in the underlying rhythm; shape of P wave changes before each ectopic
PRI: 0.12 second
QRS: 0.08 second; shape of QRS is uniform in both underlying beats and ectopics
Interp: Sinus Tachycardia with three PACs

5.8   Regularity: irregular
Rate: approximately 90 bpm
P Waves: not discernible; undulations present
PRI: none
QRS: 0.08 seconds
Interp: Atrial Fibrillation, controlled

5.9   Regularity: irregular
Rate: approximately 140 bpm
P Waves: not discernible
PRI: none
QRS: 0.06 second
Interp: Atrial Fibrillation, uncontrolled

5.10   Regularity: regular underlying rhythm interrupted by an ectopic
Rate: 65 bpm (rate changes after the ectopic because sinus firing mechanism resets itself)
P Waves: uniform in underlying rhythm; shape differs in ectopic
PRI: 0.16 second and constant; 0.20 second in ectopic
QRS: 0.10 second
Interp: Sinus Rhythm with one PAC

5.11   Regularity: irregular
Rate: atrial rate 300 bpm; ventricular rate approximately 130 bpm
P Waves: uniform; sawtooth appearance
PRI: none
QRS: 0.08 second
Interp: Atrial Flutter with variable response

5.12   Regularity: irregular
Rate: approximately 80 bpm
P Waves: not discernible
PRI: none
QRS: 0.10 second
Interp: Atrial Fibrillation, controlled

5.13   Regularity: regular
Rate: atrial rate is 332 bpm; ventricular rate is 83 bpm
P Waves: uniform; sawtooth in appearance
PRI: none
QRS: 0.08 second
Interp: Atrial Flutter with 4:1 response

5.14   Regularity: regular
Rate: atrial rate is 300 bpm; ventricular rate is 75 bpm
P Waves: uniform; there are four P waves for every QRS complex
PRI: none
QRS: 0.10 second
Interp: Atrial Flutter with 4:1 response

5.15   Regularity: irregular
Rate: 60 bpm
P Waves: morphology changes
PRI: varies
QRS: 0.08 second
Interp: Wandering Pacemaker

5.16   Regularity: irregular
Rate: approximately 80 bpm
P Waves: not visible; only undulations are present
PRI: none
QRS: 0.04 second
Interp: Atrial Fibrillation, controlled

5.17   Regularity: regular
Rate: atrial rate is 334 bpm; ventricular rate is 166 bpm
P Waves: uniform; sawtooth appearance; two P waves for every QRS complex
PRI: none
QRS: 0.10 second; slightly obscured by Flutter waves
Interp: Atrial Flutter with 2:1 response

5.18   Regularity: irregular
Rate: approximately 120 bpm
P Waves: not discernible; only undulations are present
PRI: none
QRS: 0.08 second
Interp: Atrial Fibrillation, uncontrolled

5.19 Regularity: irregular
Rate: approximately
70 bpm
P Waves: not discernible;
only fine undulations are
present

PRI: none
QRS: 0.04 second
Interp: Atrial Fibrillation,
controlled

5.20 Regularity: irregular
Rate: approximately
110 bpm
P Waves: what appear to
be P waves do not map
out; they are actually
coarse fibrillatory waves

PRI: none
QRS: 0.06 second; QRS
complexes are obscured
by fibrillatory waves
Interp: Atrial Fibrillation,
uncontrolled

5.21 Regularity: irregular
Rate: approximately
150 bpm
P Waves: unable to map
out; undulations present

PRI: none
QRS: 0.06 second (QRS
complexes are obscured
by fibrillatory waves)
Interp: Atrial Fibrillation,
uncontrolled

5.22 Regularity: irregular
Rate: 70 bpm
P Waves: morphology
changes

PRI: varies
QRS: 0.08 second
Interp: Wandering
Pacemaker

5.23 Regularity: irregular
Rate: 80 bpm
P Waves: undulations
present

PRI: unable
QRS: 0.08 second
Interp: Atrial Fibrillation,
controlled

5.24 Regularity: regular underlying rhythm interrupted
by ectopic
Rate: 50 bpm
P Waves: upright and
uniform

PRI: 0.16 second
QRS: 0.14 second
Interp: Sinus Bradycardia
(with wide QRS) with one
PAC

5.25 Regularity: irregular
Rate: atrial rate 300 bpm;
ventricular rate 80 bpm
P Waves: sawtooth
appearance

PRI: unable
QRS: 0.10 second
Interp: Atrial Flutter with
variable response

5.26 Regularity: irregular
Rate: 100 bpm
P Waves: undulations
present

PRI: unable
QRS: 0.14 second
Interp: Atrial Fibrillation,
controlled (with wide
QRS)

5.27 Regularity: regular underlying rhythm interrupted
by ectopic
Rate: 65 bpm in underlying
rhythm; 70 bpm overall
P Waves: upright and
uniform

PRI: 0.18 second
QRS: 0.11 second
Interp: Sinus Rhythm with
one PAC

5.28 Regularity: regular
Rate: atrial rate 250 bpm;
ventricular rate 125 bpm
P Waves: sawtooth
appearance

PRI: unable
QRS: 0.08 second
Interp: Atrial Flutter with
2:1 response

5.29 Regularity: irregular
Rate: 120 bpm
P Waves: none visible

PRI: unable
QRS: 0.10 second
Interp: Atrial Fibrillation,
uncontrolled

5.30 Regularity: regular
Rate: atrial rate 284 bpm;
ventricular rate 71 bpm
P Waves: sawtooth
appearance

PRI: unable
QRS: 0.08 second
Interp: Atrial Flutter with
4:1 response

5.31 Regularity: irregular
Rate: 50 bpm
P Waves: none visible

PRI: unable
QRS: 0.08 second
Interp: Atrial Fibrillation,
controlled

5.32 Regularity: irregular
Rate: atrial rate 300 bpm;
ventricular rate 150 bpm
P Waves: sawtooth
appearance

PRI: unable
QRS: 0.08 second
Interp: Atrial Flutter with
variable response,
uncontrolled

5.33 Regularity: regular underlying rhythm interrupted
by ectopic
Rate: 50 bpm in underlying
rhythm
P Waves: upright in underlying rhythm; morphol-
ogy changes in ectopic

PRI: 0.16 second
QRS: 0.14 second
Interp: Sinus Bradycardia
(with wide QRS) with one
PAC

5.34 Regularity: regular
Rate: atrial rate 272 bpm;
ventricular rate 136 bpm
P Waves: sawtooth

PRI: unable
QRS: 0.08 second
Interp: Atrial Flutter with
2:1 response

5.35 Regularity: irregular
Rate: 110 bpm
P Waves: none visible

PRI: unable
QRS: 0.08 second
Interp: Atrial Fibrillation,
uncontrolled

5.36 Regularity: irregular
Rate: 140 bpm
P Waves: undulations
present

PRI: unable
QRS: 0.08 second
Interp: Atrial Fibrillation,
uncontrolled

5.37 Regularity: regular underlying rhythm interrupted
by ectopic
Rate: 88 bpm
P Waves: upright and
uniform

PRI: 0.14 second
QRS: 0.10 second
Interp: Sinus Rhythm with
one PAC

5.38 Regularity: regular
Rate: atrial rate 272 bpm;
ventricular rate 136 bpm
P Waves: sawtooth

PRI: unable
QRS: 0.10 second
Interp: Atrial Flutter with
2:1 response

5.39 Regularity: irregular in
a pattern of grouped
beating
Rate: 80 bpm (including
ectopics)
P Waves: upright and
uniform

PRI: 0.12 second
QRS: 0.08 second (both
underlying rhythm and
ectopics)
Interp: Sinus Rhythm with
4 PACs (every other beat
is a PAC). This pattern
is called "bigeminy,"
which will be explained
in Chapter 8.

5.40 Regularity: regular
Rate: atrial rate 272 bpm;
   ventricular rate 136 bpm
P Waves: sawtooth
   appearance

PRI: unable
QRS: 0.10 second
Interp: Atrial Flutter with
   2:1 response

5.41 Regularity: regular
Rate: atrial rate 316 bpm;
   ventricular rate 79 bpm
P Waves: sawtooth
   appearance

PRI: unable
QRS: 0.08 second
Interp: Atrial Flutter with
   4:1 response

5.42 Regularity: regular underlying rhythm interrupted
   by ectopic
Rate: 65 bpm
P Waves: upright and
   uniform

PRI: 0.14 second
QRS: 0.08 second
Interp: Sinus Rhythm with
   one PAC

5.43 Regularity: irregular
Rate: 110 bpm
P Waves: none visible;
   cannot map out

PRI: unable
QRS: 0.10 second
Interp: Atrial Fibrillation,
   uncontrolled

5.44 Regularity: regular underlying rhythm interrupted
   by ectopic
Rate: 54 bpm
P Waves: upright and
   uniform

PRI: 0.16 second
QRS: 0.08 second
Interp: Sinus Bradycardia
   with one PAC

5.45 Regularity: regular
Rate: atrial rate 200 bpm;
   ventricular rate 100 bpm
P Waves: sawtooth
   appearance

PRI: unable
QRS: 0.08 second
Interp: Atrial Flutter with
   2:1 response

5.46 Regularity: irregular
Rate: 70 bpm
P Waves: none visible

PRI: unable
QRS: 0.10 second
Interp: Atrial Fibrillation,
   controlled

5.47 Regularity: regular
Rate: atrial rate 272 bpm;
   ventricular rate 136 bpm
P Waves: sawtooth
   appearance

PRI: unable
QRS: 0.08 second
Interp: Atrial Flutter with
   2:1 response

5.48 Regularity: regular underlying rhythm interrupted
   by ectopics
Rate: 65 bpm
P Waves: upright and
   uniform

PRI: 0.16 second
QRS: 0.08 second
Interp: Sinus Rhythm with
   run of three PACs

5.49 Regularity: irregular
Rate: 100 bpm
P Waves: undulations
   present

PRI: unable
QRS: 0.08 second
Interp: Atrial Fibrillation,
   controlled

5.50 Regularity: regular underlying rhythm interrupted
   by ectopic
Rate: 125 bpm
P Waves: upright and
   uniform

PRI: 0.12 second
QRS: 0.08 second (in both
   underlying rhythm and
   ectopic)
Interp: Sinus Tachycardia
   with one PAC

5.51 Regularity: regular
Rate: atrial rate 332 bpm;
   ventricular rate 166 bpm
P Waves: sawtooth
   appearance

PRI: unable
QRS: 0.11 second
Interp: Atrial Flutter with
   2:1 response

5.52 Regularity: regular underlying rhythm interrupted
   by ectopic
Rate: 65 bpm
P Waves: upright and
   uniform

PRI: 0.16 second
QRS: 0.08 second (in both
   underlying rhythm and
   ectopic)
Interp: Sinus Rhythm with
   one PAC

5.53 Regularity: regular underlying rhythm interrupted
   by ectopic
Rate: 71 bpm
P Waves: upright and
   uniform

PRI: 0.16 second
QRS: 0.08 second (in both
   underlying rhythm and
   ectopic)
Interp: Sinus Rhythm with
   one PAC

5.54 Regularity: regular underlying rhythm interrupted
   by ectopic
Rate: 68 bpm
P Waves: upright and
   uniform

PRI: 0.16 second
QRS: 0.10 second (in both
   underlying rhythm and
   ectopic)
Interp: Sinus Rhythm with
   one PAC

5.55 Regularity: irregular
Rate: atrial rate 300 bpm;
   ventricular rate 90 bpm
P Waves: sawtooth
   appearance

PRI: unable
QRS: 0.08 second
Interp: Atrial Flutter with
   variable response

5.56 Regularity: slightly irregular
Rate: 80 bpm
P Waves: changing
   morphology

PRI: varies
QRS: 0.10 second
Interp: Wandering
   Pacemaker

5.57 Regularity: regular
Rate: atrial rate 376 bpm;
   ventricular rate 188 bpm
P Waves: sawtooth
   appearance

PRI: unable
QRS: 0.08 second
Interp: Atrial Flutter with
   2:1 response

Chapter 6

6.1 Regularity: regular underlying rhythm interrupted
   by an ectopic
Rate: 107 bpm
P Waves: uniform P waves
   except one missing be-
   fore ectopic QRS

PRI: 0.16 second and
   constant
QRS: 0.08 second; QRS
   of ectopic beat is same
   size and shape as QRS
   of underlying rhythm
Interp: Sinus Tachycardia
   with one PJC

6.2 Regularity: regular
Rate: 83 bpm
P Waves: no visible
   P waves

PRI: none
QRS: 0.08 second
Interp: Accelerated Junc-
   tional Rhythm

6.3 Regularity: regular
Rate: 100 bpm
P Waves: all P waves are
   inverted

PRI: 0.10 second and
   constant
QRS: 0.06 second
Interp: Junctional
   Tachycardia

6.4   Regularity: regular
Rate: 43 bpm
P Waves: no visible
P waves

PRI: none
QRS: 0.08 second
Interp: Junctional Escape
Rhythm

6.5   Regularity: slightly irregular
underlying rhythm inter-
rupted by an ectopic
Rate: 50 bpm
P Waves: uniform, upright
P waves; one inverted
P wave before ectopic
QRS

PRI: 0.16 second and
constant for underlying
rhythm; 0.11 second for
ectopic
QRS: 0.08 second; QRS of
ectopic is same shape
and width as QRS of un-
derlying rhythm
Interp: Sinus Bradycardia
with one PJC

6.6   Regularity: regular
Rate: 71 bpm
P Waves: no visible
P waves

PRI: none
QRS: 0.10 second
Interp: Accelerated Junc-
tional Rhythm

6.7   Regularity: regular
Rate: 167 bpm
P Waves: P waves are not
visible

PRI: none
QRS: 0.06 second
Interp: Supraventricular
Tachycardia

6.8   Regularity: regular
Rate: 79 bpm
P Waves: no visible
P waves

PRI: none
QRS: 0.06 second
Interp: Accelerated Junc-
tional Rhythm

6.9   Regularity: regular
Rate: 214 bpm
P Waves: P waves are not
visible

PRI: none
QRS: 0.08 second
Interp: Supraventricular
Tachycardia

6.10   Regularity: regular underlying rhythm interrupted
by an ectopic
Rate: 81 bpm
P Waves: uniform and
upright except for one
inverted P wave in front
of ectopic QRS

PRI: 0.16 second and
constant for underlying
rhythm; 0.10 second for
ectopic
QRS: 0.08 second for both
underlying rhythm and
ectopic
Interp: Sinus Rhythm with
one PJC

6.11   Regularity: regular
Rate: 150 bpm
P Waves: P waves are not
visible

PRI: none
QRS: 0.10 second
Interp: Supraventricular
Tachycardia

6.12   Regularity: regular
Rate: 43 bpm
P Waves: P waves are not
visible

PRI: none
QRS: 0.10 second
Interp: Junctional Escape
Rhythm

6.13   Regularity: regular
Rate: 88 bpm
P Waves: inverted and uni-
form P waves

PRI: 0.11 second and
constant
QRS: 0.10 second
Interp: Accelerated Junc-
tional Rhythm

6.14   Regularity: regular
Rate: 50 bpm
P Waves: none visible

PRI: unable
QRS: 0.14 second
Interp: Junctional Escape
Rhythm (with wide QRS)

6.15   Regularity: regular
Rate: 188 bpm
P Waves: inverted follow-
ing QRS

PRI: unable
QRS: 0.08 second
Interp: Junctional
Tachycardia

6.16   Regularity: regular
Rate: 188 bpm
P Waves: unable

PRI: unable
QRS: 0.08 second
Interp: Supraventricular
Tachycardia (with base-
line artifact)

6.17   Regularity: regular (slightly
irregular)
Rate: 140 bpm
P Waves: none visible

PRI: unable
QRS: 0.08 second
Interp: Junctional
Tachycardia

6.18   Regularity: slightly irregular
Rate: 44 bpm
P Waves: none visible

PRI: none
QRS: 0.08 second
Interp: Junctional Escape
Rhythm

6.19   Regularity: regular
Rate: 75 bpm
P Waves: none visible

PRI: unable
QRS: 0.08 second
Interp: Accelerated Junc-
tional Rhythm

6.20   Regularity: regular underlying rhythm interrupted
by ectopic
Rate: 56 bpm
P Waves: upright in underlying rhythm

PRI: 0.16 second in underlying rhythm; unable to
measure in ectopic
QRS: 0.08 second
Interp: Sinus Bradycardia
with one PJC

6.21   Regularity: regular
Rate: 188 bpm
P Waves: unable

PRI: unable
QRS: 0.08 second
Interp: Supraventricular
Tachycardia

6.22   Regularity: regular
Rate: 71 bpm
P Waves: none visible

PRI: unable
QRS: 0.08 second
Interp: Accelerated Junc-
tional Rhythm

6.23   Regularity: regular
Rate: 167 bpm
P Waves: upright and
uniform

PRI: unable
QRS: 0.08 second
Interp: Supraventricular
Tachycardia

6.24   Regularity: regular
Rate: 125 bpm
P Waves: none visible

PRI: unable
QRS: 0.10 second
Interp: Junctional
Tachycardia

6.25   Regularity: slightly irregular
Rate: 58 bpm
P Waves: none visible

PRI: unable
QRS: 0.08 second
Interp: Junctional Escape
Rhythm

6.26   Regularity: regular underlying rhythm interrupted
by ectopic
Rate: 45 bpm
P Waves: upright in underlying rhythm; absent in
ectopic

PRI: 0.12 second in underlying rhythm; unable to
measure in ectopic
QRS: 0.10 second (in both
underlying rhythm and
ectopic)
Interp: Sinus Bradycardia
with one PJC

6.27 Regularity: regular
Rate: 45 bpm
P Waves: none

PRI: unable
QRS: 0.08 second
Interp: Junctional Escape Rhythm

6.28 Regularity: regular
Rate: 214 bpm
P Waves: unable

PRI: unable
QRS: 0.08 second
Interp: Supraventricular Tachycardia

6.29 Regularity: regular
Rate: 58 bpm
P Waves: none

PRI: unable
QRS: 0.08 second
Interp: Junctional Escape Rhythm

6.30 Regularity: regular underlying rhythm interrupted by ectopics
Rate: 54 bpm
P Waves: upright in underlying rhythm

PRI: 0.16 second in underlying rhythm; unable to measure in ectopics
QRS: 0.08 second (in both underlying rhythm and ectopics)
Interp: Sinus Bradycardia with two PJCs

6.31 Regularity: regular
Rate: 79 bpm
P Waves: none

PRI: unable
QRS: 0.08 second
Interp: Accelerated Junctional Rhythm

6.32 Regularity: regular
Rate: 150 bpm
P Waves: unable

PRI: unable
QRS: 0.08 second
Interp: Supraventricular Tachycardia

6.33 Regularity: regular
Rate: 150 bpm
P Waves: unable

PRI: unable
QRS: 0.10 second
Interp: Supraventricular Tachycardia

6.34 Regularity: regular
Rate: 214 bpm
P Waves: unable

PRI: unable
QRS: 0.08 second
Interp: Supraventricular Tachycardia

6.35 Regularity: irregular in a pattern of grouped beating
Rate: 100 bpm (including ectopics)
P Waves: upright in underlying rhythm; absent in ectopics

PRI: 0.14 second in underlying rhythm; unable to measure in ectopics
QRS: 0.08 second in underlying rhythm; 0.10 second in ectopics
Interp: Sinus Rhythm with bigeminy of PJCs. When every other beat is an ectopic, the pattern is called "bigeminy." It will be explained further in Chapter 8.

6.36 Regularity: regular
Rate: 100 bpm
P Waves: inverted before every QRS complex

PRI: 0.08 second
QRS: 0.08 second
Interp: Accelerated Junctional Rhythm

6.37 Regularity: regular
Rate: 150 bpm
P Waves: unable

PRI: unable
QRS: 0.12 second
Interp: Supraventricular Tachycardia

6.38 Regularity: regular
Rate: 79 bpm
P Waves: none

PRI: unable
QRS: 0.10 second
Interp: Accelerated Junctional Rhythm

6.39 Regularity: regular
Rate: 150 bpm
P Waves: unable

PRI: unable
QRS: 0.10 second
Interp: Supraventricular Tachycardia

6.40 Regularity: regular underlying rhythm interrupted by ectopic
Rate: 75 bpm
P Waves: upright in underlying rhythm; absent in ectopic

PRI: 0.16 second in underlying rhythm; unable to measure in ectopic
QRS: 0.08 second (in both underlying rhythm and ectopic)
Interp: Sinus Rhythm with one PJC

6.41 Regularity: regular
Rate: 214 bpm
P Waves: unable

PRI: unable
QRS: 0.08 second
Interp: Supraventricular Tachycardia

Chapter 7

7.1 Regularity: regular
Rate: 51 bpm
P Waves: uniform and upright; regular P–P interval

PRI: 0.24 second and constant
QRS: 0.10 second
Interp: Sinus Bradycardia with First-Degree Heart Block

7.2 Regularity: irregular with a pattern of grouped beating
Rate: atrial rate 115 bpm; ventricular rate approximately 90 bpm
P Waves: uniform; regular P–P intervals; more P waves than QRS complexes

PRI: changes; progressively lengthens from 0.20 second to 0.32 second
QRS: 0.08 second
Interp: Wenckebach (Type I Second-Degree Heart Block)

7.3 Regularity: regular
Rate: atrial rate 157 bpm; ventricular rate 33 bpm
P Waves: uniform; regular P–P intervals; more P waves than QRS complexes

PRI: P waves are not associated with QRS complexes
QRS: 0.12 second
Interp: Third-Degree Heart Block (CHB) with ventricular escape focus

7.4 Regularity: regular
Rate: atrial rate 115 bpm; ventricular rate 73 bpm
P Waves: non-conducted P waves are more apparent after mapping the P–P interal, since some P waves are hidden within the QRS complexes and T waves

PRI: P waves are not associated with QRS complexes
QRS: 0.08 second
Interp: Third-Degree Heart Block (CHB) with junctional escape focus

7.5 Regularity: regular
Rate: 88 bpm
P Waves: uniform and upright; regular P–P interval (*Note:* P wave of last complex is distorted by artifact.)

PRI: 0.26 second and constant
QRS: 0.12 second
Interp: Sinus Rhythm with First-Degree Heart Block (with wide QRS)

7.6 Regularity: irregular with a pattern of grouped beating
Rate: atrial rate 100 bpm; ventricular rate 80 bpm
P Waves: uniform; regular P–P interval

PRI: changing; progressively lengthens from 0.16 second to 0.24 second
QRS: 0.08 second
Interp: Wenckebach (Type I Second-Degree Heart Block)

7.7 Regularity: irregular with a pattern of grouped beating
Rate: atrial rate 75 bpm; ventricular rate approximately 60 bpm
P Waves: uniform; regular P–P interval; more P waves than QRS complexes

PRI: changing; progressively lengthens from 0.20 second to 0.30 second
QRS: 0.06 second
Interp: Wenckebach (Type I Second-Degree Heart Block)

7.8 Regularity: regular
Rate: atrial rate 120 bpm; ventricular rate 60 bpm
P Waves: uniform and upright; regular P–P interval; consistently two P waves for every QRS complex

PRI: 0.38 second and constant on conducted beats
QRS: 0.10 second
Interp: Type II Second-Degree Heart Block with 2:1 conduction

7.9 Regularity: irregular with a pattern of grouped beating
Rate: atrial rate 125 bpm; ventricular rate approximately 80 bpm
P Waves: uniform; regular P–P interval; more P waves than QRS complexes

PRI: changing; progressively lengthens from 0.20 second to 0.28 second
QRS: 0.12 second
Interp: Wenckebach (Type I Second-Degree Heart Block) (with wide QRS)

7.10 Regularity: irregular (see note)
Rate: atrial rate 63 bpm; ventricular rate approximately 25 bpm
P Waves: uniform; regular P–P intervals; more P waves than QRS complexes

PRI: the P waves are not associated with the QRS complexes
QRS: 0.20 second
Interp: Third-Degree Heart Block (CHB) with ventricular escape focus.

Note: The ventricular pacemaker site usually has a regular firing mechanism; but if a dangerous ventricular rhythm is allowed to continue untreated, its serious effects on the myocardium will ultimately cause the firing site to slow or die out. In this strip, the change in ventricular rate demonstrates this slowing phenomenon.

7.11 Regularity: regular
Rate: 75 bpm
P Waves: uniform; regular P–P interval

PRI: 0.30 second and constant
QRS: 0.14 second
Interp: Sinus Rhythm with First-Degree Heart Block (with wide QRS)

7.12 Regularity: regular
Rate: atrial rate 74 bpm; ventricular rate 37 bpm
P Waves: uniform; regular P–P interval; consistently two P waves for every QRS complex

PRI: 0.26 second and constant on conducted beats
QRS: 0.12 second
Interp: Type II Second-Degree Heart Block with 2:1 conduction

7.13 Regularity: irregular with a pattern of grouped beating
Rate: atrial rate 83 bpm; ventricular rate approximately 60 bpm
P Waves: uniform; regular P–P interval

PRI: changes; progressively lengthens from 0.28 second to 0.48 second
QRS: 0.06 second
Interp: Wenckebach (Type I Second-Degree Heart Block)

7.14 Regularity: regular
Rate: atrial rate 100 bpm; ventricular rate 35 bpm
P Waves: uniform; regular P–P interval; more P waves than QRS complexes

PRI: the P waves are not associated with the QRS complexes
QRS: 0.12 second
Interp: Third-Degree Heart Block (CHB) with ventricular escape focus

7.15 Regularity: regular
Rate: 65 bpm
P Waves: uniform and upright; regular P–P interval

PRI: 0.26 second and constant
QRS: 0.10 second
Interp: Sinus Rhythm with First-Degree Heart Block

7.16 Regularity: slightly irregular
Rate: atrial rate 64 bpm; ventricular rate 32 bpm
P Waves: uniform; slight irregularity of the P–P interval (see note); consistently two P waves for every QRS complex

PRI: 0.20 second
QRS: 0.12 second
Interp: Type II Second-Degree Heart Block with 2:1 conduction

Note: A rhythm with a consistent 2:1 conduction ratio usually produces a regular rhythm. In this strip, however, the presence of an underlying sinus arrhythmia results in an irregular P–P, with an ultimate irregularity of the ventricular response.

7.17 Regularity: regular
Rate: atrial rate 100 bpm; ventricular rate 24 bpm
P Waves: uniform; regular P–P interval; more P waves than QRS complexes

PRI: the P waves are not associated with the QRS complexes
QRS: 0.08 second
Interp: Third-Degree Heart Block (CHB) with a junctional escape focus

Note: The ventricular rate in this strip is slower than the usual junctional rate, but the QRS measurement of 0.08 second could not have been produced by a ventricular pacemaker; thus, the escape focus must have been junctional.

7.18 Regularity: irregular with a pattern of grouped beating
Rate: atrial rate 107 bpm; ventricular rate approximately 90 bpm
P Waves: uniform; regular P–P interval; more P waves than QRS complexes

PRI: changes; progressively lengthens from 0.20 second to 0.36 second
QRS: 0.10 second
Interp: Wenckebach (Type I Second-Degree Heart Block)

7.19 Regularity: regular
Rate: 54 bpm
P Waves: upright and uniform

PRI: 0.24 second and constant
QRS: 0.16 second
Interp: Sinus Bradycardia with First-Degree Heart Block (with wide QRS)

7.20 Regularity: regular P–P; irregular R–R
Rate: atrial rate 107 bpm; ventricular rate 90 bpm
P Waves: upright and uniform

PRI: progressively lengthens until one P wave is not conducted
QRS: 0.08 second
Interp: Wenckebach (Type I Second-Degree Heart Block)

7.21 Regularity: regular R–R; regular P–P
Rate: atrial rate 56 bpm; ventricular rate 36 bpm
P Waves: upright and uniform

PRI: not related
QRS: 0.16 second
Interp: Third-Degree Heart Block (CHB) with ventricular escape focus

7.22 Regularity: regular
Rate: 83 bpm
P Waves: upright and uniform

PRI: 0.22 second and constant
QRS: 0.10 second
Interp: Sinus Rhythm with First-Degree Heart Block

7.23 Regularity: regular
Rate: 65 bpm
P Waves: upright and uniform

PRI: 0.24 second and constant
QRS: 0.08 second
Interp: Sinus Rhythm with First-Degree Heart Block

7.24 Regularity: regular P–P; regular R–R
Rate: atrial rate 43 bpm; ventricular rate 31 bpm
P Waves: upright and uniform

PRI: unrelated; P waves "march through" QRS complexes
QRS: 0.10 second
Interp: Third-Degree Heart Block (CHB) with junctional escape focus

7.25 Regularity: regular P–P; irregular R–R
Rate: atrial rate 65 bpm; ventricular rate 40 bpm
P Waves: upright and uniform

PRI: 0.20 second and constant on conducted beats
QRS: 0.08 second
Interp: Type II Second-Degree Heart Block with variable conduction

7.26 Regularity: slightly irregular
Rate: 83 bpm
P Waves: upright and uniform

PRI: 0.24 second and constant
QRS: 0.08 second
Interp: Sinus Rhythm with First-Degree Heart Block

7.27 Regularity: regular
Rate: 65 bpm
P Waves: upright and uniform

PRI: 0.24 second and constant
QRS: 0.08 second
Interp: Sinus Rhythm with First-Degree Heart Block

7.28 Regularity: irregular
Rate: 62 bpm
P Waves: upright and uniform

PRI: 0.24 second and constant
QRS: 0.10 second
Interp: Sinus Arrhythmia with First-Degree Heart Block

7.29 Regularity: regular P–P; irregular R–R
Rate: atrial rate 79 bpm; ventricular rate 60 bpm
P Waves: upright and uniform

PRI: progressively lengthens until one P wave is not conducted
QRS: 0.08 second
Interp: Wenckebach (Type I Second-Degree Heart Block)

7.30 Regularity: regular
Rate: 65 bpm
P Waves: upright and uniform

PRI: 0.24 second and constant
QRS: 0.10 second
Interp: Sinus Rhythm with First-Degree Heart Block

7.31 Regularity: regular
Rate: 52 bpm
P Waves: upright and uniform

PRI: 0.24 second and constant
QRS: 0.08 second
Interp: Sinus Bradycardia with First-Degree Heart Block

7.32 Regularity: P–P very slightly irregular; R–R irregular
Rate: atrial rate 79 bpm; ventricular rate 70 bpm
P Waves: upright and uniform

PRI: progressively lengthens until oneP wave is not conducted
QRS: 0.12 second
Interp: Wenckebach (Type I Second-Degree Heart Block) (with wide QRS)

7.33 Regularity: regular P–P
Rate: atrial rate 60 bpm; ventricular rate 20 bpm
P Waves: upright and uniform

PRI: P waves unrelated to QRS complexes
QRS: 0.12 second
Interp: Third-Degree Heart Block (CHB) with ventricular escape focus

7.34 Regularity: regular
Rate: 88 bpm
P Waves: upright and uniform

PRI: 0.24 second and constant
QRS: 0.10 second
Interp: Sinus Rhythm with First-Degree Heart Block

7.35 Rgularity: regular
Rate: 35 bpm
P Waves: upright and uniform

PRI: 0.28 second and constant
QRS: 0.16 second
Interp: Sinus Bradycardia with First-Degree Heart Block (with wide QRS)

7.36 Regularity: regular P–P; regular R–R
Rate: atrial rate 107 bpm; ventricular rate 58 bpm
P Waves: upright and uniform

PRI: P waves unrelated to QRS complexes; more P waves than QRS complexes
QRS: 0.10 second
Interp: Third-Degree Heart Block (CHB) with junctional escape focus

7.37 Regularity: regular P–P; regular R–R
Rate: atrial rate 115 bpm; ventricular rate 65 bpm
P Waves: upright; two P waves for every QRS complex

PRI: 0.28 second and constant on conducted beats
QRS: 0.08 second
Interp: Type II Second-Degree Heart Block with 2:1 conduction

7.38 Regularity: regular P–P; irregular R–R
Rate: atrial rate 115 bpm; ventricular rate 90 bpm
P Waves: upright and uniform; more P waves than QRS complexes

PRI: progressively lengthens until one P wave is not conducted
QRS: 0.08 second
Interp: Wenckebach (Type I Second–Degree Heart Block)

7.39 Regularity: slightly irregular P–P; regular R–R
Rate: atrial rate 88 bpm; ventricular rate 32 bpm
P Waves: upright and uniform

PRI: P waves unrelated to QRS complexes; P waves "march through" QRS complexes
QRS: 0.08 second
Interp: Third-Degree Heart Block (CHB) with junctional escape focus

7.40 Regularity: regular P–P; regular R–R
Rate: atrial rate 94 bpm; ventricular rate 47 bpm
P Waves: upright and uniform

PRI: 0.24 second and constant on conducted beats; more P waves than QRS complexes
QRS: 0.06 second
Interp: Type II Second-Degree Heart Block with 2:1 conduction

7.41 Regularity: regular P–P; regular R–R
Rate: atrial rate 88 bpm; ventricular rate 68 bpm
P Waves: upright and uniform

PRI: P waves unrelated to QRS complexes; P waves "march through" QRS complexes
QRS: 0.10 second
Interp: Third-Degree Heart Block (CHB) with junctional escape focus

Chapter 8

8.1 Regularity: regular underlying rhythm interrupted by ectopics
Rate: 75 bpm
P Waves: uniform; regular P–P interval

PRI: 0.18 second
QRS: 0.12 second in underlying complex; 0.12 second in ectopics; ectopics have bizarre configuration
Interp: Sinus Rhythm (with wide QRS) with two PVCs

8.2 Regularity: regular underlying rhythm interrupted by ectopics in a pattern of grouped beating
Rate: 39 bpm according to visible P waves; true sinus rate is probably 78 bpm
P Waves: uniform; regular P–P interval

PRI: 0.18 second
QRS: 0.08 second in underlying rhythm; 0.14 second in ectopic
Interp: Sinus Rhythm with bigeminy of PVCs

8.3 Regularity: regular underlying rhythm interrupted by an ectopic
Rate: 58 bpm
P Waves: uniform; regular P–P interval

PRI: 0.20 second
QRS: 0.10 second in underlying rhythm; 0.18 second in ectopic; ectopic has bizarre configuration
Interp: Sinus Bradycardia with one PVC

8.4 Regularity: slightly irregular
Rate: approximately 170 bpm
P Waves: not visible

PRI: none
QRS: 0.12 second; configuration is bizarre
Interp: Ventricular Tachycardia

8.5 Regularity: regular underlying rhythm interrupted by ectopics
Rate: 79 bpm (underlying rhythm)
P Waves: uniform; regular P–P interval

PRI: 0.16 second
QRS: 0.06 second in underlying rhythm; 0.20 second in ectopics; ectopics have bizarre configuration
Interp: Sinus Rhythm with three unifocal PVCs (possibly trigeminy)

8.6 Regularity: totally chaotic baseline
Rate: cannot be determined
P Waves: none

PRI: none
QRS: none
Interp: Ventricular Fibrillation

8.7 Regularity: regular underlying rhythm interrupted by ectopics
Rate: 107 bpm (underlying rhythm)
P Waves: uniform; regular P–P interval interrupted by ectopics

PRI: 0.14 second
QRS: 0.10 second in underlying rhythm; 0.14 second in ectopics; ectopics have bizarre configuration
Interp: Sinus Rhythm with two unifocal PVCs and a short burst of VentricularTachycardia

8.8 Regularity: regular
Rate: 167 bpm
P Waves: not visible

PRI: none
QRS: 0.16 second; bizarre configuration
Interp: Ventricular Tachycardia

8.9 Regularity: regular underlying rhythm interrupted by ectopics
Rate: 83 bpm
P Waves: uniform; regular P–P interval

PRI: 0.16 second
QRS: 0.14 second in underlying rhythm; 0.16 second in ectopics; ectopics have bizarre configuration
Interp: Sinus Rhythm (with wide QRS) with two multifocal PVCs

8.10 Regularity: regular
Rate: 150 bpm
P Waves: not visible

PRI: none
QRS: 0.20 second; bizarre configuration
Interp: Ventricular Tachycardia

8.11 Regularity: regular underlying rhythm interrupted by ectopics
Rate: 100 bpm
P Waves: uniform; regular P–P interval

PRI: 0.14 second
QRS: 0.06 second in underlying rhythm; 0.12 second in ectopics; ectopics have bizarre configuration
Interp: Sinus Tachycardia with three unifocal PVCs

8.12 Regularity: regular
Rate: 167 bpm
P Waves: not visible

PRI: none
QRS: 0.16 second; bizarre configuration
Interp: Ventricular Tachycardia

8.13 Regularity: regular underlying rhythm interrupted by ectopics in a pattern of grouped beating
Rate: 38 bpm according to visible P waves; true sinus rate is probably 76 bpm
P Waves: uniform; regular P–P interval

PRI: 0.20 second
QRS: 0.10 second in underlying rhythm; 0.14 second in ectopics; ectopics have bizarre configuration
Interp: Sinus Rhythm with bigeminy of PVCs

8.14 Regularity: totally chaotic baseline
Rate: cannot be determined
P Waves: none

PRI: none
QRS: none
Interp: Ventricular Fibrillation

8.15 Regularity: regular
Rate: 40 bpm
P Waves: none

PRI: none
QRS: 0.20 second; bizarre configuration
Interp: Idioventricular Rhythm

8.16 Regularity: regular underlying rhythm interrupted by ectopics
Rate: 94 bpm
P Waves: uniform; regular P–P interval

PRI: 0.12 second
QRS: 0.10 second in underlying rhythm; 0.16 second in ectopics; ectopics have bizarre configuration; ectopics occur consecutively
Interp: Sinus Rhythm with a run of three PVCs

8.17 Regularity: regular
Rate: 150 bpm
P Waves: are visible through QRS complexes but do not appear related to QRS complexes

PRI: none
QRS: 0.28 second; bizarre configuration
Interp: Ventricular Tachycardia

8.18 Regularity: totally chaotic baseline
Rate: cannot be determined
P Waves: none

PRI: none
QRS: none
Interp: Ventricular Fibrillation

8.19 Regularity: regular underlying rhythm interrupted by an ectopic
Rate: 79 bpm
P Waves: uniform; regular P–P interval

PRI: 0.16 second
QRS: 0.08 second
Interp: Sinus Rhythm with one PVC

8.20 Regularity: totally chaotic baseline
Rate: cannot be determined
P Waves: none

PRI: none
QRS: none
Interp: Ventricular Fibrillation

8.21 Regularity: first part of rhythm is regular but then changes into a totally chaotic pattern
Rate: 167 bpm (first part of strip)
P Waves: not visible

PRI: none
QRS: 0.20 second in first part of strip; cannot be identified in latter part of strip
Interp: Ventricular Tachycardia changing into Ventricular Fibrillation

8.22 Regularity: regular underlying rhythm interrupted by ectopics
Rate: 79 bpm
P Waves: uniform; regular P–P interval

PRI: 0.20 second
QRS: 0.10 second in underlying rhythm; 0.14 second in ectopics; ectopics have bizarre configuration
Interp: Sinus Rhythm with two unifocal PVCs

8.23 Regularity: regular
Rate: 42 bpm
P Waves: none

PRI: none
QRS: 0.12 second; bizarre configuration
Interp: Idioventricular Rhythm

8.24 Regularity: slightly irregular rhythm interrupted by ectopic
Rate: approximately 65 bpm
P Waves: uniform; slightly irregular P–P interval

PRI: 0.18 second and constant
QRS: 0.14 second in underlying rhythm; 0.16 second in ectopic; ectopic has bizarre configuration
Interp: Sinus Arrhythmia (with wide QRS) with one PVC

8.25 Regularity: totally chaotic baseline
Rate: cannot be determined
P Waves: none

PRI: none
QRS: none
Interp: Ventricular Fibrillation

8.26 Regularity: regular underlying rhythm interrupted by ectopics
Rate: 83 bpm
P Waves: uniform; regular P–P interval

PRI: 0.14 second
QRS: 0.12 second in underlying rhythm; 0.16 second in ectopics; ectopics have bizarre configuration
Interp: Sinus Rhythm (with wide QRS) with two unifocal PVCs

8.27 Regularity: regular
Rate: 37 bpm
P Waves: none

PRI: none
QRS: 0.20 second; bizarre configuration
Interp: Idioventricular Rhythm

8.28 Regularity: totally chaotic baseline
Rate: cannot be determined
P Waves: none

PRI: none
QRS: none
Interp: Ventricular Fibrillation

8.29 Regularity: irregular underlying rhythm interrupted by an ectopic
Rate: approximately 60 bpm (underlying rhythm)
P Waves: uniform; regular P–P interval

PRI: 0.16 second and constant
QRS: 0.10 second in underlying rhythm; 0.12 second in ectopic; ectopic has bizarre configuration
Interp: Sinus Rhythm with one PVC

8.30 Regularity: regular
Rate: 188 bpm
P Waves: none

PRI: none
QRS: 0.20 second; bizarre configuration
Interp: Ventricular Tachycardia

8.31 Regularity: regular underlying rhythm interrupted by ectopics
Rate: 94 bpm (underlying rhythm)
P Waves: uniform; regular P–P interval

PRI: 0.24 second and constant
QRS: 0.10 second in underlying rhythm; 0.12–0.20 second in ectopics; ectopics occur consecutively; ectopics have bizarre configuration
Interp: Sinus Rhythm with First-Degree Heart Block, with one PVC and run of three PVCs

8.32 Regularity: regular
Rate: 167 bpm
P Waves: not visible

PRI: none
QRS: 0.14 second; bizarre configuration
Interp: Ventricular Tachycardia

8.33 Regularity: regular underlying rhythm interrupted by ectopics
Rate: 83 bpm (underlying rhythm)
P Waves: uniform; regular P–P interval

PRI: 0.16 second
QRS: 0.10 second in underlying rhythm; 0.16 second in ectopics; ectopics have bizarre configuration
Interp: Sinus Rhythm with two unifocal PVCs

8.34 Regularity: irregular underlying rhythm interrupted by ectopics in pattern of grouped beating
Rate: approximately 30 bpm (underlying rhythm)
P Waves: not discernible; undulations present

PRI: none
QRS: 0.10 second in underlying rhythm; 0.14 second in ectopics; ectopics have bizarre configuration
Interp: Atrial Fibrillation, controlled, with bigeminy of unifocal PVCs

8.35 Regularity: irregular
Rate: 100 bpm (including ectopics)
P Waves: upright in underlying rhythm; absent in ectopics

PRI: 0.20 second in underlying rhythm
QRS: 0.08 second in underlying rhythm; 0.14–0.16 second in ectopics
Interp: Sinus Rhythm with four multifocal PVCs

8.36 Regularity: totally chaotic baseline
Rate: cannot be determined
P Waves: none

PRI: none
QRS: none
Interp: Ventricular Fibrillation

8.37 Regularity: irregular underlying rhythm interrupted by ectopic
Rate: 150 bpm (including ectopic)
P Waves: none visible

PRI: unable
QRS: 0.14 second in underlying rhythm; 0.18 second in ectopic
Interp: Atrial Fibrillation, uncontrolled, (with wide QRS) and one PVC

8.38 Regularity: irregular underlying rhythm interrupted by ectopic
Rate: 180 bpm (including ectopic)
P Waves: none visible

PRI: unable
QRS: 0.10 second in underlying rhythm; 0.14 second in ectopic
Interp: Atrial Fibrillation, uncontrolled, with one PVC

8.39 Regularity: irregular in a pattern of grouped beating
Rate: 80 bpm (including ectopic)
P Waves: upright and uniform

PRI: 0.12 second in underlying rhythm
QRS: 0.10 second in underlying rhythm; 0.18 second in ectopic
Interp: Sinus Rhythm with bigeminy of unifocal PVCs

8.40 Regularity: unable to determine
Rate: ventricular rate 20 bpm
P Waves: cannot be mapped out

PRI: none
QRS: 0.18 second
Interp: Idioventricular Rhythm

8.41 Regularity: slightly irregular
Rate: 150 bpm
P Waves: none visible

PRI: none
QRS: 0.20 second
Interp: Ventricular Tachycardia

8.42 Regularity: regular underlying rhythm interrupted by ectopics
Rate: 115 bpm (in underlying rhythm)
P Waves: upright in underlying rhythm

PRI: 0.14 second in underlying rhythm
QRS: 0.10 second in underlying rhythm; 0.16 second in ectopics
Interp: Sinus Tachycardia with two multifocal PVCs

8.43 Regularity: irregular underlying rhythm interrupted by ectopic
Rate: 120 bpm (including ectopic)
P Waves: none visible

PRI: none
QRS: 0.08 second in underlying rhythm; 0.16 second in ectopic
Interp: Atrial Fibrillation, uncontrolled, with one PVC

8.44 Regularity: totally chaotic baseline
Rate: cannot be determined
P Waves: none

PRI: none
QRS: none
Interp: Ventricular Fibrillation

8.45 Regularity: irregular in a pattern of grouped beating
Rate: 100 bpm (including ectopics)
P Waves: upright in underlying rhythm
PRI: 0.14 second in underlying rhythm
QRS: 0.08 second in underlying rhythm; 0.16 second in ectopic
Interp: Sinus Rhythm with bigeminy of PVCs

8.46 Regularity: slightly irregular underlying rhythm interrupted by ectopic
Rate: 75 bpm
P Waves: upright in underlying rhythm
PRI: 0.14 second
QRS: 0.10 second in underlying rhythm; 0.20 second in ectopic
Interp: Sinus Rhythm with one PVC

8.47 Regularity: irregular in a pattern of grouped beating
Rate: sinus rate 75 bpm
P Waves: upright in underlying rhythm
PRI: 0.14 second in underlying rhythm
QRS: 0.10 second in underlying rhythm; 0.16 second in ectopic
Interp: Sinus Rhythm with trigeminy of PVCs (assuming pattern continues)

8.48 Regularity: slightly irregular underlying rhythm interrupted by ectopic
Rate: sinus rate 54 bpm
P Waves: upright
PRI: 0.14 second in underlying rhythm
QRS: 0.08 second in underlying rhythm; 0.18 second in ectopic
Interp: Sinus Bradycardia with one PVC (R on T Phenomenon)

8.49 Regularity: totally chaotic baseline
Rate: cannot be determined
P Waves: none
PRI: none
QRS: none
Interp: Ventricular Fibrillation

8.50 Regularity: regular
Rate: 140 bpm
P Waves: none visible
PRI: none
QRS: 0.16 second
Interp: Ventricular Tachycardia (slow rate range)

8.51 Regularity: irregular underlying rhythm interrupted by ectopics
Rate: 90 bpm including ectopics
P Waves: none visible
PRI: none
QRS: 0.08 second in underlying rhythm; 0.12–0.16 second in ectopics
Interp: Atrial Fibrillation, controlled, with two multifocal PVCs

8.52 Regularity: totally chaotic baseline
Rate: cannot be determined
P Waves: none
PRI: none
QRS: none
Interp: Ventricular Fibrillation

8.53 Regularity: regular underlying rhythm interrupted by ectopic
Rate: 68 bpm
P Waves: upright and uniform
PRI: 0.16 second
QRS: 0.14 second in underlying rhythm; 0.16 second in ectopic
Interp: Sinus Rhythm (with wide QRS) with one PVC

8.54 Regularity: totally chaotic baseline
Rate: cannot be determined
P Waves: none
PRI: none
QRS: none
Interp: Ventricular Fibrillation

8.55 Regularity: regular underlying rhythm interrupted by ectopics
Rate: 115 bpm
P Waves: upright and uniform
PRI: 0.14 second
QRS: 0.08 second in underlying rhythm; 0.16 second in ectopics
Interp: Sinus Tachycardia with two unifocal PVCs

8.56 Regularity: regular
Rate: 167 bpm
P Waves: none visible
PRI: none
QRS: wide and bizarre; unable to measure
Interp: Ventricular Tachycardia

8.57 Regularity: regular
Rate: 35 bpm
P Waves: none
PRI: none
QRS: 0.16 second
Interp: Idioventricular Rhythm

8.58 Regularity: regular underlying rhythm interrupted by ectopics
Rate: 75 bpm
P Waves: upright and uniform
PRI: 0.20 second
QRS: 0.08 second in underlying rhythm; 0.14 second in ectopics
Interp: Sinus Rhythm with two unifocal PVCs, possibly quadrigeminy (if pattern continues)

8.59 Regularity: slightly irregular
Rate: 130 bpm (including ectopic)
P Waves: varying shapes
PRI: varies slightly
QRS: 0.08 second in underlying rhythm; 0.14 second in ectopic
Interp: Wandering Pacemaker (tachycardia range) with one PVC

8.60 Regularity: P–P regular; regular ventricular rhythm interrupted by ectopic
Rate: atrial rate 47 bpm; ventricular rate 65 bpm
P Waves: upright and uniform
PRI: P waves unrelated to QRS complexes
QRS: 0.08 second in underlying rhythm; 0.16 second in ectopic
Interp: Third-Degree Heart Block (CHB) with junctional escape focus with one PVC

8.61 Regularity: totally chaotic baseline
Rate: cannot be determined
P Waves: none
PRI: none
QRS: none
Interp: Ventricular Fibrillation

8.62 Regularity: regular underlying rhythm interrupted by ectopics
Rate: 107 bpm
P Waves: upright in underlying rhythm; absent in ectopics
PRI: 0.14 second in underlying rhythm; no P waves preceding ectopics
QRS: 0.08 second in underlying rhythm; 0.12–0.16 second in ectopic
Interp: Sinus Tachycardia with multiple multifocal PVCs, including a run of three PVCs

8.63 Regularity: unable to determine
Rate: 10 bpm or less
P Waves: none

PRI: none
QRS: 0.24 second
Interp: Idioventricular Rhythm

8.64 Regularity: irregular in pattern of grouped beating
Rate: 80 bpm (including ectopics)
P Waves: upright in underlying rhythm; absent in ectopics

PRI: 0.16 second
QRS: 0.10 second in underlying rhythm; 0.16 second in ectopics
Interp: Sinus Rhythm with bigeminy of PVCs

8.65 Regularity: regular underlying rhythm interrupted by ectopics
Rate: 83 bpm (underlying rhythm)
P Waves: upright in underlying rhythm; absent in ectopics

PRI: 0.16 second
QRS: 0.08 second in underlying rhythm; 0.16 second in ectopic
Interp: Sinus Rhythm with multiple unifocal PVCs, possibly quadrigeminy

8.66 Regularity: regular underlying rhythm interrupted by ectopic
Rate: 75 bpm
P Waves: upright in underlying rhythm; absent in ectopic

PRI: 0.20 second
QRS: 0.08 second in underlying rhythm; 0.14 second in ectopic
Interp: Sinus Rhythm with one PVC

8.67 Regularity: slightly irregular underlying rhythm interrupted by ectopics
Rate: 94 bpm (underlying rhythm)
P Waves: upright in underlying rhythm; absent in ectopics

PRI: 0.18 second
QRS: 0.08 second in underlying rhythm; 0.14 second in ectopics
Interp: Sinus Rhythm with multiple unifocal PVCs, possibly quadrigeminy

8.68 Regularity: regular
Rate: 150 bpm
P Waves: none

PRI: none
QRS: 0.16 second
Interp: Ventricular Tachycardia

8.69 Regularity: slightly irregular underlying rhythm interrupted by ectopic
Rate: 70 bpm (underlying rhythm)
P Waves: upright in underlying rhythm; absent in ectopic

PRI: 0.14 second
QRS: 0.10 second in underlying rhythm; 0.14 second in ectopic
Interp: Sinus Rhythm with one PVC

8.70 Regularity: regular
Rate: 136 bpm
P Waves: cannot be determined

PRI: none
QRS: 0.18 second
Interp: Ventricular Tachycardia (slow rate range)

8.71 Regularity: totally chaotic baseline
Rate: cannot be determined
P Waves: none

PRI: none
QRS: none
Interp: Ventricular Fibrillation

8.72 Regularity: regular underlying rhythm interrupted by ectopics
Rate: 68 bpm
P Waves: upright in underlying rhythm; absent in ectopics

PRI: 0.16 second
QRS: 0.08 second in underlying rhythm; 0.16 second in ectopics
Interp: Sinus Rhythm with two unifocal PVCs

8.73 Regularity: unable to determine
Rate: less than 10 bpm
P Waves: none

PRI: none
QRS: 0.24 second
Interp: Idioventricular Rhythm ending in Agonal Rhythm

8.74 Regularity: slightly irregular
Rate: 160 bpm
P Waves: none

PRI: none
QRS: 0.14 second
Interp: Ventricular Tachycardia

8.75 Regularity: grossly irregular
Rate: 110 bpm (including ectopic)
P Waves: none

PRI: none
QRS: 0.08 second in underlying rhythm; 0.16 second in ectopic
Interp: Atrial Fibrillation, uncontrolled, with one PVC

8.76 Regularity: slightly irregular
Rate: 160 bpm
P Waves: none mappable

PRI: none
QRS: 0.14 second
Interp: Ventricular Tachycardia

8.77 Regularity: regular underlying rhythm interrupted by ectopics
Rate: 68 bpm in underlying rhythm
P Waves: upright and uniform

PRI: 0.20 second
QRS: 0.14 second in underlying rhythm; 0.16 second in ectopics
Interp: Sinus Rhythm (with wide QRS) with two multifocal PVCs

Chapter 9

9.1 Regularity: regular
Rate: 60 bpm
P Waves: uniform; regular P–P interval

PRI: 0.28 second and constant
QRS: 0.14 second
Interp: Sinus Rhythm (borderline bradycardia) with First–Degree Heart Block (with wide QRS)

9.2 Regularity: irregular
Rate: approximately 50 bpm
P Waves: not discernible; undulations present

PRI: none
QRS: 0.10 second
Interp: Atrial Fibrillation, controlled (bradycardia)

9.3 Regularity: regular underlying rhythm interrupted by ectopics
Rate: 79 bpm
P Waves: uniform; regular P–P interval

PRI: 0.20 second and constant
QRS: 0.08 second in underlying rhythm; 0.12 second in ectopic beats; ectopic complexes differ from normal complexes
Interp: Sinus Rhythm with two unifocal PVCs

9.4 Regularity: regular underlying rhythm interrupted
by ectopics in a pattern
of grouped beating
Rate: 50 bpm according
to visible P waves; true
sinus rate is probably
100 bpm
P Waves: uniform; regular
P–P interval

PRI: 0.20 second and
constant
QRS: 0.14 second in
underlying rhythm;
0.14 second in ectopic
beats; ectopic QRSs
have a different configu-
ration than normal QRSs
Interp: Sinus Rhythm (with
a wide QRS) with bigem-
iny of PVCs

9.5 Regularity: irregular R–R
interval; regular P–P
interval
Rate: atrial rate 300 bpm;
ventricular rate approxi-
mately 90 bpm
P Waves: uniform; saw-
tooth appearance;
regular P–P interval;
more P waves than QRS
complexes

PRI: none
QRS: 0.08 second
Interp: Atrial Flutter with
variable block

9.6 Regularity: regular underly-
ing rhythm interrupted
by ectopics
Rate: 60 bpm
P Waves: uniform; regular
P–P interval

PRI: 0.22 second and
constant
QRS: 0.08 second in un-
derlying rhythm; 0.12
second in ectopic beats;
ectopic QRSs are bizarre
Interp: Sinus Rhythm (borderline bradycardia) with
First-Degree Heart Block
and two unifocal PVCs

9.7 Regularity: regular
Rate: 48 bpm
P Waves: uniform and up-
right; regular P–P interval

PRI: 0.16 second and
constant
QRS: 0.10 second
Interp: Sinus Bradycardia

9.8 Regularity: regular underlying rhythm interrupted
by ectopics in a pattern
of grouped beating
Rate: atrial rate 300 bpm;
ventricular rate 40 bpm
P Waves: uniform; sawtooth
appearance; regular P–P
interval; more P waves
than QRS complexes

PRI: none
QRS: 0.06 second in
underlying rhythm;
0.12 second in ectopics;
ectopics have bizarre
configuration
Interp: Atrial Flutter with
bigeminy of PVCs

9.9 Regularity: irregular underlying rhythm interrupted
by ectopics in a pattern
of grouped beating
Rate: approximately 40
bpm (excluding ectopics)
P Waves: not discernible;
undulations present

PRI: none
QRS: 0.10 second in
underlying rhythm;
0.14 second in ectopics;
ectopics have bizarre
configuration
Interp: Atrial Fibrillation,
controlled, with bigeminy
of PVCs

9.10 Regularity: irregular
Rate: approximately
120 bpm
P Waves: not discernible;
undulations present

PRI: none
QRS: 0.10 second
Interp: Atrial Fibrillation,
uncontrolled

9.11 Regularity: totally chaotic
baseline
Rate: cannot determine
P Waves: none

PRI: none
QRS: none
Interp: Ventricular
Fibrillation

9.12 Regularity: regular
Rate: atrial rate 300 bpm;
ventricular rate 75 bpm
P Waves: uniform, saw-
tooth appearance;
regular P–P interval;
more P waves than QRS
complexes

PRI: none
RS: 0.10 second
Interp: Atrial Flutter with
4:1 response

9.13 Regularity: regular
Rate: 150 bpm
P Waves: not visible

PRI: none
QRS: 0.16 second; bizarre
configuration
Interp: Ventricular
Tachycardia

9.14 Regularity: slightly irregular
Rate: approximately
58 bpm
P Waves: uniform; irregular
P–P interval

PRI: 0.16 second and
constant
QRS: 0.16 second
Interp: Sinus Bradycardia
(with wide QRS) and a
slight sinus arrhythmia

9.15 Regularity: totally chaotic
baseline
Rate: cannot determine
P Waves: none

PRI: none
QRS: none
Interp: Ventricular
Fibrillation

9.16 Regularity: regular underlying rhythm interrupted
by ectopics
Rate: 100 bpm
P Waves: uniform P waves;
regular P–P interval

PRI: 0.22 second and
constant
QRS: 0.12 second in
underlying rhythm;
0.20 second in ectopics;
ectopics have bizarre
configuration
Interp: Sinus Rhythm (with
wide QRS) with First-
Degree Heart Block and
three unifocal PVCs
(possibly quadrigeminy)

9.17 Regularity: irregular
Rate: approximately
170 bpm
P Waves: not discernible;
undulations present

PRI: none
QRS: 0.08 second
Interp: Atrial Fibrillation,
uncontrolled

9.18 Regularity: regular underlying rhythm interrupted
by ectopics
Rate: 107 bpm
P Waves: uniform P waves
in underlying rhythm;
shape of P waves
changes in ectopic beats

PRI: 0.14 second
QRS: 0.08 second in both
underlying rhythm and
ectopics
Interp: Sinus Tachycardia
with two PACs

9.19 Regularity: regular underly-
ing rhythm interrupted
by ectopics
Rate: 83 bpm
P Waves: uniform; regular
P–P interval

PRI: 0.20 second
QRS: 0.08 second in un-
derlying beats; 0.16 sec-
ond in ectopics
Interp: Sinus Rhythm with
three unifocal PVCs
(possibly trigeminy)

9.20 Regularity: regular
Rate: 68 bpm
P Waves: uniform; regular P–P interval

PRI: 0.44 second and constant
QRS: 0.12 second
Interp: Sinus Rhythm with First-Degree Heart Block (with wide QRS)

9.21 Regularity: regular underlying rhythm interrupted by ectopics
Rate: 83 bpm
P Waves: uniform; regular P–P interval

PRI: 0.12 second
QRS: 0.12 second in underlying rhythm; 0.12 second in ectopics; ectopics have bizarre configuration
Interp: Sinus Rhythm (with wide QRS) with two multifocal PVCs

9.22 Regularity: regular
Rate: atrial rate 96 bpm; ventricular rate 48 bpm
P Waves: upright and uniform; regular P–P interval

PRI: 0.20 second
QRS: 0.16 second
Interp: Type II Second-Degree Heart Block (2:1)

9.23 Regularity: regular underlying rhythm interrupted by ectopics in a pattern of grouped beating
Rate: 56 bpm according to visible P waves; true sinus rate is probably 112 bpm
P Waves: uniform; regular P–P interval

PRI: 0.12 second
QRS: 0.08 second in underlying rhythm; 0.12 second in ectopics; ectopics have bizarre configuration
Interp: Sinus Rhythm with bigeminy of PVCs

9.24 Regularity: irregular
Rate: approximately 50 bpm
P Waves: not discernible; undulations present

PRI: none
QRS: 0.12 second
Interp: Atrial Fibrillation, controlled (with wide QRS)

9.25 Regularity: regular
Rate: 94 bpm
P Waves: uniform and upright; regular P–P interval

PRI: 0.20 second and constant
QRS: 0.10 second
Interp: Normal Sinus Rhythm

9.26 Regularity: irregular rhythm interrupted by ectopics
Rate: approximately 60 bpm; if ectopics are included, the rate is 90 bpm
P Waves: not discernible; undulations present

PRI: none
QRS: 0.08 second in underlying rhythm; 0.14 second in ectopics; ectopics have bizarre configuration
Interp: Atrial Fibrillation, controlled, with three unifocal PVCs

9.27 Regularity: regular underlying rhythm interrupted by ectopics
Rate: 103 bpm
P Waves: uniform in underlying rhythm; shape changes in ectopic beats

PRI: 0.16 second
QRS: 0.10 second in both underlying rhythm and ectopics; shape does not change in ectopics
Interp: Sinus Tachycardia with two PACs

9.28 Regularity: regular underlying rhythm interrupted by ectopics in a pattern of grouped beating
Rate: 54 bpm according to visible P waves; true sinus rate is probably 108 bpm
P Waves: uniform; regular P–P interval

PRI: 0.16 second and constant
QRS: 0.12 second in both underlying rhythm and ectopics; ectopics have bizarre configuration
Interp: Sinus Tachycardia (with a wide QRS) with bigeminy of PVCs

9.29 Regularity: regular
Rate: 79 bpm
P Waves: upright and uniform; regular P–P interval

PRI: 0.20 second and constant
QRS: 0.08 second
Interp: Normal Sinus Rhythm

9.30 Regularity: irregular underlying rhythm interrupted by ectopics
Rate: approximately 70 bpm; if ectopics are included rate is 110 bpm
P Waves: not discernible; undulations present

PRI: none
QRS: 0.12 second in underlying rhythm; 0.14 second in ectopics; ectopics have bizarre configurations
Interp: Atrial Fibrillation (with wide QRS) with multifocal PVCs and one PVC couplet

9.31 Regularity: irregular
Rate: approximately 60 bpm
P Waves: not discernible; undulations present

PRI: none
QRS: 0.08 second
Interp: Atrial Fibrillation, controlled

9.32 Regularity: irregular
Rate: atrial rate 300 bpm; ventricular rate 80 bpm
P Waves: uniform, sawtooth appearance; regular P–P interval; more P waves than QRS complexes

PRI: none
QRS: 0.08 second
Interp: Atrial Flutter with variable block

9.33 Regularity: irregular
Rate: atrial rate 94 bpm; ventricular rate 60 bpm
P Waves: uniform; regular P–P interval; occasional non-conducted P waves

PRI: changing; progressively lengthens from 0.20 second to 0.26 second
QRS: 0.08 second
Interp: Wenckebach (Type I Second-Degree Heart Block)

9.34 Regularity: regular
Rate: 136 bpm
P Waves: uniform and upright; regular P–P interval

PRI: 0.12 second and constant
QRS: 0.06 second
Interp: Sinus Tachycardia

9.35 Regularity: regular
Rate: 83 bpm
P Waves: uniform and upright; regular P–P interval

PRI: 0.28 second and constant
QRS: 0.08 second
Interp: Sinus Rhythm with First-Degree Heart Block

9.36 Regularity: regular
Rate: 136 bpm
P Waves: uniform; regular P–P interval

PRI: 0.14 second (partially obscured by T wave)
QRS: 0.10 second
Interp: Sinus Tachycardia

9.37 Regularity: regular underlying rhythm interrupted by ectopics
Rate: atrial rate 284 bpm; ventricular rate 71 bpm
P Waves: uniform; sawtooth appearance; regular P–P interval; consistently four P waves for every QRS complex
PRI: none
QRS: 0.10 second in underlying rhythm; 0.16 second in ectopics; ectopics have bizarre configuration
Interp: Atrial Flutter with 4:1 response and two unifocal PVCs

9.38 Regularity: regular underlying rhythm interrupted by ectopics
Rate: 100 bpm
P Waves: uniform; regular P–P interval
PRI: 0.20 second and constant
QRS: 0.12 second in underlying rhythm and in ectopics; ectopics have bizarre configuration
Interp: Sinus Tachycardia (with a wide QRS) with two unifocal PVCs

9.39 Regularity: regular
Rate: 71 bpm
P Waves: uniform; regular P–P interval
PRI: 0.14 second and constant
QRS: 0.10 second
Interp: Normal Sinus Rhythm

9.40 Regularity: regular
Rate: 300 bpm
P Waves: not visible
PRI: none
QRS: 0.16 second; bizarre configuration
Interp: Ventricular Tachycardia (Ventricular Flutter)

9.41 Regularity: irregular
Rate: approximately 70 bpm
P Waves: not discernible
PRI: none
QRS: 0.08 second
Interp: Atrial Fibrillation, controlled

9.42 Regularity: regular underlying rhythm interrupted by ectopic (rate changes following ectopic)
Rate: approximately 80 bpm
P Waves: uniform in underlying rhythm; configuration changes in ectopic beat
PRI: 0.16 second
QRS: 0.12 second
Interp: Sinus Rhythm (with wide QRS) with one PAC

9.43 Regularity: regular
Rate: 107 bpm
P Waves: uniform; regular P–P interval
PRI: 0.14 second
QRS: 0.16 second
Interp: Sinus Tachycardia (with wide QRS)

9.44 Regularity: irregular
Rate: approximately 11 bpm
P Waves: not discernible; undulations present
PRI: none
QRS: 0.06 second
Interp: Atrial Fibrillation, uncontrolled

9.45 Regularity: regular underlying rhythm interrupted by ectopics
Rate: 88 bpm
P Waves: uniform; regular P–P interval
PRI: 0.20 second
QRS: 0.10 second in underlying rhythm; 0.14 second in ectopic; ectopic has bizarre configuration
Interp: Sinus Rhythm with one PVC

9.46 Regularity: regular
Rate: 125 bpm
P Waves: uniform; regular P–P interval
PRI: 0.16 second
QRS: 0.10 second
Interp: Sinus Tachycardia

9.47 Regularity: irregular
Rate: approximately 70 bpm
P Waves: not discernible; undulations present
PRI: none
QRS: 0.10 second
Interp: Atrial Fibrillation, controlled

9.48 Regularity: regular
Rate: 52 bpm
P Waves: uniform; regular P–P interval
PRI: 0.20 second and constant
QRS: 0.08 second
Interp: Sinus Bradycardia

9.49 Regularity: irregular
Rate: atrial rate 375 bpm; ventricular rate approximately 100 bpm
P Waves: uniform; sawtooth appearance; regular P–P interval; more P waves than QRS complexes
PRI: none
QRS: 0.08 second; complexes partially obscured by Flutter waves
Interp: Atrial Flutter with variable response

9.50 Regularity: regular
Rate: 115 bpm
P Waves: none visible
PRI: none
QRS: 0.08 second
Interp: Junctional Tachycardia

9.51 Regularity: regular
Rate: 107 bpm
P Waves: uniform; regular P–P interval
PRI: 0.12 second and constant
QRS: 0.12 second
Interp: Sinus Tachycardia (with wide QRS)

9.52 Regularity: irregular
Rate: atrial rate 300 bpm; ventricular rate 80 bpm
P Waves: uniform; sawtooth appearance; regular P–P interval; more P waves than QRS complexes
PRI: none
QRS: 0.08 second (complexes partially obscured by Flutter waves)
Interp: Atrial Flutter with variable response

9.53 Regularity: regular underlying rhythm interrupted by ectopics
Rate: 103 bpm (underlying rhythm)
P Waves: uniform; regular P–P interval
PRI: 0.14 second
QRS: 0.06 second in underlying rhythm; 0.12 second in ectopics; ectopics have bizarre configuration
Interp: Sinus Tachycardia with trigeminy of PVCs

9.54 Regularity: irregular
Rate: approximately 80 bpm
P Waves: not discernible; undulations present
PRI: none
QRS: 0.08 second
Interp: Atrial Fibrillation, controlled

9.55 Regularity: regular
Rate: 167 bpm
P Waves: not visible
PRI: none
QRS: 0.20 second; bizarre configuration
Interp: Ventricular Tachycardia

9.56 Regularity: irregular
Rate: atrial rate 300 bpm; ventricular rate approximately 140 bpm
P Waves: uniform; sawtooth configuration; regular P–P interval; more P waves than QRS complexes

PRI: none
QRS: 0.08 second (complexes partially obscured by Flutter waves)
Interp: Atrial Flutter with variable response

9.57 Regularity: totally chaotic baseline
Rate: unable to determine
P Waves: none

PRI: none
QRS: none
Interp: Ventricular Fibrillation

9.58 Regularity: irregular
Rate: approximately 110 bpm
P Waves: not discernible; undulations present

PRI: none
QRS: 0.08 second
Interp: Atrial Fibrillation, uncontrolled

9.59 Regularity: regular
Rate: 107 bpm
P Waves: uniform; regular P–P interval

PRI: 0.20 second
QRS: 0.12 second
Interp: Sinus Tachycardia (with wide QRS)

9.60 Regularity: irregular rhythm is interrupted by an ectopic
Rate: approximately 70 bpm
P Waves: uniform; irregular P–P interval; shape of P wave changes in ectopic beat

PRI: 0.14 second
QRS: 0.12 second in both underlying beat and ectopic; shape of complexes consistent
Interp: Sinus Arrhythmia (with wide QRS) with one PAC

9.61 Regularity: irregular
Rate: approximately 170 bpm
P Waves: not discernible

PRI: none
QRS: 0.10 second
Interp: Atrial Fibrillation, uncontrolled

9.62 Regularity: regular underlying rhythm interrupted by ectopics
Rate: 75 bpm
P Waves: uniform in underlying rhythm; regular P–P interval

PRI: 0.20 second
QRS: 0.14 second in underlying complexes; 0.16 second in ectopics; ectopics differ in configuration from underlying complexes
Interp: Sinus Rhythm (with wide QRS) with two unifocal PVCs

9.63 Regularity: irregular
Rate: approximately 130 bpm
P Waves: not discernible; undulations present

PRI: none
QRS: 0.10 second
Interp: Atrial Fibrillation, uncontrolled

9.64 Regularity: regular
Rate: atrial rate 300 bpm; ventricular rate 75 bpm
P Waves: uniform; sawtooth appearance; regular P–P interval; consistently four P waves for every QRS complex

PRI: none
QRS: 0.08 second
Interp: Atrial Flutter with 4:1 response

9.65 Regularity: regular
Rate: 71 bpm
P Waves: uniform; regular P–P interval

PRI: 0.24 second and constant
QRS: 0.10 second
Interp: Sinus Rhythm with First-Degree Heart Block

9.66 Regularity: regular
Rate: 111 bpm
P Waves: uniform; regular P–P interval

PRI: 0.12 second
QRS: 0.08 second
Interp: Sinus Tachycardia

9.67 Regularity: irregular
Rate: approximately 90 bpm
P Waves: not discernible; undulations present

PRI: none
QRS: 0.08 second
Interp: Atrial Fibrillation, controlled

9.68 Regularity: irregular
Rate: approximately 70 bpm
P Waves: uniform; irregular P–P interval

PRI: 0.12 second
QRS: 0.08 second
Interp: Sinus Arrhythmia

9.69 Regularity: irregular underlying rhythm interrupted by ectopics
Rate: approximately 90 bpm
P Waves: not discernible; undulations present

PRI: none
QRS: 0.12 second in underlying complexes; 0.14 second in ectopics; ectopics have bizarre configuration
Interp: Atrial Fibrillation, controlled (with wide QRS) with runs of PVCs

9.70 Regularity: totally chaotic baseline
Rate: cannot be determined
P Waves: none

PRI: none
QRS: none
Interp: Ventricular Fibrillation

9.71 Regularity: regular underlying rhythm interrupted by ectopic
Rate: 88 bpm
P Waves: uniform in underlying rhythm; regular P–P interval; shape changes in ectopic beats

PRI: 0.16 second
QRS: 0.14 second
Interp: Sinus Rhythm (with wide QRS) with one PAC

9.72 Regularity: regular
Rate: 91 bpm
P Waves: uniform; regular P–P interval

PRI: 0.28 second and constant
QRS: 0.08 second
Interp: Sinus Rhythm with First-Degree Heart Block

9.73 Regularity: regular
Rate: 150 bpm
P Waves: not discernible

PRI: none
QRS: 0.08 second
Interp: Supraventricular Tachycardia

9.74 Regularity: totally chaotic baseline
Rate: cannot be determined
P Waves: none

PRI: none
QRS: none
Interp: Ventricular Fibrillation

9.75 Regularity: irregular
Rate: approximately 110 bpm
P Waves: not discernible; undulations present

PRI: none
QRS: 0.12 second
Interp: Atrial Fibrillation, uncontrolled (with wide QRS)

9.76 Regularity: regular
Rate: 56 bpm
P Waves: not visible

PRI: none
QRS: 0.16 second; configuration is bizarre
Interp: Accelerated Idioventricular Rhythm

Note: This rhythm fits all of the rules for Idioventricular Rhythm except that the rate is faster than you would expect it to be, but not as fast as you would think a Ventricular Tachycardia would be. This patient may have been in an Idioventricular Rhythm at a slower rate and then received a drug to make the rate increase and improve his or her condition.

9.77 Regularity: regular
Rate: atrial rate 260 bpm; ventricular rate 65 bpm
P Waves: uniform; sawtooth appearance; regular P–P interval; consistently four P waves for every QRS complex

PRI: none
QRS: 0.10 second
Interp: Atrial Flutter with 4:1 block

9.78 Regularity: irregular underlying rhythm interrupted by ectopic
Rate: approximately 60 bpm
P Waves: not discernible; undulations present

PRI: none
QRS: 0.10 second in underlying rhythm; 0.14 second in ectopic; ectopic has bizarre configuration
Interp: Atrial Fibrillation, controlled, with one PVC

9.79 Regularity: regular underlying rhythm interrupted by ectopic
Rate: 81 bpm
P Waves: uniform; regular P–P interval

PRI: 0.14 second
QRS: 0.12 second in underlying rhythm; 0.14 second in ectopic; ectopic has bizarre configuration
Interp: Sinus Rhythm with one PVC

9.80 Regularity: irregular
Rate: atrial rate 300 bpm; ventricular rate approximately 80 bpm
P Waves: uniform; sawtooth appearance; regular P–P interval; more P waves than QRS complexes

PRI: none
QRS: 0.10 second
Interp: Atrial Flutter with variable block

9.81 Regularity: totally chaotic baseline
Rate: cannot be determined
P Waves: none

PRI: none
QRS: none
Interp: Ventricular Fibrillation

9.82 Regularity: irregular
Rate: atrial rate 56 bpm; ventricular rate 50 bpm
P Waves: uniform; regular P–P interval; occasional non-conducted P waves

PRI: changing PRI; progressively lengthens from 0.28 second to 0.40 second
QRS: 0.08 second
Interp: Wenckebach (Type I Second-Degree Heart Block)

9.83 Regularity: irregular rhythm interrupted by ectopics
Rate: approximately 60 bpm (underlying rhythm)
P Waves: uniform; irregular P–P interval

PRI: 0.20 second
QRS: 0.08 second in underlying rhythm; 0.16 second in ectopics; ectopics have bizarre configuration; ectopics have different shapes
Interp: Sinus Arrhythmia with multifocal PVCs

9.83 Regularity: regular
Rate: atrial rate 65 bpm; ventricular rate 29 bpm
P Waves: uniform; regular P–P interval; more P waves than QRS complexes

PRI: P waves are not associated with QRS complexes
QRS: 0.20 second; bizarre configuration
Interp: Third-Degree Heart Block (CHB) with ventricular escape focus

9.85 Regularity: irregular
Rate: approximately 90 bpm
P Waves: not discernible; undulations present

PRI: none
QRS: 0.14 second
Interp: Atrial Fibrillation, controlled (with wide QRS)

9.86 Regularity: irregular
Rate: approximately 120 bpm
P Waves: not discernible; undulations present

PRI: none
QRS: 0.10 second
Interp: Atrial Fibrillation, uncontrolled

9.87 Regularity: regular
Rate: 75 bpm
P Waves: uniform and upright; regular P–P interval

PRI: 0.16 second and constant
QRS: 0.06 second
Interp: Normal Sinus Rhythm

9.88 Regularity: regular underlying rhythm interrupted by ectopics
Rate: 88 bpm
P Waves: uniform in underlying rhythm; form changes in ectopics

PRI: 0.12 second
QRS: 0.10 second in both underlying rhythm and ectopics; form does not change in ectopics
Interp: Sinus Rhythm with three PACs

9.89 Regularity: regular
Rate: 214 bpm
P Waves: not visible

PRI: none
QRS: 0.06 second
Interp: Supraventricular Tachycardia—probably Atrial Tachycardia (see note)

Note: Of all the supraventricular tachycardias, Atrial Tachycardia is the only one that can produce this ventricular rate with 1:1 conduction.

9.90 Regularity: regular
Rate: atrial rate 100 bpm; ventricular rate 44 bpm
P Waves: uniform; regular P–P interval; more P waves than QRS complexes

PRI: P waves are not associated with QRS complexes
QRS: 0.08 second
Interp: Third-Degree Heart Block (CHB) with junctional escape focus

9.91 Regularity: regular, interrupted by ectopic
Rate: 83 bpm
P Waves: uniform; regular P–P interval

PRI: 0.24 second and constant in underlying rhythm; 0.12 second in ectopic
QRS: 0.14 second in underlying rhythm; 0.14 second in ectopic
Interp: Sinus Rhythm (with wide QRS) with First-Degree Heart Block and one PJC

9.92 Regularity: regular
Rate: 188 bpm
P Waves: none visible

PRI: not discernible
QRS: 0.10 second
Interp: Supraventricular Tachycardia

9.93 Regularity: slightly irregular
Rate: atrial rate 88 bpm; ventricular rate approximately 33 bpm
P Waves: uniform; regular P–P interval; more P waves than QRS complexes

PRI: none
QRS: 0.12 second
Interp: Third-Degree Heart Block (CHB) with ventricular escape focus

9.94 Regularity: totally chaotic baseline
Rate: unable to determine
P Waves: none visible

PRI: unable to determine
QRS: none visible
Interp: Ventricular Fibrillation (Agonal Rhythm)

9.95 Regularity: regular
Rate: 50 bpm
P Waves: uniform; regular P–P interval

PRI: 0.16 second and constant
QRS: 0.14 second
Interp: Sinus Bradycardia (with wide QRS)

9.96 Regularity: slightly irregular underlying rhythm interrupted by ectopics
Rate: approximately 107 bpm (underlying rhythm)
P Waves: not discernible (see note); ectopics not preceded by P waves

PRI: none
QRS: 0.08 second in underlying rhythm; 0.12 second and 0.16 second in ectopics
Interp: Atrial Fibrillation, uncontrolled, with two multifocal PVCs

Note: Small waves precede some QRS complexes but by too short a distance to have been conducted; furthermore, these waves do not map out across the strip.

9.97 Regularity: slightly irregular
Rate: approximately 37 bpm
P Waves: uniform; regular P–P interval

PRI: 0.20 second and constant
QRS: 0.08 second
Interp: Sinus Bradycardia (with slight sinus arrhythmia)

9.98 Regularity: regular
Rate: 125 bpm
P Waves: uniform; regular P–P interval

PRI: 0.16 second and constant (obscured slightly by T waves)
QRS: 0.08 second
Interp: Sinus Tachycardia

9.99 Regularity: slightly irregular
Rate: approximately 110 bpm
P Waves: shape changes from beat to beat

PRI: approximately 0.16 second; varies slightly
QRS: 0.12 second
Interp: Wandering Pacemaker (with a wide QRS)

9.100 Regularity: slightly irregular
Rate: approximately 170 bpm
P Waves: none visible

PRI: none
QRS: 0.24 second
Interp: Ventricular Tachycardia

9.101 Regularity: irregular
Rate: approximately 130 bpm
P Waves: none visible, undulations present

PRI: none
QRS: 0.06 second
Interp: Atrial Fibrillation, uncontrolled

9.102 Regularity: totally chaotic baseline
Rate: not discernible
P Waves: none visible

PRI: none
QRS: none visible
Interp: Ventricular Fibrillation

9.103 Regularity: regular underlying rhythm interrupted by ectopics in a pattern of grouped beating
Rate: 68 bpm
P Waves: uniform; regular P–P interval in underlying rhythm; no P waves preceding ectopics

PRI: 0.16 second and constant
QRS: 0.08 second in underlying rhythm; 0.14 second in ectopics
Interp: Sinus Rhythm with bigeminy of PVCs

9.104 Regularity: regular underlying rhythm interrupted by ectopics
Rate: 100 bpm
P Waves: uniform; regular P–P interval; no P waves preceding ectopics

PRI: 0.14 second and constant
QRS: 0.12 second
Interp: Sinus Tachycardia (with a wide QRS) and two PJCs

9.105 Regularity: regular (very slightly irregular)
Rate: approximately 70 bpm
P Waves: uniform; regular P–P interval

PRI: 0.30 second and constant
QRS: 0.08 second
Interp: Sinus Rhythm with First-Degree Heart Block

9.106 Regularity: totally chaotic baseline
Rate: unable to determine
P Waves: none visible

PRI: none
QRS: none visible
Interp: Ventricular Fibrillation

9.107 Regularity: slight irregular underlying rhythm interrupted by ectopic
Rate: approximately 50 bpm
P Waves: uniform and upright

PRI: 0.08 second and constant
QRS: 0.08 second in underlying rhythm; 0.20 second in ectopic
Interp: Sinus Bradycardia with one PVC

9.108 Regularity: irregular
Rate: atrial rate 214 bpm; ventricular rate approximately 100 bpm
P Waves: characteristic sawtooth pattern

PRI: unable to determine
QRS: 0.10 second
Interp: Atrial Flutter with variable response

9.109 Regularity: regular
Rate: 75 bpm
P Waves: uniform; regular P–P interval

PRI: 0.24 second and constant
QRS: 0.08 second
Interp: Sinus Rhythm with First-Degree Heart Block

9.110 Regularity: slightly irregular
Rate: approximately 150 bpm
P Waves: none visible

PRI: none
QRS: 0.12 second
Interp: Ventricular Tachycardia

9.111 Regularity: irregular
Rate: approximately 70 bpm
P Waves: none visible; undulations present

PRI: none
QRS: 0.14 second
Interp: Atrial Fibrillation, controlled (with wide QRS)

9.112 Regularity: regular (very slightly irregular)
Rate: approximately 46 bpm
P Waves: inverted following QRS complex

PRI: none
QRS: 0.08 second
Interp: Junctional Escape Rhythm

9.113 Regularity: irregular
Rate: approximately 150 bpm initially; then 0
P Waves: none

PRI: none
QRS: approximately 0.20 second
Interp: Ventricular Tachycardia into Asystole

9.114 Regularity: irregular underlying rhythm with a pattern of grouped beating
Rate: atrial rate 125 bpm; ventricular rate approximately 80 bpm
P Waves: uniform; regular P–P interval

PRI: varies; progressively lengthens until one P wave is not conducted
QRS: 0.12 second
Interp: Wenckebach (Type I Second-Degree Heart Block)

9.115 Regularity: slightly irregular
Rate: approximately 150 bpm
P Waves: none visible

PRI: none
QRS: approximately 0.24 second
Interp: Ventricular Tachycardia

9.116 Regularity: regular underlying rhythm interrupted by ectopic
Rate: 63 bpm
P Waves: uniform; regular P–P interval

PRI: 0.20 second and constant
QRS: 0.08 second in underlying rhythm; 0.14 second in ectopic
Interp: Sinus Rhythm with one PVC

9.117 Regularity: regular underlying rhythm interrupted by ectopics in a pattern of grouped beating
Rate: 79 bpm
P Waves: uniform; regular P–P interval; no P waves preceding ectopics

PRI: 0.22 second and constant
QRS: 0.10 second in underlying rhythm; 0.16 second in ectopics
Interp: Sinus Rhythm with First-Degree Heart Block with trigeminy of PVCs

9.118 Regularity: regular
Rate: 150 bpm
P Waves: none visible

PRI: none
QRS: 0.14 second
Interp: Ventricular Tachycardia

9.119 Regularity: regular, interrupted by ectopics
Rate: 79 bpm
P Waves: uniform; regular P–P interval

PRI: 0.20 second and constant
QRS: 0.08 second in underlying rhythm; 0.12 second in ectopics
Interp: Sinus Rhythm with two unifocal PVCs

9.120 Regularity: slightly irregular
Rate: approximately 107 bpm
P Waves: none visible

PRI: none
QRS: 0.22 second
Interp: slow Ventricular Tachycardia

9.121 Regularity: regular underlying rhythm interrupted by ectopic
Rate: 83 bpm
P Waves: uniform; regular P–P interval; no P wave preceding ectopic

PRI: 0.14 second and constant
QRS: 0.08 second in underlying rhythm; 0.16 second in ectopic
Interp: Normal Sinus Rhythm with one PVC

9.122 Regularity: regular underlying rhythm interrupted by ectopic
Rate: 77 bpm
P Waves: uniform; regular P–P interval; no P wave preceding ectopic

PRI: 0.26 second and constant
QRS: 0.08 second in underlying rhythm; 0.12 second in ectopic
Interp: Sinus Rhythm with First-Degree Heart Block and one PVC

9.123 Regularity: regular
Rate: atrial rate 94 bpm; ventricular rate 47 bpm
P Waves: uniform; regular P–P interval; three P waves for every QRS complex

PRI: 0.28 second and constant on conducted beats
QRS: 0.12 second
Interp: Type II Second-Degree Heart Block with 2:1 conduction (with wide QRS)

9.124 Regularity: totally chaotic baseline
Rate: unable to determine
P Waves: none visible

PRI: none
QRS: none visible
Interp: Ventricular Fibrillation into Asystole

9.125 Regularity: regular underlying rhythm interrupted by ectopic
Rate: 88 bpm
P Waves: uniform; regular P–P interval; ectopic is preceded by upright P wave

PRI: 0.20 second and constant
QRS: 0.08 second
Interp: Normal Sinus Rhythm with one PAC

9.126 Regularity: totally chaotic baseline
Rate: unable to determine
P Waves: none visible

PRI: none
QRS: none visible
Interp: Ventricular Fibrillation

9.127 Regularity: regular
Rate: atrial rate 300 bpm; ventricular rate 60 bpm
P Waves: characteristic sawtooth pattern

PRI: unable to determine
QRS: 0.08 second (slightly obscured by Flutter waves)
Interp: Atrial Flutter with 5:1 response

9.128 Regularity: irregular
Rate: approximately 110 bpm
P Waves: configuration varies from beat to beat

PRI: varies
QRS: 0.08 second
Interp: Wandering Pacemaker

9.129 Regularity: slightly irregular
Rate: approximately 48 bpm
P Waves: uniform; regular P–P interval

PRI: 0.16 second and constant
QRS: 0.10 second
Interp: Sinus Bradyarrhythmia

9.130 Regularity: regular
Rate: 150 bpm
P Waves: none visible

PRI: none
QRS: 0.16 second
Interp: Ventricular Tachycardia

9.131 Regularity: slightly irregular
Rate: approximately 75 bpm
P Waves: shape changes from beat to beat

PRI: varies
QRS: 0.08 second
Interp: Wandering Pacemaker

9.132 Regularity: regular
Rate: 71 bpm
P Waves: uniform; regular P–P interval

PRI: 0.32 second and constant
QRS: 0.08 second
Interp: Sinus Rhythm with First-Degree Heart Block

9.133 Regularity: regular underlying rhythm interrupted by ectopic
Rate: atrial rate 300 bpm; ventricular rate 75 bpm
P Waves: characteristic sawtooth pattern

PRI: unable to determine
QRS: 0.08 second in underlying rhythm (slightly obscured by Flutter waves); 0.16 second in ectopic
Interp: Atrial Flutter with 4:1 response, with one PVC

9.134 Regularity: regular
Rate: 83 bpm
P Waves: none

PRI: none
QRS: 0.08 second
Interp: Accelerated Junctional Rhythm

9.135 Regularity: irregular in a pattern of grouped beating
Rate: atrial rate 115 bpm; ventricular rate approximately 70 bpm
P Waves: uniform; regular P–P interval

PRI: varies; progressively lengthens until one P wave is not conducted
QRS: 0.10 second
Interp: Wenckebach (Type I Second-Degree Heart Block)

9.136 Regularity: regular underlying rhythm interrupted by ectopics in a pattern of grouped beating
Rate: approximately 70 bpm
P Waves: uniform; regular P–P interval; no P wave preceding ectopics

PRI: 0.16 second and constant
QRS: 0.10 second in underlying rhythm; 0.16 second in ectopics
Interp: Sinus Rhythm with bigeminy of PVCs

9.137 Regularity: regular underlying rhythm interrupted by ectopics in a pattern of grouped beating
Rate: 79 bpm
P Waves: uniform in underlying rhythm; inverted P waves following QRS complexes of ectopics

PRI: 0.18 second and constant
QRS: 0.08 second in underlying rhythm; 0.08 second in ectopics
Interp: Sinus Rhythm with bigeminy of PJCs

9.138 Regularity: regular underlying rhythm interrupted by ectopic
Rate: 83 bpm
P Waves: uniform; regular P–P interval; ectopic is preceded by an upright P wave

PRI: 0.16 second and constant
QRS: 0.12 second in underlying rhythm; 0.12 second in ectopic
Interp: Sinus Rhythm (with wide QRS) with one PAC

9.139 Regularity: regular underlying rhythm interrupted by ectopics
Rate: 94 bpm
P Waves: uniform in underlying rhythm; no P waves preceding ectopics

PRI: 0.16 second and constant
QRS: 0.08 second in underlying rhythm; 0.16 second in ectopics
Interp: Normal Sinus Rhythm with bursts of Ventricular Tachycardia

9.140 Regularity: regular
Rate: atrial rate 75 bpm; ventricular rate 40 bpm
P Waves: uniform; regular P–P interval

PRI: none
QRS: 0.08 second
Interp: Third-Degree Heart Block (CHB)

9.141 Regularity: regular
Rate: 47 bpm
P Waves: uniform; regular P–P interval

PRI: 0.20 second and constant
QRS: 0.08 second
Interp: Sinus Bradycardia

9.142 Regularity: regular
Rate: 125 bpm
P Waves: none visible

PRI: none
QRS: 0.20 second
Interp: slow Ventricular Tachycardia

9.143 Regularity: regular
Rate: 94 bpm
P Waves: inverted preceding QRS complex

PRI: 0.12 second
QRS: 0.12 second
Interp: Accelerated Junctional Rhythm

9.144 Regularity: regular underlying rhythm interrupted by ectopics
Rate: approximately 80 bpm
P Waves: uniform in underlying rhythm; morphology changes with ectopics

PRI: 0.14 second and constant
QRS: 0.10 second in underlying rhythm; 0.10 second in ectopics
Interp: Normal Sinus Rhythm with three PACs

9.145 Regularity: regular
Rate: atrial rate 103 bpm;
ventricular rate 42 bpm
P Waves: uniform; regular
P–P interval

PRI: none
QRS: 0.16 second
Interp: Third-Degree Heart
Block (CHB) with ven-
tricular escape focus

9.146 Regularity: irregular
Rate: atrial rate 300 bpm;
ventricular rate approxi-
mately 80 bpm
P Waves: characteristic
sawtooth pattern

PRI: unable to determine
QRS: 0.10 second
Interp: Atrial Flutter with
variable response

9.147 Regularity: regular
Rate: 83 bpm
P Waves: uniform; regular
P–P interval

PRI: 0.32 second and
constant
QRS: 0.10 second
Interp: Sinus Rhythm with
First-Degree Heart Block

9.148 Regularity: regular
Rate: 38 bpm
P Waves: uniform; regular
P–P interval

PRI: 0.16 second and
constant
QRS: 0.14 second
Interp: Sinus Bradycardia
(with wide QRS)

9.149 Regularity: regular underlying rhythm interrupted
by ectopic
Rate: 115 bpm
P Waves: uniform; regular
P–P interval; no P wave
preceding ectopic

PRI: 0.16 second and
constant
QRS: 0.06 second in
underlying rhythm;
0.14 second in ectopic
Interp: Sinus Tachycardia
with one PVC

9.150 Regularity: slightly irregular
underlying rhythm inter-
rupted by ectopic
Rate: approximately
55 bpm
P Waves: uniform in underlying rhythm; no P wave
preceding ectopic

PRI: 0.16 second
QRS: 0.08 second in
underlying rhythm;
0.12 second in ectopic
Interp: Sinus Bradycardia
with one PVC

9.151 Regularity: slightly irregular
Rate: approximately
250 bpm
P Waves: none visible

PRI: none
QRS: approximately
0.16 second
Interp: Ventricular
Tachycardia

9.152 Regularity: no visible
waves or complexes
Rate: unable to determine
P Waves: none visible

PRI: none
QRS: none
Interp: Asystole

9.153 Regularity: irregular
Rate: approximately
150 bpm
P Waves: none visible

PRI: none
QRS: 0.08 second
Interp: Atrial Fibrillation,
uncontrolled

9.154 Regularity: regular
Rate: 79 bpm
P Waves: uniform; regular
P–P interval

PRI: 0.22 second and
constant
QRS: 0.10 second
Interp: Sinus Rhythm with
First-Degree Heart Block

9.155 Regularity: regular
Rate: 25 bpm
P Waves: none visible

PRI: none
QRS: 0.12 second
Interp: Idioventricular
Rhythm

9.156 Regularity: totally chaotic
baseline
Rate: unable to determine
P Waves: none visible

PRI: none
QRS: unable to determine
Interp: Ventricular
Fibrillation

9.157 Regularity: regular
Rate: 100 bpm
P Waves: uniform; regular
P–P interval

PRI: 0.14 second and
constant
QRS: 0.10 second
Interp: Sinus Tachycardia

9.158 Regularity: regular
Rate: 58 bpm
P Waves: uniform; regular
P–P interval

PRI: 0.20 second and
constant
QRS: 0.08 second
Interp: Sinus Bradycardia

9.159 Regularity: totally chaotic
baseline
Rate: unable to determine
P Waves: none visible

PRI: none
QRS: unable to determine
Interp: Ventricular
Fibrillation

9.160 Regularity: regular
Rate: 56 bpm
P Waves: uniform; regular
P–P interval

PRI: 0.16 second and
constant
QRS: 0.08 second
Interp: Sinus Bradycardia

9.161 Regularity: regular
Rate: atrial rate 63 bpm;
ventricular rate 32 bpm
P Waves: uniform; regu-
lar P–P interval; more
P waves than QRS
complexes

PRI: none
QRS: 0.14 second
Interp: Third-Degree Heart
Block (CHB) with ven-
tricular escape focus

9.162 Regularity: regular
Rate: 38 bpm
P Waves: uniform; regular
P–P interval

PRI: 0.16 second and
constant
QRS: 0.10 second
Interp: Sinus Bradycardia

9.163 Regularity: regular
Rate: 79 bpm
P Waves: uniform; regular
P–P interval

PRI: 0.20 second and
constant
QRS: 0.10 second
Interp: Normal Sinus
Rhythm

9.164 Regularity: regular underlying rhythm interrupted
by ectopic
Rate: 63 bpm
P Waves: uniform in underlying rhythm; no P waves
preceding ectopic

PRI: 0.20 second and
constant
QRS: 0.14 second in
underlying rhythm;
0.16 second in ectopic
Interp: Sinus Rhythm (with
wide QRS) with one PVC

9.165 Regularity: regular underlying rhythm interrupted
by ectopics
Rate: 63 bpm
P Waves: uniform in underlying rhythm; no P waves
preceding ectopics

PRI: 0.24 second and
constant
QRS: 0.10 second in
underlying rhythm;
0.16 second in ectopics
Interp: Sinus Rhythm with
First-Degree Heart Block
with two unifocal PVCs

9.166 Regularity: irregular
Rate: approximately 110 bpm
P Waves: none visible; undulations present

PRI: none
QRS: 0.06 second
Interp: Atrial Fibrillation, uncontrolled

9.167 Regularity: irregular
Rate: atrial rate 300 bpm; ventricular rate approximately 100 bpm
P Waves: characteristic sawtooth pattern

PRI: unable to determine
QRS: 0.10 second
Interp: Atrial Flutter with variable response

9.168 Regularity: regular
Rate: 107 bpm
P Waves: uniform; regular P–P interval

PRI: 0.14 second and constant
QRS: 0.06 second
Interp: Sinus Tachycardia

9.169 Regularity: regular underlying rhythm interrupted by ectopics
Rate: 103 bpm
P Waves: uniform in underlying rhythm; no P waves preceding ectopics

PRI: 0.14 second and constant
QRS: 0.08 second in underlying rhythm; 0.14 second in ectopics
Interp: Sinus Tachycardia with two PVCs and coupled PVCs, all unifocal

9.170 Regularity: regular underlying rhythm interrupted by ectopics in a pattern of grouped beating
Rate: visible sinus rate is 36 bpm; actual sinus rate is probably 72 bpm
P Waves: uniform in underlying rhythm; no P waves preceding ectopics

PRI: 0.16 second and constant
QRS: 0.08 second in underlying rhythm; 0.16 second in ectopics
Interp: Sinus Rhythm with bigeminy of PVCs

9.171 Regularity: totally chaotic baseline
Rate: unable to determine
P Waves: none visible

PRI: none
QRS: unable to determine
Interp: Ventricular Fibrillation (Agonal Rhythm)

9.172 Regularity: regular
Rate: atrial rate 96 bpm; ventricular rate 48 bpm
P Waves: uniform; regular P–P interval; two P waves for every QRS complex

PRI: 0.20 second and constant on conducted beats
QRS: 0.10 second
Interp: Type II Second-Degree Heart Block (2:1)

9.173 Regularity: regular underlying rhythm interrupted by ectopics
Rate: 68 bpm
P Waves: uniform in underlying rhythm; morphology changes in ectopics

PRI: 0.20 second and constant
QRS: 0.08 second in underlying rhythm; 0.10 second in ectopics
Interp: Normal Sinus Rhythm with two PACs

9.174 Regularity: irregular
Rate: atrial rate 333 bpm; ventricular rate approximately 70 bpm
P Waves: characteristic sawtooth pattern

PRI: unable to determine
QRS: 0.08 second
Interp: Atrial Flutter with variable response

9.175 Regularity: regular underlying rhythm interrupted by ectopics in a pattern of grouped beating
Rate: 83 bpm
P Waves: uniform in underlying rhythm; morphology changes in ectopics

PRI: 0.12 second and constant
QRS: 0.10 second in underlying rhythm; 0.10 second in ectopics
Interp: Sinus Rhythm with trigeminy of PACs

9.176 Regularity: regular underlying rhythm interrupted by ectopics
Rate: 75 bpm
P Waves: uniform in underlying rhythm; no P waves preceding ectopics

PRI: 0.20 second and constant
QRS: 0.08 second in underlying rhythm; 0.12 second in ectopics
Interp: Normal Sinus Rhythm with two unifocal PVCs

9.177 Regularity: regular
Rate: 60 bpm
P Waves: uniform; regular P–P interval

PRI: 0.24 second and constant
QRS: 0.08 second
Interp: Sinus Rhythm with First-Degree Heart Block

9.178 Regularity: irregular
Rate: approximately 80 bpm
P Waves: morphology changes with each beat

PRI: varies
QRS: 0.12 second
Interp: Wandering Pacemaker (with wide QRS)

9.179 Regularity: regular underlying rhythm interrupted by ectopics in a pattern of grouped beating
Rate: approximately 80 bpm
P Waves: uniform in underlying rhythm; no P waves preceding ectopics

PRI: 0.14 second and constant in underlying rhythm
QRS: 0.08 second in underlying rhythm; 0.14 second in ectopics
Interp: Sinus Rhythm with bigeminy of PVCs

9.180 Regularity: regular
Rate: 115 bpm
P Waves: none visible

PRI: none
QRS: 0.08 second
Interp: Junctional Tachycardia

9.181 Regularity: irregular in a pattern of grouped beating
Rate: atrial rate 88 bpm; ventricular rate approximately 60 bpm
P Waves: uniform; regular P–P interval; some P waves are not followed by QRS complexes

PRI: varies; progressively lengthens until a beat is not conducted
QRS: 0.10 second
Interp: Wenckebach (Type I Second-Degree Heart Block)

9.182 Regularity: regular underlying rhythm interrupted by ectopics
Rate: 107 bpm
P Waves: uniform in underlying rhythm; no P wave preceding ectopics

PRI: 0.12 second and constant
QRS: 0.08 second in underlying rhythm; 0.14 second in ectopics
Interp: Sinus Tachycardia with PVC and coupled PVCs, all unifocal

9.183 Regularity: no visible complexes; essentially straight line
Rate: not discernible
P Waves: none

PRI: none
QRS: none
Interp: Asystole (Agonal Rhythm)

9.184 Regularity: slightly irregular
Rate: approximately 70 bpm
P Waves: morphology changes from beat to beat

PRI: varies slightly (0.18–0.20 second)
QRS: 0.08 second
Interp: Wandering Pacemaker

9.185 Regularity: regular underlying rhythm interrupted by ectopics in a pattern of grouped beating
Rate: 120 bpm
P Waves: uniform in underlying rhythm; no P waves preceding ectopics

PRI: 0.12 second and constant
QRS: 0.08 second in underlying rhythm; 0.12 second in ectopics
Interp: Sinus Tachycardia with bigeminy of PVCs

9.186 Regularity: regular
Rate: 54 bpm
P Waves: inverted in front of QRS complexes

PRI: 0.12 second and constant
QRS: 0.08 second
Interp: Junctional Escape Rhythm

9.187 Regularity: regular
Rate: atrial rate 100 bpm; ventricular rate 35 bpm
P Waves: uniform; regular P–P interval; more P waves than QRS complexes

PRI: none
QRS: 0.20 second
Interp: Third-Degree Heart Block (CHB) with ventricular escape focus

9.188 Regularity: irregular
Rate: approximately 100 bpm
P Waves: none visible; undulations present

PRI: none
QRS: 0.08 second
Interp: Atrial Fibrillation, controlled

9.189 Regularity: totally chaotic baseline
Rate: unable to determine
P Waves: none visible

PRI: none
QRS: none
Interp: Ventricular Fibrillation

9.190 Regularity: irregular
Rate: approximately 90 bpm
P Waves: none visible; undulations present

PRI: none
QRS: 0.08 second
Interp: Atrial Fibrillation, controlled

9.191 Regularity: irregular
Rate: approximately 80 bpm
P Waves: none discernible; undulations present

PRI: none
QRS: 0.16 second
Interp: Atrial Fibrillation, controlled (with wide QRS)

9.192 Regularity: regular underlying rhythm interrupted by ectopics in a pattern of grouped beating
Rate: 100 bpm
P Waves: uniform in underlying rhythm; no P waves preceding ectopics

PRI: 0.14 second and constant
QRS: 0.08 second in underlying rhythm; 0.14 second in ectopics
Interp: Sinus Tachycardia with trigeminy of PVCs

9.193 Regularity: slightly irregular
Rate: approximately 136 bpm
P Waves: none visible

PRI: none
QRS: 0.16 second
Interp: Ventricular Tachycardia (slow rate range)

9.194 Regularity: regular underlying rhythm interrupted by ectopics
Rate: 83 bpm
P Waves: uniform in underlying rhythm; no P waves preceding ectopics

PRI: 0.16 second and constant
QRS: 0.12 second in underlying rhythm; 0.16 second in ectopics
Interp: Sinus Rhythm (with wide QRS) with two unifocal PVCs

9.195 Regularity: regular
Rate: atrial rate 125 bpm; ventricular rate 22 bpm
P Waves: uniform; regular P–P interval

PRI: none
QRS: 0.12 second
Interp: Third-Degree Heart Block (CHB) with ventricular escape focus

Note: You might also want to note that the atria are being depolarized at a faster than normal rate. You could call this a CHB with an underlying Sinus Tachycardia.

9.196 Regularity: regular
Rate: 125 bpm
P Waves: uniform; regular P–P interval

PRI: 0.16 second and constant
QRS: 0.10 second
Interp: Sinus Tachycardia

9.197 Regularity: regular
Rate: 94 bpm
P Waves: uniform; regular P–P interval

PRI: 0.24 second and constant
QRS: 0.10 second
Interp: Sinus Rhythm with First-Degree Heart Block

9.198 Regularity: regular
Rate: atrial rate 264 bpm; ventricular rate 88 bpm
P Waves: characteristic sawtooth pattern

PRI: unable to determine
QRS: 0.12 second
Interp: Atrial Flutter with 3:1 response

9.199 Regularity: regular underlying rhythm interrupted by ectopic
Rate: 71 bpm
P Waves: uniform; regular P–P interval; no P wave preceding ectopic

PRI: 0.16 second and constant
QRS: 0.08 second in underlying rhythm; 0.14 second in ectopic
Interp: Normal Sinus Rhythm with one PVC

9.200 Regularity: regular
Rate: 167 bpm
P Waves: none visible

PRI: none
QRS: 0.16 second
Interp: Ventricular Tachycardia

9.201 Regularity: totally chaotic baseline
Rate: unable to determine
P Waves: none visible

PRI: none
QRS: none
Interp: Ventricular Fibrillation (Agonal Rhythm)

9.202 Regularity: regular
Rate: approximately 48 bpm
P Waves: uniform; regular P–P interval

PRI: 0.20 second and constant
QRS: 0.10 second
Interp: Sinus Bradycardia

9.203 Regularity: regular underlying rhythm interrupted by frequent ectopics
Rate: 107 bpm
P Waves: uniform in underlying rhythm; no P waves preceding ectopics
PRI: 0.12 second and constant
QRS: 0.08 second in underlying rhythm; 0.14 second in ectopics
Interp: Sinus Tachycardia with three PVCs, two of them coupled

9.204 Regularity: regular
Rate: 115 bpm
P Waves: uniform; regular P–P interval
PRI: 0.14 second and constant
QRS: 0.08 second
Interp: Sinus Tachycardia

9.205 Regularity: irregular
Rate: approximately 100 bpm
P Waves: none visible; undulations present
PRI: none
QRS: 0.08 second
Interp: Atrial Fibrillation, controlled

9.206 Regularity: regular
Rate: 43 bpm
P Waves: uniform; regular P–P interval
PRI: 0.20 second and constant
QRS: 0.06 second
Interp: Sinus Bradycardia

9.207 Regularity: irregular
Rate: approximately 60 bpm
P Waves: none visible; undulations present
PRI: none
QRS: 0.08 second
Interp: Atrial Fibrillation, controlled

9.208 Regularity: regular underlying rhythm interrupted by ectopics
Rate: 94 bpm
P Waves: uniform in underlying rhythm; no P waves preceding ectopics
PRI: 0.16 second and constant
QRS: 0.08 second in underlying rhythm; 0.14 second in ectopics
Interp: Normal Sinus Rhythm with two unifocal PVCs

9.209 Regularity: regular
Rate: 143 bpm
P Waves: uniform; regular P–P interval
PRI: 0.14 second and constant
QRS: 0.08 second
Interp: Sinus Tachycardia

9.210 Regularity: regular
Rate: 47 bpm
P Waves: uniform; regular P–P interval
PRI: 0.28 second and constant
QRS: 0.10 second
Interp: Sinus Bradycardia with First-Degree Heart Block

9.211 Regularity: irregular
Rate: approximately 150 bpm
P Waves: none visible; undulations present
PRI: none
QRS: 0.12 second
Interp: Atrial Fibrillation, uncontrolled (with wide QRS)

9.212 Regularity: irregular initially, then totally chaotic
Rate: unable to determine
P Waves: none visible
PRI: none
QRS: approximately 0.16 second in initial rhythm; unable to measure in terminal pattern
Interp: Ventricular Tachycardia into Ventricular Fibrillation

9.213 Regularity: irregular
Rate: approximately 130 bpm
P Waves: none visible; undulations present
PRI: unable to determine
QRS: 0.10 second
Interp: Atrial Fibrillation, uncontrolled

9.214 Regularity: regular underlying rhythm interrupted by ectopic
Rate: 84 bpm
P Waves: uniform in underlying rhythm; no P wave preceding ectopic
PRI: 0.24 second and constant
QRS: 0.08 second in underlying rhythm; 0.12 second in ectopic
Interp: Sinus Rhythm with First-Degree Heart Block with one PVC

9.215 Regularity: irregular
Rate: approximately 110 bpm
P Waves: none visible; undulations present
PRI: none
QRS: 0.08 second
Interp: Atrial Fibrillation, uncontrolled

9.216 Regularity: irregular
Rate: atrial rate 250 bpm; ventricular rate 70 bpm
P Waves: characteristic sawtooth pattern
PRI: unable to determine
QRS: 0.08 second
Interp: Atrial Flutter with variable response

9.217 Regularity: regular
Rate: 125 bpm
P Waves: uniform; regular P–P interval
PRI: 0.16 second and constant
QRS: 0.14 second
Interp: Sinus Tachycardia (with wide QRS)

9.218 Regularity: regular
Rate: atrial rate 167 bpm; ventricular rate 22 bpm
P Waves: uniform; regular P–P interval
PRI: none
QRS: 0.14 second
Interp: Third-Degree Heart Block (CHB) with ventricular escape focus

Note: You might also want to note that the atria are being depolarized at a faster than normal rate. You could call this a CHB with an underlying Atrial Tachycardia.

9.219 Regularity: regular
Rate: 167 bpm
P Waves: none visible
PRI: unable to determine
QRS: 0.08 second
Interp: Supraventricular Tachycardia

9.220 Regularity: irregular
Rate: approximately 120 bpm
P Waves: none visible; undulations present
PRI: none
QRS: 0.10 second
Interp: Atrial Fibrillation, uncontrolled

9.221 Regularity: regular
Rate: 60 bpm
P Waves: uniform and upright
PRI: 0.22 second and constant
QRS: 0.08 second
Interp: Sinus Bradycardia with First-Degree Heart Block

9.222 Regularity: regular
Rate: 52 bpm
P Waves: upright and uniform
PRI: 0.16 second and constant
QRS: 0.10 second
Interp: Sinus Bradycardia

9.223 Regularity: very slightly irregular
Rate: 35 bpm
P Waves: none

PRI: none
QRS: 0.18 second
Interp: Idioventricular Rhythm

9.224 Regularity: regular
Rate: atrial rate 60 bpm; ventricular rate 58 bpm
P Waves: upright and uniform

PRI: none
QRS: 0.14 second
Interp: Third-Degree Heart Block (CHB) with a ventricular escape focus

Note: The nearly identical atrial and ventricular rates make it difficult to identify; however, the P waves "marching through" the QRS complexes confirms A–V dissociation.

9.225 Regularity: regular
Rate: 56 bpm
P Waves: upright and uniform

PRI: 0.20 second and constant
QRS: 0.08 second
Interp: Sinus Bradycardia

9.226 Regularity: irregular
Rate: atrial rate 375 bpm; ventricular rate approximately 60 bpm
P Waves: characteristic sawtooth pattern

PRI: none
QRS: 0.08 second
Interp: Atrial Flutter with variable response

9.227 Regularity: regular
Rate: 130 bpm
P Waves: upright and uniform

PRI: 0.12 second and constant
QRS: 0.08 second
Interp: Sinus Tachycardia

9.228 Regularity: regular
Rate: 136 bpm
P Waves: none discernible

PRI: none discernible
QRS: 0.10 second
Interp: Supraventricular Tachycardia

9.229 Regularity: regular underlying rhythm interrupted by ectopics
Rate: 68 bpm (underlying rhythm)
P Waves: upright and uniform

PRI: 0.12 second
QRS: 0.08 second in underlying rhythm; 0.16–0.20 second in ectopics
Interp: Sinus Rhythm with two multifocal PVCs

9.230 Regularity: irregular
Rate: approximately 70 bpm
P Waves: none

PRI: none
QRS: 0.10 second
Interp: Atrial Fibrillation, controlled

9.231 Regularity: irregular
Rate: approximately 80 bpm
P Waves: upright and uniform

PRI: 0.14 second and constant
QRS: 0.10 second
Interp: Sinus Arrhythmia

9.232 Regularity: irregular
Rate: approximately 100 bpm
P Waves: upright and uniform

PRI: 0.12 second and constant
QRS: 0.08 second
Interp: Sinus Arrhythmia

9.233 Regularity: regular
Rate: 59 bpm
P Anaves: none

PRI: none
QRS: 0.12 second
Interp: Junctional Escape Rhythm

9.234 Regularity: regular
Rate: 52 bpm
P Waves: upright and uniform

PRI: 0.24 second and constant
QRS: 0.08 second
Interp: Sinus Bradycardia with First-Degree Heart Block

9.235 Regularity: regular underlying rhythm interrupted by ectopics
Rate: 83 bpm (underlying rhythm)
P Waves: uniform and upright
PRI: 0.18 second

QRS: 0.08 second (underlying rhythm); 0.16 second (ectopics); ectopics have bizarre configuration
Interp: Sinus Rhythm with one PVC and a run of three PVCs, all unifocal

9.236 Regularity: slightly irregular underlying rhythm interrupted by ectopics in a pattern of grouped beating
Rate: approximately 83 bpm according to visible P waves
P Waves: upright and uniform

PRI: 0.16 second and constant (underlying rhythm)
QRS: 0.08 second (underlying rhythm); 0.16 second (ectopics)
Interp: Sinus Rhythm with trigeminy of PVCs

9.237 Regularity: regular
Rate: 48 bpm
P Waves: upright and uniform

PRI: 0.16 second and constant
QRS: 0.08 second
Interp: Sinus Bradycardia

9.238 Regularity: slightly irregular
Rate: approximately 58 bpm
P Waves: upright and uniform

PRI: 0.24 second and constant
QRS: 0.08 second
Interp: Sinus Bradycardia with First-Degree Heart Block

9.239 Regularity: slightly irregular
Rate: atrial rate 94 bpm; ventricular rate approximately 60 bpm
P Waves: uniform; regular P–P interval; more P waves than QRS complexes

PRI: P waves are not associated with the QRS complexes
QRS: 0.14 second
Interp: Third-Degree Heart Block (CHB) with a ventricular escape focus (rate accelerated, probably due to drugs)

9.240 Regularity: irregular
Rate: 30 bpm
P Waves: none

PRI: none
QRS: 0.16 second
Interp: Idioventricular Rhythm

9.241 Regularity: regular
Rate: 107 bpm
P Waves: none discernible

PRI: none
QRS: 0.20 second
Interp: Slow Ventricular Tachycardia

9.242 Regularity: regular
Rate: atrial rate 58 bpm
P Waves: upright and uniform

PRI: none
QRS: none
Interp: Ventricular Standstill

9.243 Regularity: regular
Rate: 176 bpm
P Waves: upright and uniform

PRI: 0.12 second
QRS: 0.08 second
Interp: Atrial Tachycardia

9.244 Regularity: slightly irregular underlying rhythm interrupted by ectopics in a pattern of grouped beating
Rate: 42 bpm according to visible P waves; true sinus rate is probably 84 bpm
P Waves: uniform; regular P–P interval

PRI: 0.18 second and constant
QRS: 0.08 second in underlying rhythm; 0.16 second in ectopics; ectopics have bizarre configuration and are further distorted by non-conducted P waves, making accurate measurement difficult
Interp: Sinus Rhythm with bigeminy of PVCs

9.245 Regularity: regular
Rate: atrial rate 66 bpm; ventricular rate 33 bpm
P Waves: uniform; regular P–P interval; consistently two P waves for every QRS complex

PRI: 0.28 second and constant on conducted beats
QRS: 0.10 second
Interp: Type II Second-Degree Heart Block with 2:1 conduction

9.246 Regularity: irregular
Rate: unable to determine
P Waves: none

PRI: none
QRS: 0.28 second
Interp: Idioventricular Rhythm, Asystole

9.247 Regularity: very slightly irregular underlying rhythm interrupted by two ectopics
Rate: 79 bpm (underlying rhythm)
P Waves: uniform and upright; regular P–P interval except for ectopics

PRI: 0.20 second and constant
QRS: 0.08 second
Interp: Sinus Rhythm with two PACs

9.248 Regularity: irregular
Rate: 110 bpm
P Waves: not discernible; undulations present

PRI: none
QRS: 0.10 second
Interp: Atrial Fibrillation, uncontrolled

9.249 Regularity: regular
Rate: atrial rate 352 bpm; ventricular rate 88 bpm
P Waves: uniform; sawtooth in appearance

PRI: none
QRS: 0.10 second
Interp: Atrial Flutter with 4:1 response

9.250 Regularity: regular underlying rhythm interrupted by ectopics
Rate: 58 bpm (underlying rhythm)
P Waves: upright and uniform

PRI: 0.12 second and constant
QRS: 0.10 second (underlying rhythm); 0.16 second (ectopics)
Interp: Sinus Bradycardia with two unifocal PVCs

Chapter 10

10.1 Regularity: regular
Rate: atrial rate 300 bpm; ventricular rate 75 bpm
P Waves: characteristic sawtooth pattern

PRI: unable to determine
QRS: 0.10 second
Interp: Atrial Flutter with 4:1 response

10.2 Regularity: regular
Rate: 125 bpm
P Waves: upright and constant

PRI: 0.12 second and constant
QRS: 0.10 second
Interp: Sinus Tachycardia

10.3 Regularity: regular
Rate: 125 bpm
P Waves: upright and constant

PRI: 0.24 second, constant
QRS: 0.08 second
Interp: Sinus Tachycardia with First-Degree Heart Block

10.4 Regularity: regular underlying rhythm interrupted by a single ectopic
Rate: 75 bpm in underlying rhythm
P Waves: upright in underlying rhythm; no P wave in ectopic

PRI: 0.14 second and constant
QRS: 0.08 second in underlying rhythm; 0.14 second in ectopic
Interp: Sinus Rhythm with one PVC

10.5 Regularity: regular
Rate: 188 bpm
P Waves: none visible

PRI: unable to determine
QRS: wide and bizarre
Interp: Ventricular Tachycardia

10.6 Regularity: irregular
Rate: 90 bpm
P Waves: upright and constant

PRI: 0.14 second
QRS: 0.08 second
Interp: Sinus Arrhythmia

10.7 Regularity: regular
Rate: 27 bpm
P Waves: none visible

PRI: unable to determine
QRS: 0.14 second
Interp: Idioventricular Rhythm

Note: A couple of bumps look suspiciously like P waves, but they don't map out. The area of artifact in the baseline following the second QRS is probably caused by patient movement.

10.8 Regularity: regular
Rate: 71 bpm
P Waves: upright; notched appearance

PRI: 0.24 second and constant
QRS: 0.08 second
Interp: Sinus Rhythm with First-Degree Heart Block

10.9 Regularity: regular underlying rhythm interrupted by a single ectopic
Rate: 107 bpm
P Waves: upright in front of every QRS; the ectopic probably also has a P wave superimposed on the preceding T wave

PRI: 0.20 second and constant in the underlying rhythm; impossible to measure in the ectopic
QRS: 0.10 second in both the underlying rhythm and ectopic
Interp: Sinus Tachycardia with one PAC

10.10 Regularity: very regular after the first beat or two
Rate: 188 bpm
P Waves: none visible

PRI: unable to determine
QRS: 0.06 second
Interp: Because these findings are consistent with several rhythms (Atrial Tachycardia, Sinus Tachycardia, Atrial Fibrillation, Atrial Flutter, Junctional Tachycardia), it is legitimately labeled a Supraventricular Tachycardia.

10.11 Regularity: slightly irregular
Rate: 50 bpm
P Waves: inverted following every QRS

PRI: unable to determine
QRS: 0.08 second
Interp: Junctional Escape Rhythm

10.12 Regularity: regular (first sinus beat following ectopic is slightly early)
Rate: 58 bpm
P Waves: upright and constant in front of every QRS except the ectopic

PRI: 0.18 second and constant
QRS: 0.06 second in underlying rhythm; 0.14 second in ectopic; ectopic is wide and bizarre and squeezed between two R waves without disrupting the underlying rhythm
Interp: Sinus Bradycardia with one (interpolated) PVC

10.13 Regularity: regular
Rate: 75 bpm
P Waves: upright and constant

PRI: 0.16 second
QRS: 0.10 second
Interp: Normal Sinus Rhythm

10.14 Regularity: irregular
Rate: ventricular rate 110 bpm; atrial rate 300 bpm
P Waves: sawtooth Flutter waves

PRI: none
QRS: 0.12 second
Interp: Atrial Flutter with rapid, variable ventricular response (with wide QRS)

10.15 Regularity: regular underlying rhythm interrupted by ectopics in a pattern of grouped beating
Rate: 80 bpm including ectopics
P Waves: upright P waves in underlying rhythm; no P waves in ectopics

PRI: 0.18 second in underlying rhythm
QRS: 0.08 second in underlying rhythm; 0.12 second in ectopics; ectopics have wide, bizarre configuration
Interp: Sinus Rhythm with bigeminy of unifocal PVCs

10.16 Regularity: only undulations on baseline
Rate: unable to determine
P Waves: none visible

PRI: none
QRS: none visible
Interp: Ventricular Fibrillation

10.17 Regularity: regular
Rate: 58 bpm
P Waves: upright in front of every QRS

PRI: 0.24 second and constant
QRS: 0.10 second
Interp: Sinus Bradycardia with First-Degree Heart Block

10.18 Regularity: irregular
Rate: 110 bpm
P Waves: none visible

PRI: none
QRS: 0.08 second
Interp: Atrial Fibrillation, uncontrolled

10.19 Regularity: regular
Rate: 214 bpm
P Waves: none visible

PRI: none
QRS: 0.06 second
Interp: Supraventricular Tachycardia

Note: If you argue that the tiny glitch following the QRS is a P wave, then you would call this a Junctional Tachycardia.

10.20 Regularity: regular (very slightly irregular)
Rate: 48 bpm
P Waves: upright in front of every QRS

PRI: 0.20 second and constant
QRS: 0.10 second
Interp: Sinus Bradycardia

10.21 Regularity: slightly irregular
Rate: 90 bpm
P Waves: precede every QRS, but morphology changes and P–P interval varies

PRI: varies from 0.12 to 0.20 second
QRS: 0.08 second
Interp: Wandering Pacemaker

10.22 Regularity: regular underlying rhythm interrupted by a single ectopic
Rate: 75 bpm
P Waves: upright preceding each QRS complex; the ectopic is preceded by an inverted P wave

PRI: 0.18 second in underlying rhythm; 0.12 second in ectopic
QRS: 0.08 second in both underlying rhythm and ectopic
Interp: Sinus Rhythm with one PJC

10.23 Regularity: regular atrial rhythm; irregular ventricular rhythm
Rate: atrial rate 65 bpm; ventricular rate 50 bpm
P Waves: upright; more P waves than QRS complexes

PRI: gets progressively longer until one P wave is not conducted
QRS: 0.08 second
Interp: Wenckebach (Type I Second-Degree Heart Block)

10.24 Regularity: regular
Rate: 167 bpm
P Waves: none visible

PRI: none
QRS: wide and bizarre
Interp: Ventricular Tachycardia

10.25 Regularity: irregular
Rate: 90 bpm
P Waves: none (only undulations)

PRI: none
QRS: 0.08 second
Interp: Atrial Fibrillation, controlled

10.26 Regularity: both atrial and ventricular rhythms are regular
Rate: atrial rate is 83 bpm; ventricular rate 45 bpm
P Waves: upright across strip; some P waves superimposed on QRS complexes

PRI: none
QRS: 0.10 second
Interp: Complete Heart Block with junctional escape focus

10.27 Regularity: rate is too slow to determine regularity
Rate: 12 bpm
P Waves: upright and clearly visible preceding both QRS complexes

PRI: 0.20 second and constant
QRS: 0.16 second
Interp: Sinus Bradycardia (with wide QRS) Agonal Rhythm

Note: This rate is insufficient to support perfusion and is extremely slow for a sinus pacemaker. However, P waves are clearly visible preceding both QRS complexes, with consistent PRIs, indicating that the rhythm did originate in the sinus node.

10.28 Regularity: regular (only very slightly irregular)
Rate: 60 bpm
P Waves: upright
PRI: 0.24 second and constant
QRS: 0.14 second
Interp: Sinus Rhythm with First-Degree Heart Block (with wide QRS)

10.29 Regularity: regular
Rate: atrial rate is 334 bpm; ventricular rate is 167 bpm
P Waves: sawtooth Flutter waves
PRI: none
QRS: 0.10 second
Interp: Atrial Flutter with 2:1 response

10.30 Regularity: regular
Rate: 83 bpm
P Waves: upright in front of every QRS
PRI: 0.16 second and constant
QRS: 0.10 second
Interp: Normal Sinus Rhythm

10.31 Regularity: regular
Rate: atrial rate is 60 bpm
P Waves: upright
PRI: none
QRS: none visible
Interp: Ventricular Standstill

10.32 Regularity: ventricular rhythm is regular; atrial rhythm is irregular
Rate: atrial rate 370 bpm; ventricular rate 29 bpm
P Waves: sawtooth Flutter waves
PRI: none
QRS: 0.10 second
Interp: Atrial Flutter with variable response

10.33 Regularity: ventricular rhythm is regular; atrial rhythm is irregular
Rate: atrial rate 40 bpm; ventricular rate 32 bpm
P Waves: upright
PRI: none
QRS: 0.12 second
Interp: Complete Heart Block with ventricular escape focus (atrial rate is slowing)

10.34 Regularity: irregular underlying rhythm interrupted by a burst of four ectopics
Rate: 90 bpm (excluding ectopics)
P Waves: none; fibrillatory undulations are present; some Flutter waves are visible but they can't be mapped across the entire strip
PRI: none
QRS: 0.10 second in underlying rhythm; 0.12 second in ectopics
Interp: Atrial Fibrillation, controlled, with a run of four PVCs (short burst of Ventricular Tachycardia)

10.35 Regularity: no visible waves or complexes
Rate: none
P Waves: none
PRI: none
QRS: none
Interp: Asystole (assuming that equipment is functioning properly)

10.36 Regularity: regular
Rate: 167 bpm
P Waves: none
PRI: none
QRS: 0.16 second, wide and bizarre
Interp: Ventricular Tachycardia

10.37 Regularity: irregular ventricular rhythm; regular atrial rhythm
Rate: atrial rate is 188 bpm; ventricular rate is 50 bpm
P Waves: sawtooth Flutter waves
PRI: none
QRS: 0.08 second
Interp: Atrial Flutter with variable response

10.38 Regularity: slightly irregular
Rate: 30 bpm
P Waves: upright in front of every QRS
PRI: 0.18 second and constant
QRS: 0.14 second
Interp: Sinus Bradycardia (with wide QRS) with underlying Sinus Arrhythmia (Sinus Bradyarrhythmia)

10.39 Regularity: no visible waves or complexes
Rate: none
P Waves: none
PRI: none
QRS: none
Interp: Asystole (Agonal Rhythm)

Note: The undulations in the baseline don't look like cardiac activity; they are more likely artifact such as CPR.

10.40 Regularity: regular
Rate: 115 bpm
P Waves: inverted following each QRS
PRI: none
QRS: 0.10 second
Interp: Junctional Tachycardia

10.41 Regularity: irregular underlying rhythm interrupted by ectopics
Rate: 100 bpm including ectopics
P Waves: none; undulations are visible
PRI: none
QRS: 0.10 second in underlying rhythm; 0.16 second in ectopics
Interp: Atrial Fibrillation, controlled, with two unifocal PVCs

10.42 Regularity: atrial rhythm is regular; unable to discern regularity of ventricular rhythm
Rate: atrial rate is 60 bpm; only one ventricular complex visible suggesting ventricular rate of 10 or less
P Waves: upright; not every P wave is followed by a QRS complex
PRI: none
QRS: 0.12 second
Interp: Complete Heart Block with ventricular escape focus (A–V dissociation)

10.43 Regularity: regular
Rate: 167 bpm
P Waves: upright preceding each QRS
PRI: 0.12 second and constant
QRS: 0.10 second
Interp: Atrial Tachycardia

10.44 Regularity: slightly irregular (more regular toward end of strip)
Rate: 150 bpm (measured after initial two beats)
P Waves: none visible
PRI: none
QRS: wide and bizarre
Interp: Ventricular Tachycardia

10.45 Regularity: regular
Rate: atrial rate is 61 bpm; ventricular rate is 59
P Waves: upright; march through QRS
PRI: none
QRS: 0.12 second
Interp: Third-Degree Heart Block (CHB) with ventricular escape focus

Note: The nearly identical atrial and ventricular rates make the pattern difficult to discern, especially on a short strip. With this rate, it is likely that the focus controlling the ventricles is junctional though the QRS measurement is 0.12, which suggests that it is ventricular. (The QRS should be measured on complexes that are not distorted by a P wave.) There are at least two possible explanations: focus is ventricular but rate is accelerated by drugs, or focus is junctional with an underlying wide QRS complex.

10.46 Regularity: regular
Rate: atrial rate is 352 bpm; ventricular rate is 88 bpm
P Waves: sawtooth Flutter waves

PRI: none
QRS: 0.12 second
Interp: Atrial Flutter with 4:1 response (with wide QRS)

10.47 Regularity: regular
Rate: 214 bpm
P Waves: none visible

PRI: not measurable
QRS: 0.08 second
Interp: Supraventricular Tachycardia

10.48 Regularity: regular
Rate: 250 bpm
P Waves: none

PRI: none
QRS: greater than 0.12 second; bizarre configuration
Interp: Ventricular Tachycardia

10.49 Regularity: irregular
Rate: 100 bpm
P Waves: fibrillatory waves

PRI: none
QRS: 0.06 second
Interp: Atrial Fibrillation, controlled

10.50 Regularity: regular
Rate: 107 bpm
P Waves: upright preceding each QRS

PRI: 0.12 second and constant
QRS: 0.08 second
Interp: Sinus Tachycardia

10.51 Regularity: atrial rhythm is regular; ventricular rhythm is irregular
Rate: atrial rate is 125 bpm; ventricular rate is 80 bpm
P Waves: upright

PRI: progressively lengthens until one P wave is not followed by a QRS complex
QRS: 0.14 second
Interp: Wenckebach (Type I Second-Degree Heart Block) (with wide QRS)

10.52 Regularity: unable to determine (since there are only two visible complexes)
Rate: 17 bpm
P Waves: none visible

PRI: none
QRS: 0.24 second
Interp: Idioventricular Rhythm

10.53 Regularity: regular
Rate: 188 bpm
P Waves: none

PRI: none
QRS: wide and bizarre
Interp: Ventricular Tachycardia

Note: Undulations in baseline are possibly due to CPR artifact.

10.54 Regularity: irregular
Rate: 100 bpm
P Waves: none

PRI: none
QRS: 0.08 second
Interp: Atrial Fibrillation, controlled

10.55 Regularity: regular underlying rhythm interrupted by ectopics
Rate: 88 bpm
P Waves: upright

PRI: 0.16 second and constant
QRS: 0.08 second in underlying rhythm; 0.16 second in ectopics
Interp: Sinus Rhythm with single PVC and a run of three PVCs, all unifocal

10.56 Regularity: regular
Rate: 68 bpm
P Waves: upright-preceding each QRS

PRI: 0.28 second and constant
QRS: 0.10 second
Interp: Sinus Rhythm with First-Degree Heart Block

10.57 Regularity: atrial rhythm is regular; ventricular rhythm is irregular
Rate: atrial rate 214 bpm; ventricular rate 70 bpm
P Waves: sawtooth Flutter waves

PRI: none
QRS: 0.10 second
Interp: Atrial Flutter with variable response (4:1, 2:1)

10.58 Regularity: regular
Rate: 125 bpm
P Waves: upright preceding each QRS

PRI: 0.16 second and constant
QRS: 0.06 second
Interp: Sinus Tachycardia

10.59 Regularity: irregular
Rate: 100 bpm
P Waves: one preceding each QRS, but morphology changes

PRI: varies from 0.08 to 0.16 second
QRS: 0.08 second
Interp: Wandering Pacemaker

10.60 Regularity: regular
Rate: 250 bpm
P Waves: none

PRI: none
QRS: greater than 0.12 second; wide and bizarre
Interp: Ventricular Tachycardia

10.61 Regularity: atrial rhythm is regular; unable to determine regularity of ventricular rhythm since only two complexes are visible
Rate: atrial rate is 33 bpm; ventricular rate is 19 bpm
P Waves: upright

PRI: no relationship between P waves and QRS complexes
QRS: 0.20 second
Interp: Third-Degree Heart Block (CHB) with ventricular escape focus

10.62 Regularity: irregular
Rate: 100 bpm
P Waves: none; fibrillatory undulations present

PRI: none
QRS: 0.08 second
Interp: Atrial Fibrillation, controlled

10.63 Regularity: regular
Rate: 88 bpm
P Waves: upright preceding each QRS

PRI: 0.18 second and constant
QRS: 0.12 second
Interp: Normal Sinus Rhythm (with wide QRS)

10.64 Regularity: irregular underlying rhythm interrupted by a single ectopic
Rate: 110 bpm
P Waves: none visible
PRI: none
QRS: 0.08 second in underlying rhythm; 0.12 second in ectopic
Interp: Atrial Fibrillation, uncontrolled, with single PVC

10.65 Regularity: irregular; has a pattern of every other beat being an ectopic
Rate: 90 bpm (including ectopics)
P Waves: visible preceding each QRS, and on T waves preceding ectopics
PRI: 0.16 second in underlying rhythm; not measurable in ectopics
QRS: 0.14 second in both underlying rhythm and ectopics
Interp: Sinus Rhythm (with wide QRS) with bigeminy of PACs

10.66 Regularity: regular
Rate: 214 bpm
P Waves: none visible
PRI: unable to determine
QRS: 0.06 second
Interp: Supraventricular Tachycardia

10.67 Regularity: ventricular rhythm regular; atrial rhythm slightly irregular
Rate: ventricular rate 36 bpm; atrial rate approximately 70 bpm
P Waves: upright
PRI: not associated with QRS complexes; seem to march through QRS complexes
QRS: 0.16 second
Interp: Complete Heart Block with ventricular escape focus (and underlying Sinus Arrhythmia)

10.68 Regularity: regular
Rate: 39 bpm
P Waves: inverted preceding each QRS
PRI: 0.12 second and constant
QRS: 0.08 second
Interp: Junctional Escape Rhythm

10.69 Regularity: regular underlying rhythm interrupted by ectopics
Rate: 107 bpm in underlying rhythm
P Waves: upright in underlying rhythm; ectopics have P waves on preceding T waves
PRI: 0.12 second and constant in underlying rhythm; not measurable in ectopics
QRS: 0.10 second in both ectopics and underlying rhythm
Interp: Sinus Tachycardia with a single PAC and a run of three PACs (short burst of PAT)

10.70 Regularity: regular
Rate: 231 bpm
P Waves: none
PRI: none
QRS: 0.10 second
Interp: Supraventricular Tachycardia

10.71 Regularity: regular
Rate: 33 bpm
P Waves: upright preceding each QRS
PRI: 0.22 second and constant
QRS: 0.16 second
Interp: Sinus Bradycardia (with wide QRS) with First-Degree Heart Block

10.72 Regularity: irregular underlying rhythm, which gives way to a pattern of every other beat being an ectopic
Rate: 110 bpm (including ectopics)
P Waves: none
PRI: none
QRS: 0.10 second in underlying rhythm; 0.16 second in ectopics; ectopics have bizarre configuration
Interp: Atrial Fibrillation, uncontrolled, with bigeminy of PVCs

10.73 Regularity: regular
Rate: atrial rate is 300 bpm; ventricular rate is 150 bpm
P Waves: sawtooth Flutter waves
PRI: none
QRS: 0.06 second
Interp: Atrial Flutter with 2:1 response

10.74 Regularity: regular
Rate: 167 bpm
P Waves: none
PRI: none
QRS: 0.16 second
Interp: Ventricular Tachycardia

10.75 Regularity: regular
Rate: 100 bpm
P Waves: inverted preceding every QRS
PRI: 0.10 second and constant
QRS: 0.08 second
Interp: Accelerated Junctional Rhythm

10.76 Regularity: regular
Rate: 158 bpm
P Waves: apparent on T waves
PRI: unable to measure
QRS: 0.12 second
Interp: Supraventricular Tachycardia (with wide QRS)

10.77 Regularity: regular
Rate: 52 bpm
P Waves: upright preceding each QRS
PRI: 0.18 second and constant
QRS: 0.10 second
Interp: Sinus Bradycardia

10.78 Regularity: irregular
Rate: 60 bpm
P Waves: none visible
PRI: none
QRS: 0.12 second
Interp: Atrial Fibrillation, controlled (with wide QRS)

10.79 Regularity: regular underlying rhythm interrupted by ectopics
Rate: 56 bpm in underlying rhythm
P Waves: upright before each QRS; no P waves in ectopics
PRI: 0.14 second and constant
QRS: 0.10 second in underlying rhythm; 0.14 second in ectopics
Interp: Sinus Bradycardia with two unifocal PVCs

10.80 Regularity: regular
Rate: 50 bpm
P Waves: none
PRI: none
QRS: 0.10 second
Interp: Junctional Escape Rhythm

10.81 Regularity: irregular
Rate: 80 bpm
P Waves: none; fibrillatory waves are present
PRI: none
QRS: 0.12 second
Interp: Atrial Fibrillation, controlled (with wide QRS)

10.82 Regularity: regular
Rate: 107 bpm
P Waves: upright preceding each QRS
PRI: 0.16 second and constant
QRS: 0.08 second
Interp: Sinus Tachycardia

10.83 Regularity: regular
Rate: 150 bpm
P Waves: not discernible

PRI: not measurable
QRS: 0.08 second
Interp: Supraventricular Tachycardia

10.84 Regularity: regular
Rate: 115 bpm
P Waves: none

PRI: none
QRS: 0.18 second, bizarre configuration
Interp: Ventricular Tachycardia (slow rate range)

10.85 Regularity: regular (very slightly irregular)
Rate: 45 bpm
P Waves: none

PRI: none
QRS: 0.08 second
Interp: Junctional Escape Rhythm

10.86 Regularity: irregular
Rate: ventricular rate approximately 30 bpm; atrial rate 65 bpm
P Waves: not immediately obvious because of unusually low voltage, but they do map out across strip

PRI: no relationship between P waves and QRS complexes
QRS: 0.08 second
Interp: Complete Heart Block with junctional escape focus

10.87 Regularity: irregular
Rate: 120 bpm (including ectopic)
P Waves: none visible

PRI: none
QRS: 0.08 second in underlying rhythm; 0.14 second in ectopic; ectopic has bizarre configuration
Interp: Atrial Fibrillation, uncontrolled, with one PVC

10.88 Regularity: regular
Rate: 47 bpm
P Waves: upright preceding each QRS

PRI: 0.16 second and constant
QRS: 0.10 second
Interp: Sinus Bradycardia

10.89 Regularity: regular
Rate: 214 bpm
P Waves: none discernible

PRI: none
QRS: 0.10 second
Interp: Supraventricular Tachycardia

10.90 Regularity: slightly irregular
Rate: approximately 40 bpm
P Waves: none

PRI: none
QRS: 0.08 second
Interp: Junctional Escape Rhythm

10.91 Regularity: atrial rhythm is regular; ventricular rhythm is irregular
Rate: atrial rate is 107 bpm; ventricular rate is 50 bpm
P Waves: upright; more than one P wave for each QRS

PRI: 0.24 second and constant on conducted beats
QRS: 0.14 second
Interp: Type II Second-Degree Heart Block (with variable conduction)

10.92 Regularity: no visible waves or complexes
Rate: none
P Waves: none

PRI: none
QRS: none
Interp: Ventricular Fibrillation

10.93 Regularity: regular underlying rhythm, interrupted by ectopics in a pattern by which every third beat is an ectopic
Rate: 79 bpm (including ectopics)
P Waves: upright in underlying rhythm; ectopics have no P waves

PRI: 0.16 second and constant in underlying rhythm
QRS: 0.08 second in underlying rhythm; 0.16 second in ectopics; ectopics have bizarre configuration, though all are similar to each other
Interp: Sinus Rhythm with trigeminy of unifocal PVCs

10.94 Regularity: regular
Rate: 79 bpm
P Waves: inverted preceding each QRS

PRI: 0.08 second and constant
QRS: 0.08 second
Interp: Accelerated Junctional Rhythm

10.95 Regularity: regular
Rate: 167 bpm
P Waves: none

PRI: none
QRS: 0.16 second
Interp: Ventricular Tachycardia

10.96 Regularity: regular
Rate: 167 bpm
P Waves: upright, encroaching on T waves of preceding complexes

PRI: unable to measure
QRS: 0.06 second
Interp: Atrial Tachycardia

10.97 Regularity: slightly irregular underlying rhythm interrupted by multiple ectopics
Rate: 120 bpm (including ectopics)
P Waves: none; undulations present

PRI: none
QRS: 0.08 second in underlying rhythm; 0.14 second in ectopics; all ectopics have similar wide, bizarre appearance
Interp: Atrial Fibrillation, uncontrolled, with two single PVCs and a run of three PVCs, all unifocal

Note: You might argue that the underlying rhythm is Atrial Flutter, rather than Fibrillation, since Flutter waves seem to map out. A longer strip might provide supporting evidence for this position. However, that point is less important than the ventricular irritability.

10.98 Regularity: atrial and ventricular rhythms are both regular
Rate: atrial rate is 100 bpm; ventricular rate is 38 bpm
P Waves: upright

PRI: no relationship between P waves and QRS complexes; P's march through QRSs
QRS: 0.16 second
Interp: Complete Heart Block with ventricular escape focus

10.99 Regularity: there is a single wide, bizarre complex amid chaotic fibrillatory waves
Rate: unable to determine
P Waves: none

PRI: none
QRS: unable to determine
Interp: Ventricular Fibrillation (Agonal Rhythm)

10.100 Regularity: slightly irregular
Rate: 167 bpm
P Waves: none

PRI: none
QRS: wide and bizarre
Interp: Ventricular Tachycardia

Index of Practice Strips by Rhythm Names

JUNCTIONAL RHYTHMS

Premature Junctional Complex

Junctional Escape Rhythm

Accelerated Junctional Rhythm

Junctional Tachycardia

Supraventricular Tachycardia

VENTRICULAR RHYTHMS

Premature Ventricular Complex

Ventricular Fibrillation

Idioventricular Rhythm

Asystole/Agonal Rhythm

Subject Index

Flash Cards

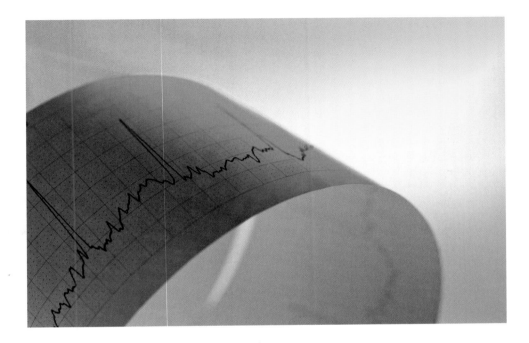

Basic Arrhythmias is a self-instructional textbook. Each chapter is carefully constructed to walk you through educational concepts, show you the skills you need, and enable you to practice applying what you have learned.

Unfortunately, some things can't be learned by reading or by practice. Some factual material, like the multiplication tables, just has to be memorized. There's no way around it.

These flash cards address all the factual material in this book that must be memorized for you to interpret basic arrhythmias. The front of each card asks the questions, and the back provides the answers. Use them in drills, alone, or with fellow students, until you have complete comfort with the information they contain.

THE CONDUCTION SYSTEM

Name the parts of the conduction system:

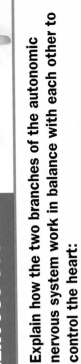

1: _____
2A: _____
2B: _____
3: _____
4: _____
5A: _____
5B: _____
6: _____

THE AUTONOMIC NERVOUS SYSTEM

Explain how the two branches of the autonomic nervous system work in balance with each other to control the heart:

SYMPATHETIC BRANCH

1. Which chambers does this branch affect?

2. When this branch is *stimulated*, what happens to heart rate, conduction, and irritability?

PARASYMPATHETIC BRANCH

1. Which chambers does this branch affect?

2. When this branch is *stimulated*, what happens to heart rate, conduction, and irritability?

THE CARDIAC CYCLE

Locate the components of a normal cardiac cycle:

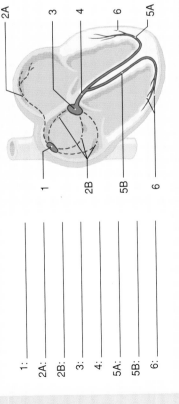

1. Waves: P, Q, R, S, T
2. PR Interval
3. PR Segment
4. QRS Complex

PRI and QRS

Explain how PRI and QRS are measured:

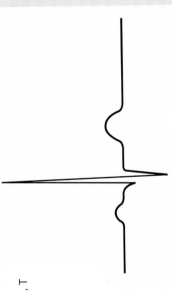

MEASURING PRI

1. The PRI is measured from which point to which point?

2. What is the normal duration for PRI?

MEASURING QRS

1. The QRS is measured from which point to which point?

2. What is the normal duration for QRS?

Innervation of the Heart by the Autonomic Nervous System

SYMPATHETIC BRANCH

1. Affects the atria and the ventricles
2. Increases:
   —heart rate
   —conduction
   —irritability

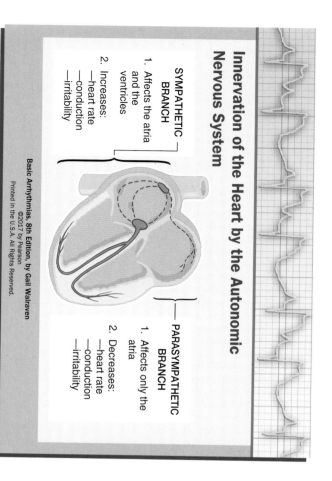

PARASYMPATHETIC BRANCH

1. Affects only the atria
2. Decreases:
   —heart rate
   —conduction
   —irritability

Measurement and Duration of PRI and QRS

MEASURING PRI

1. The PRI is measured from the beginning of the P wave to the beginning of the QRS complex.
2. The normal PRI is 0.12–0.20 second.

MEASURING QRS

1. The QRS is measured from the beginning of the Q wave to the end of the S wave.
2. The QRS is normally <0.12 second.

Electrical Conduction Through the Heart

The parts of the conduction system:

1: Sinoatrial (SA) node
2A: Intraatrial pathway
2B: Internodal pathways
3: Atrioventricular (AV) junction
4: Bundle of His
5A: Left bundle branch
5B: Right bundle branch
6: Purkinje fibers

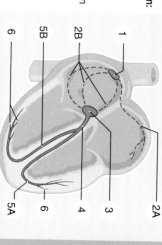

EKG Complex

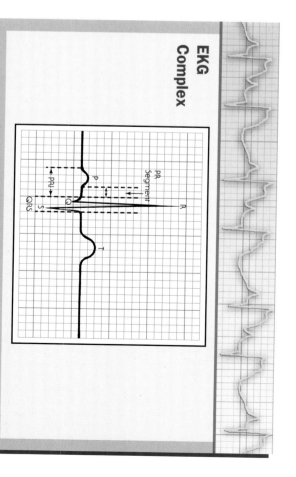

PACEMAKER SITES and RATES

The inherent rates of the three pacemaker sites are:

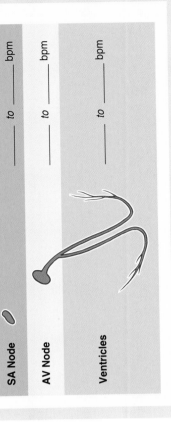

SA Node _____ to _____ bpm

AV Node _____ to _____ bpm

Ventricles _____ to _____ bpm

NORMAL SINUS RHYTHM

SINUS node is the pacemaker, firing at a regular rate of 60–100 times per minute. Each beat is conducted normally through to the ventricles.

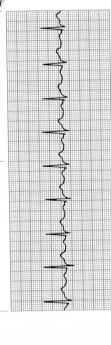

What are the rules for this rhythm? (Regularity, Rate, P wave, PRI, QRS)

EKG WAVE PATTERNS

Name each EKG wave area and explain its electrical activity:

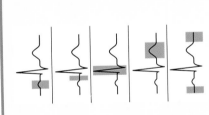

1. What are each of these areas called?

2. What cardiac electrical activity is associated with each area?

HEART RATE CALCULATION

How do you calculate heart rate...

1. ...when the rate is irregular, or you want a very quick (but rough) estimate?

2. ...when the rate is regular and you need a quick (but accurate) estimate?

3. ...when the rate is regular and accuracy is more important than speed?

Inherent Rates

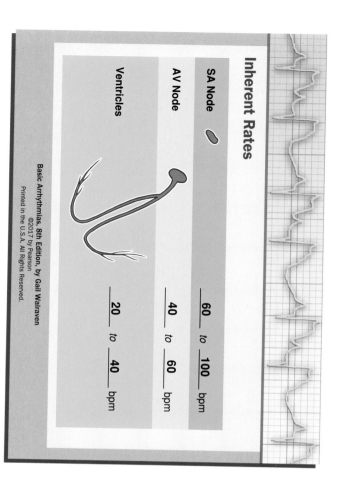

SA Node	_60_ to _100_ bpm
AV Node	_40_ to _60_ bpm
Ventricles	_20_ to _40_ bpm

Normal Sinus Rhythm

The rules for this rhythm:

REGULARITY: The R–R intervals are constant; the rhythm is regular.

RATE: The atrial and ventricular rates are equal; heart rate is between 60 and 100 bpm.

P WAVE: The P waves are uniform. There is one P wave in front of every QRS complex.

PRI: The PR interval measures between 0.12 and 0.20 second; the PRI measurement is constant across the strip.

QRS: The QRS complex measures less than 0.12 second.

EKG Wave Patterns

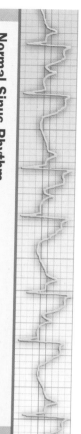

AREA	ELECTRICAL ACTIVITY
P wave	Atrial depolarization
PR segment	Delay at AV node
QRS complex	Ventricular depolarization
T wave	Ventricular repolarization
Isoelectric line	No electrical activity

Heart Rate Calculation

HOW TO CALCULATE HEART RATE

	FEATURES
1. Count the number of R waves in a 6-second strip and multiply by 10.	• Not very accurate • Used only with very quick estimate
2. Count the number of large squares between 2 consecutive R waves and divide into 300. --OR-- *memorize this scale:* 1 large square = 300 bpm 2 large squares = 150 bpm 3 large squares = 100 bpm 4 large squares = 75 bpm 5 large squares = 60 bpm 6 large squares = 50 bpm	• Very quick • Not very accurate with fast rates • Only used with regular rhythms
3. Count the number of small squares between 2 consecutive R waves and divide by 1,500.	• Most accurate • Time-consuming • Used only with regular rhythms

SINUS TACHYCARDIA

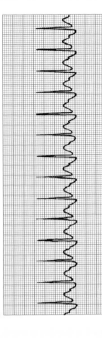

SINUS node is the pacemaker, firing regularly at a rate of greater than 100 times per minute. Each impulse is conducted normally through to the ventricles.

What are the rules for this rhythm? (Regularity, Rate, P wave, PRI, QRS)

WANDERING PACEMAKER

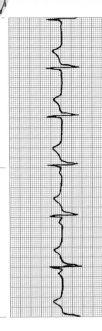

The pacemaker site wanders between the SINUS node, the ATRIA, and the AV JUNCTION. Although each beat originates from a different focus, the rate usually remains within a normal range, but can be slower. Conduction through to the ventricles is normal.

What are the rules for this rhythm? (Regularity, Rate, P wave, PRI, QRS)

SINUS BRADYCARDIA

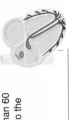

SINUS node is the pacemaker, firing regularly at a rate of less than 60 times per minute. Each impulse is conducted normally through to the ventricles.

What are the rules for this rhythm? (Regularity, Rate, P wave, PRI, QRS)

SINUS ARRHYTHMIA

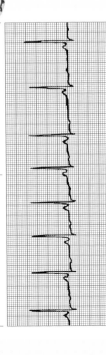

SINUS node is the pacemaker, but impulses are initiated in an irregular pattern. The rate increases as the patient breathes in and decreases as the patient breathes out. Each beat is conducted normally through to the ventricles.

What are the rules for this rhythm? (Regularity, Rate, P wave, PRI, QRS)

Sinus Tachycardia

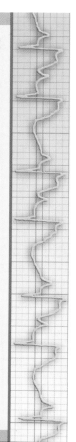

The rules for this rhythm:

REGULARITY: The R–R intervals are constant; the rhythm is regular.

RATE: The atrial and ventricular rates are equal; the heart rate is greater than 100 bpm (usually between 100 and 160 bpm).

P WAVE: There is a uniform P wave in front of every QRS complex.

PRI: The PR interval measures between 0.12 and 0.20 second; the PRI measurement is constant across the strip.

QRS: The QRS complex measures less than 0.12 second.

Basic Arrhythmias, 8th Edition, by Gail Walraven
©2017 by Pearson
Printed in the U.S.A. All Rights Reserved.

Sinus Bradycardia

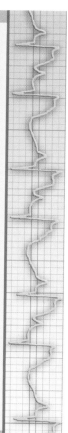

The rules for this rhythm:

REGULARITY: The R–R intervals are constant; the rhythm is regular.

RATE: The atrial and ventricular rates are equal; heart rate is less than 60 bpm.

P WAVE: There is a uniform P wave in front of every QRS complex.

PRI: The PR interval measures between 0.12 and 0.20 second; the PRI measurement is constant across the strip.

QRS: The QRS complex measures less than 0.12 second.

Basic Arrhythmias, 8th Edition, by Gail Walraven
©2017 by Pearson
Printed in the U.S.A. All Rights Reserved.

Wandering Pacemaker

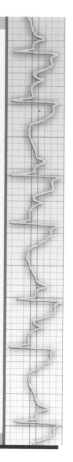

The rules for this rhythm:

REGULARITY: The R-R intervals vary slightly as the pacemaker site changes; the rhythm can be slightly irregular.

RATE: The atrial and ventricular rates are equal; heart rate is usually within a normal range (60–100 bpm) but can be slower.

P WAVE: The morphology of the P wave changes as the pacemaker site changes. There is one P wave in front of every QRS complex, although some may be difficult to see, depending on the pacemaker site.

PRI: The PRI measurement will vary slightly as the pacemaker site changes. All PRI measurements should be less than 0.20 second; some may be less than 0.12 second.

QRS: The QRS complex measures less than 0.12 second.

Basic Arrhythmias, 8th Edition, by Gail Walraven
©2017 by Pearson
Printed in the U.S.A. All Rights Reserved.

Sinus Arrhythmia

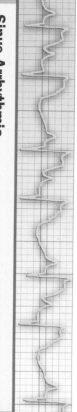

The rules for this rhythm:

REGULARITY: The R–R intervals vary; the rate changes with the patient's respirations.

RATE: The atrial and ventricular rates are equal; heart rate is usually in a normal range (60–100 bpm), but can be slower.

P WAVE: There is a uniform P wave in front of every QRS complex.

PRI: The PR interval measures between 0.12 and 0.20 second; the PRI measurement is constant across the strip.

QRS: The QRS complex measures less than 0.12 second.

Basic Arrhythmias, 8th Edition, by Gail Walraven
©2017 by Pearson
Printed in the U.S.A. All Rights Reserved.

PREMATURE ATRIAL COMPLEX

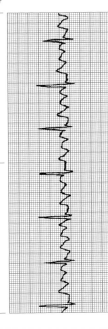

The pacemaker is an irritable focus within the ATRIUM that fires prematurely and produces a single ectopic beat. Conduction through to the ventricles is normal.

What are the rules for this rhythm? (Regularity, Rate, P wave, PRI, QRS)

ATRIAL FIBRILLATION

The ATRIA are so irritable that a multitude of foci initiate impulses, causing the atria to depolarize repeatedly in a fibrillatory manner. The AV node blocks most of the impulses, allowing only a limited number through to the ventricles.

What are the rules for this rhythm? (Regularity, Rate, P wave, PRI, QRS)

ATRIAL FLUTTER

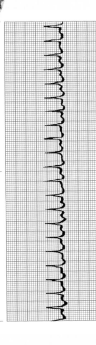

A single irritable focus within the ATRIA issues an impulse that is conducted in a rapid, repetitive fashion. To protect the ventricles from receiving too many impulses, the AV node blocks some of the impulses from being conducted through to the ventricles.

What are the rules for this rhythm? (Regularity, Rate, P wave, PRI, QRS)

ATRIAL TACHYCARDIA

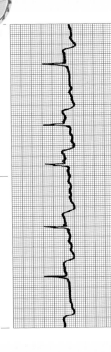

The pacemaker is a single irritable site within the ATRIUM that fires repetitively at a very rapid rate. Conduction through to the ventricles is normal.

What are the rules for this rhythm? (Regularity, Rate, P wave, PRI, QRS)

Atrial Flutter

The rules for this rhythm:

REGULARITY: The atrial rhythm is regular. The ventricular rhythm will be regular if the AV node conducts impulses through in a consistent pattern. If the pattern varies, the ventricular rate will be irregular.

RATE: Atrial rate is between 250 and 350 bpm. Ventricular rate will depend on the ratio of impulses conducted through to the ventricles.

P WAVE: When the atria flutter they produce a series of well-defined P waves. When seen together, these "Flutter" waves have a sawtooth appearance.

PRI: Because of the unusual configuration of the P wave (Flutter wave) and the proximity of the wave to the QRS complex, it is often impossible to determine a PRI in this arrhythmia. Therefore, the PRI is not measured in Atrial Flutter.

QRS: The QRS complex measures less than 0.12 second; measurement can be difficult if one or more Flutter waves is concealed within the QRS complex.

Basic Arrhythmias, 8th Edition, by Gail Walraven
©2017 by Pearson
Printed in the U.S.A. All Rights Reserved.

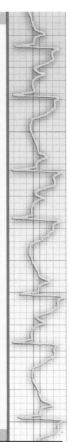

Premature Atrial Complex

The rules for this rhythm:

REGULARITY: Since this is a single premature ectopic beat, it will interrupt the regularity of the underlying rhythm.

RATE: The overall heart rate will depend on the rate of the underlying rhythm.

P WAVE: The P wave of the premature beat will have a different morphology than the P waves of the rest of the strip. The ectopic beat will have a P wave, but it can be flattened, notched, or otherwise unusual. It may be hidden within the T wave of the preceding complex.

PRI: The PRI should measure between 0.12 and 0.20 second, but can be prolonged; the PRI of the ectopic will probably be different from the PRI measurements of the other complexes.

QRS: The QRS complex measurement will be less than 0.12 second.

Basic Arrhythmias, 8th Edition, by Gail Walraven
©2017 by Pearson
Printed in the U.S.A. All Rights Reserved.

Atrial Tachycardia

The rules for this rhythm:

REGULARITY: The R-R intervals are constant; the rhythm is regular.

RATE: The atrial and ventricular rates are equal; the heart rate is usually 150–250 bpm.

P WAVE: There is one P wave in front of every QRS complex. The configuration of the P wave will be different than that of sinus P waves; they may be flattened or notched. Because of the rapid rate, the P waves can be hidden in the T waves of the preceding beats.

PRI: The PRI is between 0.12 and 0.20 seconds and constant across the strip. The PRI may be difficult to measure if the P wave is obscured by the T wave.

QRS: The QRS complex measures less than 0.12 second.

Basic Arrhythmias, 8th Edition, by Gail Walraven
©2017 by Pearson
Printed in the U.S.A. All Rights Reserved.

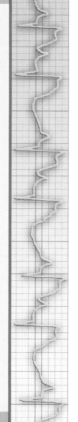

Atrial Fibrillation

The rules for this rhythm:

REGULARITY: The atrial rhythm is unmeasurable; all atrial activity is chaotic. The ventricular rhythm is grossly irregular, having no pattern to its irregularity.

RATE: The atrial rate cannot be measured because it is so chaotic; research indicates that it exceeds 350 bpm. The ventricular rate is significantly slower because the AV node blocks most of the impulses. If the ventricular rate is 100 bpm or less, the rhythm is said to be "controlled." If it is over 100 bpm, it is considered to have a "rapid ventricular response" and is called "uncontrolled."

P WAVE: In this arrhythmia the atria are not depolarizing in an effective way; instead, they are fibrillating. Thus, no P wave is produced. All atrial activity is depicted as "fibrillatory" waves, or grossly chaotic undulations of the baseline.

PRI: Since no P waves are visible, no PRI can be measured.

QRS: The QRS complex measurement should be less than 0.12 second.

Basic Arrhythmias, 8th Edition, by Gail Walraven
©2017 by Pearson
Printed in the U.S.A. All Rights Reserved.

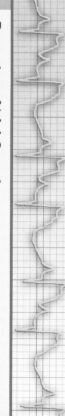

PREMATURE JUNCTIONAL COMPLEX

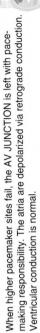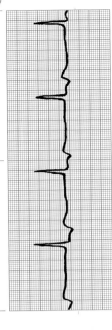

The pacemaker is an irritable focus within the AV JUNCTION that fires prematurely and produces a single ectopic beat. The atria are depolarized via retrograde conduction. Conduction through the ventricles is normal.

What are the rules for this rhythm? (Regularity, Rate, P wave, PRI, QRS)

JUNCTIONAL ESCAPE RHYTHM

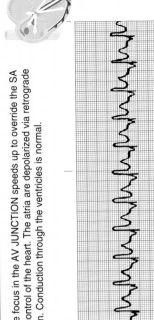

When higher pacemaker sites fail, the AV JUNCTION is left with pace-making responsibility. The atria are depolarized via retrograde conduction. Ventricular conduction is normal.

What are the rules for this rhythm? (Regularity, Rate, P wave, PRI, QRS)

ACCELERATED JUNCTIONAL RHYTHM

An irritable focus in the AV JUNCTION speeds up to override the SA node for control of the heart. The atria are depolarized via retrograde conduction. Conduction through the ventricles is normal.

What are the rules for this rhythm? (Regularity, Rate, P wave, PRI, QRS)

JUNCTIONAL TACHYCARDIA

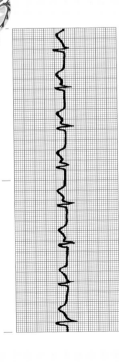

An irritable focus in the AV JUNCTION speeds up to override the SA node for control of the heart. The atria are depolarized via retrograde conduction. Conduction through the ventricles is normal.

What are the rules for this rhythm? (Regularity, Rate, P wave, PRI, QRS)

Junctional Escape Rhythm

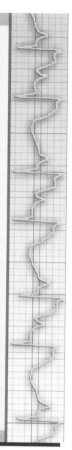

The rules for this rhythm:

REGULARITY: The R–R intervals are constant; the rhythm is regular.

RATE: Atrial and ventricular rates are equal; the inherent rate of the AV junction is 40–60 bpm.

P WAVE: The P wave can come before or after the QRS complex, or it can be lost entirely within the QRS complex. If visible, the P wave will be inverted.

PRI: If the P wave precedes the QRS complex, the PRI will be less than 0.12 second. If the P wave falls within the QRS complex or following it, there will be no PRI.

QRS: The QRS complex measurement will be less than 0.12 second.

Basic Arrhythmias, 8th Edition, by Gail Walraven
©2017 by Pearson
Printed in the U.S.A. All Rights Reserved.

Premature Junctional Complex

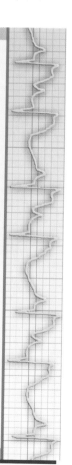

The rules for this rhythm:

REGULARITY: Since this is a single premature ectopic beat, it will interrupt the regularity of the underlying rhythm. The R–R interval will be irregular.

RATE: The overall heart rate will depend on the rate of the underlying rhythm.

P WAVE: The P wave can come before or after the QRS complex, or it can be lost entirely within the QRS complex. If visible, the P wave will be inverted.

PRI: If the P wave precedes the QRS complex, the PRI will be less than 0.12 second. If the P wave falls within the QRS complex or following it, there will be no PRI.

QRS: The QRS complex measurement will be less than 0.12 second.

Basic Arrhythmias, 8th Edition, by Gail Walraven
©2017 by Pearson
Printed in the U.S.A. All Rights Reserved.

Junctional Tachycardia

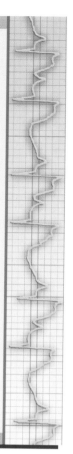

The rules for this rhythm:

REGULARITY: The R–R intervals are constant; the rhythm is regular.

RATE: Atrial and ventricular rates are equal. The rate will be in the tachycardia range, but does not usually exceed 180 bpm. Usual range is 100–180 bpm.

P WAVE: The P wave can come before or after the QRS complex, or it can be lost entirely within the QRS complex. If visible, the P wave will be inverted.

PRI: If the P wave precedes the QRS complex, the PRI will be less than 0.12 second. If the P wave falls within the QRS complex or following it, there will be no PRI.

QRS: The QRS complex measurement will be less than 0.12 second.

Basic Arrhythmias, 8th Edition, by Gail Walraven
©2017 by Pearson
Printed in the U.S.A. All Rights Reserved.

Accelerated Junctional Rhythm

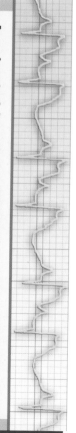

The rules for this rhythm:

REGULARITY: The R–R intervals are constant; the rhythm is regular.

RATE: Atrial and ventricular rates are equal. The rate will be faster than the AV junction's inherent rate but not yet into a true tachycardia range. It will be in the 60–100 bpm range.

P WAVE: The P wave can come before or after the QRS complex, or it can be lost entirely within the QRS complex. If visible, the P wave will be inverted.

PRI: If the P wave precedes the QRS complex, the PRI will be less than 0.12 second. If the P wave falls within the QRS complex or following it, there will be no PRI.

QRS: The QRS complex will be less than 0.12 second.

Basic Arrhythmias, 8th Edition, by Gail Walraven
©2017 by Pearson
Printed in the U.S.A. All Rights Reserved.

FIRST-DEGREE HEART BLOCK

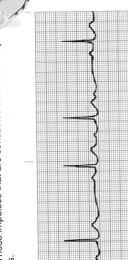

The AV NODE holds each sinus impulse longer than normal before conducting it through the ventricles. Each impulse is eventually conducted. Once into the ventricles, conduction proceeds normally.

What are the rules for this rhythm? (Regularity, Rate, P wave, PRI, QRS)

Type I Second-Degree Heart Block WENCKEBACH

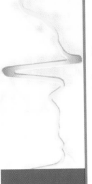

As the sinus node initiates impulses, each one is delayed in the AV NODE a little longer than the preceding one, until one is eventually blocked completely. Those impulses that are conducted travel normally through the ventricles.

What are the rules for this rhythm? (Regularity, Rate, P wave, PRI, QRS)

TYPE II Second-Degree Heart Block

The AV NODE selectively conducts some beats while blocking others. Those that are not blocked are conducted through to the ventricles, although they may encounter a slight delay in the node. Once in the ventricles, conduction proceeds normally.

What are the rules for this rhythm? (Regularity, Rate, P wave, PRI, QRS)

COMPLETE HEART BLOCK

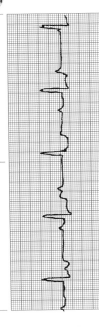

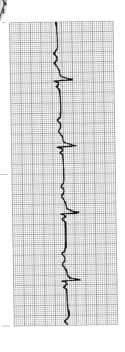

The block at the AV NODE is complete. The sinus impulses cannot penetrate the node and thus are not conducted through to the ventricles. An escape mechanism from either the junction or the ventricles will take over to pace the ventricles. The atria and the ventricles function in a totally dissociated fashion.

What are the rules for this rhythm? (Regularity, Rate, P wave, PRI, QRS)

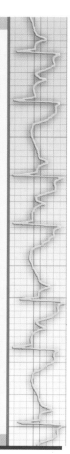

Wenckebach Type I Second-Degree Heart Block

The rules for this rhythm:

REGULARITY: The R–R interval is irregular in a pattern of grouped beating.

RATE: Since some beats are not conducted, the ventricular rate is usually slightly slower than normal (<100 bpm). The atrial rate is normal (60–100 bpm).

P WAVE: The P waves are upright and uniform. Some P waves are not followed by QRS complexes.

PRI: The PR intervals get progressively longer, until one P wave is not followed by a QRS complex. After the blocked beat, the cycle starts again.

QRS: The QRS complex measurement will be less than 0.12 second.

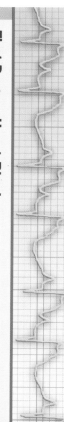

First-Degree Heart Block

The rules for this rhythm:

REGULARITY: This will depend on the regularity of the underlying rhythm.

RATE: The rate will depend on the rate of the underlying rhythm.

P WAVE: The P waves will be upright and uniform. Each P wave will be followed by a QRS complex.

PRI: The PRI will be constant across the entire strip, but it will always be greater than 0.20 second.

QRS: The QRS complex measurement will be less than 0.12 second.

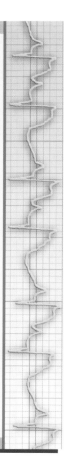

Complete Heart Block

The rules for this rhythm:

REGULARITY: Both the atrial and the ventricular foci are firing regularly; thus the P–P intervals and the R–R intervals are regular.

RATE: The atrial rate will usually be in a normal range. The ventricular rate will be slower. If a junctional focus is controlling the ventricles, the rate will be 40–60 bpm. If the focus is ventricular, the rate will be 20–40 bpm.

P WAVE: The P waves are upright and uniform. There are more P waves than QRS complexes.

PRI: Since the block at the AV node is complete, none of the atrial impulses is conducted through to the ventricles. There is no PRI. The P waves have no relationship to the QRS complexes. You may occasionally see a P wave superimposed on the QRS complex.

QRS: If the ventricles are being controlled by a junctional focus, the QRS complex will measure less than 0.12 second. If the focus is ventricular, the QRS will measure 0.12 second or greater.

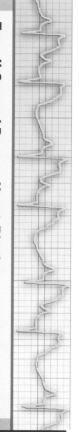

Type II Second-Degree Heart Block

The rules for this rhythm:

REGULARITY: If the conduction ratio is consistent, the R–R interval will be constant, and the rhythm will be regular. If the conduction ratio varies, the R–R will be irregular.

RATE: The atrial rate is usually normal (60–100 bpm). Since many of the atrial impulses are blocked, the ventricular rate will usually be in the bradycardia range (< 60 bpm), often one half, one third, or one fourth of the atrial rate.

P WAVE: The P waves are upright and uniform. There are always more P waves than QRS complexes.

PRI: The PRI on conducted beats will be constant across the strip, although it might be longer than a normal PRI measurement.

QRS: The QRS complex measurement will be less than 0.12 second.

VENTRICULAR TACHYCARDIA

An irritable focus in the VENTRICLES fires regularly at a rate of 150–250 bpm to override higher sites for control of the heart.

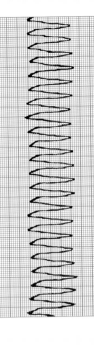

What are the rules for this rhythm? (Regularity, Rate, P wave, PRI, QRS)

IDIOVENTRICULAR RHYTHM

In the absence of a higher pacemaker, the VENTRICLES initiate a regular impulse at their inherent rate of 20–40 bpm.

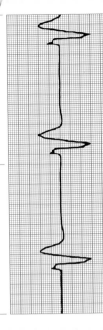

What are the rules for this rhythm? (Regularity, Rate, P wave, PRI, QRS)

PREMATURE VENTRICULAR COMPLEX

A PVC is a single irritable focus within the VENTRICLES that fires pre-maturely to initiate an ectopic complex.

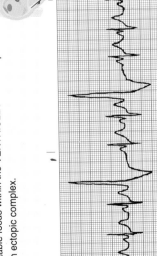

What are the rules for this rhythm? (Regularity, Rate, P wave, PRI, QRS)

VENTRICULAR FIBRILLATION

Multiple foci in the VENTRICLES become irritable and generate uncoordinated, chaotic impulses that cause the heart to fibrillate rather than contract.

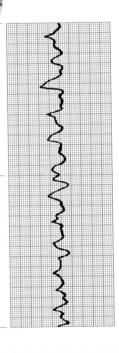

What are the rules for this rhythm? (Regularity, Rate, P wave, PRI, QRS)

Ventricular Tachycardia

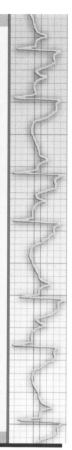

The rules for this rhythm:

REGULARITY: This rhythm is usually regular, although it can be slightly irregular.

RATE: Atrial rate cannot be determined. The ventricular rate range is 150–250 bpm. If the rate is below 150 bpm, it is considered a slow VT. If the rate exceeds 250 bpm, it is called Ventricular Flutter.

P WAVE: None of the QRS complexes will be preceded by P waves. You may see dissociated P waves intermittently across the strip.

PRI: Since the rhythm originates in the ventricles, there will be no PRI.

QRS: The QRS complexes will be wide and bizarre, measuring at least 0.12 second. It is often difficult to differentiate between the QRS and the T wave.

Basic Arrhythmias, 8th Edition, by Gail Walraven
©2017 by Pearson
Printed in the U.S.A. All Rights Reserved.

Premature Ventricular Complex

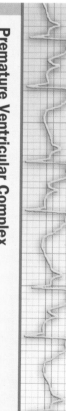

The rules for this rhythm:

REGULARITY: The underlying rhythm can be regular or irregular. The ectopic PVC will interrupt the regularity of the underlying rhythm (unless the PVC is interpolated).

RATE: The rate will be determined by the underlying rhythm. PVCs are not usually included in the rate determination because they frequently do not produce a pulse.

P WAVE: The ectopic is not preceded by a P wave. You may see a coincidental P wave near the PVC, but it is dissociated.

PRI: Since the ectopic comes from a lower focus, there will be no PRI.

QRS: The QRS complex will be wide and bizarre, measuring at least 0.12 second. The configuration will differ from the configuration of the underlying QRS complexes. The T wave is frequently in the opposite direction from the QRS complex.

Basic Arrhythmias, 8th Edition, by Gail Walraven
©2017 by Pearson
Printed in the U.S.A. All Rights Reserved.

Idioventricular Rhythm

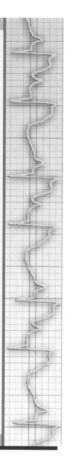

The rules for this rhythm:

REGULARITY: This rhythm is usually regular, although it is less reliable as the heart dies.

RATE: The ventricular rate is usually 20–40 bpm, but it can drop below 20 bpm.

P WAVE: There are no P waves in this arrhythmia.

PRI: There is no PRI.

QRS: The QRS complex is wide and bizarre, measuring at least 0.12 second.

Basic Arrhythmias, 8th Edition, by Gail Walraven
©2017 by Pearson
Printed in the U.S.A. All Rights Reserved.

Ventricular Fibrillation

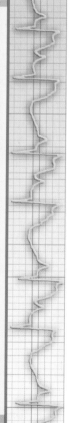

The rules for this rhythm:

REGULARITY: There are no waves or complexes that can be analyzed to determine regularity. The baseline is totally chaotic.

RATE: The rate cannot be determined since there are no discernible waves or complexes to measure.

P WAVE: There are no discernible P waves.

PRI: There is no PRI.

QRS: There are no discernible QRS complexes.

Basic Arrhythmias, 8th Edition, by Gail Walraven
©2017 by Pearson
Printed in the U.S.A. All Rights Reserved.

ASYSTOLE

The heart has lost its electrical activitiy. There is no electrical pacemaker to initiate electrical flow.

What are the rules for this rhythm? (Regularity, Rate, P wave, PRI, QRS)

Asystole

The rules for this rhythm:

REGULARITY: There is no electrical activity; only a straight line.

RATE: There is no electrical activity; only a straight line.

P WAVE: There is no electrical activity; only a straight line.

PRI: There is no electrical activity; only a straight line.

QRS: There is no electrical activity; only a straight line.

Basic Arrhythmias, 8th Edition, by Gail Walraven
©2017 by Pearson
Printed in the U.S.A. All Rights Reserved.